Seating and Wheeled Mobility

A Clinical Resource Guide

T0131030

Seating and Wheeled Mobility

A Clinical Resource Guide

Michelle L. Lange, OTR/L, ABDA, ATP/SMS
Access to Independence, Inc.
Arvada, Colorado

Jean L. Minkel, PT, ATP
ICS—Independence Care System
Minkel Consulting
New York, New York

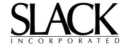
SLACK
INCORPORATED

www.Healio.com/books

ISBN: 978-1-63091-396-0

Published by: SLACK Incorporated
                  6900 Grove Road
                  Thorofare, NJ 08086 USA
                  Telephone: 856-848-1000
                  Fax: 856-848-6091
                  www.Healio.com/books

Contact SLACK Incorporated for more information about other books in this field or about the availability of our books from distributors outside the United States.

Library of Congress Cataloging-in-Publication Data
Names: Lange, Michelle L., editor. | Minkel, Jean, 1958- editor.
Title: Seating and wheeled mobility : a clinical resource guide / [edited by]
  Michelle L. Lange, Jean L. Minkel.
Description: Thorofare, NJ : Slack Incorporated, [2018] | Includes
  bibliographical references and index.
Identifiers: LCCN 2017047602 (print) | LCCN 2017048480 (ebook) | ISBN
  9781630913977 (epub) | ISBN 9781630913984 (Web) | ISBN 9781630913960
  (paperback)
Subjects: | MESH: Wheelchairs | Disabled Persons--rehabilitation | Disability
  Evaluation | Posture | Pressure Ulcer--prevention & control | Equipment
  Design
Classification: LCC RD798 (ebook) | LCC RD798 (print) | NLM WB 320 | DDC
  617.1/03--dc23
LC record available at https://lccn.loc.gov/2017047602

Printed in the United States of America.

Last digit is print number: 10 9 8 7 6 5 4 3 2

DEDICATION

For my family who keeps me grounded, you are my life. Be joyful in hope, patient in affliction, faithful in prayer.

Michelle L. Lange, OTR/L, ABDA, ATP/SMS

I can't help thinking of the saying, "We stand on the shoulders of those who came before us." I want to thank my "family" of clients, professional colleagues and mentors, and my multigenerational family, all of whom have provided me guidance, support and tons of love.

Jean L. Minkel, PT, ATP

CONTENTS

ACKNOWLEDGMENTS

The editors would like to thank the community of providers who are part of the Rehabilitation Engineering and Assistive Technology Society of North America (RESNA), and especially the Wheeled Mobility and Seating Special Interest Group. This project emerged as a solution to the challenge of how to share specialized information with a broader community of service providers. The RESNA community rallied when called and stuck with the project to see it through to the end. Each author was approached to be a contributor based on expertise and passion for a specific topic, and the end result is a text that truly covers the depth and breadth of wheelchair seating and mobility. The editors would like to thank each and every author for their time, energy, effort, perseverance, and patience.

We would also like to thank our many teachers, the persons with a disability, who challenge the status quo. These people, the end-users of the technology, share with us the successful, and not so successful, solutions that shape our practice and industry. Listen carefully to the end-user. The solution becomes easier to identify, when we are listening to understand the real need. Thank you for leading us to solutions that work for you to be as independent as possible.

ABOUT THE EDITORS

Michelle L. Lange, OTR/L, ABDA, ATP/SMS is an occupational therapist with 30 years of experience and has been in private practice, Access to Independence, for over 10 years. She is a well-respected lecturer, both nationally and internationally, and has authored numerous texts, chapters, and articles. She is the editor of *Fundamentals in Assistive Technology*, 4th edition, NRRTS Continuing Education Curriculum Coordinator, and Clinical Editor of *Directions* magazine. Michelle is on the teaching faculty of Rehabilitation Engineering and Assistive Technology Society of North America (RESNA). She is a member of the Clinician Task Force. Michelle is a certified ATP, certified SMS, and a Senior Disability Analyst of the American Board of Disability Analysts.

Jean L. Minkel, PT, ATP is a physical therapist and master clinician well recognized for her work in assistive technology. She is currently the Senior Vice President of Care Coordination and Rehabilitation Services for Independence Care System, a nonprofit, Medicaid long-term care program in New York City. Jean is also an independent consultant who provides educational and consulting service to all members of the assistive technology team—consumers, therapists, suppliers, manufacturers, and payers. Before entering the private sector, Jean was the Director of the Seating and Mobility Program at the Center for Rehabilitation Technology at Helen Hayes Hospital in West Haverstraw, NY. She produced the video series *Spending or Investing—Funding Assistive Technology*. She is coauthor of the *Wheelchair Selection Guide: How to Use the ANSI–RESNA Standards*, the *Manual Mobility Training Guide*, and the *Power Mobility Training Guide*. The assistive technology community has recognized Jean for her contributions with the RESNA Fellow award in 1995 and the Sam McFarland Mentor Award in 2012.

Contributing Authors

Atli Ágústsson, PT, MSc Bioeng (Chapter 7)
Seating and Mobility Specialist
Endurhæfing—Þekkingarsetur
Kópavogur, Iceland

Michael Babinec, OTR/L, ABDA, ATP (Chapter 10)
Invacare Corporation
Elyria, Ohio

Theresa F. Berner, MOT, OTR/L, ATP (Chapter 15)
Wexner Medical Center
The Ohio State University
Columbus, Ohio

Sheila N. R. Buck, BSc(OT), OT Reg (Ont), ATP (Chapter 14)
Therapy NOW! Inc.
Milton, Ontario, Canada

Mary Ellen Buning, PhD, OTR/L, ATP/SMS, RESNA Fellow
(Chapter 24)
Retired
Denver, Colorado

Jo-Anne Chisholm, MSc, OT (Chapter 2)
Access Community Therapists
Vancouver, British Columbia, Canada

Elizabeth Cole MSPT, ATP (Chapter 8)
ROHO, A Division of Permobil
Belleville, Illinois

Barbara A. Crane, PT, PhD, ATP/SMS (Chapter 6)
University of Hartford
West Hartford, Connecticut

Carmen P. DiGiovine, PhD, ATP/SMS, RET (Chapter 15)
The Ohio State University
Columbus, Ohio

John "Jay" Doherty, OTR, ATP/SMS (Chapter 20)
Director of Clinical Education
Quantum Rehab
Exeter, Pennsylvania

Jan Furumasu, PT, ATP (Chapter 17)
Rancho Los Amigos National Rehabilitation Center
Downey, California

Deborah A. Jones, PT, DPT, GSC, CEEAA, ATP (Chapter 18)
Board-Certified Clinical Geriatric Specialist
Providence Bridgeport Rehab
Tigard, Oregon

Guðný Jónsdóttir, PT, MSc (Chapter 7)
Seating and Mobility Specialist
Endurhæfing—Þekkingarsetur
Kópavogur, Iceland

Kay Ellen Koch, OTR/L, ATP, RESNA Fellow (Chapter 25)
The Joint Commission
Atlanta, Georgia

David Kreutz, PT, ATP (Chapter 3)
Shepherd Center
Atlanta, Georgia

Elizabeth McCarty, OTR/L (Chapter 21)
The Perlman Center
Cincinnati Children's Hospital Medical Center
Cincinnati, Ohio

Amy M. Morgan, PT, ATP (Chapter 12)
Permobil, Inc.
Lebanon, Tennessee

Anita Perr, PhD, OT/L, FAOTA, RESNA Fellow (Chapter 25)
New York University
New York, New York

Cindi Petito, OTR/L, ATP, CAPS (Chapter 23)
CHAS Group
Middleburg, Florida

Julie Piriano, PT, ATP/SMS (Chapter 16)
Quantum Rehab
Exeter, Pennsylvania

Joanne Rader, RN, MN (Chapter 18)
Rader Consulting
Portland, Oregon

Lauren E. Rosen, PT, MPT, MSMS, ATP/SMS (Chapter 9)
St. Joseph's Children's Hospital
Tampa, Florida

Jill Sparacio, OTR/L, ATP/SMS, ABDA (Chapter 5)
Sparacio Consulting Services
Downers Grove, Illinois

Sharon Sutherland, PT (Chapter 4)
Seating Solutions LLC
Longmont, Colorado

Melissa Tally, PT, MPT, ATP (Chapter 21)
The Perlman Center
Cincinnati Children's Hospital Medical Center
Cincinnati, Ohio

Stephanie Tanguay OT/L, ATP (Chapter 19)
Motion Concepts
Tonawanda, New York

Susan Johnson Taylor, OTR/L, RESNA Fellow (Chapter 22)
Numotion
Charleston, South Carolina

Kelly Waugh, PT, MAPT, ATP (Chapter 6)
Assistive Technology Partners
University of Colorado—Denver
Denver, Colorado

Joanne Yip, BSR, OT (Chapter 2)
Access Community Therapists
Vancouver, British Columbia, Canada

FOREWORD

We are honoured to have the opportunity to write the foreword to this pertinent and so relevant book. Michelle and Jean are both exceptional individuals we hold in great esteem. Through their passion and dedication they have truly made substantial contributions to the evolution of our practice. When noting the content of this book and the list of contributors, we were humbled at the depth and quality of the people involved, all of who are at the forefront of their field. This enhances the quality of this publication establishing a solid knowledge base in this complex and challenging profession.

Let's face it, seating and mobility is a challenging field. Everyday we encounter a set of circumstances that differs from what we have previously experienced, a different and new challenge that takes us back to the fundamentals of our practice, fundamentals from which we create a solution specific to the individual. There is a tremendous amount of responsibility to ensure the prescribed product is effective for the end user. As practitioners we have a profound effect on each individual's life.

The end user solution has many components to it: tissue integrity, swallowing, respiration, upper and lower body function, maintenance of symmetry, rest, mobility, communication, socialization, transportation, access, education, participation, employment…the list is endless. As seating and mobility professionals, it is our job to take all of this into consideration in our assessments and prescriptions.

Feeling challenged yet? It truly is a daunting process. However, this book provides an excellent foundation that can be utilized in everyday practice. The organization of the book, starting with essential fundamental information leading into specific topic areas, is logical and reinforces the progression from assessment to prescription.

It was enlightening to read each chapter and find a consistent method of approach to seating and mobility. The knowledge base of the previous decades has come together and has been well-consolidated.

There is much satisfaction working in this field, but it is not always easy. It can be challenging at times, regardless of your knowledge and abilities as a professional in this field. The practice of seating and mobility is always evolving, and best practice will continue to change. This book provides a solid foundation from which to work.

This book is a valuable resource to all practitioners. Use it!

Congratulations to Michelle and Jean, and all the contributors for a job well done.

David Cooper, MSc Kines, Rehab Tech
Priority Posture Systems Ltd.
Burnaby, British Columbia, Canada
Co-Chair, International Seating Symposium (Vancouver)
Vancouver, British Columbia, Canada

Maureen Story, BSR(PT/OT)
Sunny Hill Health Centre for Children
Co-Chair, International Seating Symposium (Vancouver)
Vancouver, British Columbia, Canada

FOREWORD

It is a pleasure and honor to prepare this foreword to a well-thought and well-planned compilation of the art, science, and clinical application of the many facets associated with provision of seating and wheeled mobility interventions to people with disabilities who aspire for the opportunity to function and participate with all. Many great books have been written over the decades. Most of the fundamentals remain the same; however, the field has grown as we have learned more, witnessed technology advances, and become more seasoned as investigators to assess the impact and outcomes of this technology on people and their quality of life.

Over the decades, people who use wheeled mobility and seating devices have rightfully become part of mainstream society and the number of users is growing substantially. Although civil rights legislation, such as the Americans with Disabilities Act in the United States and the United Nations Convention on the Rights of People with Disabilities, speaks to inclusion and accessibility, public policies and coverage for wheeled mobility and seating often continue to marginalize access over walking. Traditional entry-level training in the health sciences still glosses over the topic. This book will serve well as a resource to overcome these challenges.

Michelle and Jean have rallied some of the best-known subject matter experts to compile the most comprehensive, up-to-date, and one-stop reference on the topic. The chapters not only share best practices that have evolved but also support each topic with the best-available research and evidence contributed by investigators and clinicians who took the time and effort to publish their expertise.

As clinicians (both new and seasoned), this book serves as a wealth of information to learn, reference, or validate practice. As teachers and mentors, we have a comprehensive resource to supplement learning. As advocates, we have an evidence-based justification for why this technology is important and necessary that can be shared with all stakeholders. As researchers and developers, we have a resource to assess the current state of the science and identify opportunities for further investigation and innovation.

Enjoy the read. I certainly did.

Mark R. Schmeler, PhD, OTR/L, ATP, RESNA Fellow
Director, International Seating Symposium/USA
Associate Professor, Department of Rehabilitation Science & Technology
School of Health and Rehabilitation Sciences
University of Pittsburgh
Pittsburgh, Pennsylvania

INTRODUCTION

If you ask a person with a disability what "functional mobility" means, the response is often some version of "Go where I want to go, when I want to go." Although this response appears simple and straightforward, it has many implications. Mobility, ideally, should be pain-free, energy efficient, and safe. Most able-bodied people give their own functional mobility very little thought:

- Walking to the bathroom
- Driving to the store
- Getting on a plane for vacation

Functional mobility takes many forms—one foot in front of another, driving a wheeled mobility device, such as an automobile, or being a passenger in an airplane or a train. We are surrounded by messages and expressions that reinforce the value and positive images associated with *one* form of functional mobility: walking. Phrases such as "one small step for man, one great leap for mankind," "every journey begins with a single step," and "pull yourself up by your bootstraps," refer to the positive societal values associated with walking (Iezzoni, 2003).

For some people, the positive image of walking may trump *functional* mobility. To avoid the negative image of using a wheeled mobility device, persons will struggle to "keep walking," consciously or unconsciously reducing involvement in activities that require "getting out and getting around." Ultimately, the result of "still walking" is to gradually become more and more isolated. The perception may be that as long as the person has not "ended up in a wheelchair," then the disease or injury has not "taken over" and the person has "won the war."

Assistive technology of all kinds is likely to be ignored or abandoned if a person does not *recognize* a need for technology or is provided a piece of technology that does not meet his or her needs. A critical component of successful clinical intervention is to understand and meet the person where he or she is at. Do not expect a reluctant person with a mobility impairment to readily accept the clinically proven options you may think are best.

This book presents clinical assessment considerations when working with a person with a disability who may need wheelchair seating for postural support and skin integrity and a wheelchair base to best meet dependent or independent mobility needs. The effectiveness of any seating and mobility intervention will be directly related to the readiness of the person and/or the people within his or her support system to accept the intervention. Information sharing, opportunities for demonstration and trial, and patience on the part of the clinicians working with the person with a disability are all critical precursors to the actual process of making equipment recommendations.

The title of this book was quite deliberately chosen; it is a *clinical* resource guide, designed to support occupational and physical therapists, complex rehabilitation technology suppliers, and even third-party payers who are interested in wheelchair seating and mobility assessment and applications. The book is designed to provide a wide spectrum of information from foundational information for those practitioners who are new to the field to in-depth, population-specific information for practitioners who perhaps have not worked with a particular population in the past.

The book is divided into sections, each addressing a different area of clinical practice in wheelchair seating and mobility.

- The first section is an in-depth presentation of the assessment process and the critical understanding of pressure management needed by the clinical team when working with people who rely on wheeled mobility.

- The second section focuses on postural support, both in sitting and during a 24-hour period of time. The level of postural support needed varies depending on the amount of intrinsic neuromuscular activity the person can control. Three types of sitters are presented: hands-free, hands-dependent, and prop sitters. Nighttime positioning needs, in the context of a 24-hour positioning program, are addressed. This section also includes a completely updated method to measure and describe the seated person and related support surfaces needed when recommending a device.

- The third section lays the foundation for clinical decision making around the assessment for and application of the most appropriate wheeled mobility device—manual wheelchair, power wheelchair, or scooter.

- The fourth section provides in-depth clinical applications for each category of mobility device, including ultralight manual wheelchairs, power wheelchairs, and manual wheelchairs for the dependent user. The final chapter in this section addresses proper documentation to assist in the funding of these devices.

- The fifth section provides population-specific information regarding the clinical application of position, pressure management, and functional mobility as it applies to the pediatric, geriatric, and bariatric populations, as well as persons with both degenerative and complex neuromuscular impairments.

- The sixth and last section presents additional considerations when working with persons who are aging with a disability, a new population that has arisen as a result of long life expectancies among persons with a disability. Other considerations include the importance of both the environment of use and the safe transport of a wheelchair in a vehicle, as well as the application of the wheelchair standards test methods in the clinic—specifically how test data can inform product recommendation.

As a whole, the text provides the depth and breadth of the clinical practice of wheelchair seating and mobility. Individual chapters provide in-depth product and population-specific information valuable to both those who are new to the field and seasoned professionals.

If you are new to the field, invest time in the foundational sections. Build strong, person-centered assessment skills, understand the importance of pressure management, learn to measure a person in a manner that allows you to communicate with others in the industry, and, finally, become familiar with the range of mobility options available to offer those with limited or no ambulatory skills the technology to meet their daily mobility needs through wheeled mobility.

If you are a seasoned professional with strong foundational skills, you may find reading individual chapters to be helpful, especially when you are asked to assist with a person whose need is different from the population with whom you most often work.

Each author has a passion for the topic presented. Enjoy learning from, and sharing with, a group of wonderful professionals, who care so much about the people we serve.

REFERENCE

Iezzoni, L. (2003). *When walking fails: Mobility problems of adults with chronic conditions* (Vol. 8). Berkeley, CA: University of California Press.

I

Postural Support and Pressure Management
Foundational Information

Seating and Mobility Evaluations for Persons With Long-Term Disabilities
Focusing on the Client Assessment

Jean L. Minkel, PT, ATP

Wheelchair seating and mobility are interdependent clinical situations. Frequently a person with a mobility impairment may also have a postural support impairment. A full assessment of a person with a disability in need of a wheeled mobility device is a multifaceted process that includes collecting subjective and objective information about a person's mobility needs, his or her environments of use and functional abilities, his or her postural support needs, and any risk factors for skin breakdown or pressure injury that could result from sitting for long periods. This chapter presents the clinical skills needed to conduct an effective seating and mobility assessment with an emphasis on the supine (gravity eliminated) assessment, which is combined with the seated assessment. This process ideally takes place on a treatment mat and thus is often referred to as the *mat assessment*.

OVERVIEW OF THE COMPONENTS OF THE SEATING AND MOBILITY ASSESSMENT

A comprehensive seating and mobility assessment has several components, and the whole process can be analogous to solving a mystery. Information from one part of the assessment can have a large impact on the whole assessment, ultimately influencing the recommendation of products and related training needed to meet the person's functional mobility needs. The assessment is arranged into three broad categories reflecting the domains and classification structure of the *International Classification of Functioning, Disability and Health* (World Health Organization, 2001): (1) body structure and functions, (2) activities and participation, and (3) environment and current technology. The Rehabilitation Engineering and Assistive Technology Society of North America *Wheelchair Service Provision Guide* (Arledge et al., 2011) is a great reference that provides additional, detailed information regarding the clinical standards of practice developed for the wheelchair service delivery process.

When working on a jigsaw puzzle, having access to the box cover helps one see the whole picture. Likewise, in the assessment process in seating and mobility, it is helpful to see an overview of the components of the assessment:

- The interview
- Understanding the person's current mobility status
- Sitting balance assessment
- Supine assessment
- Skin inspection and assessment risk of skin breakdown or pressure injury
- Hand-supported sitting assessment
- Mobility assessment
- Trialing of potential solutions
- Recommendation of seating and mobility products
- Training, as needed
- Follow-up and determination of actual outcomes

Lange, M. L., & Minkel, J. L.
Seating and Wheeled Mobility: A Clinical Resource Guide
(pp. 3-26). © 2018 SLACK Incorporated.

Just like putting a puzzle together, each component is not always performed in a linear, step-by-step sequence. Most assessments do start with an interview and end with a follow-up outcome phone call or visit, but the steps in between may vary depending on the needs of the client and the information received as the assessment process progresses. Don't be afraid to go back and look at someone's sitting balance when he or she is not as successful pushing a manual chair as you had expected. There is interdependence between postural stability, the ability to maintain skin integrity and effective use the most appropriate mobility device in a specific environment of use.

INTERVIEW

A clinician needs to start by asking questions and listening to the answers. The only way to meet someone where he or she is at is to be truly curious about *where* he or she really is—not where you want that person to be. An essential component of any seating and mobility assessment is an initial interview. To help guide your clinical decision making later in the process, it is important to collect specific information using questions such as the following:

- What is your primary diagnosis or medical condition for which you are seeking a wheelchair?

- What do you know about your condition?

- What other conditions or diagnoses do you have or have you been treated for?

- What types of intervention/treatment have you undergone to address your medical condition(s)? Are there any treatment plans in place for the future?

- Do you have a permanent need for a wheelchair?

The Functional Mobility Assessment (FMA; Kumar et al., 2013) is a validated outcome measurement tool that helps guide a needs assessment interview. The FMA allows the consumer to rate his or her own satisfaction regarding such factors as comfort, the ability to get around indoors, and even access to transportation. By using a tool like the FMA during an initial interview, clinicians will have documented the preintervention data to use for comparison with follow-up data after delivery.

Other client-lead tools are also available, including the Canadian Occupational Performance Measure (Law et al., 1990) and the Quebec User Evaluation of Satisfaction with Assistive Technology (Demers, Monette, Lapierre, Arnold, & Wolfson, 2002). Although not specifically designed for seating and mobility interventions, both of these assessment tools offer clinicians and clients a way to identify what is important for the individual seeking a technology intervention.

Suggested Interview Questions

If a structured interview tool is not being used, several key questions should be considered as part of an interview.

Suggested Interview Questions to Assess Mobility Needs and Methods

Describe your current method of getting around:

- What is working for you?

- Has there been a change in how you get around?

  ○ If yes, what do you think are the reasons for these changes?

- Over the past year, have there been changes in where you go?

  ○ If yes, what do you think are the reasons for these changes?

- Do you have a permanent need for a wheelchair?

- What are you having trouble doing?

- Where are you having trouble maneuvering?

- Tell me how you were getting around 2 years ago during the holiday season? Tell me how you were getting around last year during the holiday season?

Asking about holidays is useful because people tend to remember where they were and with whom they spent the holidays. Some clients have photos to document themselves during the holidays, illustrating the device being used. Family members who were at the holiday celebration may be able to contribute helpful information about the person's use of mobility aid at that time. Each of these interview questions provides the clinical team with the client's subjective information. Careful interviewing will provide the clinician the client-specific information that will be important in painting a picture of this particular person when documenting the outcome of the assessment. Painting a picture is essential in providing client-specific information about why a selected piece of equipment or whole system has been recommended to meet *this* person's needs.

Suggested Interview Questions to Assess Environmental and Transportation Accessibility

Closely related to understanding a person's current mobility status is the need to understand the accessibility of the person's daily environments of use, including home, work, and other frequently used environments.

- Are there any steps leading into your home?

  ○ If yes, how many?

  ○ If yes, is there another entrance with either fewer steps or no steps?

- How do you get around in the community?
- Are there any public transportation options in your community?
- If using personal transportation, what kind of vehicle is being used?

Suggested Interview Questions to Inquire About Problems With Sitting Balance and the Need for Postural Supports

- Do you have any problems keeping your balance when you are seated?
- Do you easily lose your sitting balance?
- Can you reposition yourself if you lose your balance?

Suggested Interview Questions to Investigate Problems With Skin Integrity

- Do you have any problems with your skin—red marks, wounds, or open areas?
- Are you able to reposition yourself when you are uncomfortable?

The answers to these interview questions begin to define the scope of the full specialty assessment.

PLANNING YOUR CLINICAL ASSESSMENT

People who need a seating and mobility assessment present with a wide range of needs and clinical issues. To help categorize the type of assessment that an individual may need, it is helpful to do a quick inventory of the needs being presented by the client. The complexity of the assessment depends on the number of interdependent issues being presented.

Evaluation of Mobility Impairment

Evaluation of mobility impairment alone is indicated if the following criteria are met:

- Limited mobility range when walking due to unsteady gait, fatigue, and/or frequency of falls
- Normal sitting balance with the ability to reposition trunk once balance is disturbed
- Not at risk for skin breakdown—full sensation across seated surface and ability to reposition if uncomfortable

CASE EXAMPLE

Rosa is a 70-year-old woman living in a small one-bedroom apartment. She has been diagnosed with both congestive heart failure and type 2 diabetes. She is currently using a rollator walker when she travels outside of her apartment because she fatigues and is unsure of her balance. In her home, she does not need an assistive device and sits comfortably in the lounge chair in her living room. She no longer does her own food shopping or attends her church services because she experiences shortness of breath when she tries to walk the needed three to five blocks to the store or church. Rosa is able to easily sit on the side of the treatment mat and is able to move herself when her buttocks hurt after sitting too long. She wants to be able to leave her apartment, do her own shopping, and go to church without depending on others to take her. Rosa represents a client who needs an evaluation of mobility impairments only.

Evaluation of Mobility and Seating Impairments

Evaluation of both mobility and seating impairments is indicated if the person meets the following criteria:

- Limited mobility range—perhaps unable to walk, having difficulty effectively self-propelling a manual chair, or will need to rely on a wheeled mobility base for functional mobility because of the inability to ambulate
- Needs external support to maintain upright sitting position, especially on a mobile base (e.g., when driving a wheelchair or riding in an automobile
- Not at risk for skin breakdown—has sensation across seated surface and is able to reposition if uncomfortable

CASE EXAMPLE

Fred is a 14-year-old boy with a diagnosis of cerebral palsy, spastic quadriplegia, who is fully integrated in the ninth grade at his local high school. Fred gets around school in a power chair and has been a power-chair user since he was 3 years old. He has recently grown more than 4 inches in height and outgrown his current chair. Fred is able to verbally express his needs, with a slight speech impairment. When he speaks, there is an increase in his tone, especially on his left side, causing him to fall to the right, when sitting up and talking to anyone (that is, anyone who will listen, as

Fred is very chatty). Fred is verbally able to indicate when his buttocks, trunk, or legs are sore from sitting. He does not want anyone to change his position for him (like they did in middle school); he wants to change his own position during the school day and when at home. Fred illustrates a client who will need a seating/positioning and mobility assessment.

Evaluation of Mobility, Seating, and Skin Integrity

Evaluation of mobility, seating, and skin integrity impairments is indicated if the person meets the following criteria:

- Limited or restricted mobility—unable to walk and will rely on a wheeled mobility base for functional mobility
- Nonsymmetrical alignment of the pelvis and trunk, leading to poor sitting balance and uneven pressure distribution
- Has an active skin injury or a history of a skin injury that is now healed
- At risk for skin breakdown because of impaired sensation and/or diminished ability to reposition pelvis and trunk while in the seated position

CASE EXAMPLE

Lisa is a 32-year-old woman, who is 12 years postspinal cord injury at the midthoracic region. Lisa works full time outside of the home in an office setting. She drives her own car and is able to transfer her manual wheelchair in and out of the car without difficulty. In the past year, she has had to miss work on several occasions due to a skin injury secondary to pressure on her right buttocks. She reports that she notices, when she looks in the mirror, she is not "sitting straight" anymore. She wants to be sure she doesn't miss any more time from work due to pressure injuries. Lisa will need an assessment that integrates postural support, skin protection, and mobility.

Each case example presented illustrates the type of information that can be recorded as part of an initial assessment. Depending on the number of needs, the clinician can plan which type of assessment will address the client's concerns.

ASSESSMENT FOR MOBILITY IMPAIRMENT

For a client who has no postural support impairment and no sensory impairments, much like Rosa described in the preceding case example, the clinical team can focus on mobility needs.

Mobility assessment is needed to determine efficacy and safety to self and others while operating a wheeled mobility device. The assessment of body structures and functions includes the following:

- Review of systems (shortness of breath, reported visual and hearing functions, any other medical conditions currently being treated)
- Demonstration of sitting balance and the ability to reposition oneself in the seated position
- Documentation of range of motion (ROM) of hips, knees, and upper extremities
- Assess upper extremity ROM, strength, and coordination to determine access method for manual wheelchair, scooter, or power chair
- Assess vision to determine impairments that may affect safety of self and others when operating a wheelchair
- Assess judgment and problem-solving skills to determine suitability for power mobility

When a person first experiences difficulties with ambulation, the symptoms often include fatigue, loss of balance when walking, increased frequency of reported falls, or shortness of breath. All of these symptoms may result in decreased activity level, and thus increased isolation.

Many persons at this stage of change in mobility may have already adopted the use of an ambulation aid, such as a cane or walker. The ambulation aid may continue to be effective, especially in familiar, controlled environments, such as a person's home or even a worksite. More frequent falls may occur when the person needs to travel further distances or tries to get around in a less familiar environment outside the home and in the community.

The usual hierarchy used in clinical decision making to determine the best match for assisted mobility is referred to as the *mobility device algorithm* (Centers for Medicare & Medicaid, 2005) (Chapter 8 provides further detail on the algorithm). This algorithm asks about the client's functional mobility when using each of the following devices:

- Ambulation aide (cane, crutch, or walker)
- Self-propelling manual wheelchair

- Scooter
- Power wheelchair
- Power wheelchair with power seating functions
- Dependent mobility (a chair being pushed or otherwise operated by someone else)

When assessing a person's mobility status, a clinician is asked to determine whether the use of each device (in sequence from least to most complex) provides the assistance needed for the person to achieve functional mobility. For the purpose of this book, *functional mobility,* with or without an assistive device, is defined as follows:

The ability to move at the speed of a walking person without pain, shortness of breath, or fatigue to accomplish your life tasks. Average walking speed is measured at 1.4 m/s (4.5 feet/second).

A highly practical measure of mobility at walking speed is to determine whether the person can cross a street while the walk sign is still being displayed. If the person cannot get across the street in the time allowed, the current method of mobility can be considered, clinically nonfunctional.

Subsequent chapters in this book provide much more detailed information about the mobility algorithm and clinical indications for each type of mobility device, which might prove to be a solution for a particular person.

WHERE TO BEGIN A MOBILITY ASSESSMENT?

If you are working with a person who is currently ambulating, is able to sit on the side of a treatment mat or on a bench with no balance problems, and has full sensation and the ability to move if uncomfortable, then you can begin by introducing this person to the mobility options that will meet his or her needs—manual, power, or scooter—all covered in detail in other chapters.

CASE EXAMPLE

Let's continue to work with Rosa and address her mobility needs. She is currently able to get around her small apartment without a wheeled mobility device and wants to focus on getting around outside, "on her own." She is able to sit on the mat table and has no problem shifting her own position when she is uncomfortable. During the seated assessment, we found she has full ROM in her hips and knees, but her upper extremity strength is only fair bilaterally. She can raise her arms against gravity but is unable to sustain the position once challenged. When we introduced Rosa to a manual wheelchair, we found she was short of breath after

self-propelling with her arms shortly after she pushed outside the clinic door, a distance of 200 yards. When she tried coming back into the clinic, pushing with her feet, she was again out of breath and needed 3 minutes to recover her regular breathing pattern. Manual mobility was ruled out.

Rosa was shown a scooter as the next option to meet her mobility needs. When the seat was swiveled to the side of the scooter, Rosa had little difficulty getting into it, swiveling the seat back into the operating position and reaching up to the tiller. Rosa was able to operate the toggle switch controlling forward and reverse directions with her thumbs with no problem. Steering with the tiller was completely intuitive to her. Almost as soon as we got outside the clinic door, in the lobby area, Rosa asked if she could use the elevator to go outside and try the scooter in the neighborhood. As we headed down the block away from the clinic, Rosa mentioned, "I haven't gone this far by myself in over a year." A scooter was the right match to meet Rosa's community mobility needs.

If you are working with a person who is not currently walking, does not have the balance to sit on the side of a treatment mat, has limited sensation or limited ability to move once uncomfortable, then you should consider starting the evaluation with the mat assessment. Fred and Lisa, from our earlier case examples, illustrate clients who, when you ask them to get out of their current chair, may have difficulty sitting on the edge of the mat due to problems with postural support or may have reported to you problems with skin integrity that you will want to investigate before looking at the appropriate mobility device to trial.

ASSESSMENT FOR SEATING IMPAIRMENTS

For persons with impairments in sitting balance or skeletal alignment of the pelvis and trunk, an assessment of the person's postural support needs is essential. An assessment of sitting balance and the position of the pelvis and trunk alignment when the person is seated against gravity will guide the recommendation of products designed to provide external postural support to improve the person's functional abilities in mobility and in completing other functional activities, such as eating, grooming, and reaching.

Mat Assessment

The initial—and all too often skipped—step of a thorough seating and mobility assessment is to get the person out of any wheeled mobility device he or she may be using at the time of the assessment. Getting a person out of the current wheelchair provides critical information about the needs of this person and his or her caregivers, beginning with what is the transfer method used to get from the chair

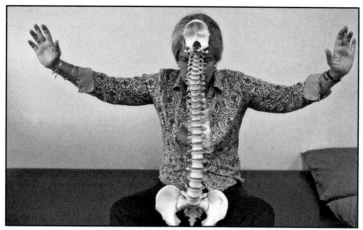

Figure 1-1. Demonstration of a hands-free sitter.

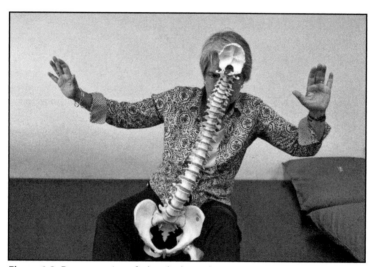

Figure 1-2. Demonstration of a hands-dependent sitter.

to another support surface. If the observed transfer method is less than ideal, additional therapy for transfer training may be indicated.

Seating Assessment: Sitting Balance Assessment to Determine the Need for Postural Support

To quickly assess the need for postural support (beyond what a standard wheelchair back support or captain's seat provides), you will to need to check the person's unsupported sitting balance. To fully assess a person's sitting balance, it is essential to conduct this assessment out of any wheelchair he or she may currently be using. Ask the person to sit over the edge of the treatment mat and lift both hands up off the support surface at the same time. This test helps to identify the person's sitting balance. The results of this assessment will help identify the person as one of the following:

- *Hands-Free Sitter*—a person who is able to lift both arms up off the surface without changing the position of the trunk. This ability indicates voluntary muscle control of the intrinsic muscles of the trunk to hold an upright sitting position, against gravity. A person with this type of trunk control can also shift his or her position off of a centered sitting position and come back into a balanced seated position. Most often a hands-free sitter requires only a minimal amount of trunk support, often in the form of a posteriorly mounted back support (Figure 1-1).

- *Hands-Dependent Sitter*—a person who often uses one or both hands to maintain sitting balance while seated. When asked to lift both hands off the mat at the same time, you will observe the trunk collapse to compensate for the loss of arm support, indicating the person's inability to use the intrinsic muscles of the trunk for support against gravity. For a hands-dependent sitter, posterior and lateral supports may be needed to support the trunk for the upper extremities to be free to engage in functional activities (Figure 1-2).

- *Prop Sitter*—a person with significant loss of sitting balance. A prop sitter is unable to maintain sitting balance, even if permitted to use his or her upper extremities for support and will fall if not provided maximum external support in the seated position. The seating system for prop sitters is designed to provide maximal support—posteriorly, anteriorly and laterally. This type of support is often custom-made and may include custom-molded supports for the seat and the backrest (Figure 1-3).

Note: If you are being asked to do a sitting balance assessment in a person's home or someplace other than a clinic setting, look for a seating support surface that has a firm seat and no backrest. Options in a home environment might include a shower chair, tub stool, or a picnic table bench. Beds are not ideal because the surface under the person is not firm enough to support the pelvis and he or she is likely to sink into the mattress when seated over the edge; thus, you will not have an accurate representation of the person's sitting balance.

Understanding the client's sitting balance as hands-free, hands-dependent, or prop sitting will allow you to focus on the type and location of supports that will be needed to provide the external support most appropriate to match your client's need. Chapters 3 through 5 provide focused, in-depth clinical information about meeting the needs of each of these types of clients. This chapter provides the specifics to perform the mat assessment across groups of clients, regardless of the extent of their need for postural support.

Once the person's sitting balance is recorded, he or she is placed in a supine position for the mat evaluation (you have the option to view the mat assessment in video format for a demonstration, through the following links):

- Part 1: http://bit.ly/2ygyzrc
- Part 2: http://bit.ly/2xUIAOX

Supine Assessment: Gravity-Eliminated Position

As the person moves from a seated to a supine position on a mat, the person's relationship with gravity is also changing. In the seated position, gravity is pushing down on the head and trunk, making the body work against gravity to sit up. In the supine position, gravity helps the person who is lying down achieve a skeletal alignment consisting of:

- The head and shoulder aligned over the trunk
- The trunk in alignment with the pelvis with both the upper and lower extremities in a relaxed position of full extension

In supine, gravity is your friend!

Before beginning the supine assessment, observe the position assumed by the person who is lying down in front of you. If the person lies down and his or her head is several inches above the mat surface, this may be the sign of a curve in his or her back. Wait just a minute or so to see whether gravity can assist in bringing his or her head down closer to

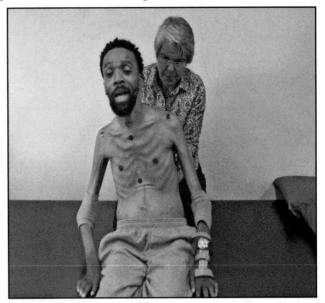

Figure 1-3. Demonstration of prop sitter who requires support.

the mat. If gravity is not an assist, give the person a pillow for comfort and note that the trunk assumes a curved, or *kyphotic*, position (Figure 1-4).

One of the main purposes of doing a mat assessment to assess pelvic mobility—is the pelvis able to be positioned in a posture that meets the following criteria?

- *Neutral in terms of tilt*: When the pelvis is in a position of *neutral* tilt, the person is able to weightbear, evenly, on the ischial tuberosities (Figure 1-5). When the pelvis is in a position of a *posterior* tilt, the person is weightbearing on the sacrum. This position is often referred to as *sacral sitting*. When the pelvis is in an *anteriorly* tilted position, he or she is weightbearing on pubic area of the pelvis.

- *Level in terms of obliquity*: When the pelvis is *level*, the person is equally weightbearing on the left and right IT. When the pelvis has an *obliquity*, one side of the pelvis is higher than other, resulting in uneven weightbearing on the ischial tuberosities (Figures 1-6 and 1-7).

- *Flat in terms of rotation*: When the pelvis is flat in terms of rotation, then both the right and left posterior pelvis crest are in contact with the back support. When the pelvis is rotated, one side of the pelvis is rotated forward of the other (Figures 1-8 and 1-9). From the rear of the person, you will observe that there is uneven weightbearing on the back support; one pelvic crest is in contact with the back support, and the other crest is forward of the back support. From the front view of the person, there is an appearance of a leg length discrepancy. If the right side of the pelvis is rotated forward, then the right leg appears to be longer than the left leg.

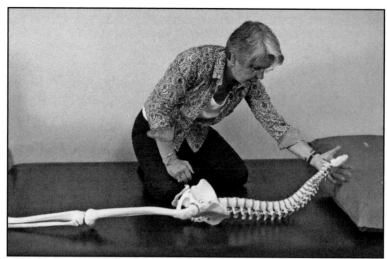

Figure 1-4. Demonstration of kyphotic posture in supine position.

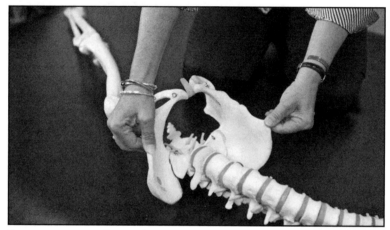

Figure 1-5. Location of anterior superior iliac spine (ASIS)—neutral pelvic tilt.

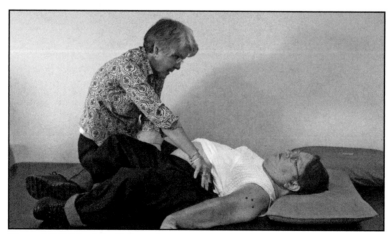

Figure 1-6. Pelvic obliquity in supine.

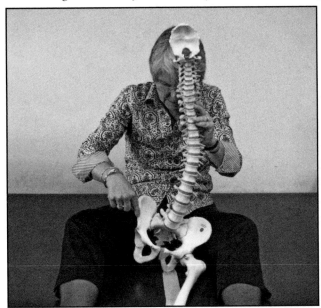

Figure 1-7. Pelvic obliquity in sitting. Note the uneven weightbearing on the lower ischial tuberosity.

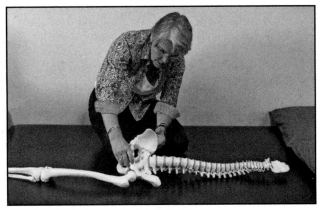

Figure 1-8. Demonstration of pelvic rotation.

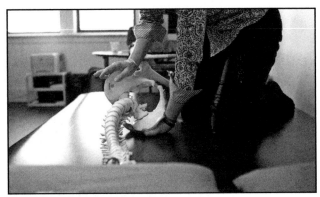

Figure 1-9. Hand position to derotate the pelvis.

The pelvis is the foundation of the seated person. The ideal position of the pelvis to support the seated person is neutral, level and flat. If the pelvis cannot be placed in this "ideal" position, the next section will guide you through how to assess and record the actual position of the pelvis. The position of the pelvis, if not in the ideal position, may need to be accommodated once the person is re positioned in sitting.

Assessing Pelvic Mobility

To check for available pelvic mobility, the person being assessed should be comfortably positioned in supine on a treatment mat. A massage table is an excellent alternative when working in someone's home. Once the person is lying down, the therapist should try to passively align the person's head, shoulder, trunk, and legs in as straight a line as possible.

Following is a description of one method used to palpate and feel anterior and posterior pelvic mobility.

Pelvic Tilt

Begin by locating the bumps on the left and right side of the pelvis, known as ASIS, with your thumbs. These bumps are used as landmarks during the mat assessment to assist you in understanding the position of the pelvis. To be able to describe pelvic tilt, you will need to passively move the pelvis, from a posteriorly tilted position into an anteriorly tilted position. We are going to begin with moving the pelvis into a posterior tilt.

Posterior tilt: Position yourself by kneeling on one side of the person. Using your thumb, locate the ASIS and use your hand to hold the pelvic crest closest to you. Using your other arm, closest to the person's feet, hold both legs under the knees. Flex the hips and knees at the same time until the thighs rest on the stomach and the buttocks have rocked up off the mat surface. The person is being rolled up into a ball, the lumbar spine is rounded, and the pelvis is posteriorly tilted. This is the starting position to assess the passive mobility of pelvic tilt (Figures 1-10 through 1-12). We now move to the anterior tilt.

Anterior tilt: Starting with thighs on chest position, keep your hand on the ASIS. With the other arm behind the knees, slowly move the hips into extension. Initially you are likely to feel the ASIS rock forward toward the feet, as the pelvis is moving from a posteriorly tilted position, toward a more anteriorly tilted position.

As you to extend the hips and knees, you are not likely to feel any further movement of the ASIS because the motion of hip extension is taking place at the ball and socket joint of the hip and the pelvis is not moving (Figure 1-13). The pelvis usually does not move again until the last few degrees of hip and knee extension, when the legs are fully straightening.

During the last degrees of full hip extension, you may feel the pelvis tilt even more anteriorly. The pelvis will move

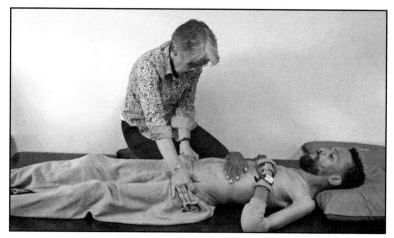

Figure 1-10. Locating the ASIS as a pelvic landmark.

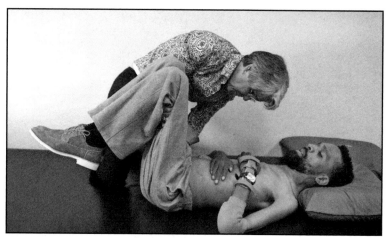

Figure 1-11. Using femurs as a lever arm to tilt pelvis into a posterior tilt.

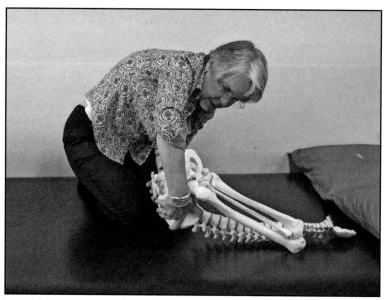

Figure 1-12. Fully posteriorly rotated pelvis.

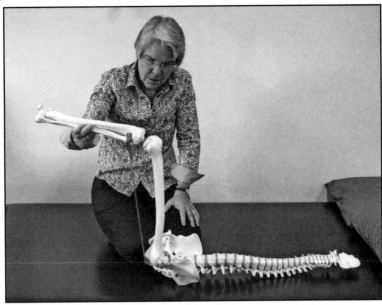

Figure 1-13. Hip extension takes place at the ball-and-socket joint of the hip.

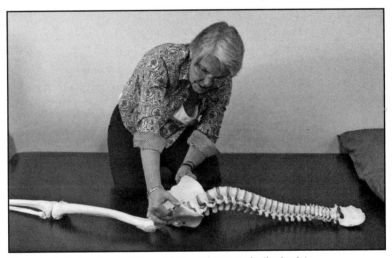

Figure 1-14. Fully extended hip and knee with anteriorly tilted pelvis.

into a more anteriorly tilted position at full hip extension because the hip flexor muscles are pulling on the pelvis, into an anterior tilt, as the muscles are stretched into hip extension (Figure 1-14).

To further assess the anterior mobility of the pelvis, take your arm out from under the knees and reach across the person's body; slide your palm under the pelvic crest on the opposite side of the body. Move your hand that was on the ASIS under the pelvic crest on the side closest to you. To gain leverage, if you are kneeling next to the client, you will need to assume a half-kneeling position and turn your body to face the top half of the person's body. Rock your own body back pulling on both of the posterior pelvic crests to create an exaggerated lumbar lordosis (arching the low back) and rock the pelvis into a maximally anteriorly tilted position. Note the ASIS will be oriented (or pointed) toward the person's toes. This is not a comfortable seated position

but will reveal to you those persons with a highly flexible lumbar lordosis.

Reposition to neutral tilt: When the pelvis is passively moved from a posterior tilt into an anteriorly tilted position, we can note two things. First, the pelvis is mobile, and second, it can be positioned in a neutral tilt.

In a supine position, when the hips and knees are moved to a flexed position (relieving any stretch from tight hip flexors or hamstring muscles), then the pelvis can be passively moved into a position with the ASIS pointed straight up toward the ceiling (Figure 1-15). In a seated person, when the pelvis is in a neutral tilt, the ischial tuberosities are in a position to be bear the person's weight.

RECORD YOUR FINDINGS

As you move through the assessment process, in both the supine and seated position, you will want to develop a

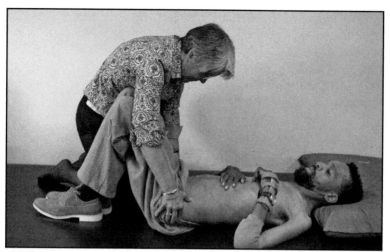

Figure 1-15. Pelvic position: neutral (tilt), level (no obliquity), and flat (no rotation).

method for recording your findings. The following section will you guide through a systematic process to assess the mobility the pelvis and the lower extremities and assess the alignment of the trunk and head. At the end of each section, there is suggested method of recording your findings because these findings are critical to planning the postural support interventions to be offered in response to the needs of the client.

Pelvic tilt: The pelvis creates the foundation of seating. Understanding the position of the pelvis is one key outcome of the mat assessment. A mobile pelvis can be passively moved from a position of posteriorly tilted through to an anteriorly tilted position. The goal is to determine if a neutral tilt, resulting in weightbearing on the ischial tuberosities, can be achieved.

Posterior pelvic tilt—pelvis stays in a posterior tilt, also known as sacral sitting: If the person is able to be easily rolled into a ball, placing the pelvis in a posterior tilt, but upon extension of the hips and the knees, you do not feel any movement of the ASIS, this reveals that the pelvis cannot be reduced from a position of being in a posterior tilt. When you place your hands behind the pelvic crests, try to rock the pelvis forward, and if there is no movement, then you need to note that the pelvis is in a posterior pelvic tilt and neutral tilt cannot be achieved. Persons who cannot move out of posterior tilt will be largely weightbearing on the sacrum when you position them in a seated position. The seating system will have to be designed to accommodate the sacral pressure to avoid increased weightbearing on this one bony area.

Anterior pelvic tilt—pelvis stays in an anterior tilt: If, when the person assumes a supine position, there is a large arch in the low back (referred to as a *lumbar lordosis*) and the person cannot be rolled into a ball because the arch does not flatten, then you need to note the pelvis is in an anterior tilt and a neutral tilt position cannot be achieved (Figure 1-16).

Most people who sit with an anteriorly tilted pelvis will have an exaggerated lumbar lordosis and will sit, leaning forward, resting either on the armrests of a chair, or by resting their arms on top of their thighs.

Neutral Tilt Can Be Achieved

If the person has a tendency to sink into a pelvic tilt (posterior tilt is much more common than anterior tilt) but is able to be passively moved to a neutral position, then we record that a neutral pelvis was achieved in supine and should be a goal in the seated position against gravity.

If you are creating a form to capture your mat assessment findings, you may find the following format an easy method for documentation:

Pelvic Tilt—check one:

_____ Neutral tilt, achieved

_____ Posteriorly tilted

_____ Anteriorly tilted

Pelvic Obliquity

The next pelvic motion we evaluate is pelvic obliquity. Again, we use the ASIS as our landmark. If, after positioning the person in supine and palpating the ASIS, you find that your right and left thumbs are even (one is not higher than the other), note that the person has a level pelvis and no further evaluation is needed. When the ASIS are level, then the ischial tuberosities will be level when the person is seated and there is equal weightbearing on the left and right side of the buttocks.

If upon palpation of the ASIS, you find one thumb is higher than the other when the person is positioned in supine, then note the presence of an obliquity. Part of the mat assessment is to determine whether the pelvis can be passively moved out of the obliquity to achieve a level pelvis. When the pelvis can be passively moved to a level position, this is referred to as a *flexible* or *reducible* pelvic obliquity.

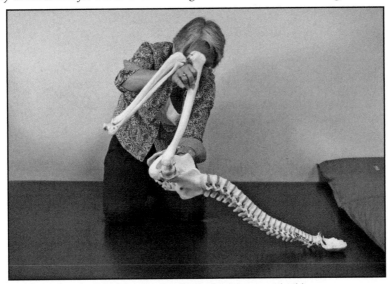

Figure 1-16. Demonstration of anteriorly tilted pelvis: non-reducible.

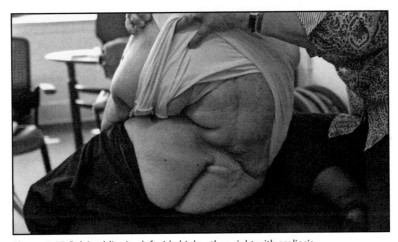

Figure 1-17. Pelvic obliquity: left side higher than right with scoliosis.

If one side of the pelvis is higher than the other and you are not able to passively change the position of the pelvis, then the position is often described as a *fixed* or *non-reducible* pelvic obliquity. Pelvic obliquity is described by referring to which side of the pelvis is higher than the other. For example, "The person presents with a pelvic obliquity, the right side higher than the left." The pelvis may assume an oblique position secondary to muscle tightening in the trunk due to asymmetrical muscle tone. A pelvic obliquity is often seen in conjunction with a spinal curve, known as a *scoliosis*—the C- or S-shaped curving of the spine. When the spine curves, the trunk muscles on the inside of the curve (the concave side of the curve) tend to tighten up compared with the muscles on the outside of the curve (the convex side of the curve). This muscle tightness pulls the pelvic crest closer to the ribs on the concave side and results in one side of the pelvis sitting higher than the other side (Figure 1-17).

To assess the passive mobility of the pelvis that is in an oblique position, place each of your thumbs on the person's ASIS. Rest the web space of your hand and your index finger on the pelvic crest. Note the resting orientation of the pelvis. Kneeling next to the person, place one arm under the knees and support the legs in a flexed position. You are going to use the long bones (femurs) of the legs as a lever to help you in passively moving the pelvis from side to side.

Pull both legs toward you, flexing the trunk on the side closest to you and extending the opposite side. Maintaining this laterally flexed position of the trunk, let the feet rest on the mat and repalpate the ASIS. The side closest to you should be higher than the opposite side. Move yourself to the other side and repeat the procedure. Can you return the pelvis to a midline position? If not, which side is higher than the other?

Observe the mobility of the trunk, as you passively move the pelvis. There should be an equal amount of

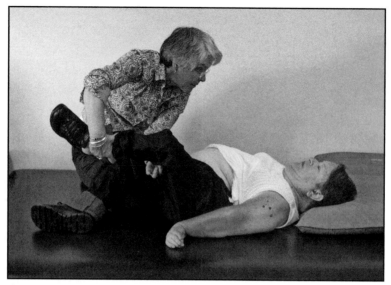

Figure 1-18. Non-reducible pelvic obliquity: no lateral trunk extension available.

lateral extension on both sides of the trunk. As you bring the person's legs toward you, observe the opposite side of the trunk, which should be elongating (stretching the muscles between the lower ribs and the pelvic crest). When you try to passively move the pelvis, if the opposite side of the trunk does not elongate, note that there is little to no change in the position of the pelvis. If one side of the pelvis stays higher than the other, this is a non-flexible, non-reducible, or fixed pelvic obliquity (Figure 1-18).

Record Your Findings

Clinicians will frequently document the presence of a pelvic obliquity as "Ms. Smith presents with a right obliquity." The challenge with this style of documentation is that the reader may not clearly understand the actual position of the pelvis. Does this documentation indicate the right side of the pelvis is high or low? A clearer method of documentation is to write out your actual findings: "Ms. Smith presents with a pelvic obliquity, right side higher than the left, and is not flexible to a level position."

If you are creating a form to capture your mat assessment findings, you may find the following format is an easy method to document your findings:

Pelvic Obliquity:

_____ None, pelvis is level, or

_____ side higher than the _____ side.

(Right or Left)   (Right or Left)

_____ Flexible/reducible to achieve level position

_____ Not flexible/non-reducible to achieve level position

Pelvic Rotation

The third axis of movement of the pelvis to be assessed is pelvic rotation. In addition to using the ASIS to assess rotation, we also use the posterior crests of the pelvis. With the person positioned in supine, if both posterior crests of the pelvis are in contact with the mat surface, then the pelvis is not rotated, and no further assessment is needed. If the pelvis is rotated, one side of the pelvic crest will be in contact with the mat surface, and the other side will be lifted off the surface. When palpating the ASIS, you will notice one thumb is closer to you and the other thumb is further back.

If, after positioning the person in supine, you find that the pelvic crests are in equal contact with the mat surface, you can note that the person has a flat pelvis, and no further evaluation is needed. When the pelvis is flat (not rotated), the pelvic crests are in a position to make equal contact (right and left side) on a back support when the person is seated.

To assess pelvic rotation, if the pelvis is not flat in a supine position, position yourself in a half-kneeling position next to the person. Place your palm on the ASIS that is raised on the raised side. With your other hand, place your hand under the posterior pelvic crest. At the same time, push down on the ASIS and pull up on the posterior pelvic crest to try to rotate the pelvis (see Figures 1-9 and 1-19). If the pelvis can be passively moved (with no movement at the shoulders), try to position the pelvis with both posterior pelvic crests resting against the mat. If the pelvis can be passively moved, then the rotation is reducible to a flat position.

When evaluating pelvic rotation, be observant of a log-rolling response. If, as you push down on the ASIS and pull up on the pelvic crest to derotate the pelvis, and you note the shoulders begin to rotate, then stop the movement. This pelvis is not able to rotate separately from the trunk. The pelvis assumes, and will maintain, a rotated position when the person is moved into a seated position. The pelvis is rotated, and the position is non-reducible.

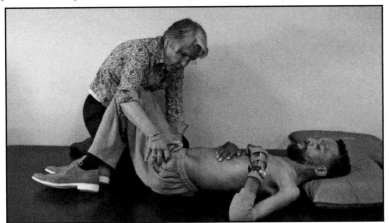

Figure 1-19. Preparing to assess pelvic rotation. Note the pelvis rotated off of mat surface.

RECORD YOUR FINDINGS

If you are creating a form to capture your mat assessment findings, you may find the following format is an easy method to document your findings:

Pelvic Rotation:

_____ Not rotated, or

_____ side rotate forward of the _____side.

(Right or Left)   (Right or Left)

_____ Flexible/reducible to achieve flat position

_____ Not flexible/non-reducible to achieve flat position

When a person with a rotated pelvis is seated against a flat backrest, only one pelvic crest will contact the back support. The side of the pelvis that is rotated forward will not be in contact with the back support. From a frontal view of the person, it may appear that the person has a leg-length discrepancy, with the posteriorly rotated pelvis appearing to be the shorter leg.

Pelvic Positioning: Putting It All Together

Before moving on in the mat assessment, stop and align the pelvis in the most ideal position possible. The ideal pelvic position we are trying to achieve when the person is in supine is as follows:

- Neutral tilt—ASIS are pointing toward the ceiling.
- Level side to side—ASIS are even, and there is no obliquity.
- Flat rotation—both pelvic crests are in contact with the mat.

If the pelvis cannot be positioned in this ideal alignment, record the actual position of the pelvis that will need to be accommodated once the person is repositioned in sitting.

Lower Extremity Range of Motion

The next phase of the mat assessment is to evaluate the ROM of the lower extremities, with the pelvis in a neutral position.

Hip Flexion With a Neutral Pelvis: Assessing the Trunk to Thigh Angle

Passive ROM of the hip joint is regarded to be within normal limits when the hip moves from full extension (0 degrees of flexion) to roughly 120 degrees of hip flexion. To achieve full range of hip flexion, a combination of movements occurs, including flexion at the hip joint and posterior pelvic rotation.

When assessing hip flexion with a neutral pelvis, the goal is to assess only the movement of the ball-and-socket joint, not pelvic rotation. As soon as the pelvis starts to rock back into a posterior pelvic tilt, flexion of the hip should be stopped. For this reason, the following procedure is used to determine the thigh to trunk angle of a seated person (Waugh & Crane, 2012), which is related to, but not the same as, the hip flexion ROM. By palpating the ASIS while flexing the hip, you will be able to detect pelvic tilt as you reach the end of the ROM of the ball-and-socket joint. This end range defines the seated thigh to trunk angle to be achieved, without allowing the pelvis to tilt back into posterior tilt to achieve greater hip ROM.

Determining the Thigh to Trunk Angle of a Seated Person

Passive ROM of the hip joint is influenced by the hamstring muscle. The hamstring is a two-joint muscle, meaning it crosses two joints from its origin to its insertion: the hip joint and the knee joint. When determining the thigh to trunk angle of the seated person, it is best to keep the knee flexed while passively flexing the hip joint to keep the hamstring muscle loose behind the knee.

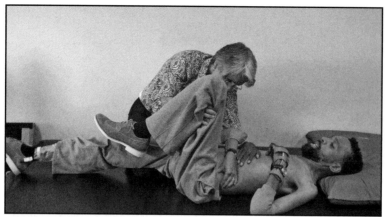

Figure 1-20. Determining trunk to thigh angle.

The thigh to trunk angle may be very different from the right to left side. The assessment of thigh to trunk angle should be done separately on each leg to determine any differences.

To assess the thigh to trunk angle:

- Assess the ball-and-socket motion of the hip joint on the left and right sides separately.

- To get a true thigh to trunk angle measurement, keep the knee bent so that the hamstring does not limit hip flexion.

- Test only the motion of the ball and socket at the hip, not the full hip flexion ROM, which includes posterior rotation of the pelvis.

- Stop flexing the hip when the pelvis begins to rotate backward (indicating pelvic motion rather than hip flexion), and record the angle between the trunk and the thigh.

Supine Procedure

While the person is in supine, align the pelvis in as neutral a position as possible. It is helpful to have the hips and knees slightly flexed to prevent muscle pull in any direction. Position yourself on the side of the hip that is being measured. Place one hand on the ASIS to palpate and detect any pelvic rotation with hip flexion. Place your other hand behind the bent knee. Your hand should be holding the distal end of the femur, closest to the knee joint. The knee joint should be bent so that the lower leg is covering your hand. Slowly flex the hip joint until you feel resistance or until you feel the pelvis (ASIS) begin to rotate back into a posterior tilt, under your thumb (Figure 1-20). Stop when the pelvis begins to move. Slowly repeat the end range of the ball-and-socket movement to determine the end point, which defines the person's thigh to trunk angle.

Many people will be able to easily achieve a thigh to trunk angle of 90 degrees, without any tilt of the pelvis. Others who are highly flexible will have a tighter thigh to trunk angle, measuring 80 or 85 degrees without any

movement of the pelvis, especially if the person's lower extremity muscles are flaccid.

If, however, the ball-and-socket motion of the hip joint is limited to less than 90 degrees when the pelvis starts to rock backward, the person will have a more open thigh to trunk angle, often measuring 100 or 110 degrees. This open angle will have an impact on the person's seated position. The angle between the seat cushion and the back support will also need to be opened to match the thigh to trunk angle.

The recorded thigh to trunk angle from the mat assessment is often a good starting point to determine the seat to back angle of the postural support system and wheelchair. To sit in a standard chair with a 90-degree seat to back support angle, a person will need at least a 90-degree thigh to trunk. Persons with an open thigh to trunk angle, greater than 90 degrees, will need specialized postural supports to match the thigh to trunk angle resulting from reduced motion in the ball-and-socket joint.

Hip Flexion With Knee Extension: Assessing the Thigh to Lower Leg Angle

As noted earlier, the hamstring muscle is a two-joint muscle. When the hip is flexed, the portion of the hamstring muscle that crosses the hip joint is stretched. When seated, we are flexed at the hips, and our knees are extended to rest on the foot pedals.

Because a person sits with flexed hips, we want to assess the flexibility of the hamstring muscle at the distal end, as it crosses the knee joint. Tightness of the hamstring muscle when the hip is flexed will impact the position of the lower leg. The following procedure helps determine the thigh to lower leg angle and the position of the feet to rest on the footplates.

To assess the thigh to lower leg angle:

- Test the right and left legs separately because hamstring tightness may differ side to side.

- The testing of hamstring tightness starts with the hip flexed (without pelvic tilt) and stops when there

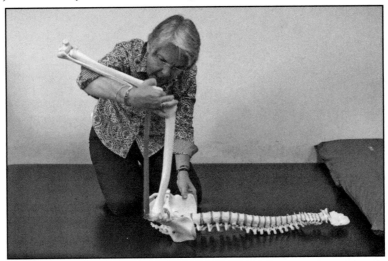

Figure 1-21. Demonstration of tight hamstring muscle on the thigh to lower leg angle.

is resistance to further knee extension. Stop passively moving the lower leg at the start of first sign of resistance and record the thigh to lower leg angle. This is referred to as the *popliteal angle* in orthopedic literature.

Supine Procedure

Position yourself on the side of the leg that is being measured. Keep one hand on the ASIS to feel for any movement of the pelvis as you flex the hip. Slowly flex the hip, as you did when testing for the thigh to trunk angle, keeping the knee fully flexed. Slowly extend the knee into extension, noting any significant tightness at the back of the knee (Figure 1-21). Stop moving the knee when you feel resistance. Allow the knee to go back into flexion and repeat slowly to determine the desired thigh to lower leg angle.

Persons with no hamstring tightness (again, those who are highly flexible) can be passively moved to a thigh to lower leg angle of 100 degrees or more. Persons with tight hamstrings, however, may only get to 90 degrees. Persons with significant hamstring tightness will have a tighter or smaller thigh to lower leg angle, resulting in an 85- to 80-degree angle. A tight thigh to lower leg angle requires a specialized foot support placement to prevent pulling on the hamstring, which pulls on the pelvis and results in sacral sitting. The most common impact of not respecting tight hamstrings in a seated person is the person sliding out of the chair to reduce the pull on the hamstring muscles. Remember the two-joint muscle? When there is not flexibility for the knee to extend to let the feet rest on a standard footplate, the lower leg is stretched to fit the foot onto the footplate. Without the needed flexibility, the hamstring muscle is being stretched at both the knee joint and the hip joint. Stretching the hamstring across the knee joint to get the feet on the footplates results in pulling the pelvis into a posterior tilt. Pulling the pelvis into a posterior tilt shifts

the person into a sacral-sitting position and results in the person sliding out of the chair.

Hip Abduction and Adduction

If you are able to easily flex and extend the hip during the assessment of hip flexion, then it is most likely that the ball-and-socket joint of the hip is intact, and there is no apparent reason to test hip abduction and adduction. If, however, when positioned in supine, the person assumes a frog-legged or a windswept position, it will be important to test the integrity of the ball in the socket.

When the legs are in a frog-legged position, the hips are both abducted. When the legs are windswept (i.e., it looks as though the wind came and swept the legs in the same direction, one hip is in abduction [positioned away from the body], and the other hip is adducted [positioned across the body]).

The goal for testing hip abduction and adduction during a mat assessment is to see whether the hips and knees can be positioned in line with each other when the hips are flexed. A hip, which is positioned in *ab*duction, will need to be moved toward the midline of the body to determine whether the knee can be positioned in line with the hip. This movement may be limited by tight hip abduction muscles—muscles on the outside of the hip joint. An abducted hip is most often in a position where the ball is in the socket, and the hip is not dislocated or subluxed. An abducted hip, which cannot be moved to neutral in the seated position, will affect the overall width of the seated surface.

An *ad*ducted hip will need to be moved toward the outside of the body, away from the midline, to determine whether the knee can be positioned in line with the hip. This movement may be limited by tight hip adductor muscles (muscles on the inside of the leg in the groin area) or by a subluxed or dislocated joint. Persistent positioning in hip adduction can result in the ball "sliding" out of the socket (being subluxed) or the ball being completely out of the socket (which is referred to as dislocated hip).

Supine Procedure

To passively test hip abduction and adduction, perform the following procedures.

Abducted Hip

Position yourself on the side of the leg that is being assessed. Slowly flex the hip, as you had done to determine the thigh to trunk angle, keeping the knee fully flexed. If the hip is frog-legged, slowly try to bring the leg toward the midline of the body (flexing and adducting the hip) until the knee is in line with the hip. If the leg can be moved toward midline (is able to be adducted) and the knee can be aligned with the hip, then the findings are recorded as "abducted, hip can be positioned into a neutral position." If the leg is highly resistant to moving into a neutral position (difficulty trying to adduct the hip), then the findings are recorded as "hip positioned in abduction."

If the hips are in a windswept position, the abducted hip is tested, as indicated earlier, and the most corrected position of the hip is recorded.

Adducted Hip

The adducted hip is tested by slowly trying to bring the leg to the outside of the body (away from the midline) until the knee is in line with the hip.

Caution: If there is significant resistance to movement of the leg to the outside of the body, then stop. The hip may be dislocated, and trying to abduct this hip will be painful. The hip position should be noted as being in adduction.

Position yourself on the side of the leg that is being assessed. Slowly flex the hip, as you did to determine the thigh to lower leg angle, keeping the knee fully flexed. If the hips are windswept, you will note that one hip is abducted and should be tested as previously described; the other hip will be adducted and should be tested using the following procedure.

Slowly try to bring the adducted leg *away from* the midline of the body (flexing and abducting the hip) until the knee is in line with the hip. If the leg can be moved away from midline (is able to be abducted), aligning the knee with the hip, then the findings are recorded as "adducted hip can be positioned into a neutral position." If the leg is highly resistant to moving into a neutral position (difficulty trying to abduct the hip), then the findings are recorded as "hip positioned in adduction."

If the hips are in a windswept position and cannot be passively moved to a neutral position, then one leg will be in an adducted position and the other will be in an abducted position.

Note: If during the seating assessment, an orthopedic finding, like a hip subluxation or dislocation, is suspected,

consult with the client and family to determine whether the person is being followed by an orthopedic specialist. A referral to an orthopedic surgeon may be indicated for long-term management of any pelvic and lower extremity alignment and pain issues.

Position of the Feet

One last observation while the person is in supine on the mat is mobility of the ankle and the position of the feet. We assess whether the bottom of the foot can be passively moved into a weightbearing position on a footplate. The sole of the foot should be flat to allow for safe weightbearing. Passively move of the foot, to determine the lower leg to foot angle.

- When the lower leg to foot angle is 90 degrees, the ankle is in a neutral position, and the sole of the foot is able to sit on a standard footplate.

- When the lower leg to foot angle is smaller than 90 degrees and the person is able to be positioned with the toes are pointing up, the ankle is in a *dorsiflexed* position.

- When the lower leg to foot angle is greater than 90 degrees and the person is only able to be positioned with the toes pointing down toward the ground, the ankle is in a *plantar flexed* position.

- When the foot is resting on the lateral side of the foot, weightbearing on the little-toe side, the foot is *inverted*.

- When the foot is resting on the inside of the foot, weightbearing on the big-toe side, the foot is *everted*.

If the foot cannot be passively moved into a position close to neutral, then adjustable-angle footplates may be indicated.

For clients with significant orthopedic foot impairments, it is often more effective to have the person be seen for an ankle-foot orthosis to be used to position and protect the feet when sitting in the wheelchair.

RECORD YOUR FINDINGS: LOWER EXTREMITIES

If you are creating a form to capture your mat assessment findings, you may find the following format is an easy method to document your findings:

Thigh to trunk angle:

Right side _____   Left side _____

Thigh to lower leg angle:

Right side _____   Left side _____

Thigh/upper-leg positioning:

_____ Hips and knees aligned bilaterally

_____ Frog-legged (both hips in abduction)

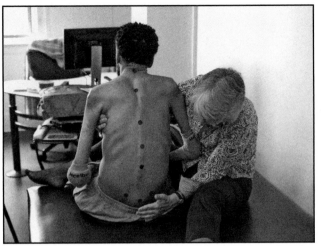

Figure 1-22. Rear view: posterior pelvic tilt and kyphosis that requires anterior support to be upright in sitting.

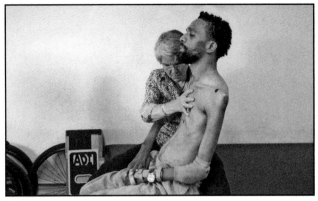

Figure 1-23. Pelvis supported in neutral tilt, trunk supported in open trunk to thigh angle.

_____ Able to reposition in alignment

_____ Not able to position in alignment

_____ Windswept to the _____ (Right or left)

_____ Able to reposition in alignment

_____ Not able to position in alignment

_____ Hip is abducted (Right or left)

_____ Hip is adducted (Right or left)

_____ Adducted, bilaterally

_____ Able to reposition in alignment

_____ Not able to position in alignment

Right hip is positioned in _____ (Adduction or alignment)

Left hip is positioned in _____ (Adduction or alignment)

Foot Position

Right foot: Left foot:

Lower Leg to foot angle: _____   Lower Leg to foot angle: _____

_____ Everted   _____ Everted

_____ Inverted   _____ Inverted

Moving From Supine to Sitting

Before asking the person to move, or assisting the person to move, from supine to sitting, observe and record the position of the head over the trunk and the trunk over the pelvis. If the head, trunk, and pelvis are not in alignment, try to passively realign the person. In this supine position, with gravity eliminated, a person with no spinal asymmetries should be able to be aligned passively in the desired position of the head and trunk in line with the pelvis. If you are not able to passively align the head, trunk, and pelvis, note the asymmetries because these same challenges will

be present when you move the person into a seated position over the edge of the mat.

Upright Seating Assessment: Hand Simulation of Postural Support

After the supine assessment and collection of information about pelvic mobility and the angular relationships between the trunk, thigh, and lower extremity, the next step is to assess the person in the upright seated position.

For hands-dependent and prop sitters, you may need assistance to provide additional postural support to maintain the person in a seated position. As you are settling the person into a seated position over the edge of the mat, be mindful of the need to respect the thigh to trunk angle to support an upright sitting position. A person with a thigh to trunk angle of 100 degrees will need to be supported in a slightly reclined position when seated over the edge of the mat. In addition, the thigh to lower leg angle also needs to be respected. For persons with tight hamstrings, allow the knees to flex under the mat to accommodate the tight thigh to lower leg angle (this angle will be <90 degrees). If the knees are allowed to flex under the person, the pelvis will be more easily supported in a neutral position, allowing for a stable base of support.

Once the person is sitting up, position the pelvis in a neutral position, if possible, and support the trunk manually using your hands. Through the use of careful positioning of your hands, you can further assess the person's need for external postural supports that may be needed to sit against gravity. This part of the mat assessment is referred to as *hand simulation*. You are using your hands (and often other body parts) to simulate the postural supports needed to allow the person to sit against gravity in a functional and comfortable position (Figures 1-22 and 1-23).

Trunk/Spine Mobility

When assessing the spinal alignment in the seated position, it is critical to have an unobstructed view of the trunk. This view can be achieved by positioning yourself behind the person and asking the person to either remove his or her shirt (or asking him or her to look under the shirt) or,

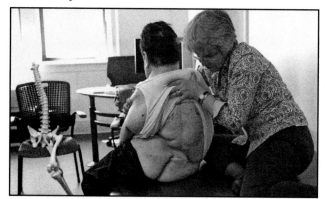

Figure 1-24. Rear view: non-reducible pelvic obliquity and scoliosis.

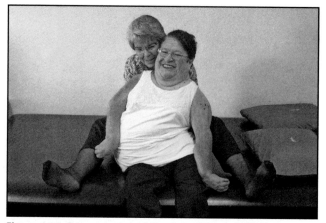

Figure 1-25. Demonstration of hand simulation of postural support for non-reducible obliquity and scoliosis. Support provided under left ischial tuberosity (higher ischial tuberosity) and right lower rib cage.

ideally, put on an examination gown to preserve modesty while allowing you to view the spinal alignment directly.

Before assessing the trunk, position the pelvis in the best corrected position you were able to achieve during the supine assessment. Support the pelvis as needed to provide a base of support, which enables the person to sit up against gravity.

Positioning Yourself to Provide Hand Simulation

If you are working with a person on a treatment mat or table, you will need to transition the person from supine to a sitting position over the edge of the mat. To continue with the seating assessment, you may find it useful to position yourself in a long-sitting position behind the person to have an unobstructed view of the spine and trunk.

If you are not able to conduct the assessment on a treatment mat, look for a stool or a bench on which the person can sit, ideally with no integrated back support, to allow you visual access to the trunk and an observation of unsupported sitting balance.

If the person is a hands-dependent or prop sitter, it is helpful to have a second set of hands available to assist in providing support, as you direct, to allow you to observe the pelvis, trunk, and head response to being supported against gravity.

Flexible/Reducible Lateral Trunk Curve

If a person leans to one side more than the other when sitting up, be sure to start at the pelvis and that it is level. If the pelvis has a flexible/reducible obliquity, you can use your legs to provide support under the low side to support and level the pelvis. When the pelvis is level, use your hands to manually provide the needed trunk support by placing your hands on either side of the trunk to realign the spine in a straight line. Observe the alignment of the spinous processes to watch the alignment move from a curved spine into a straight line. If the spine is realigned with this maneuver, properly positioned lateral trunk and pelvic supports will be needed to support the trunk when the person is seated in a wheelchair.

Non-Flexible/Non-Reducible Lateral Trunk Curve

If the person leans to one side and trunk alignment is not fully achieved when you provide external support using your hands, a skeletal asymmetry is indicated. Lateral trunk muscle shortening between the pelvis and the lower ribs will result in a non-reducible pelvic obliquity and a non-reducible spinal curve. If the pelvic obliquity is non-reducible and you attempt to level the pelvis, the result will be an increase in the lateral lean. If you cannot realign the spinous processes with your hands into an upright sitting position, then you should treat the pelvis a non-reducible obliquity. You can support a non-reducible pelvic obliquity with your leg, this time placing your leg under the high side of the pelvis, acting as a lift you would put on a shoe if there is a leg-length discrepancy. Filling in this space to support the high side of the pelvis will help in increasing the weightbearing on the high side ischial tuberosity, resulting in improved pressure distribution across both ischial tuberosities when the person is sitting in the wheelchair cushion (Figures 1-24 and 1-25).

Other Trunk Alignment Presentations

Kyphotic Trunk Position

If the person sits with a posterior pelvic tilt, rounded back, and forward head, it is important to check the flexibility of both the pelvis and the kyphotic curve of the trunk.

If the pelvis can easily be moved out of the posterior tilt, into a neutral position, start there. You will need to support the pelvis in the neutral position, perhaps with one of your legs, and then assess the flexibility of the kyphosis (see Figure 1-22). Position your hands with one just below the apex of the kyphosis and the other brought forward onto the sternum. Use gentle pressure to try to reduce the amount of forward trunk flexion by bringing the forwardly leaning upper trunk back in alignment with the pelvis.

If the trunk easily straightens, this is a flexible/reducible kyphotic curve, which can be supported by firm posterior pelvic support and a firm backrest mounted onto the wheelchair in an open angle (> 90 degrees) between the seat and back support, which allows gravity to assist in positioning of the trunk. Anterior trunk support may be required to support the trunk against the backrest.

If the pelvis and trunk do not easily move to a corrected position, then the most corrected posture needs to be accommodated. For relatively small kyphotic curves, accommodation can be made with a contoured back support mounted on the wheelchair in an open seat to back support angle that allows the kyphotic curve to rest against the backrest when the head is in a neutral position over the pelvis. For significantly larger curves, a tilt chair is useful in accommodating a non-reducible kyphotic curve because the system can be tilted until the head is balanced over the pelvis. A combination of an open seat to back angle and a tilt may be required.

The goal of hand simulation over the edge of the treatment mat is to determine the desired supported sitting position to be achieved in the wheelchair. Ideally, there is an exchange of information at this point, checking with the person being supported about her comfort and desire to remain in that position. *Listen carefully to this feedback.* If the person is comfortable and likes the supported position, then a rehabilitation technology supplier can facilitate the translation of this hand simulation into wheelchair seating products to replicate the amount and type of support being provided by the therapist. Chapters 3 through 5 will give you more specific intervention strategies for each type of sitter. Depending on the population you work with most frequently, you may find these chapters a great next step in synthesizing your seating assessment findings and translating your hand simulation into product trials.

Skin Integrity

For persons who rely on wheeled mobility full time, there may be an increased risk of skin breakdown, largely due to poor pressure distribution or ineffective pressure relief, resulting in pressure injury to the skin. The Braden Scale (Bergstrom, Laguzza, & Holman, 1987) is an excellent tool to assess a person's risk factors for pressure injury development. The scale addresses a variety of risk factors, including nutrition, mobility, sensation, and exposure to moisture. For therapists working with persons who are unable to shift their own position while sitting in a wheelchair, the biggest risk factors to address are mobility and sensation.

Impaired Sensation

When administrating the risk scale, you will be asking about level of sensation, especially on the seated surfaces (the buttocks, back of legs and back of trunk) and whether the person ever has the sensation of being uncomfortable when sitting for long periods of time.

- A person who reports discomfort while seated for a period of time likely has adequate sensation and, if able to adjust his or her own position, is not at high risk.

- A person who reports he or she does not experience any discomfort after sitting for a long period of time is likely to have impaired sensation. Due to impaired sensation, he or she is unlikely to shift position to interrupt continuous pressure, especially under the ischial tuberosities and greater trochanters, and thus is at higher risk for pressure injury development.

Impaired Mobility

With or without impaired sensation, a person who is not able to adequately shift his or her own position when sitting in the chair is at increased risk for developing pressure injuries due to immobility.

While the person is out of the chair and on the mat, it is a convenient time to visually inspect the skin, especially on the weightbearing areas of the buttocks and trunk. In addition to observing any areas of skin that are at risk due to scar tissue or persistent redness, the visual inspection verifies the presence or absence of any existing injuries. The skin can contribute a lot of information if you look closely. Ask about any surgical scars you may notice because these could lead to information not previously shared (see Figures 1-24 and 1-26).

Chapter 2 provides you with more detailed information about pressure management and measurement when working with persons who are relying on wheeled mobility as their primary means of mobility.

CASE EXAMPLES: PUTTING IT ALL TOGETHER

Rosa: Mobility Limitations Only

Rosa came to the clinic to review the options available to address her mobility needs. While sitting on the treatment mat, Rosa was able to lift both arms (hands-free sitter) and shift her own position on the mat, and she reported full sensation. She was able to maintain an upright sitting position during our interview, requiring minimal external postural support.

Rosa walked over to the scooter and was able to swivel the seat into the driving position independently. The scooter was equipped with a captain's seat, much like an automobile seat. Rosa reached down to the lever at the bottom of the backrest and adjusted the seat to back angle

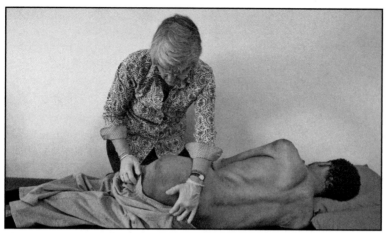

Figure 1-26. Skin assessment of left buttock and greater trochanter. Note changes in pigmentation marking healed wounds.

to 100 degrees (open), which she found more comfortable for both her lower back and head position. Her feet rested comfortably on the deck of the scooter, and Rosa reported being both comfortable and functional because she could now drive herself around her neighborhood, regaining her independence in shopping and participating in her community life at church.

Fred: Postural Support and Mobility Needs

Fred is heading into the second half of his freshman year in high school with his new chair. When he came to the clinic, we found the increased tone on the left side of his trunk, combined with his growth spurt, had caused tightening of the left trunk muscles and a tendency for him to assume a pelvic obliquity with the left side higher than the right. The obliquity is still reducible, so his new cushion is equipped with a right-side obliquity pad, which gently shifts his weight to the left side, balancing the pressure distribution under each ischial tuberosity. With the obliquity pad in place, his pelvis is level, and he can position himself against the back support of the wheelchair to be in a neutral tilt with no pelvic rotation. Fred asked for small, bilateral trunk supports for his chair because he needs to use his hands to drive, access his phone, and manage things in his life other than holding up his trunk against gravity, especially as the day goes on and he gets tired.

Fred can assume and maintain a 90-degree trunk to thigh angle using a 90-degree seat to back support angle in his chair. He does, however, need to change the orientation of his seating system throughout the day. When eating at the cafeteria, Fred brings his seat to a full upright position for easy access to the table and his food. When he is driving through the hallway, he tilts his seat 5 to 10 degrees for comfort and ease of driving. Several times during the day between classes, he will tilt the chair all the way back 45 degrees to shift the weight off his buttocks to the back support and headrest.

Fred's new chair is a power wheelchair equipped with a postural support seat cushion, back support, and lateral trunk supports for additional postural support. He has a power tilt system that allows him independence in pressure distribution and repositioning, and thus he can stay in his chair for the 14 to 16 hours needed to get through his day.

Lisa: Skin Integrity, Postural Supports, and Mobility Needs

Lisa is now 12 years postinjury and has been experiencing more frequent pressure injuries. During her mat assessment, we found both a non-reducible posterior pelvic tilt and a pelvic obliquity, with the left side higher than the right. This has resulted in higher pressure distribution under the right ischial tuberosity where she has been having the persistent injury, currently a Stage 3 healed wound. When seated over the edge of the mat, Lisa needed to support herself with her right arm. When she lifts her arms, she falls to the right side of the mat. During hand simulation, we provided support under the left ischial tuberosity to even the pressure distribution; this increased Lisa's base of support, but she still needed lateral support at her pelvis and trunk to allow her to be a hands-free sitter and continue to self-propel. We discussed the option of moving to a power chair with power seating for pressure relief, but Lisa just bought a new car and wanted to try to manage her skin with a new manual chair with proper postural supports and a pressure distribution cushion. Her new ultralight manual chair is equipped with a back support, supporting her to the midthoracic level of her trunk, an open seat to back angle of 95 degrees to accommodate her posterior pelvic tilt, and her pressure distributing cushion provides additional support under the left ischial tuberosity to balance the weightbearing between her ischial tuberosities. The new back support has integrated lateral pelvic and trunk support, which supports her pelvis and trunk when she pushes her chair. Lisa is now able to self-propel faster than walking speed without leaning to the right side of the chair and can transfer the chair in and out of the car without additional assistance. A smaller pressure distribution cushion was also added to her vehicle's seat, and she has now successfully managed her skin for the last 10 months, not missing another day at work.

SUMMARY: AN INTRODUCTION AND AN INVITATION

This chapter has given you the basic instructions on how and why to conduct a mat assessment as an essential step in the seating and mobility assessment process. The subsequent chapters are designed to build on this information with a focused view on how to address typical findings that you are likely to document within each group of sitters. We invite you to read the subsequent chapters to determine how to best address the postural support needs of the hands-free , hands-dependent, and prop sitter.

In addition, we hope that as you continue to review this book, you keep the following pointers in mind:

- A careful interview is always important to identify the person's desired goals and intentions for improved mobility and postural support. Learning to interview is the most important tool in a practitioner's skill set.

- After the interview, a supine mat assessment and hand simulation of postural support for hands-free, hands-dependent, and prop sitters will assist all team members (client, therapist, and supplier) to understand the goals for supported seating position.

- As appropriate seating supports are identified, address the risk factors that may affect skin integrity. To maintain skin integrity, the person must have adequate sensation and be able to shift position independently to redistribute pressure on the seated surface. A lack of sensation or a lack of ability to change one's position needs to be addressed using a pressure relief method.

- The final choice of a particular mobility device—manual chair, scooter, or power chair—depends on the information received and documented during the interview, mat assessment (including hand simulation), assessment of risks to skin integrity, and the person's choice depending on environment of use and personal preference.

- Ultimately, the most effective intervention with regard to seating and mobility is a device that is comfortable and will be used by the person who is experiencing mobility limitations.

- Optimal interventions are the result of a team of people working together, keeping the client at the center of the decision-making process.

 All photos in this chapter by Justo Diaz.

REFERENCES

Arledge, S., Armstrong, W., Babinec, M., Dicianno, B. E., DiGiovine, C., Dyson-Hudson, T.,...& Schmeler, M. (2011). RESNA wheelchair service provision guide. Retrieved from https://www.resna.org/sites/default/files/legacy/resources/position-papers/RESNAWheelchairServiceProvisionGuide.pdf

Bergstrom, N., Braden, B. J., Laguzza, A., & Holman, V. (1987). The Braden Scale for predicting pressure sore risk. *Nursing Research, 36,* 205-210.

Centers for Medicare & Medicaid. (2005). National coverage determination for mobility assistive equipment. Retrieved from https://www.cms.gov/medicare-coverage-database/details/ncd-details.aspx?NCDId=219&ncdver=2&NCAId=143&ver=25&NcaName=Mobility+Assistive+Equipment&bc=BEAAAAAAEAAA

Demers, L., Monette, M., Lapierre, Y., Arnold, D. L., & Wolfson, C. (2002). Reliability, validity, and applicability of the Quebec User Evaluation of Satisfaction with assistive Technology (QUEST 2.0) for adults with multiple sclerosis. *Disability and Rehabilitation, 24(1-3),* 21-30.

Kumar, A., Schmeler, M. R., Karmarkar, A. M., Collins, D. M., Cooper, R., Cooper, R. A.,...& Holm, M. B. (2013). Test-retest reliability of the functional mobility assessment (FMA): A pilot study. *Disability and Rehabilitation: Assistive Technology, 8,* 213-219.

Law, M., Baptiste, S., McColl, M., Opzoomer, A., Polatajko, H., & Pollock, N. (1990). The Canadian Occupational Performance Measure: An outcome measure for occupational therapy. *Canadian Journal of Occupational Therapy, 57,* 82-87.

Waugh, K., & Crane, B. (2013). *A clinical application guide to standardized wheelchair seating measures of the body and seating support surfaces.* Aurora, CO: University of Colorado School of Medicine.

World Health Organization. (2001). *International classification of functioning, disability and health: ICF.* Geneva, Switzerland: World Health Organization.

SUGGESTED READINGS

Batavia, M. (2010). *The wheelchair evaluation: A clinician's guide.* Sudbury, MA: Jones & Bartlett Learning.

Iezzoni, L. I. (1996). When walking fails. *Journal of the American Medical Association, 276,* 1609-1613.

Iezzoni, L. (2003). *When walking fails: Mobility problems of adults with chronic conditions* (Vol. 8). Berkeley, CA: University of California Press.

Minkel, J. L. (2000). Seating and mobility considerations for people with spinal cord injury. *Physical Therapy, 80,* 701-709.

Minkel, J. L. (2012). *Clinical bulletin: Seating and mobility evaluations.* Retrieved from http://www.nationalmssociety.org/NationalMSSociety/media/MSNationalFiles/Brochures/Clinical-Bulletin-Seating-and-mobility-evaluations.pdf

Paralyzed Veterans of America. (2005). *Preservation of upper limb function following spinal cord injury: A clinical practice guideline for health-care professionals.* Retrieved from https://www.ncbi.nlm.nih.gov/pmc/articles/PMC1808273/

Zollars, J. A. (2010). *Special seating: An illustrated guide.* Chicago, IL: Prickly Pear Publications.

Please see video on the accompanying website at

www.healio.com/books/mobility

2

Pressure Management for the Seated Client

Jo-Anne Chisholm, MSc, OT and Joanne Yip, BSR, OT

Everybody has a degree of risk for developing skin breakdown from prolonged pressure on an area of the body. The resultant skin damage is termed a *pressure injury* (National Pressure Ulcer Advisory Panel [NPUAP], 2016), previously termed *pressure ulcer*. Risk of developing a pressure injury increases exponentially with time spent in a single body position; therefore, an individual who sits in a wheelchair is at higher risk. For this reason, management of pressure is a key consideration in wheelchair seating.

Managing pressure effectively requires an interprofessional team approach (Houghton, Campbell, & the CPG Panel, 2013). The clinician responsible for wheelchair seating is one member of this health care team. The role of the wheelchair seating clinician is to do a thorough seating assessment that identifies and scales risk of developing a pressure injury. On the basis of assessment findings, the clinician prescribes a seating and mobility system designed to prevent sitting-acquired pressure injuries or, where a pressure injury already exists, to heal it and prevent recurrence.

In this chapter, determination of pressure risk and strategies to manage pressure through posture, position change, and sitting surface in the wheelchair seating system are discussed. An interprofessional pressure management model that encompasses prevention, treatment, and lifetime management is presented with specific reference to wheelchair seating.

Pressure management in general terms as well as in the context of wheelchair seating provision includes the following best clinical practices:

- Interprofessional team management

- Specialized training of team members

- Comprehensive seating assessment, including skin health factors

- A 24-hour positioning approach

- Skin observation as part of physical assessment

- Use of outcome measures and screening tools

- Use of specialized tools, such as pressure mapping

- Education, both general and targeted to the individual

- Teaching the client critical skin protection behaviors:

  ○ Skin check of at-risk areas morning and night—can be accomplished with a long-handled mirror, camera (smart phone), or by knowledgeable assistant

  ○ Effective weight shift—every 15 to 30 minutes for 1 to 2 minutes minimum and can be forward lean, side to side lean, tilt back, or by other method

  ○ Equipment maintenance, including cushion(s) and all weightbearing surfaces as well as wheelchair and other mobility devices

  ○ Awareness of local health resources: who to call or how to get help when needed

- Scheduled follow-up

Lange, M. L., & Minkel, J. L.
Seating and Wheeled Mobility: A Clinical Resource Guide
(pp. 27-46). © 2018 SLACK Incorporated.

INTERPROFESSIONAL PRESSURE MANAGEMENT MODEL

Pressure injuries are caused primarily by pressure and shear, and influenced by microclimate (moisture and temperature). Underlying conditions, such as poor nutrition, incontinence, systemic health concerns, lifestyle choices, and socioeconomic status, can all predispose to pressure problems. Pressure management best practice stipulates an interprofessional team approach and for team members to have specialized knowledge (Houghton et al., 2013). Clear understanding of the scope and skills of the team members, including points of intersection and overlap, enhances the collaborative process and ultimately leads to better outcomes. The use of a 24-hour approach is recommended to clearly understand all the risks to skin integrity (NPUAP, 2014). It is not enough to consider only wheelchair positioning and mobility, because time spent in bed, on a toilet, in a car, on a sofa, using a recreational device, or lying on an emergency department stretcher all have implications for skin health.

Use of a pressure management practice model (Figure 2-1) helps define the role of the seating clinician (occupational and physical therapists) and wound nurse, as well as seating individual, supplier, and other professions, in prevention, treatment, and monitoring of persons at risk for pressure injuries also termed wounds (Chisholm & Yip, 2016).

This model has three traffic circles containing the seated client, seating clinician, and nurse. The changing size of the players in the model reflects the shifting role emphasis. The direction of arrows illustrates that it is possible to stay in the green pre-wound (prevention) phase forever; however, once an open pressure injury (Stages 2 to 4) occurs, the client moves into the wound phase. Although they can leave the wound phase for the post-wound (lifetime management) phase, they can never return to the optimal pre-wound phase. This is because a pressure injury that is healed achieves just 80% tensile strength, leaving the area forever more vulnerable.

The overarching goal is therefore to keep our high-risk clients (think spinal cord injury, palliative, older bedbound adult) from ever moving out of the safe pre-wound phase. The seating clinician has a key role to play in prevention, however, including the following responsibilities:

- Identification of higher risk clients
- Education and training to develop proven pressure prevention habits (skin check, weight shift)
- Prescription of medical equipment, including wheelchair seating and mattresses
- Optimal positioning in bed and wheelchair
- Environmental modifications

- Teaching safe methods in transfers, repositioning, mobility, and other functional activities
- Ensuring the seating client knows the local resources

The expanded team can include health professionals and non-health professionals, including the family doctor, dietitian, orthotist, psychologist, and social worker, as well as family members, paid assistants, the medical equipment supplier, and others as relevant.

If the seating client has an open pressure injury (ulcer/wound) and moves into the wound phase, then the role emphasis shifts to nursing treatment to heal the wound. In this phase, the seating clinician continues to work in prevention of future wounds but also has a critical role in determining the cause of the wound and remedying it. Unfortunately, it is often not until someone develops a wound that the seating clinician is called in, whereas, if the clinician had been involved in the pre-wound phase, the wound might have been prevented. In the wound phase, the plastic or orthopedic surgeon could be called in if the pressure injury does not improve with local treatment. The dietitian plays an important role in ensuring the client has adequate nutrition to heal the pressure injury.

In the post-wound, lifetime management phase the role emphasis shifts to empowerment of the seated client to ensure that he or she does not develop another wound. The seating clinician continues to maintain the prevention/monitoring role with the understanding that risk can change with age, illness, weight change, progression of postural asymmetry, or other life events. Seated clients' needs change over their lifetimes, and aging increases the risk of pressure injury, as does the length of time that the client has been in a wheelchair (see Chapter 22). The seating clinician, with the knowledge of both the effects of aging and the expected trajectory of illness or disability, schedules assessment and implements interventions accordingly for clients. For example, it might be necessary to move from a nontilting to a tilting wheelchair or to change from manual to power operation. Because aging skin is more vulnerable to breakdown, the seating clinician might choose a seat with a greater level of protection.

A proactive approach of scheduled follow-up is best practice in the post-wound phase. Maintaining healthy skin over the seated client's lifetime will always involve the seating clinician together with other team members, depending on health need.

Changes to wheelchair seating are prescribed in all phases of this model. It is important for the funder to understand that money spent in the prevention phase is absolutely worthwhile and will save money if a wound is prevented in a high-risk individual.

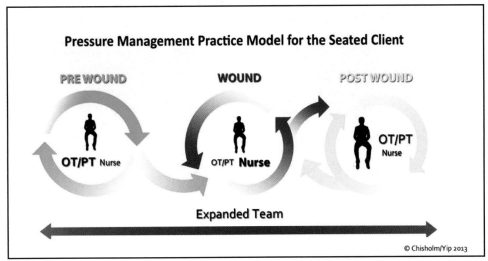

Figure 2-1. Pressure management practice model for the seated client. (OT = occupational therapist; PT = physical therapist.)

MECHANISMS OF PRESSURE INJURY DEVELOPMENT

Understanding how and why pressure injuries develop assists the seating clinician in effective prevention. Pressure management is a wide and well-researched health topic, and there is an abundance of scientific information and clinical best practice guidelines to reference (e.g., the NPUAP 2014 Clinical Practice Guidelines). The presented information is intended to provide accepted definitions on commonly used pressure terms, and the reader is encouraged to become further educated on the topic.

NPUAP (2016) stated that the term *pressure injury* would henceforth replace pressure ulcer because this more accurately describes a pressure injury to both intact (Stage 1 and deep tissue injury) and ulcerated (Stage 2 to 4 and unstageable) skin.

The new NPUAP definition of a pressure injury is as follows:

Localized damage to the skin and/or underlying soft tissue usually over a bony prominence… The injury can present as intact skin or an open injury and may be painful. The injury occurs as a result of intense and/or prolonged pressure or pressure in combination with shear (The Joint Commission, 2016).

Staging

Pressure injuries are staged by the extent of tissue damage. If a seating clinician observes any open pressure injury, a nurse is required to provide local treatment.

Stage 1 Pressure Injury: Nonblanchable Erythema of Intact Skin

Skin observation that reveals any redness or a Stage 1 pressure injury (redness that does not disappear on finger pressing) is an opportunity for the seating clinician to identify the source of the pressure and fix the problem before the skin opens (pre-wound phase). The redness may be more difficult to distinguish in darkly pigmented skin (Figure 2-2). Generally no local treatment is required other than removing the source of pressure.

Stage 2 Pressure Injury: Partial-Thickness Skin Loss With Exposed Dermis

The wound bed is viable, pink or red, moist, and may also present as an intact or ruptured blister. Fat and deeper tissues are not visible. These injuries often result from adverse microclimate and shear in the skin overlying the pelvis and shear in the heel (Figure 2-3).

In this wound phase, the seating clinician will be looking for causality, including adverse microclimate and shear conditions. Consultation with a wound nurse for local treatment as well as feedback regarding equipment or behavior changes and the effect on the wound is beneficial.

Stage 3 Pressure Injury: Full-Thickness Skin Loss

Fat is visible in the injury, and granulation tissue and rolled wound edges are often present. Undermining and tunneling may occur. Fascia, muscle, tendon, ligament, cartilage, and bone are not exposed (Figure 2-4).

The seating clinician makes changes regarding 24-hour positioning to reduce or eliminate pressure on the pressure

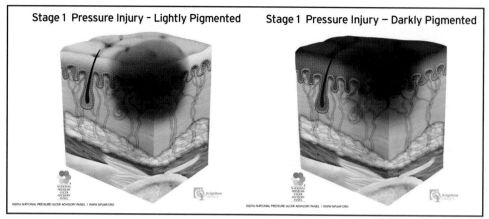

Figure 2-2. Stage 1 pressure injury. (Used with permission of the National Pressure Ulcer Advisory Panel, July 5, 2016.)

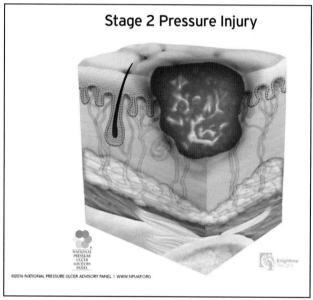

Figure 2-3. Stage 2 pressure injury. (Used with permission of the National Pressure Ulcer Advisory Panel, July 5, 2016.)

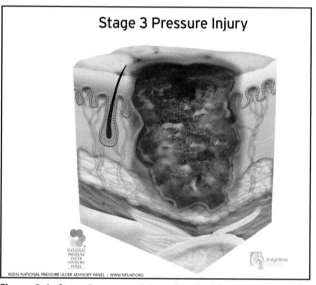

Figure 2-4. Stage 3 pressure injury. (Used with permission of the National Pressure Ulcer Advisory Panel, July 5, 2016.)

injury site and prescribes equipment (purchase or rental) to promote healing. Collaboration with the wound nurse may be required for safe positioning with alternative local treatments, such as negative pressure therapy. Nutrition for wound healing becomes more important.

Stage 4 Pressure Injury: Full-Thickness Skin and Tissue Loss

Exposed or palpable fascia, muscle, bone, tendon, ligament or cartilage can be visualized in the injury. Rolled edges and undermining/tunneling often present (Figure 2-5). The seating clinician continues to support solutions that enable the seated individual to mobilize as prolonged bedrest has negative systemic and emotional consequences. An ongoing dialogue among the seating clinician, wound nurse, and other health professionals can improve health outcomes.

Unstageable Pressure Injury: Obscured Full-Thickness Skin and Tissue Loss

Extent of tissue damage cannot be confirmed because it is obscured by slough or eschar. Stable eschar on an ischemic limb or the heels should not be removed. An unstageable pressure injury will declare as either a Stage 3 or 4 once the slough and eschar is gone. As per other stages, the seating clinician works to determine and remove the cause, and provide equipment solutions that address pressure, microclimate, and shear.

Deep Tissue Pressure Injury: Persistent Nonblanchable Deep Red, Maroon, or Purple Discoloration

Intact or nonintact skin with localized area of persistent, nonblanchable discoloration or epidermal separation revealing a dark wound bed or blood filled blister. The injury results from intense and/or prolonged pressure and

Stage 4 Pressure Injury

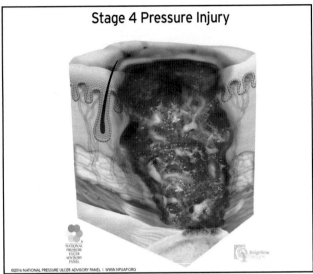

Figure 2-5. Stage 4 pressure injury. (Used with permission of the National Pressure Ulcer Advisory Panel, July 5, 2016.)

Deep Tissue Pressure Injury

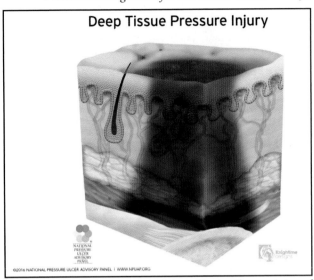

Figure 2-6. Deep tissue pressure injury. (Used with permission of the National Pressure Ulcer Advisory Panel, July 5, 2016.)

shear forces at the bone/muscle interface. Discoloration may appear differently in darkly pigmented skin (Figure 2-6).

This injury may either evolve to reveal a Stage 3 or 4 pressure injury and require nursing treatment, or it may resolve without tissue loss. The seating clinician, with the recognition that either a trauma (single incident) or prolonged pressure and shear caused the deep tissue injury, will look for the specific causative factor(s). Some examples of a deep tissue injury caused by trauma include a poor transfer in which the seated individual bumped his or her hip on the wheel of the wheelchair or an incident where he or she hit his or her heel on the edge of a metal footplate. It could also have been caused by prolonged pressure at the underlying tissues where the damage starts at the bone-tissue interface and moves outward. The seating clinician must investigate both possibilities to ensure that causation is effectively addressed.

Rules of Staging

- You can only stage a pressure injury, not a surgical wound, burn, or other skin opening.
- You can only stage up (1, 2, 3, 4) and never back: A Stage 2 can become a Stage 3, but a Stage 3 can never become a Stage 2 pressure injury.
- You cannot stage if you cannot see the wound bed, hence the term *unstageable*.
- A single pressure injury is staged by the worst damage present.

- Even when healed, a closed injury is referred to by its deepest level of tissue injury. For example, a "healed Stage 3 pressure injury."

Shear

The distortion of a body by two oppositely directed parallel forces. A pressure injury results when tissue is shifted against bone—for example, sliding down in a wheelchair such that the ischial tuberosities shift forward and the soft tissue remains in place (Figure 2-7).

Friction

Friction is superficial scraping of the skin, as when you skin your knee. It can indicate that there is shear below, but not always. Friction without shear does not cause a pressure injury (NPUAP, 2016).

Microclimate

This refers to the local conditions of temperature and moisture that can contribute to pressure injury.

Temperature

Wound healing benefits from a normal body temperature. Too much heat causes sweating, which causes moisture. Cooling can interfere with healing a pressure injury by dropping body temperature out of optimal healing range.

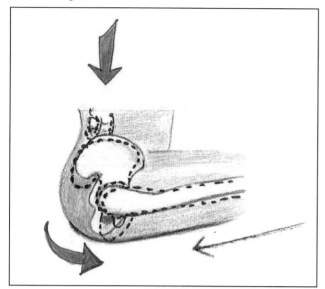

Figure 2-7. Shear.

Moisture

Skin that is too moist or too dry increases the likelihood of pressure injury when combined with pressure. Skin that has had prolonged exposure to moisture becomes macerated.

RISK EVALUATION

Effective pressure management requires a comprehensive understanding of the client's level of risk. Everybody has some level of risk for skin breakdown. A healthy, young, able-bodied athlete can develop a pressure injury under extreme conditions—for example, if he or she lies unconscious on a concrete floor for an extended period.

Accurate determination of risk is the combined result of both standardized measurement and clinical assessment, including pressure mapping. The seating clinician weighs all findings and makes a clinical judgment on the client's risk of developing a pressure injury.

Standardized Risk Assessment Scales

A standardized tool is helpful in screening for risk on initial assessment and to evaluate treatment efficacy ongoing. The Braden Scale (Bergstrom, Braden, Laguzza, & Holman, 1987) is the most widely used and tested and its scoring from low to very high risk is understood across health disciplines. It includes six subscales rating sensory perception: moisture, activity, mobility, nutrition, friction, and shear. Other standardized scales, such as the Waterlow, contain similar categories with the addition of more specific information, including gender, age, body mass index, and skin condition by visual inspection (Mortensen &

Miller, 2008). The Spinal Cord Injury Pressure Ulcer Scale (Salzberg et al., 1996) is specific to persons with spinal cord injury and includes risk factors pertinent to this population.

Clinical Risk Assessment

The assessment of physical health, functional abilities, psychosocial factors, and the environment all help the seating clinician formulate pressure injury risk for a client. Each component of the seating assessment provides opportunity to learn about the individual in terms of his or her pressure risk. In the preliminary information gathering via document review and interview, the clinician gains knowledge of diagnosis, health comorbidities (medications/hospitalizations), history of skin issues (previous wounds, surgeries) nutrition, smoking and other substance use, environment, and socioeconomic situation. Liaison with other health professionals regarding medical management promotes fuller awareness of the health picture and results in improved pressure outcomes. Sensory status is a key indicator of pressure risk and can be partially inferred via diagnosis (e.g., spinal cord injury, multiple sclerosis).

Awareness of how a client performs day-to-day functional activities provides the seating clinician with important data. The multitude of occupations performed throughout the day from dressing, bathing, transfers, and toilet hygiene to driving, employment, and recreational pursuits are all relevant in the building of a risk profile. Although not all activities can be directly observed, at a minimum, it is important to observe wheelchair mobility and transfers, ideally in the environment of use. Skin protection behaviors, such as skin checks and weight shifts, are recorded in terms of method and frequency. The seating clinician also gathers information about 24-hour positioning, time spent in any one position, and the equipment and surfaces used.

Where the client lives, works, and plays are factors in pressure risk. Evaluation in the home or workplace provides the most accurate contextual information. If a client can't take his wheelchair up the stairs into his home, he might be forced to get out of his chair and "bum" up the stairs to get in. An inaccessible bathroom could require a client to wear incontinence protection, which causes moist skin. Another client might rarely use the wheelchair you assessed her in, preferring to use her ATV with the saddle seat because there are no paved roads where she lives.

The physical assessment encompasses sensory status, posture in and out of the wheelchair, wheelchair mobility, gravity eliminated supine assessment (mat evaluation), upright seating assessment including level of sitting balance (hand-free, hands-dependent, prop), and sitting simulation with hands (see Chapter 1). When observing the client in his wheelchair, postures that flag pressure risk include any asymmetry (e.g., pelvic obliquity), poor distribution of load (e.g., no loading of thighs because footrests too high), or heavy loading of a body part (e.g., lower leg pressed on foot hanger). The clinician confirms his or her visual findings by palpation of the client to determine where and how heavily the person is weightbearing, effectiveness of the seating surfaces (cushion, back support, head support), accuracy of sensory perception, and boniness.

Visual skin inspection is done as part of the mat assessment and provides invaluable information about the current condition of the skin as well as historical issues, typically revealed by wound or surgical scars or skin discoloration. Redness on any area indicates loading regardless of whether it is transient or a Stage 1 pressure injury. Location of the redness needs to be correlated with the causative factor (where on the equipment the redness corresponds to). When a pressure injury is present, it is important to see it, stage it, and palpate (gloved) the bony prominence it is related to. A pressure injury provides clues as to its causation and phase of healing:

- An injury with feathered edges might indicate there is some movement cause, such as transfers or sliding down in a wheelchair.

- An injury that has defined edges might indicate that a more direct pressure cause exists.

- An injury that presents at a distance from a bony prominence could indicate that tunneling or undermining is present, and this should be confirmed via consultation typically with a wound nurse.

- The presence of undermining can indicate movement in the direction of the undermining, which can help determine causality. For example, sliding forward in the wheelchair or sideways when transferring.

Taking a close-up and long-view picture, with consent, is a valuable documentation strategy. Pictures can be shared with other health professionals and can help you to determine whether your seating interventions are working.

Assessment of posture with gravity eliminated (supine) enables the seating clinician to determine to what degree postural correction is possible. Corrective forces add concentrated pressure where force is applied and this must be monitored. Postural correction can also decrease pressure risk by creating a more symmetrical body posture, which improves pressure redistribution on the weightbearing surface. For example, in the case of a flexible pelvic obliquity, providing external posture supports to maintain a neutral pelvis will result in more even pelvic pressure redistribution side to side. If a pelvic obliquity is nonreducible, then pressure might be managed by seat surface accommodation of the asymmetry, contouring the seat surface to equally contact the high and low sides.

In the upright seating assessment, the placement of external supports is determined by hand simulation. This is further translated into equipment setup for client trial. During this portion of the seating assessment, pressure risk can be further evaluated by interface pressure mapping.

Interface Pressure Mapping

Interface pressure mapping is a clinical tool (like a tape measure or a goniometer) used to collect objective data about pressure risk by providing a two-dimensional (2D) color or three-dimensional (3D) topographical visual display of a client's distribution of pressure on a surface. A component of a comprehensive seating assessment, it assists the clinician to assess existing equipment, analyze posture, compare seating surfaces, and adjust wheelchair configurations. Pressure mapping is also a compelling biofeedback or educational tool for encouraging positive pressure management behaviors, such as effective weight shifts and equipment maintenance.

A protocol that ensures infection control and the collection of consistent and comparable data should be used (Chisholm & Yip, 2016). These data are only useful if correctly interpreted by a clinician. Key parameters for visual interpretation (an ongoing dynamic clinical process) include the following:

- Peak pressure: Pressure map area of highest pressure(s). There can be more than one peak pressure within a map. The map in Figure 2-8 with individual cell readings in millimeters mercury (mm Hg) shows a peak pressure at the left ischial tuberosity as determined by hand palpation in conjunction with visual interpretation.

- Pressure gradient: The difference between the highest to the lowest pressure with the objective in pressure redistribution of attaining the lowest gradient possible (gentle slope, no peaks and valleys). In pressure off-loading a high gradient is acceptable. Figure 2-9 shows a 2D and a 3D pressure map of an off-loading cushion where the load is being taken through the proximal femurs and cantle area with the ischial tuberosities, greater trochanters, and coccyx off-loaded.

- Symmetry: Comparison of the left and right sides of the pressure map for overall symmetry with the goal being even weight distribution side to side. In Figure 2-10, because the client is sitting primarily on the right side of his pelvis, the pressure map indicates this asymmetrical presentation with the peak pressures located at the right greater trochanter and right ischial tuberosity, less pressure at the left ischial tuberosity, and no pressure over the left greater trochanter.

- Posterior-anterior (P-A) dispersion: Distribution back to front; ideally loading fully from buttocks to thighs. In Figure 2-11, the 3D pressure map shows poor P-A dispersion with the weight entirely over the pelvis and no loading of the thighs. In Figure 2-12 the 3D pressure map P-A dispersion is improved with a shift of load from pelvis to thighs.

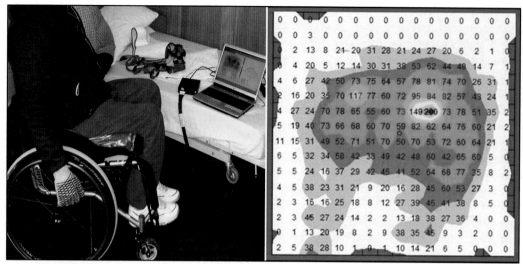

Figure 2-8. Peak pressure.

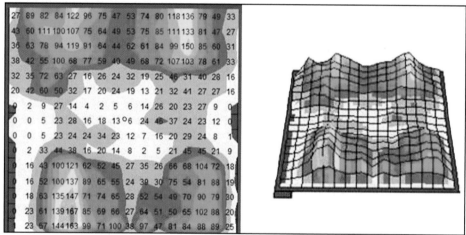

Figure 2-9. Pressure gradient.

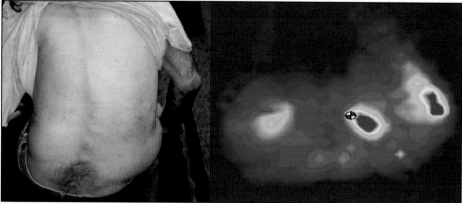

Figure 2-10. Symmetry.

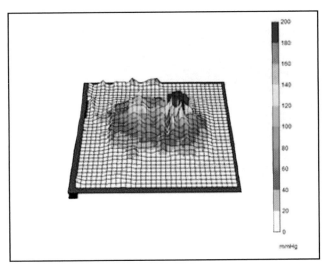

Figure 2-11. Poor P-A dispersion.

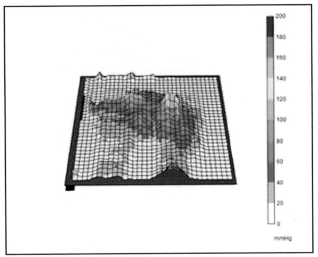

Figure 2-12. Improved P-A dispersion.

- Total contact area: Evaluation of the total number of sensors loaded (sensors that show on the pressure map). The goal is usually the maximum number to achieve the largest surface area possible for pressure redistribution.

Visual interpretation of peak pressure, symmetry, dispersion, gradient, and total contact area is done within the context of the entire pressure mapping session. These are useful terms to describe the pressure mapping session but do not in themselves define individual client need or the recommendations that will arise from the session.

In addition to visual interpretation, the clinician may choose to use metrics available in pressure mapping (Crane, Hetzel, & Sonenblum, 2016). Measures used include the following:

- Peak pressure index: Peak and surrounding values
- Average pressure
- Contact area
- Dispersion index: Ratio of ischial tuberosity/sacral loading to total loading

Clinical Judgment of Risk

The clinician uses both standardized risk measurements and clinical assessment findings including pressure mapping to form an overall clinical judgment about the client risk of developing a pressure injury "regardless of how the risk assessment is structured, clinical judgment is essential" (NPUAP, 2014). High-risk findings, such as absent sensation, are weighed against positive mitigating factors, such as good skin protection behaviors, to determine whether the overall estimation of risk is low, medium, high, or extremely high. Each client has unique circumstances, and scoring with standardized risk tools does not provide the whole picture. For example, a client with absent sensation, no mobility, incontinence, and shear potential could mitigate these negative factors with excellent skin protection behaviors, good nutrition, accurately prescribed equipment, and well-trained paid assistants such that his or her clinical risk is effectively lowered.

SEATING INTERVENTIONS FOR PRESSURE MANAGEMENT

In wheelchair seating, pressure management is addressed through the following:

- Postural modifications
- Facilitating position change
- Surface selection
- Microclimate management

Postural Modifications

There are many benefits to optimizing sitting posture, and pressure management is one. Performing a thorough mat assessment is the foundation to understanding client posture, and therefore, also foundational to pressure management. The clinician translates physical findings, including body dimensions and joint range of motion (ROM), into the wheelchair seating configuration. For example, if hip flexion range is limited to 75 degrees, resulting in a trunk to thigh angle of 105 degrees (neutral hip angle is 90 degrees), then the seat back angle is typically set at an open angle of 105 degrees to accommodate this fixed body position. If this angle is not correctly matched to the person's body, then the mismatch will result in pressure and shear forces that can lead to a pressure injury.

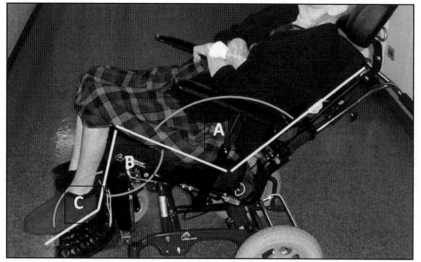

Figure 2-13. Posture modifications. (A) an open seat to back angle to accommodate hip flexion; (B) a closed seat to lower leg support angle to accommodate tight hamstrings; (C) an open lower leg to foot support angle to accommodate plantarflexion deformity.

In addition to getting a good fit (matching body and seating angles correctly), the following postural strategies are used to minimize pressure, shear, and friction.

Optimize Distribution of Pressure

When pressures are distributed over the greatest surface area possible, peak pressure in any one location (e.g., an ischial tuberosity) is minimized. This concept is used in postural support systems where it is understood that improving symmetry, dispersion, and overall surface contact will optimize pressure distribution. For example, if a client tends to lean to the right and this posture is correctable, then correcting this lean will lead to a reduction in pressure over the right side of the pelvis and right hip by shifting some body weight to the left side.

Symmetry refers to symmetrical or even side to side weight distribution in sitting for all body parts in contact with the postural support system. In the pelvic region, this refers to equal loading of the ischial tuberosities and greater trochanters (seat) as well as posterior superior iliac spines (back support) and anterior superior iliac spines anterior pelvic controls). Other at-risk areas include the elbows (arm support), scapulae (back support), feet (foot support), and occiput (head support).

P-A dispersion refers to the back-to-front distribution of weight on a weightbearing surface. In the seat, this refers to the distribution of weight of the pelvis compared with the amount of weight of the thighs with the usual goal of spreading the weight from the back of the seat to the front. Other supports this might apply to include arm supports (including trays) and foot supports. Examples of using posture modification to improve P-A dispersion would be lowering a footrest to increase thigh contact or angling a footrest to improve overall foot contact.

Use of Orientation in Space

In wheelchair seating, orientation in space is the selective tipping of the whole body in a forward, rearward, or lateral position to achieve specific postural goals, including greater or more even distribution of pressure. This is particularly helpful when nonreducible, or difficult-to-correct, body postures are present. Using tilt (nondynamic) to orient a client backward in space will redistribute load from buttock only to buttock and sacrum using the back support as a weightbearing surface.

An example of posture modifications is shown in Figure 2-13. The client has limited hip flexion, tight hamstring with less than 90 degrees of knee extension and plantarflexion asymmetries that are accommodated for through matching of these angles in her wheelchair. In addition, pressure is distributed symmetrically and there is full contact from head to toe. A rearward orientation in space shifts weight from seat to back.

Facilitating Position Change

Evolution of wheelchair technology has been driven in part by the recognition that position change is good for the body. Position change includes the concept of getting out of the wheelchair entirely or changing position within the wheelchair. Before there were tilt-in-space wheelchairs, practical clinicians educated their clients or assistants on how to achieve a rearward tilt position change by tipping the chair back onto a bed (brakes on). However, today a bed is not required because the wheelchair itself can be tilted in space through power or manual operation.

Dynamic tilt is the ability of a chair to be tilted backward, forward, or to the side so that the load is shifted from one area of the body to another. Manual chair dynamic tilt

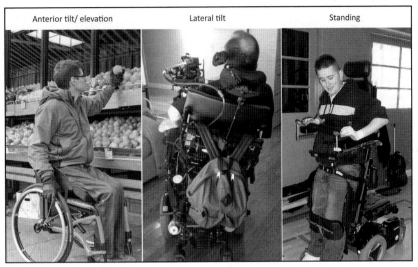

| Anterior tilt/ elevation | Lateral tilt | Standing |

Figure 2-14. Position change.

systems are generally operated by an assistant, and power chair dynamic tilt is set up for independent operation; however, the reverse is true for both. A rearward tilt greater than 30 degrees is the minimum requirement to adequately redistribute pressure from the seat to the back and increase blood flow (Houghton et al., 2013), and this change of position should be held as individual skin response dictates. Although more tilt is generally better, clinicians determine the optimal amount of tilt required to achieve an adequate weight shift for their clients and educate them regarding this important pressure protection behavior.

Anterior tilting and lateral tilting are less common dynamic position features but are effective depending on individual posture needs. Anterior or forward tilt shifts weight from the buttocks to the thighs and feet (Figure 2-14). Although more often used to facilitate transfers and foot propelling, it can also be a pressure management strategy. Lateral tilt shifts weight from one side of the body to the other and is usually used where a nonreducible lateral orthopedic asymmetry causes excessive weightbearing on one side of the body. For example, a side-flexion neck contracture that causes increased pressure on one side of the head or a fixed lateral curvature of the spine that results in heavy loading of the one trunk support or asymmetrical weightbearing on the seat. As per other dynamic tilt options, you are shifting weight off one area to differentially load another area (see Figure 2-14).

Dynamic recline is another wheelchair function that can be used in pressure management. In the recline position, body contact area is greatly increased, and pressure redistribution is over the seat, and back, head, and lower leg support. Dynamic recline is available with manual or power operation and can be specified on its own or as part of a group of dynamic features including recline, tilt, and leg elevation. Recline (alone or in combination) must be used with caution because it can cause shear due to sliding of the

buttocks forward on the seat. Power recline is often paired with a low-shear back feature. Clinicians must always weigh the individual risk-benefit factors. For example, recline would be contraindicated for a client with strong hip extensor spasm. When appropriately prescribed, an additional benefit of recline is the change of total body position from seated to lying.

Combined tilt and recline allows the greatest weight transference from the seat to the back support (Aissaoui, Lacoste, & Dansereau, 2001) and may be more effective than either function on its own. To minimize the friction and shear that may occur when a seated individual reclines, it is recommended to tilt the chair before reclining (Houghton et al., 2013). A position of 25 degrees of tilt combined with 120 degrees of recline is effective in enhancing both muscle and skin perfusion at the ischial tuberosities (Jan, Jones, Rabadi, Foreman, & Thiessen, 2010).

Standing wheelchairs enable the individual to go from sitting to standing supported by the chair. Standing has numerous benefits, including pressure management (Sprigle, Maurer, & Sorenblum, 2010); however, it is not as commonly used for this purpose because the individual must have adequate range and bone density for safe standing. Standing wheelchairs shift the weight from the seat to the foot support and anterior supports, such as a tray. Dynamic standing can be a feature of a manual or power wheelchair, and although its roots are with the manual wheelchair; but it is now more usual to find it paired with power. Power operation does not require as much upper body strength and function, and the additional weight of the standing feature does not affect mobility in power as it does in manual wheelchairs. As with most aspects of wheelchair seating prescription, the decision to prescribe standing in a wheelchair would involve more factors than solely that of pressure management (see Figure 2-14).

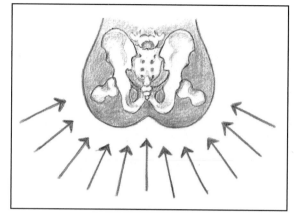

Figure 2-15. Pressure redistribution.

Other dynamic features include a manual wheelchair that will facilitate independent partial standing and dynamic "dump" adjustment over a preset range and will also enable the user to manually adjust back recline (Borisoff & Mitchell, 2015). Dynamic spring-loaded backrests, footrests, and headrests can reduce shear in particular for people with extensor spasticity.

Position change encompasses individual solutions for getting in and out of the wheelchair and weight shifting within the wheelchair. It is the clinician's responsibility to ensure that his or her clients or the clients' assistants can easily manage these activities as part of a comprehensive approach to pressure management. Education about pressure injury prevention includes the importance of position change and weight shift in general, as well as targeting information specific to the client's needs and abilities. For example, the best method to weight shift for an individual might be pushing up with his or her elbows. To make this possible, the armrest height, surface area, and padding would be specified to this purpose. The best method to transfer out of the chair might be to do a low pivot lateral transfer and the front edge of the seat would therefore be firm, noncontoured, and long enough to facilitate this. There are myriad individual solutions for one-off client scenarios to facilitate position change. Some unique modifications are the following:

- Custom anti-tippers that are intended to weightbear in a tilt-back position

- Trunk supports that are power swing-away to facilitate independent operation

- Pelvic laterals that flip down to become a surface for independent transfers

- A power-up system to enable a transfer from floor to seat

Wheelchair seating solutions can be as varied as the people who need them.

Surface Selection

Seating surfaces are any and all surfaces that the client may sit on. This commonly includes wheelchair cushions, but also includes toilets, commodes, bathing surfaces, vehicle seats, alternate positioning equipment, and furniture of all kinds. When an in individual spends time sitting up in bed for any reason, then this surface needs to be evaluated as a seat surface as well. For example, a mattress that has been set up for supine or side-lying may not be safe for sitting. Every surface can be modified to reduce the risk of skin breakdown, and any time a surface is changed, skin inspection is recommended. When selecting a seat surface there are three general principles to keep in mind:

1. Pressure redistribution

2. Force isolation (or off-loading)

3. Alternating pressure

Pressure Redistribution

Pressure redistribution refers to the spreading of pressure over as much surface area as possible to reduce loading of any one area. Generally, this is done through immersion in fluid, air, or foam or through contouring to match body shape. Cushions that use the principle of pressure redistribution are the most frequently prescribed cushion for pressure management. The classic air cushion uses this principle where less air/inflation equals greater immersion and so greater pressure redistribution, until too little air leads to bottoming out, at which point the benefit is lost. Cushions constructed of varying types of foams, thermoplastics, gels, fluids and hybrid products that use a combination of these are all based on the principle of pressure redistribution. Custom-molded systems allow for pressure redistribution through exact matching of body contour, and there are a variety of techniques and materials used in their fabrication (Figure 2-15).

Force Isolation

Force isolation (or off-loading) refers to the total removal of pressure from a select area of the body onto another designated area of the body that is better able to tolerate it. This principle is used in orthotic insoles, for example, where the metatarsal heads are fully off-loaded by selectively loading the arch of the foot. Pressure relief boots are a commonly prescribed pressure management device that off-load the heels and load either the sole of the foot (walking boot) or the calf (bed positioning) dependent on body position.

In seating, we off-load bony prominences that are at risk of skin breakdown, including ischial tuberosities, coccyx, greater trochanters, spinous processes, and scapulae, but also as the situation demands, ears, heels, toes, and elbows. Off-loading can be accomplished by shape capture or by

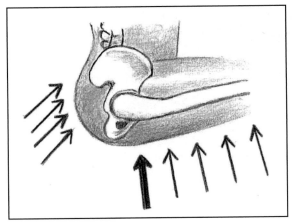

Figure 2-16. Force isolation.

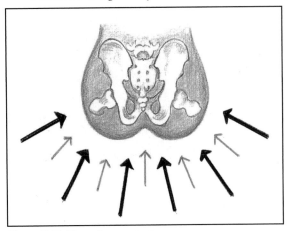

Figure 2-17. Alternating pressure.

carving out or building up an area on an existing surface. As off-loading, by definition, requires loading, it is important to educate your client to check skin on body parts that are loaded.

Seats that use the principle of force isolation can be firmer than other seat bases and must be carefully sized and fitted to ensure that the bony prominences of concern are truly off-loaded. Some cushions off-load the ischial tuberosities and coccyx by selectively loading the greater trochanters and thighs, and other cushions off-load coccyx, ischial tuberosities, and greater trochanters by loading the proximal femurs and posterior buttock area surrounding the coccyx (cantle). Either option can be effective dependent on the individual need (Figure 2-16).

Alternating Pressure

Alternating pressure surfaces actively shift pressure from one area of the body to the other through differential inflation and deflation of segments/air bladders. A cushion with this feature requires a power source and so would usually be found on a power chair, but could also use a portable battery carried on a manual wheelchair. Such cushions are less commonly used, possibly because of the lack of availability for trial and/or because they are expensive and efficacy is unclear (Figure 2-17).

Coverings

Coverings of seating surfaces affect pressure management properties. For example, where the principle of pressure redistribution is being used, a cover must be loose and resilient so that the client can sink into the surface. In force isolation, covers are designed not to hammock, which could reduce the off-loading property. Thick, soft covers can add cushioning; slippery covers can reduce friction, especially during transfers; double covers (or a cover with two layers of material) can help reduce the impact of shear. At times, a cover that has friction or nap is used to prevent sliding and potential shear, such as a one-way slide, which allows movement in only one direction.

Microclimate Management

Close contour and multiple areas of body contact are common features of posture control systems. As a result, the system itself can cause microclimate problems of heat and moisture buildup on the skin. A narrow body temperature range is optimal for healing pressure injuries, and moisture increases the risk of skin breakdown exponentially (NPUAP, 2014). Excess heat, incontinence, and wound drainage all contribute to an undesirably moist environment. Microclimate management should always be considered in seating.

Microclimate management of heat and temperature is generally addressed through the following:

- Material choices for the internal structure of the seat, back support, and other posture components. Foams of various kinds are typically used in fabrication and are often heat retentive. Other materials, such as air, gel, or fluid, have different thermal characteristics and can be used instead of, or in combination with, foam to improve heat dispersion.

- Material choices for coverings. How a system is covered has major implications for microclimate management as well as pressure management in general. A cover that is too tight or does not allow for envelopment can negate the pressure properties of a seat or cushion. Addressing issues of incontinence is a two-pronged problem, because both the client and the seating require protection from moisture. Protecting the seat surface can mean using a moisture-repellant, less stretchy cover, which can then create heat buildup and reduce immersion. Another approach is to use a seat surface product that allows moisture to penetrate without damaging it. A breathable cover can then be used, as the product does not require moisture protection. A cover that has a degree of breathability and cushioning, such as spacer mesh or pile, can provide airflow to

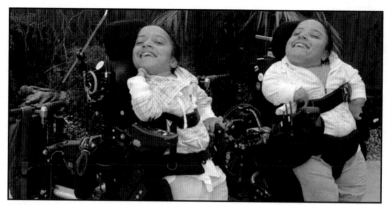

Figure 2-18. Twins: Jotti and Deepi. (Deepi is on the right.)

help reduce heat buildup and wick moisture away from skin. Clothing is basically another "seat covering" that can be helpful or problematic. Snug, seamless, stretchy clothing can be protective, whereas clothing with seams and buttons at weightbearing areas can cause added pressure and shear. The addition of incontinent pads can interfere with surface properties.

- Design features incorporated into the seating system to provide air flow and ventilation include such simple measures as leaving a gap between seat and back support, minimizing contact by only providing support where specifically required, and adding holes to a back support or using a grid base under a cushion.

- Powered ventilation and cooling/heating can be used in seating as in mattress technology. A computer fan can be wired under a grid base and powered by a battery where excessive sweating is an issue. Cushions that have low air loss feature will reduce moisture buildup and can keep skin cooler. Heating components can also be included if keeping warm is a problem.

CASE EXAMPLES

Case examples help to illustrate how pressure management and seating are interrelated. Three cases are presented here, each in a different phase of the Pressure Management Practice Model for the Seated Client. Clinical estimation of risk and seating interventions are described.

Pre-Wound Phase (Prevention)

Deepi has metatropic dwarfism, a skeletal disorder characterized by short stature, spine asymmetries, joint

contractures, and painful restricted joints. Deepi's identical twin sister has the same condition (Figure 2-18).

Risk Evaluation

Standardized risk assessment: Deepi has a score of 14 on the Braden Scale, indicating moderate risk of pressure injury. Her clinical risk assessment is as follows:

- Physical: Deepi has nonreducible asymmetries, including limited ROM at the head/neck, upper extremities, spine, pelvis, and lower extremities. She has minor skin issues from wheelchair seating: Stage 1 pressure injuries at anterior pelvis and symphysis pubis (weightbearing locations when upright in wheelchair); recent issues with respiratory function and swallowing. Vision is limited due to fixed side-flexed and rotated head position. Sensation is normal. She is able to feel discomfort and knows when position change is needed

- Functional: Deepi has normal cognition and attended university. She can independently operate a power wheelchair and seat functions using her right hand only. She is fully dependent for all activities of daily living and has access to her computer only when lying on her day bed.

- Socioeconomic: Deepi works part time as a journalist and with a radio network. She requires use of the computer for writing projects, which means being out of her wheelchair. She has both paid assistance with morning care and supportive family who assist other times. She has support to assist her with going out during the day 3 or 4 times/week.

- Environment: She lives in a non–wheelchair-accessible home, and her power wheelchair is left at the entrance to the family room after transfer to a firm, flat day bed. She is always on the day bed when at home.

Interface pressure mapping was not done because Deepi has normal sensation. She is fully aware of when she is uncomfortable or positioned incorrectly and able to weight

TABLE 2-1	
DEEPI'S RISK EVALUATION	
DEEPI'S NEGATIVE RISK FACTORS	**DEEPI'S POSITIVE (MITIGATING) FACTORS**
Stage 1 pressure injuries	Intact sensation
Negligible active movement	Aware of incorrect positioning in wheelchair
Physically dependent for all activities of daily living	Competent to direct her own care; strong communication skills
Dependent for physical movement including transfers and repositioning	Consistent, capable paid assistance and family support
Nonreducible asymmetries	Custom-molded seating system that matches her contours perfectly
Cannot assume a seating position and is supported in a modified standing posture	Continent and has good nutrition
In her wheelchair for long hours	Can independently use her dynamic wheelchair seat functions: forward and rearward tilt, lateral tilt both directions

shift using the power seat functions. She directs her own repositioning within the seat when needed.

Clinical Judgment: Overall, Deepi presents as being at low risk for pressure injuries, although her Braden Scale indicates moderate risk. Her serious risk factors are mitigated by her personal attributes, excellent care, and equipment as illustrated in Table 2-1.

Equipment to Help Deepi Remain in Pre-Wound Phase

- Posture support: Deepi's custom-molded seating system (Figure 2-19) completely matches her angles and contours; weightbearing is distributed over as great a surface area as possible; rigid pelvic saddle support with off-loading contours (contact at sub-anterior superior iliac spine) to reduce sliding; and off-loaded at symphysis pubis for comfort.

- Facilitating position change: Her custom wheelchair has multiple seat functions. Anterior tilt enables upright positioning to drive. Posterior tilt is a position used for rest and repositioning, because she will slide down when in the upright position. Lateral tilt allows for alternate pressure weight shifting side to side when in upright position. Seat elevation facilitates caregiver assistance to position and reposition in the wheelchair. Custom seating features include swing-away trunk supports and foot support to allow easy transfers in and out of the wheelchair.

- Surface selection: Foam in box molding technique used with medium soft SunMate foam (Dynamic Systems Inc.); Neoprene covers to allow contour matching and for additional cushion.

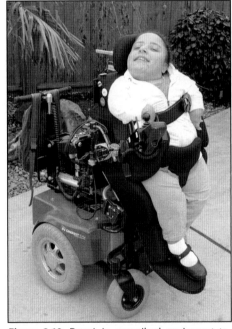

Figure 2-19. Deepi: in prescribed equipment to remain in pre-wound phase.

- Shear: Deepi has a rigid anterior pelvic support to prevent sliding forward on the seat surface when in upright position. She also weightbears through her feet as tolerated.

- Microclimate: Heat and moisture are not an issue for Deepi, and a warm system is preferable. Custom sun/rain protection is fabricated to fit the wheelchair.

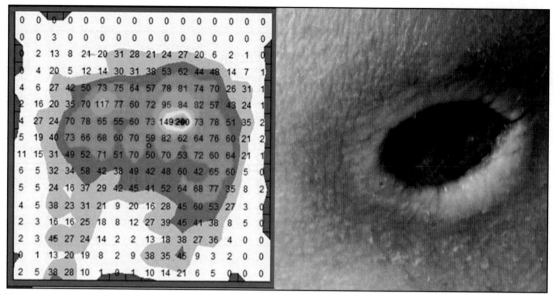

Figure 2-20. Clint: pressure map and pressure injury in wound/treatment phase.

Wound Phase (Treatment)

Clint has a low thoracic paraplegia secondary to a spinal cord injury, multiple orthopedic traumas, and an acquired brain injury sustained when a tree fell on him. He has a Stage 3 pressure injury on his left ischial tuberosity.

Risk Evaluation

Standardized risk assessment: Braden score of 15 (moderate risk)

Clinical risk assessment is as follows.

- Physical: T10 paraplegia with absent sensation and motor abilities below level of injury. Clint sustained a crush injury with multiple fractures of the pelvis and spine with spinal fusion from lower thoracic spine to pelvis. Secondary complications include acquired brain injury with mild cognitive impairment, left side visual field deficit, and left hemiparesis. No hip, knee, ankle limitations in range to limit sitting in a wheelchair. Nonreducible pelvic positioning; obliquity high on the right by 1 inch; severe anterior tilted pelvis. Torso lateral shift to the left secondary to spinal fusion. Clint has chronic back and neuropathic pain and is on opiates.

- Functional: Clint lives alone and is independent with his self-care but requires some assistance with activities outside the home. He is not able to drive because of his visual deficit. He enjoys taking his dogs walking, and hunting and fishing when he can find a buddy to take him out.

- Socioeconomic: Clint has his own home with a shop where he enjoys his woodworking hobby. He has paid assistants for homemaking and driving his

wheelchair-accessible van. His dogs go everywhere with him.

- Environment: Clint lives in a fully wheelchair accessible single-level detached home with a yard near a shopping mall in a small town. He has a home gym.

Interface Pressure Mapping

Clint was pressure mapped on his manual wheelchair with pressure redistribution air cushion. The map shows high peak pressure (> 200 mm Hg) at his left ischial tuberosity confirmed by palpation. This is the location of the existing pressure injury (Figure 2-20).

Clinical Judgment: Although Clint scores as just moderate risk on the Braden Scale, he presents as extremely high risk because of poor pressure readings, current Stage 3 pressure injury, and a history of other pressure injuries. On the plus side, he has good funding and a supportive family. Table 2-2 outlines the positive and negative risk factors.

Equipment That Successfully Moved Clint From Wound to Post-Wound Phase

- Posture support: Clint has a rigid-frame wheelchair that is well-fitted (Figure 2-21); it is set in 2 inches of fixed tilt, with a rigid backrest with shallow midline lower trunk supports that is offset to the left to accommodate for his trunk lateral shift. A firm seat provides pelvic support and thigh support in conjunction with rigid pelvic side guards.

- Facilitating position change: A firm front cushion edge facilitates independent transfers and forward leaning for effective weight shift. He has reinforced antitippers to enable him to tilt back for a position change.

TABLE 2-2	
CLINT'S RISK EVALUATION	
CLINT'S NEGATIVE RISK FACTORS	**CLINT'S POSITIVE (MITIGATING) FACTORS**
Stage 3 pressure injury and history of pressure injuries to his sacrum and right greater trochanter	Uses skin protection behaviors including skin checks and weight shifts
Absent sensation	Has a supportive family and paid assistants
Paralyzed below the waist	Good funding for care support and equipment
Cognitive impairment with decreased judgment	Motivated to heal the pressure injury because he wants to enjoy his leisure interests.
Extremely high pressure over his left ischial tuberosity (location of wound) in current seating	Physically fit and works out regularly; walks his dogs
Nonreducible pelvic and spine asymmetries	Able to do an independent safe transfer
Opiate use for chronic pain	
In his wheelchair for 12 hours a day minimum	
Lives alone; nutrition inadequate	

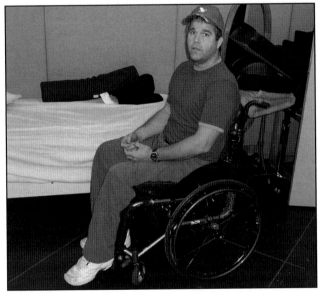

Figure 2-21. Clint: in prescribed equipment to move from wound to post-wound phase.

- Surface selection: He is positioned on a custom force isolation cushion that off-loads his ischials and greater trochanters.

- Shear: Clint used to slide backward in his chair, and his current cushion and backrest prevent this. The cushion has a rear boundary, and the backrest contacts the upper edge of the cushion limiting rearward shift.

- Microclimate: Clint's cushion is breathable with a double spacer fabric cover to further enhance air movement.

Post-Wound Phase (Lifetime Management)

Bill sustained a quadriplegia as a teenager when he fell out of a tree. Since his spinal cord injury, he has had multiple pressure injuries and many plastic surgeries that failed because the cause of the pressure injuries was not adequately addressed. He recently healed his last Stage 3 wounds without surgery and is now pressure injury free.

Risk Evaluation

Standardized risk assessment: Braden score of 12 (high risk)

Bill's clinical risk assessment is as follows.

- Physical: Bill has a C7 quadriplegia motor and sensory complete. He presents with a severe collapsing scoliosis of the spine, which is partially reducible; forefoot amputation secondary to pressure injury; and multiple scars from previous surgeries and recently healed wounds on his right rib cage and right greater trochanter. He has a nonreducible pelvic obliquity 4 inches high on the left with overlapping rib cage. Bill has many comorbid health conditions including diabetes. His ROM limitations in his hip, knees, and ankles require accommodation in his seating system.

- Functional: Bill lives independently with paid assistance in the morning only. He is able to transfer independently from his chair to his bed and undress independently. Bill prepares his own meals and directs his care.

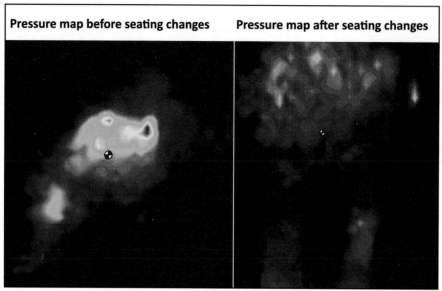

Figure 2-22. Bill: pressure map before and after seating changes.

TABLE 2-3	
BILL'S RISK EVALUATION	
BILL'S NEGATIVE RISK FACTORS	**BILL'S POSITIVE (MITIGATING) FACTORS**
History of multiple pressure ulcers	Does routine skin checks with a mirror and does dynamic weight shifts in his power wheelchair
Absent sensation	Healed his pressure injuries without surgery
Severe postural asymmetries	Pressure map shows full contact and no peak pressures with good pressure redistribution in his new seating system.
Comorbid health concerns	Motivated to stay pressure injury free and has ongoing community health supports in place
Lives alone and does not have many care hours	Careful about not staying in his wheelchair for too long
Limited funding for care and equipment	Able to do an independent safe transfer
	Paid assistance and connected to his community
	Lifetime management attitude and behavior established

- Socioeconomic: He has limited funding and retired from his job some years ago due to continual health issues and pressure injuries. Bill's mom remains involved in his life, and he is connected in his small rural community.

- Environment: Bill rents a small apartment that is not fully wheelchair accessible and does not drive.

Interface Pressure Mapping

Bill was pressure mapped (Figure 2-22) while he had a wound and since he healed his wound; these pressure maps are dramatically different. In the pressure map before seating changes were made, the peak pressure is on the right greater trochanter and the right leg; there is no weight-bearing on the left side of the pelvis or the left leg. On the pressure map after seating changes, there is symmetrical weightbearing, good P-A dispersion from pelvis to thighs, and no peak pressure evident.

Clinical Judgment: Overall, Bill still presents as high risk (Braden Score provides a clinical estimation) due to his postural asymmetries, health concerns, and history of multiple pressure injuries. However, this is now mitigated by naturally healed wounds, a positive pressure map, and a wheelchair and seating system that meets his posture, pressure, and functional needs as shown in Table 2-3.

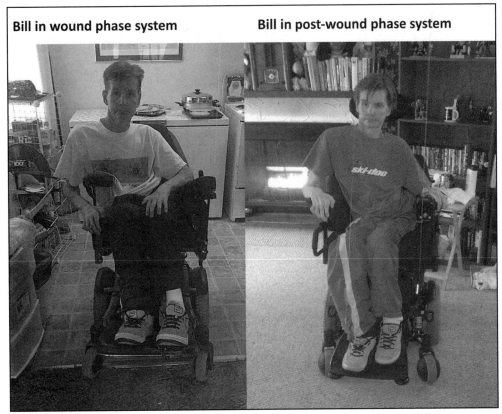

Figure 2-23. Bill: in old seating system and in prescribed equipment to remain in post-wound phase.

Equipment That Enables Bill to Remain in the Post-Wound Phase

- Posture support: Molded foam in box custom seat and back support with full contour to support Bill in his optimal posture (Figure 2-23). Lateral and rearward tilt used for positioning and weight shift and to maintain a more neutral head position.

- Facilitating position change: Dynamic lateral tilt, rearward tilt to facilitate position change while in chair. Powered right trunk lateral used in conjunction with laterally tilting away from right side to enable independent transfer on and off his bed.

- Surface selection: Embedded air cushion in pelvic well and air overlay on right trunk lateral. Molded surfaces fabricated of medium SunMate foam. Neoprene covers for warmth and additional cushioning.

- Shear: Bill uses dynamic features of his chair to minimize sliding. Good foot support and arm support to provide further block to sliding in chair.

- Microclimate: Bill is always cold and appreciates the warmth of the encompassing system. The neoprene covers protect the foam from any moisture.

SUMMARY

Pressure injuries are preventable. Keeping seated clients free of pressure injuries throughout their lives is a fundamental seating and mobility goal. A comprehensive seating and pressure assessment includes skin inspection, pressure mapping, and clinical estimation of pressure risk. This chapter describes an interprofessional pressure management model and provides some global pressure terminology. It identifies what a seating clinician can do to prevent and manage pressure problems through a systematic process to ensure postural fit, facilitate movement and position change, optimize weight distribution, define surface properties, and select microclimate materials and coverings to promote positive pressure outcomes.

ACKNOWLEDGMENT

The authors thank Donna Chisholm for the original artwork in Figures 2-7 and 2-15 through 2-17.

REFERENCES

Aissaoui, R., Lacoste, M., & Dansereau, J. (2001). Analysis of sliding and pressure distribution during a repositioning of persons in a simulator chair. *IEEE Transactions on Neural Systems and Rehabilitation Engineering, 9*, 215-224. doi: 10.1109/7333.928581

Bergstrom, N., Braden, B. J., Laguzza, A., & Holman, V. (1987). The Braden Scale for predicting pressure sore risk. *Nursing Research, 36.* doi: 10.1097/00006199-198707000-00002

Borisoff, J., & Mitchell, S. (2015). Dynamic wheeled mobility: Next chapter in the ultralight evolution. Proceedings of the 31st International Seating Symposium (pp. 99-104), Pittsburgh, PA.

Chisholm, J., & Yip, J. (2016, March). Prescribing the right pressure management equipment. Proceedings of 32nd International Seating Symposium (pp. 222-224), Vancouver, Canada.

Crane, B., Hetzel, T., & Sonenblum, S. (2016, March). Clinical application of the dispersion index. Proceedings of the 32nd International Seating Symposium (pp. 47-50), Vancouver, Canada.

Houghton, P. E., Campbell, K. E., & the CPG Panel. (2013). *Canadian best practice guidelines for the prevention and management of pressure ulcers in people with spinal cord injury: A resource handbook for clinicians.* Retrieved from http://www.onf.org/system/attachments/168/original/Pressure_Ulcers_Best_Practice_Guideline_Final_web4.pdf

Jan, Y., Jones, M. A., Rabadi, M. H., Foreman, R. D., & Thiessen, A. (2010). Effect of wheelchair tilt-in-space and recline angles on skin perfusion over the ischial tuberosity in people with spinal cord injury. *Archives of Physical Medicine and Rehabilitation, 91*, 1758-1764. doi: 10.1016/j.apmr.2010.07.227

The Joint Commission. (2016). Preventing pressure injuries. *Quick Safety.* Retrieved from www.jointcommission.org/assets/1/23/Quick_Safety_Issue_25_July_20161.PDF

Mortenson, W. B., & Miller, W. C. (2008). A review of scales for assessing the risk of developing a pressure ulcer in individuals with SCI. *Spinal Cord, 46*, 168-175. doi: 10.1038/sj.sc.3102129

National Pressure Ulcer Advisory Panel. (2014). 2014 Prevention and treatment of pressure ulcers: Clinical practice guideline. Retrieved from http://www.npuap.org/resources/educational-and-clinical-resources/prevention-and-treatment-of-pressure-ulcers-clinical-practice-guideline/

National Pressure Ulcer Advisory Panel. (2016). Pressure injury stages. Retrieved from http://www.npuap.org/resources/educational-and-clinical-resources/npuap-pressure-injury-stages

Salzberg, C. A., Byrne, D. W., Cayten, C. G., Niewerburgh, P. V., Murphy, J. G., & Viehbeck, M. (1996). A new pressure ulcer risk assessment scale for individuals with spinal cord injury. *American Journal of Physical Medicine & Rehabilitation, 75*, 96-104. doi: 10.1097/00002060-199603000-00004

Sprigle, S., Maurer, C., & Sorenblum, S. E. (2010). Load redistribution in variable position wheelchairs in people with spinal cord injury. *Journal of Spinal Cord Medicine, 33*, 58-64. doi: 10.1080/10790268.2010.11689674

II

Postural Support and Pressure Management
Clinical Applications

Postural Support and Pressure Management Considerations for Hands-Free Sitters

David Kreutz, PT, ATP

ASSESSMENT TOOLS

Standardized assessment tools provide the clinician with objective data about a person's baseline, progression of symptoms, and effectiveness of the interventions. In addition, the assessment aids in appropriate goal development. Ultimately, these clinical finding and goals lead to specific equipment recommendations. The following assessment tools aid the clinician in identifying clients' baseline status.

Visual Assessment of Seated Posture

A person's posture affects his or her sitting balance, reach, and function. Optimal reach and function is achieved when the person is able to sit with good posture. It is well-documented that the position of the pelvis is key to good posture. Pelvic position is known to effect spinal and head alignment. A person who sits with a level pelvis that is in a slight anterior tilt and has erect spinal and head alignment will have improved proximal stability and an improved reach. A person can further improve his or her base of support by having a slightly abducted hip position. This will further improve his or her sitting balance and reach.

Balance Assessment

Sitting balance among wheelchair users varies greatly. Balance may range from hands-free to completely dependent. Sitting hands-free on the side of a mat table describes only static sitting balance. It does not adequately describe the ability of the person to maintain balance while pushing

a manual wheelchair, driving a power wheelchair, the ability to react to external forces, or the extent of one's reach. A number of balance assessment tools have been developed to assess balance in older adults and individuals with neurologic deficits (Duncan, Weiner, Chandler, & Studenski, 1990). Boswell-Ruys et al. (2009) adapted and modified standing balance tests for assessing unsupported sitting in individuals with spinal cord injury. These tests can provide information about the client's ability to maintain his or her balance over a timed period, maximal range of reach in different directions, coordinated stability, seated reach distance, and information about how quickly a client can perform a functional task, such as donning and doffing a T-shirt.

Range of Motion

To achieve hands-free sitting balance a client must have the available range of motion (ROM), strength, muscle tone and sensation to maintain an erect sitting posture. Transferring the client to a therapy mat and performing an evaluation will provide the clinician with information regarding the client's ROM, muscle tone, skin condition, and sensory status. This is essential for establishing an appropriate plan of treatment.

ROM of the hip joints and flexibility of the lumbar spine are crucial to achieving a pelvic position that is level, in neutral rotation and in a neutral to slight anterior pelvic tilt to achieve an erect and symmetrical sitting posture. When assessing the pelvic alignment in the frontal plane view, the anterior superior iliac spines (ASIS) of the pelvis should be level. In the transverse plane view, the ASIS of the pelvis

Lange, M. L., & Minkel, J. L.
Seating and Wheeled Mobility: A Clinical Resource Guide
(pp. 49-59). © 2018 SLACK Incorporated.

should be equidistant from a fixed backrest. In the sagittal plane view the ASIS and posterior iliac spine of the pelvis should be level or tilted so that the anterior iliac spines are slightly lower than the posterior iliac spines. Flexibility of the pelvis on the lumbar spine should be equal in opposite directions in all three planes of motion.

Hip flexion ROM should be greater than 90 degrees to achieve the pelvic position previously described. Hip joint contractures that limit hip flexion can result in pelvic alignment asymmetries, such as a posterior pelvic tilt, pelvic obliquity, and pelvic rotation. It is possible for individuals with hip contractures to achieve a symmetrical sitting posture and a neutral pelvic tilt if provided a seating system that accommodates the contracture. Possible seating system modifications used to accommodate this contracture would include adjusting the seat to back support angle or using cushion materials or custom shapes to accommodate the lack of hip flexion.

Lack of knee ROM does not significantly affect a client's ability to sit with hands-free balance, provided that the contracture is adequately accommodated by the seating and mobility base. For example, a knee flexion contracture greater than 90 degrees would require the seat depth and foot support placement accommodate the lost ROM. If this contracture were not accommodated by allowing the knee to bend to the available range, then the hamstring muscle group, a two-joint muscle, would cause the pelvis to rotate posterior and also lead to a reduction of the natural lumbar lordosis. Sixty- and 70-degree swing-away leg supports with heel loops or elevating leg supports with calf supports are examples of leg supports that do not accommodate this knee flexion contracture.

Limitations in upper extremity joint ROM may also affect posture, transfers, wheelchair propulsion, joystick access, reaching, and activities of daily living (ADL). Asymmetry in range and strength can greatly affect a client's ability to propel a manual wheelchair. Numerous studies have been performed on upper extremity ROM during wheelchair propulsion (Corfman, Cooper, Boninger, Koontz, & Fitzgerald, 2003; Newsam et al., 1999). A study by Newsam et al. (1999) showed slight differences between paraplegics and quadriplegics in upper extremity ROM primarily based on strategies used to contact the hand rim. Wheelchair propulsion is complex and requires movement in multiple planes of motion. Adequate ROM and strength is essential for wheelchair propulsion. A client must have the ROM for proper hand placement on the handrim, an efficient push stroke, and recovery cycle. Wheelchair propulsion will be covered in greater detail in a later chapter.

Manual Muscle Test

Muscle Strength and the Functional Independence Measure

Muscle testing should be performed to determine current strength and distribution of muscle weakness. Muscle testing provides the clinician with an understanding of the client's baseline strength. Periodic testing will provide information regarding the disease progression Reassessment can provide the clinician with information as to whether the treatment is effective. In conjunction with manual muscle testing, some form of functional tests, such as the functional independence measure (FIM), can provide the clinician a better understanding of the client's progress toward independence in ADL. The FIM evaluation includes self-care activities (eating, dressing, grooming, bathing, and toileting), sphincter control (bowel and bladder management), mobility (transfers to bed, wheelchair, toilet, and tub), locomotion (ambulation, wheelchair mobility), communication (comprehension and expression), and social cognition (social interaction, problem solving, and memory). Functional testing identifies the level of assistance required to perform each task. In addition, wheelchair skills testing will help the clinician determine whether a client is best suited for manual or power wheelchair mobility.

Sensory Status

Sensory testing provides the clinician with information about the client's ability to sense pain, pressure, temperature, position, and balance. Impaired sensation can lead to decreased awareness of painful stimuli. Clients with impaired sensation are at increased risk of pressure injury, burns, and other injuries to their skin. For example, a client with complete paraplegia will have loss of deep pressure and pain sensation, which will place him at greater risk of pressure injury and burns. Loss of proprioceptive awareness in a client with incomplete quadriplegia will affect her control of movement and position sense. Assessment of the sensory system can be achieved with formal testing (proprioceptive testing, two-point discrimination, balance tests, or more informally with interview-style questioning).

Self-Assessment

Educating clients on proper positioning and postural awareness should precede functional training especially for individuals with hands-free balance. Client and caregiver education regarding proper positioning in the wheelchair will reduce the risk of developing asymmetries and pain caused by habitual tendencies and poor body awareness.

Clients should be instructed in palpation of bony landmarks and encouraged to periodically assess their seated wheelchair posture in front of a mirror. Working on symmetrical sitting posture and stability will provide improved balance and function.

GOALS FOR THE CLIENT WITH HANDS-FREE SITTING BALANCE

- To maximize the client's reach by using compensatory strategies or components of the wheelchair and seating system: The client should be able to balance and reach for items on the floor, countertops, and possibly shelves above his or her head given adequate upper extremity strength.
- To achieve maximal independence in as many ADL as the client desires, such as transfers, dressing, bathing, cooking, and cleaning
- To prevent the development of asymmetrical postures with clients who have a progressive condition
- To perform independent pressure relief or weight shifts to maintain intact skin

FUNCTIONAL ACTIVITIES

Stability

Stability of the wheelchair user and wheelchair can be improved by providing a pelvic positioning belt, proper adjustment of the foot support, appropriate seat width that allows slight abduction of the legs, and a cushion that provides lateral stability. Improving reach outside the base of support requires educating the client how to properly orient the mobility base and how to use the environment to improve reach. For example, forward-reaching stability can be increased in a manual wheelchair by rotating the casters so that the caster wheel is forward facing prior to setting the wheel locks. This will increase the wheel base and stability of the wheelchair, and help to prevent forward tipping of the wheelchair. Additional range is possible by teaching clients to use the frame of the wheelchair for stability. Hooking around a push handle or propping one's forearm on his or her thighs are two methods of increasing one's stability while reaching forward. Using the opposite wheel or push handle allows one to reach further to the side without loss of balance. Using the surrounding environment for stability is another method used to extend ones reach. For example, a client will grasp a steering wheel with one hand while bending to reach and lift his or her wheelchair for self-loading in a vehicle.

Clients are able to participate in more numerous and challenging activities if they have hands-free balance, feel stable in their seating and mobility base, and can reach beyond the limits of their arm length. Independence in bathing, dressing, cooking, cleaning, and hygiene should be attainable functional goals for the client with hands-free sitting balance. Clients should also be made aware of the numerous manual and power wheelchair skills that allow them greater independence and safety if attained. Activities such as managing doors and thresholds, ramps and curbs, maneuvering in tight spaces, and side slopes are just a few of the functional mobility goals and skills that should be discussed and taught. The ability to lean forward and backward allows one to shift his or her center of gravity and improve the stability of the mobility base as he or she ascends and descends ramps. Learning how to shimmy or hop a manual wheelchair sideways in tight spaces may make the difference in one's ability to access a small bathroom stall or kitchen. More detailed lists of mobility skills can be found in Chapters 9 and 10.

Functional Reach

It is well-documented that proximal stability improves distal functions. Activities that require little movement of the center of mass relative to the base of support can be achieved with relative ease by the person with hands-free balance and functional upper extremity strength and ROM. Improving reach can be achieved by working on balance and by reducing the footprint of the seating and mobility device to allow a person to get closer to the desired object. To reduce the length of the wheelchair, use the available knee and ankle ROM to tuck the feet and legs as much as possible, and position the client's feet so that the toes are directly under the knees, if possible. In addition, order a power mobility base with a center mount foot support vs swing-away leg supports. On manual rigid-frame wheelchairs, this can be achieved by ordering a rigid-frame wheelchair with a tighter frame angle that results in a more tucked position of the lower extremities. Consideration should also be given to minimizing the width of the seating system and mobility device to improve reach in the lateral direction. The overall width of manual wheelchairs can be narrowed by prescribing a minimal seat width, using short tab handrims, narrowing the wheel spacing, and tapering the leg support of the rigid-frame wheelchair.

Transfers

The preferred type of transfer will depend on the client's physical strength, ROM, sensation, and coordination. Stand-pivot, depression, scooting, and sliding board transfers are the most common options for the person with hands-free balance. Some clients will use several of different transfer techniques depending on the environment. Uneven surfaces or large gaps between surfaces may result in a person opting to use a sliding board for improved

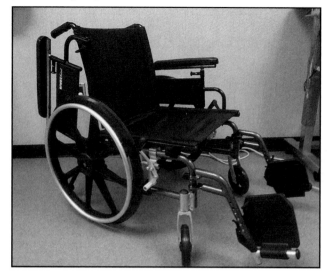

Figure 3-1. Sling seat in a manual wheelchair.

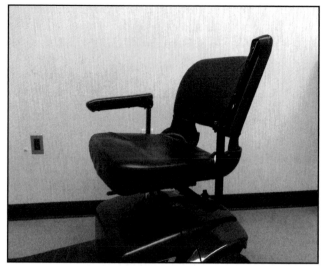

Figure 3-2. Fish-on seat on power-operated vehicle (scooter) base.

safety. Other clients may experience fatigue and resort to a different transfer method for safety. For example, clients with a diagnosis of multiple sclerosis may report performing stand-pivot transfers in the morning and relying on a sliding board and assistance in the evening. Clients with lower-level paraplegia may be able to perform depression transfers. A client with bilateral above-knee amputations may perform stand-pivot, scoot, or sliding board transfers depending on whether he or she is able to use prosthetic limbs. The ability of the person to transfer and the type of transfer will influence both the seating system and mobility base. One example, if a person cannot perform an independent stand-pivot transfer, it might preclude the use of a power operated vehicle (scooter) because of safety issues.

POSTURAL SUPPORTS AND SEATING CONSIDERATIONS

Sling Seats and Back Supports

Manual wheelchair seating systems vary considerably in their shape, orientation, and materials. The primary support surfaces of a wheelchair are the seat and back surfaces. The seat is composed of either a sling or solid seat surface. Manual wheelchairs typically have sling seats made of nylon or vinyl, but may be replaced with a solid seat (Figure 3-1). The adverse affects of a sling seat and back on a wheelchair user's posture is well-documented throughout the literature (Shaw & Taylor, 1991). Sling seats and backs contribute to a posterior pelvic tilt and a kyphotic sitting posture. Back support options that provide improved postural support over the standard sling back support include tension adjustable upholstery and replacement contoured back supports. In addition to affecting one's posture, sling seats can also adversely affect one's balance and reach.

Amos et al. (2001) determined that elderly participants in their study had a statistically significant greater forward reach when using a wheelchair with a wedge cushion and solid seat insert compared with the sling seat. The seat and back upholstery can be replaced with solid seats and cushions as well as contoured adjustable back support to provide the client with improved postural support. Seat and back support options are discussed in detail later in this chapter.

Fish-On Seat

Power-operated vehicles (scooters) and basic light-duty power wheelchairs have either a fish-on seat or a captain's seat. The fish-on seat is a basic plastic molded seat and back that is covered with a flat or gently molded foam cushion and vinyl covering (Figure 3-2). It is mounted to the mobility base by a single post that allows the seat to be swiveled for easier access. The post also allows for mechanical seat height adjustment of just a few inches. The backrest does fold to allow easier transport. These fish-on seats are limited in size and postural support. A client should have good sitting balance to consider this type of seating. Having good static and dynamic sitting balance is necessary for safe mobility on uneven terrain and side slopes when using a power operated vehicle. It is important to discuss pain when considering these minimally adjustable seating systems. Making sure that the client can tolerate sitting for long periods of time may become an issue for clients with arthritis or chronic lower back pain. A power seat elevator may be an option for improving reach, transfers, and function when performing activities of daily living.

Captain's Seat

A captain's seat comes standard on Medicare-coded Group 2 power wheelchairs (Figure 3-3). The captain's seat provides greater leg support and back support than the

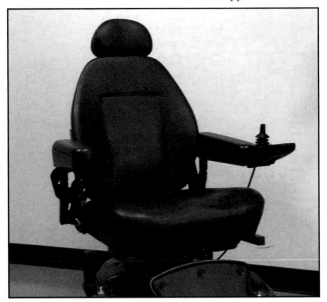

Figure 3-3. Captain's seat on Group 2 power wheelchair.

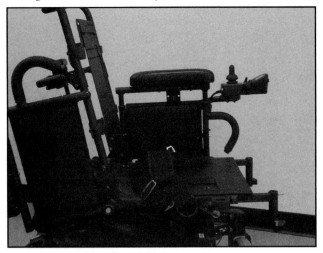

Figure 3-4. Rehab seat.

fish-on seat. The captain's seat has more supportive contours and a much larger array of sizes. This captain's seat comes with limited seat height and back angle adjustment. Although the range of adjustment will meet the majority of client's needs, those with very short or long leg lengths may find the adjustment range inadequate. The backrest of a captain's seat allows for limited angle adjustment and folds forward to allow easy transport in a vehicle. One of the downsides to the Medicare-competitive bid program is that the manufacturers have reduced the number of seat dimension options.

Captain's seat are most commonly prescribed with basic power wheelchairs, the Medicare-coded Group 2 power wheelchairs. The client should be able to sit in a symmetrical and erect posture, and have normal sensation and the ability to change positions and transfer independently. The captain's seat has a gentle contour, nonremovable vinyl cover, and is permanently affixed to the seat frame of the mobility device, much like an automobile seat. One advantage of this seating system is that it provides easy access and a stable base of support for function and transfers. For example, a client with bilateral below-knee amputations would find the cushion very stable when scooting forward or laterally during transfers. Disadvantages include minimal contours for postural support, limited envelopment and immersion for pressure distribution, limited seat size options, and limited seat height and foot support height adjustments. For clients who fall outside of the limited seat height and leg-length range adjustments, it becomes difficult to provide adequate postural support and comfort.

A captain's seat can be an option on Medicare-coded Group 3 power wheelchair. Group 3 power wheelchairs have a longer range and higher speed and can accept multiple power seat functions. Funding authorization for a

Group 3 power wheelchair with a captain's seat may be a challenge unless the client has a progressive condition and is expected to decline in function and require power seating in the future. A power seat elevator is also an option on some Group 3 power wheelchairs with a captain's seat. Clients can use the power seat elevator to improve their reach and transfers.

Rehab Seating

Rehab seating is available for both light duty (Group 2) and power wheelchairs (Group 3). A rehab seat is essentially a seating frame structure with a solid seat pan and adjustable backrest canes that will accept a cushion and back support (Figure 3-4). The seat frame is mounted on four seat posts or side panels that allow it to be mechanically raised and tilted to improve a client's stability in the wheelchair. The backrest canes are also angle adjustable. One of the chief justifications for selecting a rehab seat over the captain's seat is the client's need for a skin protection or skin protection and postural support cushion. Clients who have impaired sensation or a history of pressure injuries will require a rehab seat and skin protection cushion. Another reason would be to address the need for postural supports that cannot be accommodated with a captain's seat. For example, a client with lower extremity paralysis may require lateral thigh supports to maintain proper lower extremity positioning. These lateral thigh supports can be mounted to the solid seat pan or multipurpose track on the sides of the rehab seat frame. Examples of secondary postural supports that can be added to the frame might include lateral pelvic, lateral thoracic, and medial and lateral thigh supports. Finally, it may not be possible to provide the seat dimensions needed to support a client with the limited options of a captain's seat. The rehab seat comes in a large array of seat widths and depths to fit most clients.

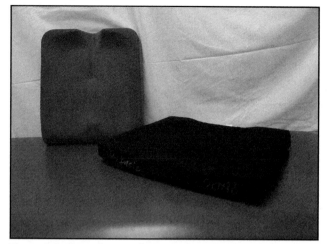

Figure 3-5. General use cushions: Synergy Simplicity (left) and Jay Basic (right).

Seat Cushions

Manual wheelchairs and power wheelchairs with rehab seating require the provision of a seat cushion and back support. There are hundreds of types of cushions. Materials used in seat cushions include foam, gel, viscous fluid, honeycomb plastic, and air. Stability on the cushion is crucial for balance. Most cushions that allow movement of the air or movement of a viscous fluid for pressure distribution, are segmented to isolate the right and left sides as well as the front and rear quadrants to improve stability. The clinician and client must consider many factors when selecting a cushion, such as shape, dimensions (e.g., thickness), weight, cushion materials, cushion cover options, cost, durability, ease of care, maintenance, and warranty. Client considerations might include the client's weight, width, and length needs; postural support needs; pressure distribution needs or risk; transfer method; and continence, among others. Cushions are classified into different categories by Medicare based on dimension, postural support, immersion for skin protection, adjustability, custom manufacturing, and power alternating.

The Centers for Medicare & Medicaid Services and the Statistical Analysis Durable Medical Equipment Regional Carrier created a classification system for wheelchair support surfaces (cushions) that includes the following categories:

- General use cushions
- Skin protection cushion
- Positioning seat cushion
- Skin protection and positioning seat cushion
- Custom fabricated cushion
- Adjustable skin protection and positioning
- Powered seat cushions

All cushions are classified into one of these eight categories. Qualification criteria for each of category are available via the Medicare policy referred to as the Local Coverage Determination for wheelchair seating (NHIC Corp., 2013). Coverage criteria for each category varies depending on the diagnosis, existence of a pressure injury, sensory status, postural asymmetries, and clinical documentation by a health care professional as to why a prefabricated cushion cannot meet the needs of the client. The primary characteristics used for categorizing cushions have to do with skin protection and postural support. It is impossible to look at a cushion and identify its respective category. From a clinician's standpoint it is critical that the clinician identify the most appropriate cushion for an individual based on his or her knowledge, experience, and tools available for comparing cushions. It is important that he or she verifies that the client's diagnosis and skin condition and postural support needs qualify him or her for the cushion selected. Following is a general description of the categories and the qualification requirements. Captain's seats that are typically provided by the manufacturer of consumer power chairs, and scooters are not included in any of the preceding categories. They come standard on certain power mobility devices.

General Use Cushion

General use cushions are similar to a captain's seat in contour (Figure 3-5). They are 1 to 2 inches thick, flat or gently contoured, and have a removable cover. The shape of the cushion is gently contoured and provides minimal postural support. General use cushions are recommended for clients who use a manual or power wheelchair and have full sensation as well as the ability to change positions frequently. They may be made of foam, air, gel, thermoplastics, or some combination of these materials. General use cushions provide improved client comfort when sitting in a wheelchair, especially if the person has been sitting the sling seat upholstery of the wheelchair.

Skin Protection Cushion

Skin protection cushions, otherwise known as *pressure distribution cushions*, are designed to redistribute the sitting pressures away from the ischial tuberosities and sacrum, thereby decreasing the magnitude of the pressure on these bony prominences (Figure 3-6). Skin protection cushions must be at least 3 inches thick. Manufacturers use materials such as air, viscous fluid, thermoplastics, and foam to redistribute the pressure. Foam cushions are designed using different contours and densities to redistribute the pressure. Thermoplastic urethane cushions are made of a honeycomb-shaped plastic material that deforms to redistribute pressure. Air and fluid cushions use the flow of the cushion's material to redistribute the load, when the person sits on the cushion. Under Medicare coverage criteria, to qualify for a skin protection cushion, a client

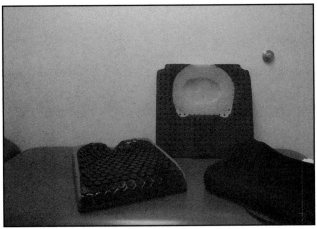

Figure 3-6. Skin protection cushions: Synergy Solution 1 (left) and Jay Lite (right).

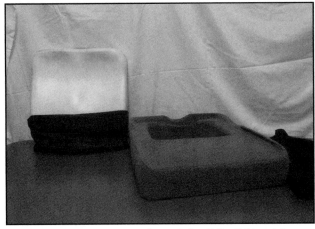

Figure 3-7. Positioning seat cushions: Roho Airlite (left) and Synergy Spectrum Gel (right).

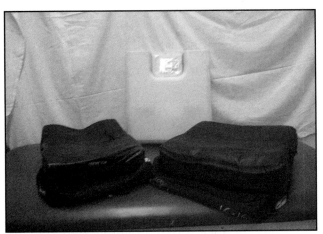

Figure 3-8. Skin protection and positioning cushions: clockwise from top: Span America Isch Dish, Jay Union, and Ride Forward.

must use a manual or power wheelchair and meet one of the following criteria:

- Have a pressure injury currently or in the past

- Have absent or impaired sensory status in the area of contact with the cushion

- A qualifying *International Classification of Diseases* (9th edition) diagnostic code

- Be unable to perform a functional weight shift due to of the diagnosis

Some off-loading cushions also fall into this category of cushions. These are cushions that are designed and shaped to off-load the area of the ischial tuberosities and sacrum; most often by creating a cutout or nonweightbearing area under the ischial tuberosities and sacrum and loading the

person's weight onto the posterior thighs, trochanters, and gluteal tissue.

Positioning Seat Cushions

Positioning seat cushions would not typically be needed for an individual with hands-free balance unless the client also presents with severe lower extremity weakness or paralysis (Figure 3-7). A positioning cushion is shaped or can be modified with components such as hip guides, lateral thigh supports, and medial thigh supports to address postural support needs of the client. Common structural modifications or components would include a pre-ischial shelf or antithrust component to reduce the tendency to slide forward and accommodate the ischial and sacral prominences in sitting relative to the femur. Other modifications include lateral pelvic supports, lateral thigh supports, and a medial thigh support. This classification of cushion is covered under Medicare only if the client meets the criteria for a manual or power wheelchair and has significant postural asymmetries due to one of the diagnosis codes listed in the Medicare coverage criteria.

Skin Protection and Positioning Seat Cushions

The cushions in this category have characteristics of both the skin protection and positioning cushions (Figure 3-8). The criteria for qualification is similar in that the client must qualify for a manual or power wheelchair, have a history of or current pressure injury, and significant postural asymmetries due to one of the diagnosis codes listed in the Medicare coverage criteria.

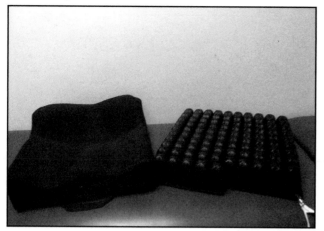

Figure 3-9. Custom cushions: Ride custom cushion and Roho custom cushion.

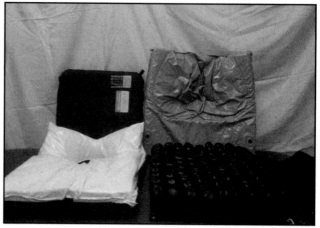

Figure 3-10. Adjustable skin protection and positioning cushions: clockwise from top left: Varilite Evolution, Jay 2 deep contour, Roho High Profile, Ride Java.

Custom Fabricated Cushions

Custom fabricated cushions are custom made to meet the needs of a client who requires a custom size and custom-molded shape that is not available in an off the shelf product. Custom-molded cushions are designed to accommodate or correct a postural asymmetry or off-load specific bony prominences (Figure 3-9). It is important that the prescribing health care professional consider custom molded or off-loading cushions as options for clients with significant pelvic asymmetries or leg-length discrepancies, or who are at high risk of pressure injury. Clients with hands-free sitting balance do not typically require custom fabricated cushions. However, clients with a chronic history of pressure injury or those who are at high risk of pressure injury due to immobility, postural changes, or significant muscle atrophy or weight loss may benefit from a custom molded or off-loading cushion. For example, in clients with a spinal cord injury, the occurrence of severe weight loss, muscle atrophy, and the development of a pelvic obliquity or posterior pelvic tilt may contribute to the development of a pressure injury. One option for addressing the high risk of sacral and ischial pressure injury is provide a custom fabricated cushion designed to off-load areas of very high pressures. The provision of a cushion in combination with education regarding sitting tolerance and an increased frequency of pressure relief will reduce the risk of pressure injury and allow the client to improve his or her sitting tolerance. This cushion requires custom fabrication and possibly alteration to achieve total off-loading of the area with the pressure injury. Care must be taken to gradually build sitting tolerance and to monitor the remaining areas of contact at the cushion interface. Qualification for a custom fabricated cushion requires a comprehensive therapy evaluation explaining why a prefabricated cushion will not work, a history of pressure ulcers or current pressure injury, absent or impaired sensation, and significant postural asymmetries due to a specific qualifying diagnosis.

Adjustable Skin Protection and Positioning Cushions

Adjustable skin protection and positioning cushions have all the characteristics that are required for the skin protection and positioning cushion (Figure 3-10). However, cushions in this category must also be adjustable by the addition or removal of air, liquid, gel, or other fluid medium in physiologically appropriate areas of the cushion to promote pressure reduction (Noridan Healthcare Solutions, 2017).

Pressure-Alternating Cushions

A cushion category that has been touted for pressure injury prevention is the power seat cushion that alters the distribution of pressure using a battery-powered pump and a segmented air bladder. These cushions regulate the pressure in the pelvic area of the seat cushion by either pumping air into a chamber or allowing a chamber to deflate for a given period of time. The duration and pressure can be adjusted by changing the settings. These cushions are designed to prevent pressure injury by continuously changing the interface pressures. However, according to the local coverage determination, power seat cushions are not covered by Medicare because the effectiveness of these cushions has not yet been established.

BACK SUPPORTS

Back supports for manual wheelchairs and rehab seats come in nearly all sizes and shapes and allow for varying degrees of angle adjustment. Clinicians and clients will select a back support based on the client's height, shape, and need for postural support. A client with hands-free balance will generally use a backrest that is below the scapula to allow freedom of movement of the upper torso and upper extremities and not interfere with propulsion of a manual wheelchair. Clients whose goal it is to become proficient at high-level manual wheelchair skills may use a lower back support height to allow greater trunk movement. This increased range allows for improved wheelchair skill, reaching laterally or behind the wheelchair, and dressing in the wheelchair. Back support contours for the person with hands-free balance should be mild so as not to restrict movement or reach. Examples of back supports might include adjustable tension upholstery, general use backs, or an array of solid back supports that vary in height and adjustability.

SECONDARY SUPPORTS

Secondary supports are postural components that may be added to the seating system to improve posture, balance, and function. These include foot supports, arm supports, amputee stump supports, pelvic positioning belts, lateral pelvic and thoracic supports, and medial and lateral thigh supports. The client with hands-free sitting balance would rarely require more than a pelvic positioning belt and possibly lateral thigh support or amputee stump support. The purpose and function of these secondary supports is addressed in Chapters 4 and 5.

ORIENTATION OF THE SEATING SYSTEM ON THE MOBILITY BASE

Adjustment of the overall seating system and mobility base is critical to the client's stability, balance, and function. Anatomical measurements of the client are necessary to achieve appropriate postural support and function. Measurements of the client should include hip width, upper and lower leg length, chest width and depth, shoulder height and width, and elbow height. These measurements must then be converted to dimensions of the wheelchair and seating system. Once the dimensions of the wheelchair are finalized, the therapist and supplier must determine the optimal orientation of the seating system on the mobility base for function. Orientation of the seating system (Figure 3-11) will effect footrest ground clearance, the stability and balance of the user, transfers, knee clearance under tables, reach, turning radius, and visual field. The orientation of the seating system is determined by the front and rear seat height, seat to backrest angle, and seat to legrest angle. The

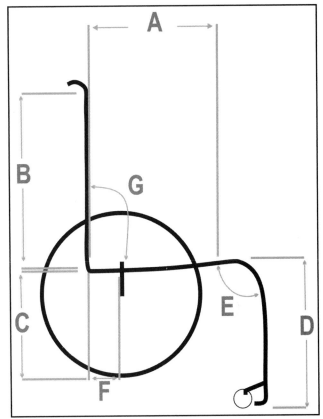

Figure 3-11. Seating system orientation. (A) Seat depth, (B) back support height, (C) rear seat to floor height, (D) front seat to floor height, (E) seat to leg support angle, and (F) rear axle position relative to the plane of the back support.

available dimensions and adjustability will vary from one product to the next. The front seat to floor height (Figure 3-11, D) and the rear seat to floor height (Figure 3-11, C) are critical measurements. The clinician and supplier must determine the ideal seat height, front and rear, and determine whether it is available on a particular mobility base. The seat height will affect the ease of transfers, stability of the client, ground clearance of the footrest, and access to the ground for a person who propels with his or her feet. There are many other issues to consider when determining the ideal seat height. On manual wheelchairs, the seat height can be adjusted by adjusting the axle position of the front and rear wheels or changing the size of the front and rear wheels. In scooters and basic power wheelchairs, there may only be the ability to raise or lower the seat height and not the ability to change the seat slope. Backrest angle adjustment is primarily used for balance and postural support of the client with hands-free balance. Back angle adjustment can be done through adjustable angle back canes on the wheelchair frame or through the mounting hardware of the back support.

PRESSURE MANAGEMENT CONSIDERATIONS FOR THE HANDS-FREE SITTER

Contributing Factors

Many contributing factors place an individual at risk of pressure injury. The etiology of pressure injury includes unrelieved pressure, shear, friction, moisture, poor nutrition, immobility, and psychological, social, and economic factors (Krouskop, Noble, Garber, & Spencer, 1983). Sitting balance, or the lack thereof, is not a good indicator of one's risk for pressure injury development. For example, a client with a diagnosis of T12 paraplegia who has hands-free sitting balance may be at high risk of pressure injury due to his lack of sensation, incontinence, and poor nutrition. Numerous risk assessment scales exist for predicting pressure injury, such as the Braden Scale, Norton Scale, Salzberg Scale, and the Pressure Injury Risk Assessment Scale for the Spinal Cord Injury (SCIPUS), to name a few (Consortium for Spinal Cord Medicine, 2001). Risk factors are slightly different in each of these tools. The Braden Scale assessment includes sensory perception, moisture, activity, mobility, nutrition, shear, and friction (Ayello & Braden 2002). The SCIPUS is more focused for individuals with spinal cord injuries and includes the following areas: level of activity, level of mobility, severity of the spinal cord injury, urine incontinence or constantly moist, preexisting conditions (e.g., age, tobacco use, pulmonary disease, cardiac disease, diabetes, or blood glucose > 110, renal disease, impaired cognitive function), residence in a nursing home or hospital, nutrition, albumin < 3.4, T protein level < 6.4, and hematocrit < 36% (Salzberg et al., 1996). Resulting scores from each test are then used to place individuals in different categories of pressure injury risk. Although these tools provide general guidance for assessing a client's risk for pressure injury, they do not address all risk factors. For example, in the area of seating and mobility, factors such as asymmetry in posture, sudden weight loss, poor transfer technique, and inappropriately fitted and adjusted equipment are just a few examples of all contributing factors to the development of pressure injury.

Prevention strategies while seated in the wheelchair include good postural alignment, an appropriate skin protection cushion, the ability to change positions effectively, frequent redistribution of sitting pressures, and twice-daily inspection of one's own skin. Morning and evening skin inspections alert the individual to areas of risk and potential causes of the pressure injury. Keep in mind that risk of pressure injury development varies widely among diagnoses and from one individual to the next, and recommendations must be tailored to each individuals needs.

Pressure Relief or Weight Shifts: Methods of Unloading the Pressure on the Seat Surface

Best practice in a variety of clinical settings and publications have touted the need for wheelchair users to perform pressure relief to prevent pressure injury. Current clinical practice guidelines recommend a weight shift every 30 minutes for 30 seconds or every 60 minutes for 1 minute (Consortium for Spinal Cord Medicine, 2001). Other researches have recommended maintaining the weight shift for longer periods of time (up to 4 minutes) to achieve full recovery of tissue oxygenation. Clinicians continue to educate and encourage clients to perform pressure reliefs or weight shifts of varying frequency and duration. It is well-documented in the research that risk of pressure injury increases with increased pressure, increased sitting duration, and decreased blood flow. Individuals with hands-free balance have several options for redistributing or relieving sitting pressures. Pressure relief methods that have been found to be effective in relieving or redistributing pressure include a full or partial forward lean, side leans to both sides, and depression where the person either fully or partially unloads the ischial tuberosities and sacrum. Sonenblum, Vonk, Janssen, and Sprigle (2014) also found that each of these methods was effective in reducing interface pressures and increasing blood flow to the ischial region regardless of the three different types of cushion that the individual with a spinal cord injury used during the study. The effectiveness of each of these techniques should be carefully assessed by the clinician.

Best practice for pressure injury prevention includes education regarding weight shifts and the prescription of a pressure distribution cushion. It is well-documented that soft tissue areas underlying bony protuberances in supine and sitting are at greatest risk of pressure injury development. Pressure distribution cushions work by increasing the surface area or contact between the person and the cushion. This is typically achieved by the cushion enveloping or conforming to the shape of the bony prominences. There are numerous classifications and types of wheelchair cushions available today. It is important that the clinician have a good understanding of the client's pressure distribution, positioning, and transfer needs before selecting a cushion to meet his or her needs.

SUMMARY

Performing a thorough evaluation is key to determining the seating and mobility needs of the client. Determining a client's sitting balance is just one of the many clinical findings that needs to be assessed during the evaluation process. The clinical findings outlined in this chapter help to establish client goals, the type of equipment that is prescribed, and the setup and fit of the seating and mobility system. Identifying the client's physical impairments, establishing goals to compensate for the impairments, and addressing those impairments and goals through simulation and trial of the equipment will lead to specific equipment recommendations that achieve the best functional outcomes. It is important that the clinician carefully consider the medical diagnosis and secondary complications that could result in changes in posture, development of pressure injury, or changes in function over time. Progressive conditions, such as muscular dystrophy, amyotrophic lateral sclerosis, multiple sclerosis, and orthopedic changes that may occur in the growing child with a disability, are just a few examples of conditions when periodic review of the postural supports is recommended.

REFERENCES

Amos, L., Brimner, A., Dierckman, H., Easton, H., Grimes, H., Kain, J.,...& Moyers, P. A. (2001). Effects of positioning on functional reach. *Physical & Occupational Therapy in Geriatrics, 20,* 59-72.

Ayello, E. A., & Braden, B. (2002). How and why to do pressure ulcer risk assessment. *Advances in Skin & Wound Care, 15,* 125-131.

Boswell-Ruys, C. L., Sturnieks, D. L., Harvey, L. A., Sherrington, C., Middleton, J. W., & Lord, S. R. (2009). Validity and reliability of assessment tools for measuring unsupported sitting in people with spinal cord injury. *Archives of Physical Medicine and Rehabilitation, 90,* 1571-1577.

Consortium for Spinal Cord Medicine. (2001). Pressure ulcer prevention and treatment following spinal cord injury: A clinical practice guideline for health-care professionals. *Journal of Spinal Cord Medicine, 24*(Suppl. 1), S40-S101.

Corfman, T. A., Cooper, R. A., Boninger, M. L., Koontz, A. M., & Fitzgerald, S. G. (2003). Range of motion and stroke frequency differences between manual wheelchair propulsion and pushrim-activated power-assisted wheelchair propulsion. *Journal of Spinal Cord Medicine, 26,* 135-140.

Duncan, P. W., Weiner, D. K., Chandler, J., & Studenski, S. (1990). Functional reach: a new clinical measure of balance. *Journal of Gerontology, 45,* M192-M197.

Krouskop, T. A., Noble, P. C., Garber, S. L., & Spencer, W. A. (1983). The effectiveness of preventive management in reducing the occurrence of pressure sores. *Journal of Rehabilitation R&D, 20,* 74-83.

Newsam, C. J., Rao, S. S., Mulroy, S. J., Gronley, J. K., Bontrager, E. L., & Perry, J. (1999). Three dimensional upper extremity motion during manual wheelchair propulsion in men with different levels of spinal cord injury. *Gait & Posture, 10,* 223-232.

NHIC Corp. (2013). Local Coverage Determination (LCD) for Manual Wheelchair Bases (L11465). Retrieved from http://www.medicarenhic.com/viewdoc.aspx?id=1683

Noridian Healthcare Solutions. (2017). Local coverage determination: wheelchair seating (L33312). Retrieved from https://med.noridianmedicare.com/documents/2230703/7218263/wheelchair%2bseating%2bLCD%20%2band%2bPA/78eccd60-ce13-40db-8127-a3aec591e176

Salzberg, C. A., Byrne, D. W., Cayten, C. G., van Niewerburgh, P., Murphy, J. G., & Viehbeck, M. (1996). A new pressure ulcer risk assessment scale for individuals with spinal cord injury. *American Journal of Physical Medicine & Rehabilitation, 75,* 96-104.

Shaw, G., & Taylor, S. J. (1991). A survey of wheelchair seating problems of the institutionalized elderly. *Assistive Technology, 3,* 5-10.

Sonenblum, S. E., Vonk, T. E., Janssen, T. W., & Sprigle, S. H. (2014). Effects of wheelchair cushions and pressure relief maneuvers on ischial interface pressure and blood flow in people with spinal cord injury. *Archives of Physical Medicine and Rehabilitation, 95*(7), 1350-1357.

Postural Support and Pressure Management Considerations for Hands-Dependent Sitters

Sharon Sutherland, PT

The process of sitting is itself a challenging one! To sit, we must flex our hips so that we can get our buttocks as far back as possible on the seat we are sitting on in an effort to bear weight through both ischial tuberosities, posterior thighs, and feet with the knees flexed. Ideally the trunk and head will be upright and balanced above the pelvis. This action, even with intact neuromuscular control, is a lot of work. If the client lacks an intact neuromuscular system to provide internal postural support, the goal of a seating and mobility system is to provide that support externally. In the absence of this external support, the client will be unable to function efficiently or safely from the seated position without postural compensation and skin integrity compromise (Arledge et al, 2011). This chapter reviews the following:

- What benchmark is being used to describe optimal sitting posture and why?
- What do we mean by hands-dependent sitters?
- What type of client might fit this profile?
- What challenges related to function are faced by the hands-dependent sitter?
- What challenges related to skin integrity are faced by the hands-dependent sitter?
- How are potential challenges translated into optimal generic seating solutions?

BENCHMARKS FOR OPTIMAL SITTING POSTURE

When looking at a person sitting in optimal sitting posture from the side, three natural curves should be observed: a concave curve at the neck, a convex curve spanning the chest and midback, and another concave curve at the lower back known as the *lumbar lordosis*. This spinal stacking is instrumental for balancing the head and trunk above the pelvis (Figure 4-1). In the seated position, the pelvis is making contact with the seating surface on a very narrow ischial base of support.

The benchmark for optimal sitting posture is initially set when a 6- to 7-month-old baby reaches the final, mature stage of sitting. Babies cannot sit without the support of another person until age 4 months, when they begin sitting by using their hands to support themselves. This is primarily because their trunk and abdominal muscles have not yet developed sufficiently to support the trunk against gravity. After 6 months of age, a baby is able hold his or her head up, while the trunk muscles, along with the abdominal muscles, stabilize him or her to permit rotation, leaning, reaching, and so on in sitting. He or she can play with both hands while sitting independently. This important milestone is known as *hands-free sitting*.

Lange, M. L., & Minkel, J. L.
Seating and Wheeled Mobility: A Clinical Resource Guide
(pp. 61-72). © 2018 SLACK Incorporated.

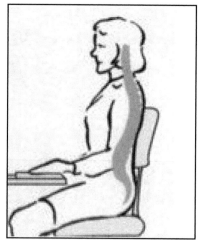

Figure 4-1. Example of spinal stacking.

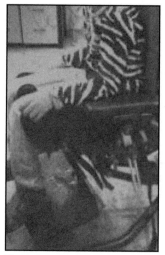

Figure 4-2. Forward trunk lean.

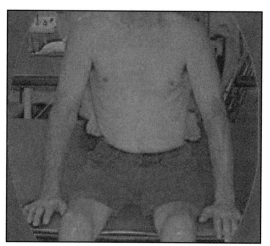

Figure 4-3. Hands needed for support.

HANDS-DEPENDENT SITTING: WHAT IS THE CLIENT PROFILE?

Any client who presents with impaired neuromuscular control of the trunk and abdominal muscles or who presents with asymmetry in the pelvis or pelvic-hip relationship may need to use his or her hands for support when attempting to sit over the side of a mat table or plinth. In the absence of using hands for support, such a person will collapse. This is what we are referring to as *hands-dependent sitting.*

To picture this client's sitting posture, imagine that the pelvis is in an upright-oriented position loading through both ischial tuberosities with both posterior thighs and feet fully supported. Visualize this lower body posture paired with trunk collapse. This could be forward in a kyphotic alignment with flattening of the lumbar lordosis in combination with an open thigh to trunk angle (Waugh & Crane, 2013) known as *sacral sitting* (Figure 4-2), or the person

could collapse laterally in a scoliotic alignment (leaning laterally) while leaning on one or both hands to stay upright against gravity (Figure 4-3).

For the client to maintain an upright seated position, a very tall structure, consisting of the trunk, neck, and head, must be in balance over the pelvis, which requires coordinated symmetrical muscle control. The adult head weighs approximately 10 to 12 pounds (that's a lot of weight perched on the neck). Trying to stay balanced in the seated position without adequate trunk and abdominal muscle control translates into compensatory patterns and dependence on hand support in an effort to achieve trunk and head stability while maintaining the position against gravity. In the absence of external supports, this makes it challenging for the client to use his or her hands for functional activities, such as propelling a manual wheelchair, eating, or reaching for objects.

When positioned on the mat in supine lying, this client will often have a flexible pelvic-spinal relationship (lumbar lordosis can be achieved passively and without resistance) and a flexible lumbar-thoracic relationship (lumbar-thoracic extension can be achieved passively and without resistance). This client will be able to sit hands-free with external support provided at the posterior lateral aspect of the pelvis and the posterior lumbar thoracic area; sometimes accommodating inferior support will be required as well.

These types of clients may be at moderate to high risk for skin integrity issues if they are sitting for long periods of time without doing consistent, effective, independent weight shifts, and/or if they have presence or history of Stage 1 or above pressure injury on any of the sitting surfaces (National Pressure Ulcer Advisory Panel, 2016).

WHAT CLIENT PROFILES OR DIAGNOSTIC GROUPS FIND THEMSELVES DEPENDING ON HAND SUPPORT WHILE TRYING TO FUNCTION FROM AN UPRIGHT SITTING POSTURE?

The following process is used for each of the following case studies:

- How does this client present in the existing wheelchair and seating system?
- What are the findings from the supine and sitting mat evaluation with regard to postural and skin analysis?
- What possible generic features might be needed in the new seating and mobility system?

CASE EXAMPLE

Client Presentation in Existing Equipment

This client is 4 years post-C6/7 spinal cord injury. He presents in his manual wheelchair, off-the-shelf seat cushion, and tension adjustable back upholstery, which provides low thoracic support. He sits with a posterior pelvic tilt, thigh to trunk angle of 120 degrees (sacral sitting), zero lumbar contour depth (flattened lumbar lordosis), and a compensatory thoracic kyphosis. The client complains of instability requiring frequent hooking of his arm over the wheelchair back post, with fatigue and neck pain after 1.5 hours of sitting. The client also has a history of Stage 2 pressure injury on his sacrum.

Mat Evaluation: Supine

Upon supine evaluation, this client presents with reducible postural deviations. Using a systematic approach to the supine evaluation, extension is evident during passive palpation of available movement in the midthoracic area. In the lumbar/thoracic and pelvic/lumbar areas, passive extension is achievable; this indicates that the client has a flexible spine and pelvic relationship, which is very positive. The pelvis thigh relationship is also flexible (at least 90 degrees hip flexion with a neutral pelvis can be achieved) and within normal limits for sitting as is the lower leg to thigh flexibility. A skin check reveals a healed Stage 2 pressure injury on the sacrum with residual skin changes.

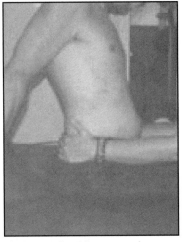

Figure 4-4. Providing external support to the pelvis.

Mat Evaluation: Sitting

While seated over the edge of the mat table with both feet supported on the floor or another support, the client can sit with equal loading through both ischial tuberosities and through both trochanters/posterior thighs. He can tolerate a neutral thigh to pelvic angle for sitting (at least 90 degrees of hip flexion with a neutral pelvis) and being passively moved from a flat lumbar posture into one of lumbar/thoracic extension without resistance. However, because of much decreased spinal and abdominal muscle group strength (T6-12 innervation), this client cannot actively hold himself up against gravity. In the absence of external posterolateral pelvic and trunk support, his pelvis and trunk collapse into an open pelvic thigh angle, with a flattened lumbar curve and exaggerated kyphotic thoracic and/or scoliotic curve. He must use his hands for support. This hands-dependent position leaves the client with compromised function when trying to sit upright against gravity. When posterolateral pelvic support in combination with lumbar/thoracic extension and mild lateral low thoracic support is provided by the assessing therapist, the client can now sit hands free. The external support provided by the therapist compensates for the lack of intrinsic muscle control, secondary to the cervical level spinal cord injury (Figure 4-4).

The client is able to demonstrate that with the support described above he is able to do an effective and independent weight shift using a push up method, as well as a forward lean/side to side method. In the forward and side leaning position he can eliminate load bearing through his ischial tuberosities and sacrum for the necessary time; therefore, these positions are recommended as the preferred method. This will reduce the likelihood of trauma to the wrists and shoulder joints that can often lead to overuse injuries while doing push up weight shifts.

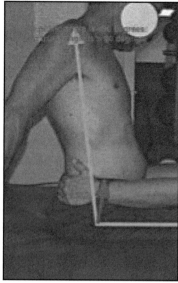

Figure 4-5. Impact of posterior pelvic support on spinal alignment.

What to Do? Translating Findings Into Generic Product Parameters and Solutions

I refer to a systematic order of hierarchy as the *sitting footprint*. One must consider where all body segments of the wheelchair-seated person are primarily bearing weight. Consider the inferior, posterior, lateral, and anterior aspects of the seated body and think about the following:

- What is the impact of gravity?
- How can the sitting footprint be maximized?
- What is the optimal sitting footprint for each individual client based on findings from the mat evaluation?

The inferior and posterior load-bearing areas are primary with lateral and anterior support surfaces regarded as secondary. In other words, anterior and lateral surfaces were never intended to be our primary supports for sitting but may be necessary to assist in supporting the trunk against gravity for a hands-free sitting position. With this process in mind, a useful hierarchy for thinking about possible solutions follows.

Inferior Support Surfaces: The Stable Foundation

- Consider using a seat cushion that is designed to offer potential for immersion and envelopment. Such a cushion allows the client to sink into the support surface with equalized loading throughout the

posterior thighs, undersurface of the trochanters, and ischial tuberosities (Brienza & Geyer, 2005). The cushion cover will need to permit this optimal immersion and envelopment without resistance so that the client is sitting in his cushion as opposed to sitting on it.

- Provide a foot support system, allowing the feet to bear weight equally.
- Arm supports, if used on the chair, should be adjusted to support the undersurface of the forearms while the trunk maintains correct/optimal alignment when a resting position is needed. The client may choose not to have arm supports.

Posterior Support Surfaces

- Back support should offer the potential for posterior stabilization of the pelvis (keeping the thigh to pelvis angle at approximately 85 degrees) in combination with upper lumber/lower thoracic extension (maintaining the thigh to trunk angle at approximately 100 degrees). In essence, this supports the spinal stacking that we know the client can tolerate based on the evaluation findings (Figure 4-5).
- If the client had an injury level or trauma affecting head control, offering suboccipital head support would be the next posterior consideration. In this case, it is not necessary.

Gravity Assist: Improve Effectiveness of Posterior Loading

Mobility base frames can offer 5 to 10 to 15 degrees of fixed tilt-in-space (seat slope) that is achieved through adjustment of the wheelchair frame as appropriate for a particular client. Less is often best. Imagine rear seat to floor height 1 inch lower than front seat to floor height while maintaining the desired pelvic, thigh, and trunk angles. This can also be achieved through adjustment of the seating system, if appropriate or necessary. For example, if a new wheelchair cannot be funded, alternative-seating components can be identified and set up to create a similar degree of tilt (seat slope) as described, by mounting an adjustable angle backrest and solid seat insert.

Changing the orientation in space or seat slope, in this case, will help overcome the negative impacts of gravity and fatigue (Paralyzed Veterans of America Consortium of Spinal Cord Medicine, 2005). This client is struggling to balance his 10- to 12-pound head over a spine with limited to no muscle assistance available for stacking of the spine. This is essential for balance and to free his hands for function while preserving his ability to transfer.

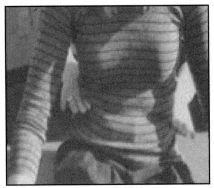

Figure 4-6. Anterior view of pelvic obliquity and collapsing spine.

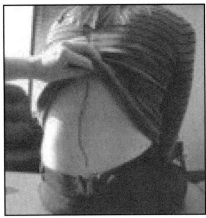

Figure 4-7. Posterior view of pelvic obliquity and collapsing spine.

Lateral Support

Mild to moderate thoracic lateral support will ensure that balance is maintained to free the hands but that function is not compromised.

For some high-functioning clients, no change to orientation in space is applicable or acceptable. For such individuals, integrating lateral supports either as part of the back support or as an added component in combination with pelvic stabilization and supporting lumbar thoracic extension will promote the client's ability to sit hands free and function from a seated position.

CASE EXAMPLE

The client is age 27 and 10 years post-T12 incomplete spinal cord injury with a past history of left partial ischial removal. This client presents in a high-performance rigid manual wheelchair, off-the-shelf cushion, and off-the-shelf back support that provides midthoracic posterior and mild lateral support. She presents in this system with an open thigh to trunk angle (110 degrees), pelvic obliquity (left side low), compensatory low thoracic scoliosis convex to her left, collapsed and flattened lumbar lordosis, mild thoracic kyphosis, and forward head posture. She complains of neck and upper thoracic pain. She has a history of flap surgery 8 years ago and partial left ischial removal secondary to a pressure injury and infection on her left side.

Mat Evaluation: Supine

Upon evaluation in supine lying on the mat, this client presents with no fixed postural deviations. Using a systematic approach, while palpating passively for movement in the midthoracic region, extension is evident. In the lumbar/thoracic area and in the pelvic/lumbar area, passive extension is achievable, which translates to a very positive finding that the client has a flexible spine and spine/

pelvic relationship. There is no pelvic obliquity or scoliosis observable or palpable in supine. Her pelvic thigh relationship is also very flexible and within normal limits for sitting as is the lower leg to thigh flexibility.

A skin check reveals a healed scar over and running laterally from her left ischial tuberosity toward her left hip joint with residual skin changes. This means that she is at high risk for skin integrity problems secondary to her past history, in combination with increased protrusion of bony prominences related to muscle atrophy as well as impaired sensation and high activity level.

Mat Evaluation: Sitting

When seated over the edge of the mat table with both feet supported on the floor, the client sits hands-dependent and collapses into a left pelvic obliquity, compensatory scoliosis convex to her left, open thigh to pelvic angle, and mild kyphosis (Figures 4-6 and 4-7).

During the evaluation, the client can tolerate a neutral thigh to pelvic angle for sitting without resistance as well as passive lumbar thoracic extension. However, because of her left ischial and buttock asymmetry, she continues to fall into a left pelvic obliquity and resultant scoliosis. She cannot actively maintain upright sitting posture against gravity without the use of her hands. Building up support beneath her left buttock can substitute for muscle and bone mass that is lacking, and external posterolateral pelvic and low trunk support can be added to assist her in maintaining upright posture against gravity. When a lift is positioned under the client's left buttock and the therapist provides her with posterior/lateral pelvic and thoracic support, she can now sit hands free and with a level pelvis (Figure 4-8).

The client demonstrates that, with the previously described support, she is able to do an effective and independent weight shift using a push up as well as a forward lean, side to side method. As noted earlier, in the forward or side-leaning position, she can get her ischial tuberosities and sacrum clear of load bearing for the necessary time;

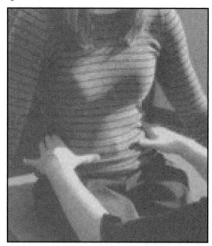

Figure 4-8. Impact of lift under left buttock to level the pelvis.

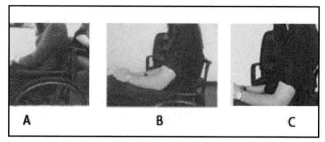

Figure 4-9. Progression on interventions: before change, inferior support only; inferior and posterior supports provided. (A) Before change. (B) Inferior footprint improved. Posterior aspect now needs change. (C) Inferior and posterior contact area addressed.

therefore, this is recommended as the preferred method for weight shifting. This client is also skilled and reliable in carrying out daily skin checks.

What to Do? Translating Findings Into Generic Product Parameters and Solutions

Inferior Support Surface: Seat Support

For this client to sit with the symmetrical pelvic spine alignment she needs to function efficiently and safely, she must have at least one of the following:

- A cushion or seat support that provides optimal immersion and envelopment for skin protection and postural stability and includes a built up surface under the left buttock to substitute for the loss of muscle and bone mass. This will result in a level pelvis, while distributing weight equally over the inferior load bearing areas that can tolerate it.

- Another option is a seat cushion that off-loads the more bony prominences by supporting the client through the inferior aspect of the greater trochanters and femurs instead of the ischial tuberosities, which are asymmetrical. As long as the client can tolerate this distribution of load, this too should result in a level pelvis without requiring buildup of the cushion on the left side.

- If a trial shows this results in excessive stress to scar tissue over the left ischial tuberosity, a combination of both is recommended. This combination could include adding a lift under the left buttock using skin-protecting materials, while redistributing weight laterally to the undersurface of the

trochanters and femurs. This will provide lateral stability for the pelvis as well as more equalized loading beneath the entire inferior aspect of the buttocks and posterior thighs.

Posterior Support Surface: Back Support

To facilitate sitting with a neutral pelvis and lumbar thoracic extension (spinal stacking), this client will need a back support that provides posterior pelvic support together with lumbar/low thoracic support; this will allow her to extend over the top of the back support. This could be achieved through contouring of the back support itself or through angle adjustability in the design of the mounting hardware (or both). It should be noted that the client will likely be able to function hands-free with a lower level back support than she presented in originally because her ischial asymmetry is now accommodated. She will no longer sit with collapsed posture, so she will have enhanced ability to function safely and efficiently from her seated position. See Figure 4-9 for progression of postural alignment

Wheelchair Setup

The client continues to use her existing chair, which works well for her, but whenever seating changes are made, it is likely that alterations to the wheelchair configuration will be required. For example, with her newly acquired level pelvis and spinal stacking, the client's shoulder-hand-wheel relationship will be different because her sitting posture could be described as taller. Thus, the vertical axle plate may require adjustment for optimal performance to bring the push rim higher and closer to the hand of the client (Paralyzed Veterans of America Consortium of Spinal Cord Medicine, 2005). During trial of the seating modifications, it must be established that propulsion on all terrains, transfers, and weight shifts are optimized and necessary adjustments are made. It is good to remind yourself that "every time we change one thing, everything changes." We therefore must check all aspects of function, especially when we have introduced a change in postural alignment.

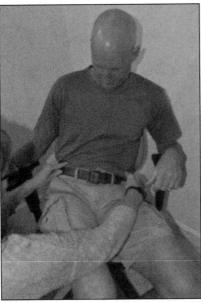

Figure 4-10. Lower extremities, windswept to the left.

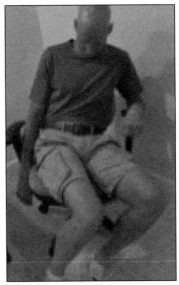

Figure 4-11. Pelvic obliquity, right side higher than the left side.

CASE EXAMPLE

This client with progressive multiple sclerosis has progressed to using a power chair with power seat functions including tilt-in-space, elevating legrests, and recline. He presents seated in his chair in a sacral sitting position. He has a large thoracic kyphosis, leans to his left side, and holds on with his left hand for balance. The inferior support surface area is minimal at his posterior thighs with more loading beneath his left ischial tuberosity and trochanter than his right. Both legs are windswept toward the client's left side. His feet touch the foot supports but with minimal weightbearing. Posteriorly, he contacts the back support only in the lower sacral/low lumbar area, with more contact on his left side than on the right. The client complains of respiratory complications, digestive complications, and constant fatigue. He also presents with chronic pain in his upper trunk and neck and has a history of Stage 1 pressure injury on his sacrum and the apex of his thoracic curve. Figures 4-10 and 4-11 demonstrate what this presenting posture may look like.

Mat Evaluation: Supine

Upon evaluation in supine lying, there is passive flexibility in the pelvis-spine relationship and potential for lumbar lordosis with thoracic extension. The client's head can lie flat on the mat table indicating no fixed kyphosis (Figure 4-12).

Approximately 5 degrees of fixed lateral curvature in the thoracic spine convex to the client's left is noted. There is no pelvic obliquity or rotation, and his hips are within normal limits bilaterally with regard to flexibility for sitting. The client's lower extremities are not windswept in supine; both knees can be positioned in line with the hip without being abducted or adducted. When his lower extremities are extended with his hips flexed to an approximate 90-degree pelvic thigh angle, it is revealed that the hamstrings are very limited bilaterally (Figure 4-13).

To maintain a pelvic/lumbar lordosis, and a healthy open space between the lower ribs and pelvis, the client's knees cannot be extended to 90 degrees with his hips flexed; the bilateral thigh to lower leg angle must be 75 to 80 degrees (Figure 4-14).

To understand this posture, picture a person sitting with his feet under the seat, rather than extended in front of the seat—a closed thigh to lower leg angle.

Mat Evaluation: Sitting

When seated over the edge of the mat table with posterior thighs and feet supported, the mat table design often forces the client's lower legs to extend closer to 90 degrees at his knees (Figure 4-15).

To compensate for his hamstring limitation, he assumes sacral sitting with kyphosis and lateral leaning to his left. He uses both hands to stabilize himself in an effort to

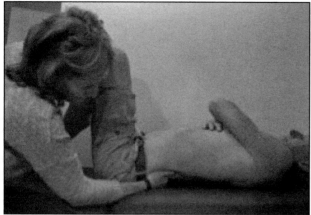

Figure 4-12. Supine alignment: pelvis in neutral position.

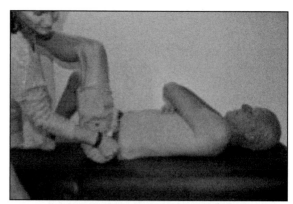

Figure 4-13. Trunk to thigh angle and impact of tight hamstring muscle on pelvic position.

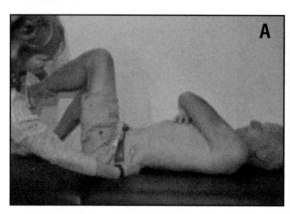 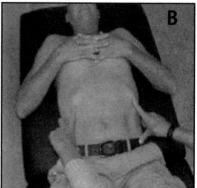

Figure 4-14. (A) Reducing the thigh to lower leg angle to accommodate tight hamstring muscle. (B) Rib cage to pelvis (anterior superior iliac spine) alignment.

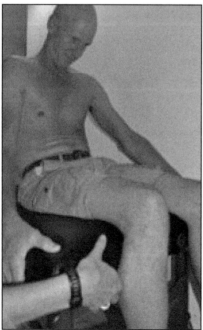

Figure 4-15. Impact of front edge on mat: knees extended, resulting in posterior pelvic tilt.

remain upright. His breathing is labored; the space between his lower ribs and pelvis is now reduced.

If he sits closer to the edge of the mat table, the client's tight hamstrings are accommodated; this allows closing of his thigh to lower leg angle to approximately 75 degrees (Figure 4-16).

When the assessing therapist, while accommodating the tight hamstrings, provides posterolateral pelvic and lateral midthoracic support, the client can sit hands-free. There is open space again between his lower ribs and pelvis. His breathing pattern is notably relaxed, and the client reports he is "feeling much better."

What to Do? Translating Findings Into Generic Product Parameters and Solutions

Respecting the hamstrings means supporting the client's feet so that the thigh to lower leg angle (75 degrees) is maintained where the hamstrings tendon is not taut or being pulled. By maintaining the distal end of the hamstrings at a relaxed angle, the proximal end can allow the pelvis to remain in neutral alignment, thereby maintaining a natural lordosis and lumbar/thoracic extension.

Inferior Support Surface

The recommended seat cushion must accommodate the sharp angle at the posterior aspect of the knee by beveling back (undercutting) the front edge of the cushion or by shortening/compromising seat depth to avoid interference with the client's lower leg, as his feet will be under the seat.

Posterior Loading Surfaces

The back support must provide posterior pelvic stabilization together with upper lumbar/lower thoracic extension, as well as moderate midthoracic lateral support.

Lower Extremity Support

The power elevating legrests on this client's chair will not be appropriate in this situation because each time his lower legs are extended, the ischial tuberosities are pulled forward, causing loss of lordosis and spinal stacking, trunk collapse, and return to sacral sitting. This not only leaves the client in a hands-dependent sitting posture, but also returns him to a position of respiratory, digestive, and skin integrity compromise.

Another option can be considered, especially if the chair configuration will not allow support of the feet at the necessary thigh to lower leg angle (75 degrees). This strategy would be to relax the hamstrings proximally by opening the thigh to trunk angle. There are many ways to accomplish this. One example is to raise the hips and buttocks higher than the knees by about 1 inch. In other words, open the thigh to trunk angle approximately 10 degrees (from 90 degrees to an angle of 100 degrees) by introducing an anterior slope in the seat such that the rear seat to floor height is 1 inch higher than the front seat to floor height (including cushion). This will translate into more forgiveness in the thigh to lower leg angle, allowing the client's feet to be positioned closer to the front edge of the chair rather than under it, while maintaining the desired trunk/gravity alignment (Figure 4-17).

Still another way to accomplish relaxation of the hamstrings proximally can be done by opening the seat to back angle to 105 to 110 degrees, while maintaining and supporting the established lumbar lordosis and lumbar thoracic extension. This will, however, place the client's body mass behind the sitting center of gravity, which will create instability and a tendency to slide. To overcome this, we must then add approximately 10 degrees of tilt-in-space. From a functional standpoint, this may or may not be acceptable to the client while driving and engaging in activities from his power chair. Ultimately, conducting a trial or simulation of each setup is necessary when establishing which of these proposed solutions would be best. During this process, while asking the client for feedback and making

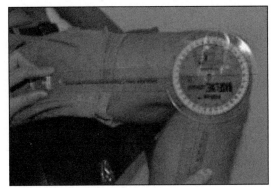

Figure 4-16. Accommodating tight hamstring, allows knee to flex, thigh to lower leg angle of approximately 75 degrees.

observations, the question is, "Can he sit hands-free and function in all necessary areas of life when optimally set up and supported?"

CASE EXAMPLE

This 26-year-old client with spinal muscular atrophy presents using a power wheelchair with power seat functions, including recline, tilt-in-space, and elevating legrests with off-the-shelf seating. The client presents seated in his chair with a thigh to pelvic angle of 50 degrees, his trunk collapsing forward, and his cervical spine in a hyper extended posture (Figure 4-18).

To drive the power chair with a standard joystick, which requires at least one hand to be free, this client must also apply a tightly fitting chest strap. The head support is adjusted forward from the back support by at least 10 inches; no contact is made with the back cushion other than in the sacral area. Removing the chest strap leaves the client totally hands-dependent while sitting, preventing him from using the joystick. Even while the client is reclined and tilted in his chair, minimal contact is made with the back cushion because the head support in its forward position prevents his spine from contacting the back support. The client uses these power features often to ease pain and provide alternate positioning throughout the day.

Mat Evaluation: Supine

Upon evaluation on the mat lying supine, this client presents with very tight hip flexors. His hips are fixed (non-reducible) in a flexed position, which can be measured as a 50-degree thigh to pelvic angle. His sacrum is extremely bony with sharp protrusions on palpation; the client expresses feeling discomfort on contact or loading. The ischial tuberosities are very palpable, but to date there is no history of skin integrity issues. Surgically placed,

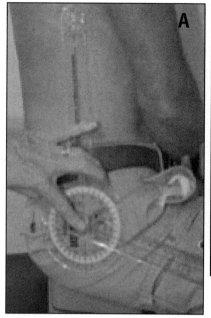
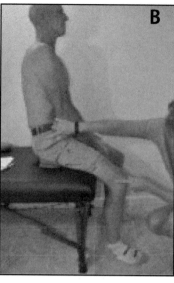

Figure 4-17. (A) Measuring an open trunk to thigh angle of 100 degrees. (B) Anterior slope of the seat and thigh.

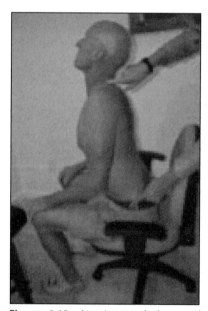

Figure 4-18. Anterior trunk lean and resulting hyperextension of the head and neck.

spinal fixation rods stabilize the entire thoracic and lumbar spine. The cervical spine and head relationship is flexible.

Mat Evaluation: Sitting

When seated over the edge of the mat table, the client cannot sit without the support of both hands. He is able to sit hands-dependent, working hard to hold his head up against gravity (Figure 4-19).

Lifting his flexed knees higher than his hips (visualize knees up) demonstrated improved potential for bringing the client's spine and head into contact with a posterior support, while maintaining an upright orientation and feeling able to free his hands for a short period of time (Figure 4-20).

The client's goal is to remain independent, but he would also like to have more contact with the back support to reduce the work involved with sitting. He cannot function in a tilted position; he is unwilling to accept anything more than a maximum of 5 to 10 degrees of tilt during functional activities; however, he will use tilt or recline frequently for weight shifting and change of position. The client cannot do a functional, independent weight shift, so he is at high risk for skin integrity issues. He is not ready to accept alternative drive mechanisms at this time.

What to Do? Translating Findings Into Generic Product Parameters and Solutions

The dilemma in this situation is that the only ways to bring the client's trunk in contact with and loading on a back support while respecting the pelvic to thigh angle at 50 degrees are to:

- Position and support the knees substantially higher than the hips

- Allow the trunk to lean forward such that the pelvic thigh angle remains at 50 degrees

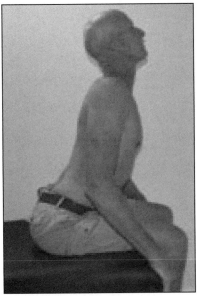

Figure 4-19. Hands-dependent sitting with anterior pelvic tilt and cervical hyperextension.

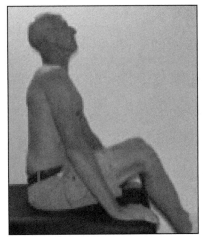

Figure 4-20. Demonstration of knees-up position, shifting the pelvis and trunk posteriorly.

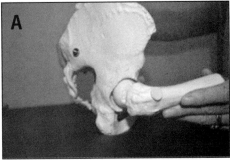

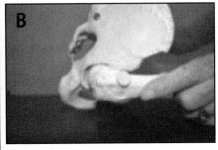

Figure 4-21. (A) Weightbearing on the ischial tuberosities in a neutral pelvic tilt. (B) Anteriorly tilted pelvis, weightbearing shifted to the pubis.

Either situation is challenging. Supporting the knees so much higher than the hips substantially increases loading on the sacrum and ischial tuberosities, which puts the client at high risk for skin integrity and bladder issues, as well as pain (Figure 4-21A). Remember, this client has not had any problems with his ischial tuberosities and skin integrity to date. It would be interesting to explore why this might be. In the forward trunk/pelvis position he sits in every day, he is assuming a posture much like forward leaning for weight shifting, meaning that the ischial tuberosities are off-loaded and have therefore been safe (Figure 4-21B).

By allowing the client to continue sitting in the forward-flexed trunk position, much loading on the chest strap remains together with head and neck control challenges and ongoing need for hands dependency.

A compromise may be possible by trial molding the client in approximately 20 degrees of tilt, with the head support aligned appropriately for a more neutral head and neck position while capturing the shape of the client's posterior trunk. Once the shape is captured, allow the client to resume the tilt angle he desires for driving (more upright) and support his posterior thighs such that his knees are approximately 1 inch higher than his hips. If more posterior spinal contact and a healthier head and neck alignment can be achieved without compromising function or skin integrity, this is a win-win situation. It is a fine balancing of angles, shapes, and orientation; it will likely take the work out of sitting for this client, who needs to have his hands free for function while managing a continuously progressing condition. This client will likely become a fully dependent sitter in the future.

Regardless of the seating approach taken, this client cannot accomplish a consistent, independent, and effective weight shift. From a skin integrity perspective, he is at high risk for pressure injuries while seated in his chair as well as in bed, toileting, and bathing. Weight shifting, through technology, such as tilt, in combination with his forward-lean sitting position, has kept his sitting surfaces safe to date.

There are additional considerations and options for a client with spinal muscular atrophy whose condition has not progressed quite as far as this client. Many individuals have successfully used abdominal bindings and soft orthoses to take the work out of sitting and free their hands for function when they have sufficient hip joint flexibility to allow more neutral alignment of the pelvic to thigh angle and make spinal stacking possible. When tolerated by the client, this solution can reduce the need for otherwise necessary changes in orientation in space—changes that are often rejected by this very functional type of client.

SUMMARY

When presented with clients who must support themselves with their hands to sit over the edge of a mat table or plinth for a seating, positioning, and mobility evaluation, it is helpful to remember that the process of sitting is itself challenging. Trying to stay balanced in the seated position without adequate trunk and abdominal muscle control translates into compensatory patterns and dependence on hand support in an effort to achieve trunk and head stability while maintaining the position against gravity. In the absence of external supports, this makes it challenging for the client to use his or her hands for functional activities, such as propelling a manual wheelchair, eating, or reaching for objects.

The hands-on evaluations described in this chapter for each client included both supine and sitting components that were critical for our success in helping these clients achieve their goals for function and inclusion independence. The findings from our detailed hands-on assessments, when translated into product parameters, are what will drive our ability to provide optional solutions. There is never just one solution, but understanding the needs and priorities of the individual client allows us to present realistic options, especially when both the positive and the potential negative consequences of each option are clearly communicated. Trialing the proposed options will then provide the necessary confidence to our clients and provide us with the essential documentation that is important as we navigate the reimbursement path for the chosen solutions.

 Figures 4-11 through 4-20 are reprinted with permission. Model demonstrating postures is Scott Sutherland. Photographs taken by Sarah Mckee.

REFERENCES

Arledge, S., Armstrong, W., Babinec, M., Dicianno, B. E., DiGiovine, C., Dyson-Hudson, T.,...& Schmeler, M. (2011). *RESNA wheelchair service provision guide.* Arlington, VA: Rehabilitation Engineering & Assistive Technology Society of North America. Retrieved from https://www.resna.org/sites/default/files/legacy/resources/position-papers/RESNAWheelchairServiceProvisionGuide.pdf

Brienza, D. M., & Geyer, M. J. (2005). Using support surfaces to manage tissue integrity. *Advances in Skin & Wound Care, 18,* 151-157.

National Pressure Ulcer Advisory Panel. (2016). *Pressure injury stages.* Retrieved from http://www.npuap.org/resources/educational-and-clinical-resources/npuap-pressure-injury-stages

Paralyzed Veterans of America Consortium of Spinal Cord Medicine. (2005). Preservation of upper limb function following spinal cord injury: a clinical practice guideline for health-care professionals. *Journal of Spinal Cord Medicine, 28,* 434-470.

Waugh, K., & Crane, B. (2013). *A clinical application guide to standardized wheelchair seating measures of the body and seating support surfaces.* Aurora, CO: University of Colorado School of Medicine.

SUGGESTED READINGS

Minkel, J. L. (2000). Seating and mobility considerations for people with spinal cord injury. *Physical Therapy, 80,* 701-709.

Waugh, K., Crane, B., Saftler Savage, F., Davis, K., Johnson Taylor, S., Cwiertnia, S....Christie, S. (2013). *Glossary of wheelchair terms and definitions.* Aurora, CO: Assistive Technology Partners, University of Colorado. Retrieved from https://www.ncart.us/uploads/userfiles/files/glossary-of-wheelchair-terms.pdf

5

Postural Support and Pressure Management Considerations for Prop Sitters

Jill Sparacio, OTR/L, ATP/SMS, ABDA

DEFINITION

Clients who are unable to actively support themselves in an upright and aligned position are frequently referred to as *prop sitters*. They rely on the provision of imposed external support for the maintenance of an upright, but often compromised, seated posture. The provision of external support can facilitate their ability to actively participate in functional tasks. Other key benefits can include improved visual orientation and oral motor and respiratory function, as well as maintaining skin integrity. Many factors influence what type of support and contact is needed, often distinguishing between the need for total contact versus key points of control.

TYPICAL DIAGNOSES AND PRESENTATION

Prop sitters can be divided into two distinct groups: those who present with little or no postural asymmetry and those who present with significant, uncorrectable or non-reducible asymmetries.

Those persons described as prop sitters who have little or no asymmetrical postures are most often completely flaccid in their trunk, meaning there is no asymmetrical muscle control, tone, or spasms, which can result in asymmetrical postures. Through the provision of external support, these clients can be positioned in and maintain a symmetrical

sitting posture against gravity, even if they cannot achieve the position through voluntary muscle control.

Those prop sitters with significant postural asymmetries also need external support to be positioned in and maintain a sitting posture against gravity. The biggest difference is these sitters are not in a symmetrical sitting position. They are being supported in a *personal posture,* supported against gravity in a functional position where the head is in a midline position even if the pelvis and spine are asymmetrical.

Various groups of clients can benefit from the provision of total support designed into a seating system. Although each person presents with unique characteristics, some generalizations can be made. Those with both orthopedic and neurological impairments can benefit from total support seating systems. From a neurological perspective, individuals with little or no voluntary trunk control, such as a person with a spinal cord injury resulting in quadriplegia or a person with advanced amyotrophic lateral sclerosis (ALS), can benefit from the external support provided by the seating system. As a result of long-standing loss of intrinsic muscle support of the trunk, persons with muscular dystrophy and those with a diagnosis of cerebral palsy resulting in spastic quadriplegia may present with a combination of neurological and orthopedic impairments that lead to asymmetrical alignment of the trunk and pelvis. This presentation can be accommodated, supporting the asymmetry, to provide a functional seated position using a total support seating system. The common theme among these diagnoses is the inability to functionally support oneself in an upright seated position with active trunk control like a hands-free sitter or with the ability to prop with one's arms

Lange, M. L., & Minkel, J. L.
Seating and Wheeled Mobility: A Clinical Resource Guide
(pp. 73-84). © 2018 SLACK Incorporated.

like a hands-dependent sitter (Sutherland, 2015). Other diagnostic groups who might benefit from total support seating systems include multiple sclerosis, cerebral vascular accident, traumatic brain injury, and intellectual disabilities. The need for these systems is based on presentation, not simply a diagnosis.

Rather than limiting seating applications to diagnostic criteria, specific evaluation presentations must be addressed. A disease process can be better described by presentation than by label. Variations of muscle tone, range of motion (ROM), and the type and presentation of skeletal asymmetries must be evaluated and considered. It is safe to say that prop sitters traditionally have multiple issues with mobility, sensation, and alignment. Although the individual may have started as a hands-free sitter, progression of the disease process or aging issues may result in a loss of function, requiring the need for more support.

As noted earlier, clients who present as prop sitters will fall into one of two groups: those who present with little to no skeletal asymmetry and those who present with skeletal asymmetry. The first group includes clients with newly acquired injuries or diagnoses (spinal cord injuries, ALS). Findings from the mat evaluation will typically reveal no skeletal issues, but a lack of intrinsic support to maintain an upright seated posture against gravity. The second group includes those who, in addition to lacking intrinsic trunk support, present with pelvic and spinal asymmetries, often leading to poor head positioning. This group can include clients with cerebral palsy and muscular dystrophy, as well as those with intellectual disabilities. Clients with extremes of muscle tone (moderate to severe hypotonicity as well as hypertonicity) have the same need for total support built into a seating system. When there is a lack of balanced muscle tone over time, tonal issues often lead to the development of skeletal asymmetries. Moderate to severe orthopedic complications can also result in the need for significant external support.

EVALUATION PROCESS

As with any seating and mobility evaluation, goals must be identified. When clients require significant external support, they typically have many needs leading to the generation of many goals. The multidisciplinary team must consider all of the individual's needs and then prioritize according to consensus (Arledge et al., 2011). During this process, the client and caregiver goals should be given priority; if this is not done, the client may not "buy into" the recommended equipment. Basic functional requests should be addressed before less significant ones. Life sustaining and vital functions, such as promoting cardiopulmonary health, should be the ultimate priority. Goals addressing other basic functions, such as eating and promoting an appropriate visual field and pressure redistribution, are

next in line. For example, if a person eats by mouth, optimal alignment for safe oral motor skills is imperative compared with color options for upholstery.

During the mat evaluation, the approach for a dependent sitter can be a bit different from that for more active sitters. Obviously, a person who requires total support for sitting cannot sit on the edge of the mat table without significant help. The prop sitter with no skeletal asymmetries will be much easier to assist while sitting on the edge of a mat table than a client with significant asymmetries.

Fixed Versus Flexible

Although commonly used, there should be reluctance to use the term fixed *asymmetry* to describe the postural asymmetries found when evaluating clients (Hetzel, 2015a). Fixed limitations imply that there is no movement available at a joint. A better description of seating asymmetries may be noncorrectable or non-reducible. This describes an asymmetrical sitting posture that cannot be corrected or realigned into a symmetrical position. With some asymmetrical sitting postures, an exaggeration into greater asymmetry can occur. The exaggeration of the posture may be a result of tone patterns, the influence of gravity or the need to recruit active movement on an unopposed muscle, at the cost of further asymmetry.

Clients with postural asymmetries who require total support for sitting may present with limitations of mobility throughout the trunks and extremities. It is important to distinguish among fixed, non-reducible, and flexible asymmetries. During the mat evaluation, specific joint mobility limitations must be identified to help determine orientation and angles of support surfaces. The difference between fixed and flexible asymmetry must be understood as part of the treatment planning process.

A fixed asymmetry has no movement available in any direction or plane. For example, a fused hip joint due to a previous surgical intervention might present without any movement, with the hip fixed at 75 degrees of flexion, resulting in a trunk to thigh angle of 105 degrees.

A flexible asymmetry has movement available. This should not imply that the asymmetry can be corrected or that full range is available. If the hip joint is unable to flex to 90 degrees but movement is present to 75 degrees of flexion, this is considered a flexible asymmetry. The hip joint moves, but not into a position to create a 90-degree trunk to thigh angle, the angle most often associated with an upright sitting posture.

If the trunk to thigh angle to 90 degrees is not achievable, the seat to back angle must be altered to accommodate the trunk to thigh angle that is available. Successful use of supportive seating for prop sitters often fails because incorrect angles of support are used in the system. If the supportive seating surfaces are not set at an angle to accommodate the available trunk to thigh angle, then the overall system will not be successful. Through the simulation process these support surface angle adjustments can easily be determined, and recorded, and then used during the setup of the final product.

Information about the necessary support surface angles (e.g., seat to back support, seat to foot support) is essential when product choices are being made, ensuring that the recommended items can be setup to meet the prop sitter's postural support needs. A mobility base without seat to back angle adjustability will not be appropriate for a client who requires a seat to back angle orientation of 105 degrees because she has only 75 degrees of hip flexion, resulting in a 105-degree trunk to thigh angle. Note that when the client is supine on the mat and maximum available hip flexion range is 75 degrees (from full extension at 0 degrees to 75 degrees of flexion), the resulting angle between the trunk and thigh is 105 degrees. To fit this person to a chair, the angle between the back support and seat must also be set at 105 degrees.

Importance of the Pelvis

When conducting the mat evaluation, it is important to understand how one body part can influence another. A number of typically seen patterns may influence a client's posture. All seating interventions must start at the pelvis (Hetzel, 2015b); individuals who require imposed external support are no different than others in this regard. If the pelvis is not in optimal alignment, the desired body position cannot be obtained.

A posterior pelvic tilt results in general trunk flexion and a forward head position. The influence of a posterior pelvic tilt in the lower extremities can either be internal rotation and adduction at the hips or external rotation and abduction.

An anterior pelvic tilt results in extension of the trunk, usually with an exaggerated lumbar curve and retraction through the shoulders. The client's head has no option other than to follow the cervical spine in an extended manner. Lower extremities usually move into hip adduction and internal rotation.

Not all dependent sitters exhibit a symmetrical anterior or posterior pelvic posture. Instead, an asymmetrical orientation of the pelvis is present. One side might be in posterior tilt with the other side of the pelvis anteriorly oriented. This will result in a spine with multiple curves. Other asymmetries associated with the pelvis include obliquity and rotation.

A person's pelvis is described as oblique when one side is higher than the other. A left pelvic obliquity (left side lower than right) results in right trunk collapse. A right pelvic obliquity (right side lower than left) results in left trunk collapse.

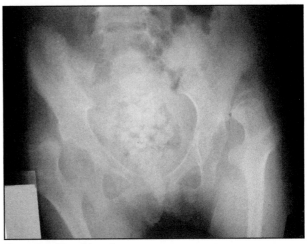

Figure 5-1. Hip subluxation on x-ray.

When pelvic rotation is present, the lower extremities orient toward the side the pelvis facing, this is commonly called a *windswept* posture. A left pelvic rotation (right side of the pelvis forward of the left with the front of the pelvis facing left) results in left windswept orientation of the hips. A right pelvic rotation (left side of the pelvis forward of the right with the front of the pelvis facing right) results in right windswept orientation of the hips.

When a person's hips are in windswept posture due to changes in the femoral head to acetabulum orientation, there is often loss of hip joint integrity as well as loss of ROM. The hip that moves into adduction is often pulled out of the very shallow acetabulum, resulting in hip subluxation (Figure 5-1). Hip subluxation can be a partial or a fully dislocated hip.

Spinal Influences

The natural curves of the spine are often exaggerated in those who require total support in sitting. This is a key factor for prop sitters who have not yet developed skeletal asymmetries. The preservation of a neutral pelvic position is vital in maintaining an upright trunk and head position when seated. When approaching this type of client, attention to the support of the pelvis is critical to help orient the upper trunk and head into the desired position. As these individuals lack the intrinsic motor function for trunk alignment, external support is needed to maintain an upright pelvic posture. The thoracic spine requires support to maintain full elongation leading to an upright head position. Prop sitters who present without skeletal asymmetries can be supported in an upright position against gravity, especially when the orientation of the seat and backrest are carefully chosen to promote a balanced upright sitting posture.

Prop sitters who have developed skeletal asymmetries can present with multiple curves in a scoliotic pattern (Figure 5-2). The initial C-curve that can be heavily

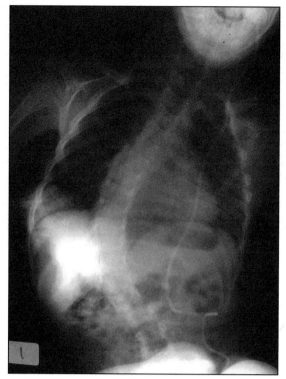

Figure 5-2. Scoliotic spine on x-ray.

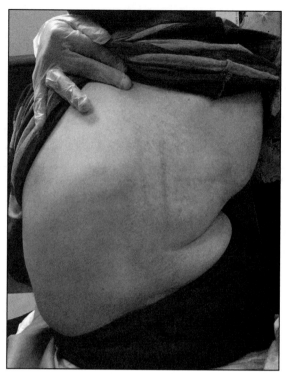

Figure 5-3. Scoliosis with rib cage rotation.

influenced by a pelvic obliquity is further complicated by natural righting reactions to help hold one's head over the shoulders. In addition to lateral curves, anterior and posterior curves can influence trunk patterns, adding to the overall asymmetry of the person's seated posture. Thoracic kyphosis and lumbar lordosis can be observed independent of lateral curves as well as with them. An oblique and rotated pelvic posture with scoliosis of the spine may present with exaggerated lumbar lordosis on the side of the anterior pelvic rotation, migrating into thoracic kyphosis on the posteriorly rotated side. Although scoliosis is thought to be a single plane disorientation, it is often heavily influenced by a rotational component. This changes the intimate placement of the vertebrae resulting in greater curvature and rib cage misalignment (Figure 5-3).

Head Control

The assumption and maintenance of an upright head position is a typical goal for dependent sitters. During the evaluation, it must be noted that if a client lacks active head control out of the seating system, he will be unable to maintain his head position when upright and against gravity in a seating system. Head alignment is dictated by the orientation of the cervical spine.

Prop sitters without asymmetries have more flexibility to maintain an upright head position if given external, proximal support that maintains alignment. If, as noted with pelvic and spinal asymmetries, there is misalignment

of the proximal structures in the neck required for an upright head posture, the head has no other option but to follow the curve of the neck or spine below. In an upright position, gravity will exaggerate a lack of active head control and result in greater asymmetry. Caregivers may tend to focus on head positioning without realizing the many related factors, involving the neck, trunk, and pelvis below.

Head position must be discussed in detail during the mat evaluation, demonstrating the client's abilities up front. As a rule, prop sitters do not show improvement in motor control as the result of using a supportive seating system. A seating system should not be used as a therapeutic tool for this purpose but should be designed to provide necessary support for the person to assume and maintain an agreed-on position. The person should not be expected to work on holding his or her head or trunk up while sitting in the system. Additionally, the client's preferred head position may result in asymmetrical alignment of his trunk and pelvis. In this case, all should agree that asymmetries will be accommodated to support the person's choice of head position.

Accommodation Versus Correction

The question of accommodation vs correction of skeletal and postural asymmetries should be addressed early in the evaluation process. Prop sitters without skeletal asymmetries or those who are flexible to midline correction should be provided with seating components that will protect and maintain their alignment. Prop sitters who are flexible but not fully reducible to symmetrical posture may benefit

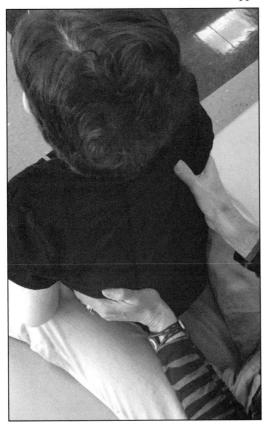

Figure 5-4. Use of therapist's dynamic hands at key points of control.

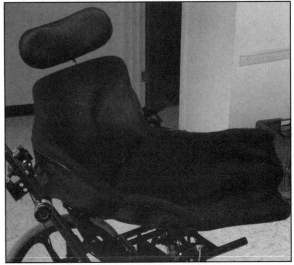

Figure 5-5. Seating system providing optimal support for a client's personal posture, being respectful of skeletal and postural needs, as well as orientation in space.

from a seating system incorporating a mixed approach of accommodation and correction. Although some correction may be available, one has to ask how it will affect the person's comfort and ability to function. Even if asymmetry can be minimized, can the position be maintained for sitting? Simulation is a great way to begin addressing this question. Using your hands and body as the simulation tool along with a mirror and client feedback will provide vital information about how much correction can be tolerated, as well as when to back off correction to achieve function and comfort.

The evaluator can use his or her body to simulate the external support necessary to find a position of balance that works for the client. Through graded movements from the therapist, posture can be altered and evaluated to determine what type of contact and support might be needed. Key points of support can be identified as well as the need for total contact (Figure 5-4). The distribution of pressure should be considered at this time, especially when determining what type of control will be most beneficial. The aim is to find a balanced, functional position for *this* client while keeping in mind the prioritized goals. For example, if an appropriate visual field is a priority, upright head orientation is needed. If a visual impairment is present, the gauge should be a comfortable head position without regard to

traditional pelvic or trunk position. When the client indicates the head is in a functional position that is this client's personal posture. For many nonverbal individuals, finding the personal posture during this hands-on simulation period can be determined when the client relaxes into your hands. You may note a significant change in tone as the person's arms and hands relax from a high guard position.

When trying to identify the balanced position, certain assumptions are often made. One frequent assumption is that the client's posture must be a traditional, symmetrical sitting posture. *Traditional seated posture* refers to positioning the head over the shoulders over the pelvis, all in alignment and held upright against gravity. In the past, the clinical goal for a seating system was to preserve alignment. The trend has swung away from focusing strictly on alignment. All too often, using this approach was not effective, and seating was abandoned by the client. Clients abandoned the supports forcing them to sit in perfect alignment, due to discomfort and, in many cases, a loss in function or sitting tolerance. Seating clinic practices have evolved and now focus on the facilitation of function. Optimal posture for a client includes accommodation of skeletal asymmetries, a balance of muscle tone (inhibiting hypertonicity, activating hypotonicity, or balancing fluctuating tone), and stable positioning of the head and extremities. In other words, respecting asymmetries is an important step in the identification of a person's personal posture (Figure 5-5).

Another assumption is the need for intentional support of all body parts. Focus should be not only on the primary seating surfaces (seat and backrest) but also how the extremities, including the head, will be supported.

After using your body as a tool to provide external support during the mat assessment, the use of a simulator is

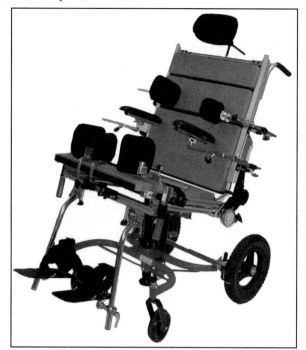

Figure 5-6. Planar simulator: effective evaluation tool to help determine angles and orientations.

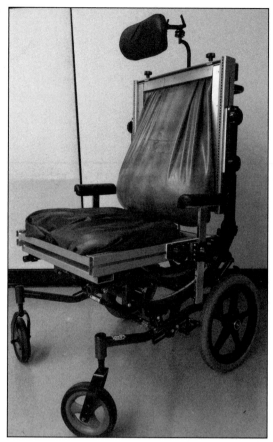

Figure 5-7. Shape simulator: effective evaluation tool to determine necessary shapes and contours of seating components as well as angles and orientations.

often the next step in the assessment process. There are two types of simulators used in seating clinics: planar simulators and molding simulators.

Planar simulators (Figure 5-6) provide planar support and offer adjustability for orientation in space, angles of support surfaces and the dimensions of these surfaces. On a planar simulator the support surfaces remain flat with no contour other than the addition of seat cushions that may have contoured surfaces as part of the cushion design. Prop sitters without skeletal asymmetries can benefit from planar simulation; it is a great tool for identifying key points of contact and the necessary angles of orientation in space to achieve the desired posture, leading to more accurate recommendation of seating components. Planar simulators also offer ancillary support surfaces for trial use including medial and lateral thigh supports and lateral thoracic supports. Because the prop sitter does not have motor control of the intrinsic trunk muscles to activate and hold the trunk in alignment against gravity when seated, simulation of needed support is an effective evaluation tool.

Molding simulators (Figure 5-7) offer similar adjustments for orientation in space and changing angles between support surfaces as a planar simulator; however, the contour and shape of the support surface can be altered to offer varying levels of contact and support. Once a person's shape is captured, the amount of contact and support can be modified during the simulation process, helping to identify where and how much is needed. When the client is transferred out of the simulator, the shape can be examined to gain a better understanding of the postural needs. The shape can be preserved in some simulators, allowing transfer of the individual back into the mold. This provides an opportunity to assess the client's performance of functional tasks while being supported in the simulated seating system.

Key Points of Control Versus Total Contact

When imposed external support is provided to improve a client's seated posture, a decision must be made regarding how much is needed. Total contact or key points of control can be provided. Throughout the evaluation process, care should be taken to ensure pressure redistribution is done effectively, eliminating potential for skin breakdown over bony prominences. Total contact seating systems can

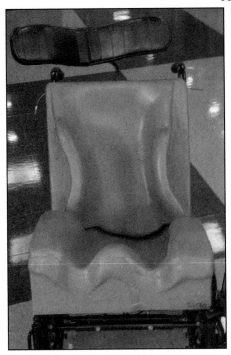

Figure 5-8. Custom-molded seating system, without covers, can offer total contact for postural support and alignment.

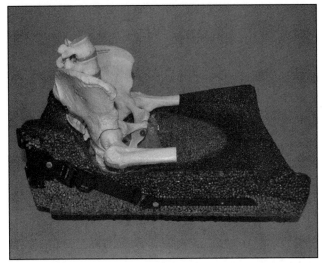

Figure 5-9. Custom-molded seat cushion that offers off-loading for ischial tuberosities while loading safe areas of the body (femurs, buttocks behind ischial tuberosities).

provide optimal pressure management; greater contact area within the system results in more surface area across which the pressure can be redistributed (Figure 5-8). Use of a total contact seating system assumes that the client's body will remain relatively calm and accurately seated in the desired alignment. During the mat evaluation and simulation, the therapist's hands can help determine where and how much support is needed. With all imposed external support, contact is needed proximal and distal to each joint requiring stabilization. For example, to stabilize a desired hip angle, contact is needed at three locations:

1. The seating surface beneath the pelvis and upper leg
2. A back cushion supporting the posterior pelvis across the pelvic crest and low back
3. A strap at the anterior pelvis helping prevent forward displacement of the pelvis

Eliminating any one of these three locations will compromise the chances of success in seated positioning. This type of decision-making process will also address whether the seating system should be symmetrical or asymmetrical. As mentioned previously, clients with skeletal asymmetries are rarely symmetrical; therefore, symmetry should not be expected in the final supports.

Use of contact at key points of control in seating systems can lead to increased pressure at those areas. Only safe parts of the body can be loaded. For example, the long bones of the upper legs are loaded, as a planned key point of contact, to unload the ischial tuberosities (Figure 5-9).

In this example, shifting weight from a prominent ischial tuberosity to the midfemur can help protect that ischial tuberosity from excessive weightbearing while loading an area that can tolerate the increased pressure. The posture is supported by more anterior contact on the long bones of the upper leg to help maintain the seated position. Key points of contact may also be used on the trunk or for the head, especially for prop sitters with no postural asymmetry. For example, a client with a cervical level spinal cord injury may just need a tall back support, head support, and lateral thoracic supports to be positioned in and maintain an upright sitting posture for long periods of time. There is no need for total contact if the key points of contact at the trunk and head are appropriate.

Proximal Support for Life-Sustaining Activities

Proximal stability leads to distal mobility in the developmental process, as most clinicians are aware. For example, try putting your socks on while standing; as you lift one foot from the floor, your balance is challenged. Maintaining a standing position becomes very difficult while trying to execute a more controlled fine motor task with your hands. Proximal stability has been disrupted by lifting one foot. If you sit down to complete the task, your trunk and pelvis are much more stable, allowing for the ease of controlled distal mobility in your arms. Development of trunk control is an important milestone for the development of controlled extremity and head movement. The fact that proximal stability is required for basic life-sustaining movements is often overlooked. The rib cage must have a stable surface to facilitate respiratory function. The client who requires total support for sitting lacks postural

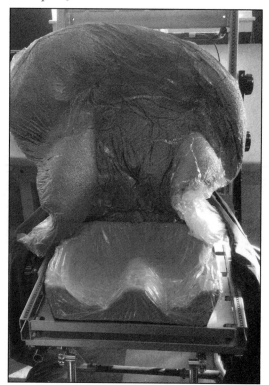

Figure 5-10. Simulated shapes for new custom-molded seating components.

control, a key component of proximal stability. A prop sitter lacks motor control of the intrinsic trunk muscles that activate and hold the trunk in alignment against the force of gravity when placed in a seated position. These are the same muscle groups that undergird the respiratory process. When stability is not present for trunk control, respiration will be affected. Providing total support offers stability for the rib cage, allowing the respiratory muscles to function more effectively. The same is true for the gastrointestinal system, because those organs also depend on the role of the postural support muscles. Therefore, imposed external support from a seating system can improve respiration and gastrointestinal function.

Extremes of Muscle Tone

Tonal asymmetries can be addressed through imposed external support. Individuals with hypertonicity and preferred patterns of extension can be positioned in a more flexed sitting posture and supported through a total contact seating system. If range of movement is available, increasing hip flexion and abduction can be effective in controlling the client's tendency to adduct and extend at the hips; this eliminates a common trigger for the extensor pattern. Total posterior contact is needed across the pelvis to help block it from tilting more posteriorly. Once the pelvic posture is secure, total contact supports can be lessened more distally according to what the client needs.

Prop sitters with extreme hypotonicity of the trunk and head can benefit from the use of fairly rigid (not soft) support surfaces with total contact. This offers increased sensory feedback regarding the location of the client's body in space, which has been found to be helpful in maintaining a more symmetrically aligned seated position. The use of softer surfaces (thick foam or air-based cushioning products) tends to increase the dynamic nature of the support surfaces, giving the hypotonic prop sitter less stability.

Solutions

Shape Capture

Successful simulation of the client requiring total support when seated is not only an evaluation tool but a means to create the contoured surfaces for the definitive supports. Once all goals have been prioritized and determination of the necessary angles and orientation in space is completed, the location of the support surfaces must be determined.

Use of a planar simulator for prop sitters will aid in determining angles and orientation of support surfaces, ensuring that optimal configuration is planned in the products recommended. A planar simulator can also be beneficial when ascertaining the location and orientation of ancillary seating supports. Care must be taken to provide support only where necessary with regard to pressure redistribution as well as the agreed-on position of alignment.

Use of a molding frame offers the opportunity to capture and change, as needed, the shapes and contours for the seating system. Intimate contact between the client and the molding surface is the key to success. Molding should initiate with stabilizing the pelvis and then proceed more distally. Nontraditional orientations can be accomplished for clients who present with severe asymmetries. With most simulators, the client can spend additional time in the captured shape to ensure that optimal support has been created (Figure 5-10). Functional tasks can be performed to ensure that the placement of support does not interfere with the client's ability to participate in necessary activities. After the client spends time in the simulator, skin checks should be done to evaluate the effectiveness of pressure redistribution. If function is limited or redness occurs, resimulation should be done to alleviate the problem. Capturing a person's shape can take some time; however, the long term benefit is well worth the time investment. More than one attempt at simulation may be necessary, with the amount of time spent as well as the number of attempts dependent on many factors. These factors can include the team's familiarity with the individual's physical presentation, including tone patterns and unexpected needs (time of day, bowel and bladder habits and timing, seizure activity). They may also include drastic changes in a person's presentation since the evaluation, and the process can be lengthened by inaccurate awareness of predetermined goals. For instance, a caregiver may express concern that the individual's head is not upright even though head position was thoroughly discussed during the evaluation process. The plan and execution of the shape capture must be carefully choreographed with all participants understanding their roles, as well as the anticipated result. All team members must be in agreement on the final shape; if not, starting over or rescheduling might be the best option.

The final contour and set up of a seating system need not be symmetrical; instead, many dependent sitters present with asymmetry and matching support must be provided (Figure 5-11). Care must be taken to ensure that all support surfaces play a role in positioning. If the surface is not serving a purpose, it should be eliminated. For example, if a client has had spinal fusion and has no potential to drift to his or her right, the right side molded lateral thoracic support can be minimized because it will not serve a function. This is true for custom-molded seating as well as premade seating with components (a back support with additional lateral thoracic supports). Although caregivers and clients might prefer a symmetrical look, they can be educated throughout the process as to why asymmetry is needed to achieve agreed-on goals regarding sitting comfort, decreased skin irritation related to uneven pressure distribution, or increased sitting tolerance.

Angles and Orientation

As noted earlier, the angles and orientations of support surfaces for prop sitters must be considered throughout the evaluation process. These can be identified in more specific terms through the mat evaluation and use of simulation. For instance, as noted previously, if a seat to back angle greater than 90 degrees is required due to limited hip flexion, this need must be identified before the selection of equipment.

When considering angles, the following must be discussed:

- Seat to back support angle—related to hip ROM into flexion (thigh to trunk angle), left and right sides

- Seat to lower leg support angle—related to the knee ROM (popliteal angle, thigh to calf angle)

- Lower leg support to foot support angle—related to the ankle, including dorsiflexion and plantarflexion range of movement (calf to foot angle)

Seat to back support angles must support and accommodate hip and pelvis angles. The assumption should be made that nontraditional angles might be necessary for prop sitters with nonsymmetrical postures. Seat to back angles should directly correlate to hip and pelvis angles. Thigh to lower leg angles correspond to seat to foot support orientation; hamstring tightness will dictate foot placement. Lower leg to foot angle dictates the orientation of

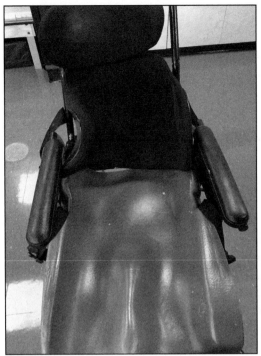

Figure 5-11. Examples of custom-molded seating. Note the asymmetry built into the system designed specifically for one person's needs.

the footplate to the leg support assembly (see Chapter 6 for more specific information regarding measurements of body and supports).

Angles and orientation of selected ancillary support surfaces must be determined so that positioning goals will be met. For prop sitters with no skeletal asymmetries, orientation of lateral thoracic or lateral thigh support might be symmetrical and used as a guide for positioning and maintaining a well-aligned seated orientation.

Prop sitters with skeletal asymmetries require ancillary supports to be asymmetrically integrated, ensuring proper contact and direction of support. If a lateral thoracic support is necessary to prevent further lateral trunk collapse, use of a flat pad pushing toward the body will be ineffective. A curved pad applying force toward the direction of correction is needed instead. The head support may require mounting more laterally than midline to offer better support for an individual with scoliosis. A medial thigh support can be mounted in a midline position for a prop sitter without asymmetries. If any type of pelvic rotation or obliquity is present, however, medial thigh support hardware may need to be mounted away from the seat center to accommodate the person's asymmetry.

Orientation in Space

Orientations in space must be considered throughout the evaluation process (Rehabilitation Engineering & Assistive Technology Society of North America, 2015).

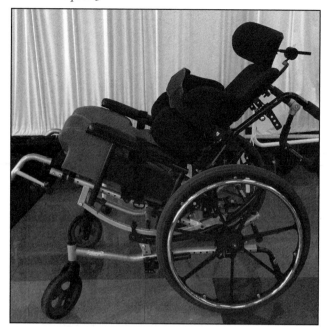

Figure 5-12. Use of posterior tilt in a mobility base offers postural assistance for upper trunk and head positioning.

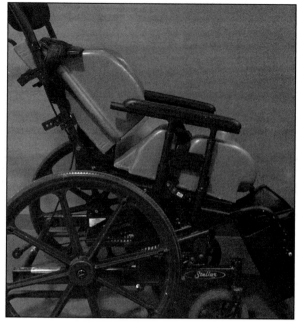

Figure 5-13. Use of anterior tilt in a mobility base can help provide an appropriate head position for functional tasks when hip flexion limitations are present.

These features offer stability of the desired seat to back angle while allowing rotation in space of the entire seating system. Three different options can be considered: posterior, anterior, and lateral. All tilt options can be provided in manual or power combinations.

Posterior tilt (Figure 5-12) is the most commonly used option. Traditional use of a tilt-in-space chair set up in a posterior position offers gravity-assisted posture for improved upper trunk and head control/positioning. A client with some head control skills may experience greater success with a bit of gravity assistance through the use of posterior tilt rather than sitting in a fully upright position.

Anterior tilt (Figure 5-13) of the chair frame is beneficial in assisting with head control for periods of focus. The anterior orientation can be used for short periods of time when attending to a specific task, whether it is work, school, or eating related. Combining use of posterior and anterior tilt can effectively optimize alignment and function by offering alternative positions for rest and more active head positioning.

A less frequently used orientation option on a wheelchair base is *lateral tilt* (Figure 5-14). Lateral tilt can be successful for a client whose trunk is collapsing with his head following. When it is engaged, lateral tilt shifts the person in the seating system to bear weight more on the left (or alternatively the right) side of his trunk. Options may include a single tilt to either the right or left, accommodating a scoliotic trunk and head position, or the tilt can move to both sides to provide pressure redistribution and comfort. Lateral tilt can assist in maintaining an upright and properly oriented head position in a person with a multicurve scoliosis and pelvic obliquity that requires accommodation.

Laterally tilting bases are becoming more popular and should not be overlooked.

Types of Seating for Prop Sitters

Many types of seating products are available for clients who rely on extensive, externally imposed support for the maintenance of an upright posture. These options include varying levels of custom seating, such as clientized seating, customized seating, custom-made seating, and custom-molded seating. In the last category, there are two different approaches: direct molding and indirect molding.

Clientized seating includes use of off-the-shelf seating products that offer key points of control. Through the use of ready-made seating and ancillary supports that are integrated into a clientized seating system, prop sitters with or without skeletal asymmetries can be given the support they require. Often times ready-made supports, when appropriately combined and assembled, provide the support system within which a person's body can be seated.

Customized seating refers to modification or adaptation of ready-made seating, such as altering leg length or accommodating a pelvic obliquity. This seating is premade with set dimensions, materials, and coverings. Modifications can often be made in the field; frequently this occurs at the time of delivery. However, there are limitations in terms of how many changes can be made. For example, if very significant changes are made in the cushion shape itself, the fit of its cover may be compromised.

Custom-made seating is fabricated per specific dimensions and specifications, as determined during the mat evaluation. In addition to the unique client measurements,

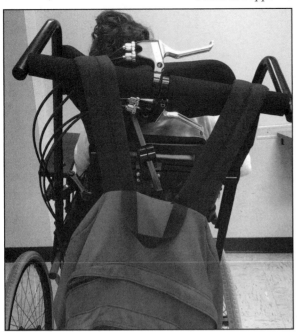

Figure 5-14. Use of lateral tilt to help reorient upper trunk and head alignment.

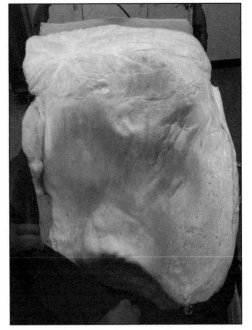

Figure 5-15. Foam in place customization in a back support (without cover).

specific types of support materials (foam, air, gel), surface coverings and shapes can be specified to meet the postural needs and seating goals. Shape of the support surfaces can be dictated through the evaluation findings and accomplished through use of specific materials that will accommodate asymmetry. Custom-made seating systems are usually ordered from a specific seating support manufacturer or, in some cases, a facility-specific shop with the supplies and fabricators to build custom seating systems.

Custom-molded seating offers two options, direct and indirect molded seating. With the direct molding technique, the actual cushion is created around the individual, using her body to create the shape. This type of direct molding is commonly referred to as *foam in place* (Figure 5-15). Direct molding offers an advantage in that the actual support surfaces are completed with the pouring of the foam. Modifications can be made to the components; however, if the desired position is not achieved, the process must be done again; and this will add additional cost to the finished product. When using the direct molding approach, the plan to ensure the fabrication of surface coverings is an additional consideration. Some kits include a cover, but the final shape will dictate the specific cover needed.

Indirect molding requires use of some type of simulation and shape capture. This can be done using a variety of simulators, usually specific to the manufacturer of the finished system. The shape can also be captured directly against the client's body. Once the shape is captured and saved through some means (e.g., electronic digitizing, plaster casting), the data are sent to the manufacturer for production. The shape that is sent to the manufacturer is used to create a mold of the client's sitting position. The mold is then used throughout the manufacturing process to relay the individual's shape for the creation of the definitive seating support. There is a delay in obtaining the final product when indirect molding is used. Time must be allowed for the cast or data to be sent to the manufacturer, the cushions to be fabricated and then delivered to the client. Custom-molded seating requires skill and a cohesive team with clearly defined goals. If focus is lacking during the shape capturing process, the client may be deprived of the expected benefits in the final product. Some indirect molded seating options allow for modifications at the time of fitting. If modifications might be necessary, an interim or initial fitting before the final covering may be an essential step in the delivery process.

Orthotic-based seating (body splints) and one piece, total contact seating systems offer minimal adjustability. Two-piece systems can allow seat to back angle changes as well as seat depth and back height adjustability, depending on their installation. Most manufacturers offer remake policies to ensure that the system will be successful. Custom-molded seating is often used as the last resort; however, some professionals believe this approach should be explored earlier in the seating process for certain individuals in an attempt to minimize the impact of worsening asymmetrical postural tendencies over time.

SUMMARY

The evaluation and provision of seating and wheeled mobility components for individuals who require imposed external support (prop sitters) is similar for clients needing other levels of support. Prop sitters fall into two distinct groups: those who lack control of their bodies who do not have skeletal asymmetries, and those who lack control but also have skeletal asymmetries. The need for varying levels of support is driven by presentation, not by specific diagnostic groups. Current trends have recently shown benefits from the use of custom seating for those with minimal to moderate skeletal asymmetries. Evaluation of the asymmetries is needed to determine whether these are fixed/non-reducible or reducible. If reducible, the evaluation determines how that is accomplished and maintained. Once determined, the focus of the evaluation moves to the generation of recommendations. Use of simulation is useful at this point to help determine the type and location of needed support. Given this information, options might include ready-made, custom-made, or custom-molded options. Other factors include angles and orientation of the seating components. Ultimately, consideration of the individual's personal posture and its impact on function needs to be addressed through the shape, contour, and the amount of contact from the support surfaces, the angles of support, and orientation in space. Prop sitters offer an added challenge to the seating and mobility evaluation process because each individual is unique.

REFERENCES

Arledge, S., Armstrong, W., Babinec, M., Dicianno, B. E., Digiovine, C., Dyson-Hudson, T.,...& Schmeler, M. (2011). *RESNA wheelchair service provision guide.* Arlington, VA: Rehabilitation Engineering & Assistive Technology Society of North America. Retrieved from https://www.resna.org/sites/default/files/legacy/resources/position-papers/RESNAWheelchairServiceProvisionGuide.pdf

Hetzel, T. (2015a). *Destructive postural tendencies: Identification and treatment.* Retrieved from http://www.ridedesigns.com/resource/destructive-postural-tendencies-identification-and-treatment

Hetzel, T. (2015b). *Understanding and caring for the posterior and anterior pelvic tilt.* Retrieved http://www.ridedesigns.com/resource/understanding-and-caring-posterior-and-anterior-pelvic-tilt

Rehabilitation Engineering & Assistive Technology Society of North America. (2015). *RESNA Position on the Application of Tilt, Recline, and Elevating Legrests for Wheelchairs.* Arlington, VA: Author.

Sutherland, S. (2015). The hands dependent sitter. *Seating Solutions LLC.* Retrieved from http://www.seatingsolutionsllc.com.

BIBLIOGRAPHY

Cook, A., & Polgar, J. (2008). *Cook and Hussey's assistive technologies: Principles and practice* (3rd ed.). St. Louis, MO: Mosby Elsevier.

Cook, A., & Polgar, J. (2012). *Essentials of assistive technologies.* St. Louis, MO: Elsevier.

Hetzel, T. (2016). Custom Sooner = More meaningful and lasting outcomes. Retrieved from http://www.ridedesigns.com/resource/custom-sooner-more-meaningful-and-lasting-outcome

6

Standardized Measures of the Person, Seating System, and Wheelchair

Kelly Waugh, PT, MAPT, ATP and Barbara A. Crane, PT, PhD, ATP/SMS

A NEED FOR STANDARDIZED TERMINOLOGY AND MEASUREMENT

The field of wheeled mobility and seating has undergone a revolution over the past 20 years or more. The industry has been heavily influenced by the development of new technologies and product performance standards, as well as funding opportunities and constraints. Increased research into the science of wheelchair seating is creating a body of knowledge that, in turn, supports an emerging specialty area of practice for clinicians and suppliers of complex rehabilitation technology. Additionally, individuals with disabilities are living longer than ever enjoying more active and productive lives. Objective measurement and consistent use of terminology related to the wheelchair occupant's body, the seating system and the wheelchair have become much more important as this evolution has occurred. Accurate measurement of the person's body and seated posture is critical to ensuring appropriate fit and function of the seating system. Being able to measure the posture of a wheelchair-seated person in a standardized manner is also critical to documenting outcomes related to wheelchair seating intervention. Consistent use of terminology regarding measures of the person, the seating system and the wheelchair promotes accuracy in prescription and communication of key features among team members, maximizing efficiency in service delivery and effectiveness in outcomes.

To this end, the International Organization of Standardization (ISO) and the Rehabilitation Engineering and Assistive Technology Society of North America

(RESNA) partnered to develop a set of standardized terms and measures related to wheelchair seating. The result of this decade-long effort was the international standard titled *ISO 16840-1: Wheelchair Seating, Part 1—Vocabulary, reference axis convention and measures for body posture and postural support surfaces* (ISO, 2006). In the United States, RESNA Assistive Technology Standards Board adopted the ISO standard and published the U.S. version, titled *RESNA WC-3:2013, Section 1: Wheelchair Seating—Vocabulary, reference axis convention and measures for body posture and postural support surfaces* (RESNA, 2013).

Although both the ISO and RESNA standards are available for purchase, they are difficult to understand and not very "clinician-friendly." To address this, a group of expert clinicians with funding support from the Paralyzed Veterans of America developed two resource manuals to assist in the implementation of these standards into clinical practice. The first of these, *A Clinical Application Guide to Standardized Wheelchair Seating Measures of the Body and Seating Support Surfaces, Revised Edition*, contains a simplified but detailed explanation of the foundational concepts presented in the standard as well as the correct term and definition for 130 angular and linear measurements of the seated person's body and the seating support system (Waugh & Crane, 2013a). For each term, the guide explains the purpose of the measure and its clinical relevance, a sample measurement procedure, and one or two illustrations to clarify each measure. Soon after, a companion resource titled *Glossary of Wheelchair Terms and Definitions, Version 1.0* was published by the same lead authors (Waugh & Crane, 2013b). This glossary includes a searchable list of more than 550 defined terms related to

Lange, M. L., & Minkel, J. L.
Seating and Wheeled Mobility: A Clinical Resource Guide
(pp. 85-119). © 2018 SLACK Incorporated.

wheelchairs, wheelchair seating, and wheelchair seated posture. Most of the terms come from a published international or national standard. For common terms for which there is no adopted standard, the authors propose a term and definition based on an extensive review of sources.

We mention these two resources because this chapter is based on their content, yet they contain a breadth of information and detail that is beyond the scope of this book. Therefore, we encourage complex rehabilitation technology (CRT) professionals to seek out and use these resources to support the goal of universal adoption and implementation of the terminology and measures described therein. Throughout the rest of this chapter, we refer to these two resources as the *Clinical Application Guide* (Waugh & Crane, 2013a) and the *Glossary of Terms* (Waugh & Crane, 2013b) for brevity.

Types of Measurements

Body, Seating System, and Wheelchair Measures

With the ongoing development of wheelchair technologies as well as seating system components designed to interface with both the client and the wheelchair, it is critical to use terms and measures that both differentiate and relate the three parts of the wheelchair system to each other: the person, seating support system, and wheelchair. The *person* refers to the occupant of the wheelchair. The *seating support system,* or *seating system,* refers to those parts of the wheelchair system that are intended to contact the person's body, such as the seat, back support, head support, arm support, lower leg support, and/or foot support (Waugh & Crane, 2013b). The *wheelchair* refers to the wheeled mobility base or wheelchair frame, excluding the seating support system.

The wheelchair occupant's body interacts directly with the seating system through surface contact; however, there is also significant interaction between the client and the wheelchair (e.g., handrims for propulsion). Additionally, any seating system components added to the wheelchair must interface properly with both the client and the wheelchair frame, making all three sets of measures (body, seating system, and wheelchair) critical in putting it all together. Wheelchair seating is a unique field in the use of many seating system products that are not produced by the wheelchair manufacturer (i.e., not original equipment manufacturer) but rather are added to the wheelchair by the CRT supplier. These components are specifically intended to meet postural support or pressure management goals for the client, but their ultimate success is heavily dependent on the fit of the entire system. After all, what good is optimizing posture for propulsion efficiency if in the process the client cannot access the handrim of the wheelchair or

get his or her feet on the floor if he or she is relying on foot propulsion?

It is critically important to differentiate terms for similar measures that relate to the body vs seating vs wheelchair because, although related, they are not the same. For example, we measure the person's buttock/thigh depth to determine the appropriate desired seat depth of the seat cushion. However, these dimensions are not the same, and there may be reasons to specify a seat depth that is significantly shorter than a person's buttock/thigh depth (e.g., to allow foot propulsion). Similarly, the depth of a seat cushion is not necessarily the same as the depth of the wheelchair frame and we need differentiating terms for these two related, but different, dimensions. Being clear in the use of terms for different measurements supports efficient and accurate communication of key parameters of the wheelchair system, leading to positive outcomes for the consumer.

Linear and Angular Measures

There are two main types of measurements: linear and angular. Linear and angular measurements need to be documented for each of the three components of the wheelchair system: the person, seating system, and wheelchair frame. Terms for these measurements must be different to differentiate the three sets of measurements, but they must follow the same measurement conventions so that they can be correlated for proper prescription and setup.

Linear measures of the seated person's body are used to specify the desired linear dimensions of the seating support system. Collectively, these linear measures help to determine the size, selection and setup of seating and wheelchair frame components. For example, the person's shoulder height will help determine the size and placement of the back support as well as the style and length of the wheelchair back posts necessary for attachment of the back support at the proper height. Linear measures of the body include such things as shoulder height and hip width. Linear measures of the seating system include such things as back support length and seat width. Linear measures of the wheelchair frame include such things as seat frame depth and width, and rear and front seat frame height.

Angular measures of the seated person's body provide an objective, standardized way of describing the client's wheelchair seated posture. These angular measures are called *body segment angles.* Corresponding angular measures of the seating support system define the orientation of seating support surfaces and are called *support surface angles.* The angular orientation of the support surfaces in a seating system is a key feature that helps to support the person's body in the desired posture. Identifying the desired seating support surface angles will help to determine the selection and setup of wheelchair frame components necessary to achieve the desired body position and posture.

Describing and Measuring Wheelchair-Seated Posture

Joint Range of Motion Versus Body Segment Angles

Traditionally, practitioners in the field of wheelchair seating have used joint range of motion (ROM) terminology to describe a person's wheelchair seated posture. For example, a therapist may say that a person is sitting in 80 degrees of hip flexion with the right hip abducted and extended, left hip adducted, trunk leaning to the left. This method of describing wheelchair-seated posture using terms for joint motion is not adequate for our field, for the following reasons:

- Joint ROM terms are frequently used inaccurately.
- Joint ROM terms do not provide a measure of orientation in space.
- Joint ROM terms do not help with the prescription of corresponding seating support surface angles.

The new, standardized angular body measures provide an alternate way to describe and quantify seated posture that is more accurate and relevant for our field, addressing the three preceding inadequacies. First, the new terms for body segment angles accurately describe the static position of body segments, avoiding the common errors that occur when using joint ROM terminology to describe seated posture. Saying that a person sits with his or her right hip abducted is only accurate if you have taken into consideration the alignment of the pelvis in addition to the thigh, because hip abduction is a measure of the femur relative to the pelvis. If you are using this term to describe a position of outward rotation of the thigh on the seat, it is not accurate if the pelvis is also rotated. The standard provides a term that accurately specifies the angular position of the thigh relative to the seat, which is relevant for seating. Second, in the new set of measures, the same conventions are used to measure the body and the seating support surfaces; this helps to translate the desired sitting position into prescriptive angles of the seating system. Third, the new measures provide a way to quantify orientation in space, which joint ROM measurements cannot do. The new terms do not replace joint ROM terminology but rather augment them in a manner that is useful for our field. Clinicians need to understand the relationship between joint ROM measurements and seated body segment angles to translate mat examination findings into a desired sitting position and posture.

Why Measure Seated Posture?

Taking linear measurements of the person's body to prescribe an appropriately fitting wheelchair and seating system is basic standard practice. Measuring body segment angles to objectively describe the seated position and posture of the wheelchair occupant is a no less important, but not yet common, practice. As clinicians and researchers gain knowledge and expertise in this growing specialty area of practice, the importance of objectively quantifying posture for clients who use wheelchairs has moved to the forefront.

Therefore, we discuss the five main reasons for measuring and documenting wheelchair seated posture:

1. To identify postural problems and set postural alignment objectives
2. To help determine product feature requirements
3. To document postural outcomes before and after seating intervention
4. To measure postural change over time
5. To facilitate research

To Identify Postural Problems and Set Postural Alignment Objectives

Objectively measuring posture (rather than subjectively describing posture) has become critical to the practice of complex wheelchair seating, because it allows clinicians to quantify the problems experienced by the client. Taking measurements of the person's existing position and posture in his or her wheelchair during assessment prompts you to notice specific aspects of the person's alignment that may need addressing. Identifying a set of specific postural measures that reflect the person's primary postural problems allows you to quantify the problem and set measurable postural objectives. For example, there is a new body angle measurement called the *frontal sternal angle* that quantifies the degree that a person's upper trunk is leaning to the left or right. Measuring this deviation quantifies a postural problem. An objective can then be set to reduce this angle to a very specific degree based on assessment findings and simulation.

To Help Determine Product Feature Requirements

In addition to quantifying problems and allowing appropriate goal setting, objective measures help a clinician and supplier work together to identify appropriate technology dimensions and features. For example, if you have a client with a fixed pelvic obliquity, you can assess the magnitude of the obliquity by measuring the *frontal pelvic angle*. Knowing the magnitude of the obliquity informs the choice of seat surface shape, seat materials, and seat thickness needed under the pelvis to accommodate the asymmetry. This in turn helps with product selection. As another example, measuring the angle between the client's thigh and trunk when he or she is seated in the desired position (called the *thigh to trunk angle*), helps determine the

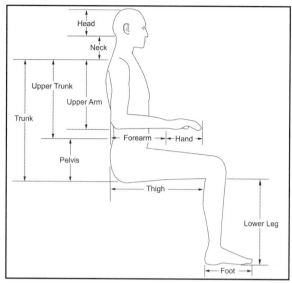

Figure 6-1. Body segmentation scheme.

corresponding *seat to back support angle* and wheelchair frame features required to support this sitting position.

To Document Postural Outcomes Before and After Seating Intervention

Clinicians are increasingly required to objectively demonstrate outcomes related to interventions. One of the primary outcomes associated with wheelchair seating and positioning is the impact on posture and ultimately on function. Measuring your client's existing seated posture at the time of assessment establishes a baseline so you can show change after a seating intervention. If you have set specific measurable objectives related to the person's postural alignment, these can be remeasured at a fitting or delivery of new seating equipment to document outcomes. Without this critical step, outcomes cannot be demonstrated or optimized, and high-quality clinical practice cannot be achieved.

To Measure Postural Change Over Time

In addition to measuring the initial outcomes of specific seating interventions, objective measurement of posture can help monitor postural changes that may occur over a longer period of time. Many clients who use wheelchairs use them for long durations or for their lifetimes. This is particularly true of clients with postural support needs, such as clients with spinal cord injury, cerebral palsy, muscular dystrophy, or progressive conditions, such as multiple sclerosis or amyotrophic lateral sclerosis. Over time, the effects of gravity on the body in a sitting position, combined with changes from skeletal growth, abnormalities in muscle tone, or orthopedic complications can produce profound changes in a person's seated posture. Being able to track this change can inform goal setting and affect a clinician's choices with respect to seating strategies, product selection, and other treatment options.

To Facilitate Research

Finally, objective quantification of posture has a multitude of research applications. Research in the field of wheelchair seating is expanding with a significant focus on outcomes related to technology interventions. However, one of the areas least studied is the impact of seated posture on the health, comfort, and function of clients who use wheelchairs. Posture is not just an aesthetic property, but affects many other body structures and functions (e.g., digestion, respiration, swallowing), as well as functional interactions of a client with his or her environment (e.g., reaching) or his or her wheeled mobility device (e.g., effects of posture on propulsion). To investigate the relationship between posture and health or function, researchers need to be able to measure seated posture in a manner that is accurate and repeatable. Standardizing the measurements used to quantify seated posture is a necessary first step. Uniformity in both measurements and terminology also fosters the ability to compare postural outcomes related to the application of different features or products. Application of research to practice hinges on the ability of clinicians to understand and apply laboratory or real-world research. Researchers, clinicians, and product manufacturers using uniform terminology and a standardized measurement system will foster the development of effective products and the appropriate application of the products in clinical practice settings.

TERMINOLOGY CONVENTIONS

Consistent use of specific terms for measurements of the body, the seating system, and the wheelchair is vital to accurate translation of body measurements into seating system and wheelchair prescription, as well as accurate setup of the equipment in preparation for delivery. To facilitate this translation, a consistent methodology of naming (or labeling) segments of the body and parts of the seating system was developed through the development of national and internationals standards (RESNA, 2009b). These same names for body segments and seating supports are then used in the terms for linear and angular measurements. This helps to both differentiate and correlate like measures of the body, seating, and wheelchair. In what follows, we provide a brief summary of these labeling conventions, which are explained in greater detail in Chapter 1 of the previously mentioned *Clinical Application Guide* (Waugh & Crane, 2013a).

Labeling Terminology for the Body

The body is divided into segments, and a consistent term is assigned to each segment (Figure 6-1). This term is then used in naming all measures related to that body segment, and it is used to label the support surface that is intended to contact that segment of the body, in most cases. For example, the upper part of the leg is called the *thigh*, and the part of the body above the pelvis is labelled the *trunk* segment. The angle between these two segments is therefore called the *thigh to trunk angle*. The segment below the knee is designated the lower leg, and the length of this body segment is therefore called the *lower leg length*.

Labeling Terminology for the Seating Support System

Components of a seating system are designed to contact and support specific segments of the body. Therefore, a support surface term is determined on the basis of the body segment it is intended to contact and the side (e.g., medial, lateral) of that body segment where it is placed. For example, a postural support device (PSD) designed to contact the lateral side of the trunk is designated a *lateral trunk support*, and a support placed behind the lower leg is called a *posterior lower leg support* (Waugh & Crane, 2013b).

Labeling Terminology for Wheelchair Components

Although much work has been completed to standardize the terms for labeling the body and seating system components (RESNA, 2009b), similar efforts have not been made to standardize terminology for labeling components of the wheelchair mobility base or frame. Some wheelchair frame measures are incorporated into Section 7 of the ISO 7176 wheelchair standards (ISO, 1998) and the RESNA WC 1 standard (RESNA, 2009a); however, there are many frame components of modern day wheelchairs for which there is no standardized terminology. The *Glossary of Terms* (Waugh & Crane, 2013b) represents a first attempt to develop a comprehensive set of wheelchair terms and definitions and as such is an excellent reference.

LINEAR MEASURES

Linear measures of the person's body in the sitting position are used to determine desired linear size and placement dimensions of seating support surfaces. These are then used to select the appropriately sized wheelchair and ensure that all components are set up or configured for optimum fit and function of the occupant. The *Clinical Application Guide* contains detailed descriptions and sample measurement methodologies for all linear measures and should be referred to for greater detail (Waugh & Crane, 2013a).

General Principles

The following terminology convention for linear measures was developed by ISO and adopted by RESNA, and is illustrated in Figure 6-2. It is based on how a postural

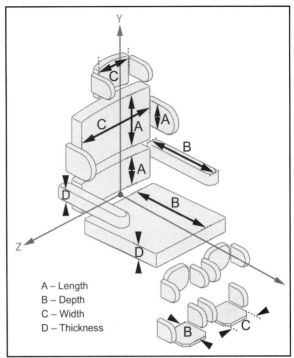

Figure 6-2. Terminology convention for linear measures.

support device is typically oriented in a wheelchair seating system.

- The term for dimensions measured in the up/down direction is either *length* or *height*:
  - *Length* is a dimension of *size*, measured parallel to the support surface or body segment.
  - *Height* is a dimension of *placement*, usually (but not always) measured vertically.
- The term for dimensions measured in the forward/backward direction is *depth*.
- The term for dimensions measured in the side to side direction is *width*.
- The term for dimensions measured perpendicular to the contact surface of a support is *thickness*.

As discussed previously, it is important to differentiate linear measures of the person's body from the linear measures of the seating system and wheelchair; therefore, different terms should be used for each to avoid confusion, while following the preceding conventions. For example, the term *seat depth* is often used to document the length of the person's thigh in sitting, but this same term is also used to describe the depth of the seat cushion, as well as the depth of the wheelchair frame. How do you know which measurement this term is referring to? The three differentiating terms in this example are *buttock/thigh depth* (person), *seat depth* (seating), and *seat frame depth* (wheelchair):

- *Buttock/thigh depth*: The distance from the back of the buttocks all the way to the popliteal fossa, measured in the desired seated position. This measure is used to prescribe the desired seat depth (of the seat cushion) and the wheelchair seat frame depth (Waugh & Crane, 2013a, 2013b).

- *Seat depth*: The distance from the back edge to the front edge of the seat surface intended to contact the person's buttocks and thighs. This is usually shorter than the buttock/thigh depth of the person (Waugh & Crane, 2013a, 2013b).

- *Seat frame depth*: The distance from the front of the back post to the front of the seat rail (Waugh & Crane, 2013b).

Although the terms buttock/thigh depth and seat depth are defined in published ISO and RESNA standards, the corresponding term for the wheelchair frame has not been defined in any standard. *Seat frame depth* is the term proposed in the *Glossary of Terms* (Waugh & Crane, 2013b).

Specific Principles Related to Linear Measures of the Body

There are some important principles and conventions to keep in mind when taking linear body measures. Following these basic principles ensures consistency and repeatability of measurement, as well as relevance to seating and wheelchair prescription.

Linear Measurements Are Taken in the Desired Seated Posture

One of the most important principles to keep in mind is that how the client is sitting affects many of the measurements. For example, shoulder height will be affected by the posture of the pelvis and spine. As the pelvis posteriorly tilts and the spine flexes, shoulder height will decrease. Similarly, as the pelvis posteriorly tilts, buttock/thigh depth increases. Therefore, the client should be supported in a sitting position that simulates the expected or desired resting sitting posture when measuring these body dimensions. This can be done by sitting the person on a firm mat table with feet on the floor or another firm platform under their feet at the appropriate height. If the person cannot sit unsupported or has significant abnormal movement or postural deviations, it may take several sets of hands to support the client in the desired sitting position for measurement. For more accurate measurement in these situations, it is recommended that the person be supported in the desired posture using an adjustable wheelchair or seating simulator.

Measurements of the Body Include Soft Tissue

Linear measures of the person's body in sitting are taken directly on the body surface without compressing the soft tissue and without adding any allowances for planned spacing between the body and seating or frame components.

Measurements Are Straight Linear Dimensions

Linear measures of the body are straight, as opposed to curved, dimensions. In other words, do not follow the natural contours of the body when taking a linear dimension.

The exception to this rule is when taking circumferential measurements of a body segment, such as head or ankle circumference.

Specific Principles Related to Linear Measures of Postural Support Devices

For consistency and repeatability of linear measurements of PSDs, Waugh and Crane (2013a) developed the following conventions, which are necessary because not all PSDs have uniform dimensions on all sides.

Measurements Are Taken on the Contact Surface Side of the Support

Unless otherwise stated, all linear dimensions of seating support surfaces are measured on the contact surface side of the support component. This makes sense clinically because this is the side of the support that will interface with the person's body. This facilitates accurate translation of the body dimension into its corresponding seating dimension.

Measurements Are Taken at the Center of the Support

Some PSDs are not rectangular, such as most off-the-shelf back supports, and therefore a rule, or convention, is necessary as to where a dimension is taken. For example, a back support may have many widths on the contact surface side at the top or bottom. A seat cushion may be deeper at the center than the sides. Therefore, the terms for linear dimensions are defined as measures taken at the centerline of the support surface. If it is clinically relevant to take alternate or additional measures at points other than centerline, it is important to note where the measurement was taken in documentation for clarity.

Measures Are Taken in an Unloaded State

All linear dimensions are defined as measures taken in an unloaded condition. This differs from some of the standardized testing methodologies that have been developed to measure seat cushions for coding purposes in the United States. It is important to understand that some linear dimensions (such as seat depth, width, and thickness) will be different in loaded and unloaded conditions, particularly when the support is made of very soft or compliant materials. However, the final loaded dimension will vary depending on the weight and characteristics of the wheelchair occupant. Therefore, the only way that practitioners in the field can measure a PSD product consistently and obtain the same measurement is to have it measured in an unloaded state. When it is clinically useful to take a measurement in a loaded state, the word "loaded" can be added to the measurement to indicate this condition.

Measurements Are Straight Linear Dimensions

Similar to the body, all linear seating dimensions are straight linear measures. For contoured PSDs, the measurements remain linear; do not follow along the curve with your tape measure. If it is clinically useful, a curved dimension can be noted separately.

Linear Measures of the Body

There are 36 linear body measures defined and described in detail in the *Clinical Application Guide* (Waugh & Crane, 2013a). Figure 6-3 shows 15 of the most commonly used measures. Which of the many possible linear measurements to take depends on the complexity of the planned seating system. For example, if the planned seating system includes lateral trunk supports, it would be useful to have a measure of the client's trunk depth. However, if the person has no need for lateral trunk supports, it is not necessary to take this measurement.

Basic Measurement Set for the Hands-Free Sitter

For a person who sits symmetrically with simple seating needs (i.e., the hands-free sitter), the following basic set of linear measures should be taken:

- Hip width
- Chest width
- Shoulder width
- External knee width (if wider than hip width)
- Buttock/thigh depth
- Lower leg length
- Elbow height
- Shoulder height (Scapula height or axilla height can be taken as an alternative to shoulder height, depending on the planned style of back support, to help determine desired back support length and height.)
- Maximum sitting height

Measurement Set for Person With More Complex Seating Needs

For a person with moderate to complex seating needs (i.e., prop sitters), additional dimensions may need to be measured. In addition to the basic set of measures, the following measures may be needed:

- Trunk depth
- Ischial depth
- Foot depth
- Posterior superior iliac spine height
- Scapula height
- Axilla height
- External thigh or knee width
- Internal knee width

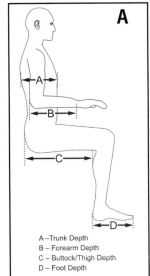
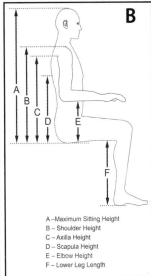

A – Trunk Depth
B – Forearm Depth
C – Buttock/Thigh Depth
D – Foot Depth

A – Maximum Sitting Height
B – Shoulder Height
C – Axilla Height
D – Scapula Height
E – Elbow Height
F – Lower Leg Length

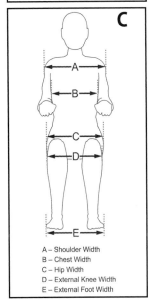

A – Shoulder Width
B – Chest Width
C – Hip Width
D – External Knee Width
E – External Foot Width

Figure 6-3. Common linear body dimensions include (A) depth measures, (B) height and length measures, and (C) width measures for linear measures.

If the client has fixed/non-reducible asymmetries or contractures and will sit with body segments in a nonsymmetrical position (such as a windswept thigh position), it is critical that additional measures are taken to help specify the placement of secondary postural support devices, such as medial or lateral knee supports, or to determine the maximum width of the wheelchair frame required. These measurements, defined in detail in the *Clinical Application Guide* (Waugh & Crane, 2013a) could include the following:

- Medial knee to centerline
- Lateral knee to centerline
- Maximum lower body width
- Maximum sitting width

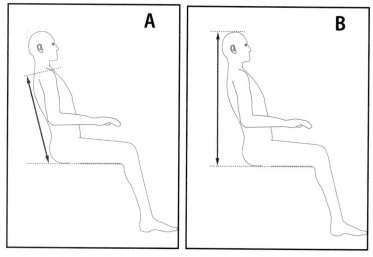

Figure 6-4. Two body height dimensions: (A) shoulder height and (B) maximum sitting height.

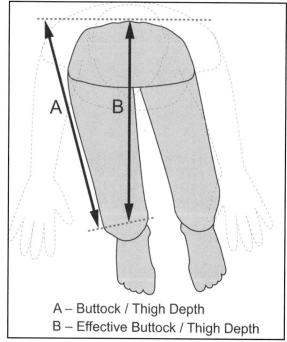

A – Buttock / Thigh Depth
B – Effective Buttock / Thigh Depth

Figure 6-5. Buttock/thigh depth vs effective buttock/thigh depth.

Special Circumstances: Effective Linear Body Measures

Most linear body measures are dimensions of a particular body segment, and they reflect the actual dimension of that segment regardless of how it is oriented. When a body segment is deviated from a neutral orientation in the desired seated posture, it is sometimes hard to know whether to follow the segment in its deviated position when taking a linear measurement. The standardized definitions of each linear measure in the *Clinical Application Guide*

(Waugh & Crane, 2013a) will indicate if a measurement is taken parallel to a body segment or whether the measurement is always a vertical or horizontal dimension regardless of the orientation of the segment.

For example, when measuring shoulder height, you should stay parallel to the trunk in the sagittal plane (side view) if the person's planned sitting position is with a reclined trunk (Figure 6-4A). This makes sense clinically because you will be using the shoulder height measurement to help determine back support length and back support height, and the back support will presumably be placed parallel to the person's trunk. Conversely, the maximum sitting height measurement is always a vertical measurement, taken perpendicular to the ground (Figure 6-4B). This is because the purpose of this measure is to help determine the overall vertical distance that the person will occupy, for clearance and access issues.

Sometimes, however, it is more clinically useful not to stay parallel to the body segment when taking a measurement, even though the term is defined as a parallel to the body segment measurement. In this situation, the word *effective* can be added to the measurement term to indicate that the dimension was not taken parallel to the body segment being measured. For example, the *buttock/thigh depth* measurement as defined is taken parallel to the thigh segment. However, if the desired sitting position of the client is with her thighs windswept to the right or left, it is more useful to take an *effective buttock/thigh depth* measurement to document how much functional depth the thighs will take up on a seat surface for the purpose of determining an appropriate seat depth (Figure 6-5). Similarly, Figure 6-6 shows the difference between *lower leg length* and *effective lower leg length*.

Linear Measures of the Seating Support System

Size and Placement Dimensions

There are two types of linear measures used to specify the dimensions and setup of postural support devices in a seating support system: size dimensions and placement dimensions.

Size dimensions include length, width, depth, and thickness. These linear measures define the size of an individual PSD and are not altered by how they are adjusted or where they are placed within the seating or wheelchair system.

Placement dimensions include such things as back support height, head support height, and seat surface height at front edge. These dimensions are altered by how and where a support is mounted or adjusted within the seating system or wheelchair frame.

There are 32 linear support surface measures described in detail in the *Clinical Application Guide* (Waugh & Crane, 2013a). An additional set of linear dimensions called *support surface location measures* are defined in the ISO and RESNA standards that are not included in the current version of the *Clinical Application Guide*. These location measures provide a standardized method for specifying the precise X, Y, Z coordinate location of any PSD within a wheelchair system and are not presented in this chapter. Waugh's team chose to provide an alternative six placement measures using the term *height* that are more commonly used in practice and easily measured.

Basic Measurement Set of Linear Seating Dimensions

Figures 6-7 through 6-10 show 19 of the most common linear seating dimensions. The type and number of seating supports needed for an individual will dictate which measurements must be specified. Note that the term for the measure is consistent with both the convention established for use of the words length, width, depth, and thickness, and the conventions established for labeling postural support devices.

It is important to remember that although these linear measurement terms have been established through a collaborative international and national standards development process, they have not yet been universally adopted by manufacturers. Unfortunately, at present, manufacturers of seating products use varying terms and methods for defining the linear dimensions of their products. Therefore, until we achieve the goal of universal adoption of measurement terminology in our field, practitioners must refer to each manufacturer's product literature and guidelines for accurate product size selection.

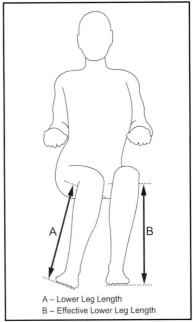

A – Lower Leg Length
B – Effective Lower Leg Length

Figure 6-6. Lower leg length vs effective lower leg length.

Length Versus Height

The difference between back support length and back support height deserves additional attention because of the ubiquitous, although erroneous, use of the term *back support height* by most practitioners and manufacturers. This has led to confusion and prescription errors. Comparing measure B in Figure 6-9 with measure B in Figure 6-10 will highlight the difference between back support length and back support height.

Back support length is the actual dimension of the back support contact surface from top edge to bottom edge. This is a size dimension that does not change unless the product's contact surface is altered. *Back support height* is the distance from the seat surface to the top of the back support, representing the vertical location or placement of the back support relative to the seat. Understanding the difference between these two measurements has serious implications on the proper fit of a back support, especially one with contours. Adjustment of an off-the-shelf back support up or down on the back canes of the wheelchair will change the back support height and alter where the surface contact is on the client's trunk. However, the back support length would not change with this adjustment.

Special Circumstances: Effective Support Surface Measures

The functional contact surface of a PSD can be altered by how adjacent supports are placed next to it. As stated in the *Clinical Application Guide*: "The word 'effective' can be added to any length, depth or width measure to indicate that the useable contact surface has either been increased or

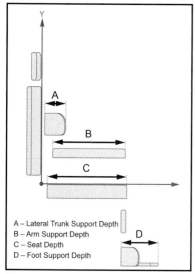

Figure 6-7. Common linear seating dimensions: depth measures.

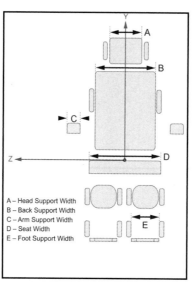

Figure 6-8. Common linear seating dimensions: width measures.

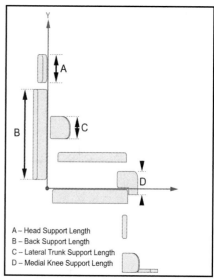

Figure 6-9. Common linear seating dimensions: length measures.

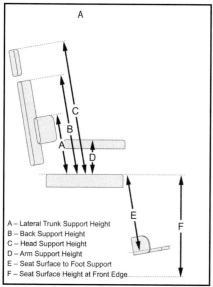

Figure 6-10. Common linear seating dimensions: placement measures.

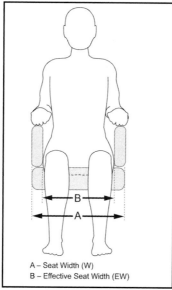

Figure 6-11. Seat width vs effective seat width.

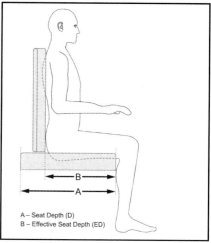

Figure 6-12. Seat depth vs effective seat depth.

reduced by the location of a separate, adjacent or attached component" (Waugh & Crane, 2013a, p. 258).

The most common example of this is when the useable seat depth has been reduced in a pediatric seating system by placing the contact surface of the back support in front of the back edge of the seat cushion. In this situation, the CRT supplier must specify and document two dimensions: the actual and the effective seat depths. Figures 6-11 and 6-12 show examples of effective seat measures.

Clinically, it is the *effective* dimension that will influence the fit of the system and often the posture of the wheelchair occupant. It is, therefore, prudent to note whether there is a difference in actual vs effective dimensions during the assessment, because this might provide clues as to the source of troublesome postural deviations. The following example illustrates the importance of distinguishing between these two measures.

CASE EXAMPLE

Mr. Smith's buttock/thigh depth when he is seated in the desired posture is 19 inches. The team recommends a seat depth of 18 inches, and a cushion that is 18 inches wide x 18 inches deep is selected and provided. However, at a follow-up appointment, the clinician notes that Mr. Smith's posture is not as expected. The clinician notes that although

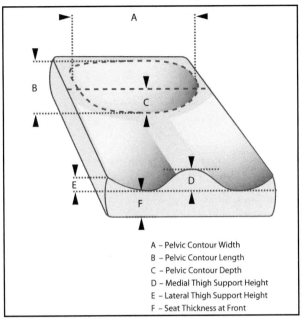

Figure 6-13. Seat cushion contour dimensions.

the seat cushion depth is 18 inches (correctly ordered), the back support placement is such that the plane of the back support's contact surface is actually 2 inches behind the back edge of the seat. The effective seat depth is thus too long at 20 inches, pulling the client into a posterior pelvic tilt and kyphotic sitting posture. The solution is to readjust the back support horizontal location to reduce the effective seat depth to 18 inches.

If all members of the team (clinician, CRT supplier, and CRT technician) understand and use consistent measurement terminology, these types of setup errors can be prevented, or at least the recommended solution can be efficiently communicated and resolved.

Additional Measures for Contoured and More Complex Postural Support Devices

The ISO and RESNA standards that define basic terms for linear dimensions did not address additional measures needed to describe contoured surfaces or more complex shapes. For example, the single measure provided for *back* support width may not adequately describe the width of an off-the-shelf back support with deep contour, which could be measured at different locations both on the inside of integrated lateral trunk support surfaces, as well as the outside of the shell itself. The *Glossary of Terms* (Waugh & Crane, 2013b) proposes several additional measures that can be used to more fully describe a contoured back support, including the following:

- Inside back support width
- Outside back support width
- Overall back support width
- Back support assembly width

- Back support contour depth

This glossary also proposes several additional measures that were not defined in ISO or RESNA standards, which can help describe the linear dimensions of a contoured seat cushion (Figure 6-13). These include the following:

- *Pelvic contour width, length, and depth*: These measures define the dimensions of the pelvic contour area of a seat cushion.
- *Lateral and medial thigh support height*: These measures define the height of the walls of the thigh troughs at the front of a seat cushion.

Linear Measures of the Wheelchair Frame

One of the final and most critical steps in the process of measuring the client and prescribing a wheelchair and seating system is ensuring that it will all fit together. Wheelchairs come in many different configurations: power or manual, highly adjustable or configurable, modular or integrated. Accurate prescription of wheelchair frame dimensions is critical to ensuring that the seating system interfaces properly with the wheelchair frame in a manner that accommodates the dimensions, body posture, and functional needs of the client.

There is a small set of wheelchair frame dimensions defined in ISO and RESNA wheelchair standards; however, many needed measures are as yet undefined and not standardized. The *Glossary of Terms* proposes several terms for basic frame dimensions to differentiate them from similar seating dimensions (Waugh & Crane, 2013b). Work still needs to be done to standardize these and other wheelchair

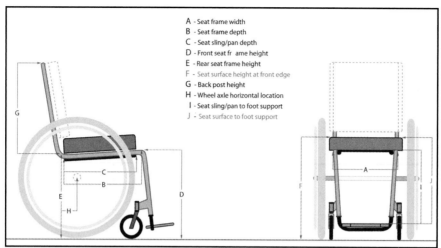

Figure 6-14. Basic linear measures of the wheelchair frame. *Note*: Dimensions F and J are related seating dimensions with seat cushion in place.

frame measures, and to promote universal adoption of measurement terms by wheelchair manufacturers.

Basic Measurement Set

The following are the most critical, basic frame dimensions that need to be specified as part of a final wheelchair recommendation (Figure 6-14):

- Seat frame width
- Seat frame depth
- Front seat frame height
- Rear seat frame height
- Wheel axle horizontal location
- Back post length
- Seat sling or pan to foot support

Seat Frame Width

The width of a wheelchair seat frame may be different from the width of the seat surface that is intended to support the person's buttocks and thighs, depending on the type and configuration of the wheelchair and the seat. Although all wheelchairs have seat structures, most are intended to be used with the addition of a seat cushion. What is frequently reported as wheelchair seat width by manufacturers is the width of the integrated wheelchair seat sling, the width of the wheelchair seat pan (if that is standard on the wheelchair), or the width of the frame itself from the outermost edges of the seat rail on each side.

To avoid confusion, we recommend the use of two terms to differentiate the width of the seating support surface from the width of the wheelchair seat frame. As defined in ISO and RESNA seating standards and clarified in the *Clinical Application Guide* and *Glossary of Terms*, the term *seat width* is used to describe the width of the seat surface intended to contact the person, whether this is a separate seat cushion, an integrated wheelchair solid seat, or an

integrated sling seat (Waugh & Crane, 2013a). Using this convention, it would not be appropriate to call the width of a wheelchair seat pan seat width because the seat pan is not intended to be sat on but rather is a support structure on which to place a seat cushion. We recommend use of the term *seat frame width* (as proposed in the *Glossary of Terms*) to describe the width of the wheelchair seat frame and to differentiate this dimension from the width of the seat support surface, because they may not be the same.

- *Seat frame width*: Distance between the lateral outside edges of the seat rails, measured in the front. (Waugh & Crane, 2013b)

Many wheelchair frames have an additional 1 to 2 inches of available width between the insides of the arm support structures beyond the reported seat frame width. Although not included in the *Glossary of Terms*, this dimension could be called *effective seat frame width*. The effective seat frame width of a wheelchair may be clinically relevant, as it indicates the space available for a wider seat cushion or for the addition of lateral pelvic or thigh supports. Similarly, it is important to understand that because seat frame width is measured from the outside of the seat rails, the space available for the occupants lower legs in between the lower leg support structure is typically 2 inches less than the seat frame width in a standard configuration. For example, if a client's external knee width is 14 inches when he or she is seated in the desired sitting posture, a 16-inch seat frame width would likely be required to allow adequate space in between the lower leg support assembly or front frame structure for the client's lower legs and feet.

A wheelchair seat frame that is excessively wide may negatively affect body alignment in the wheelchair (e.g., the buttocks or trunk may not be centered properly in the wheelchair) or propulsion efficiency, if the client is manually propelling the wheelchair using the handrims. A wheelchair seat frame that is too narrow may not properly accommodate the hip width or maximum sitting width of the client, potentially affecting his or her seated posture or causing pressure injuries on the lateral surface of the hips.

Seat Frame Depth

Most manufacturers will report a wheelchair seat depth based on the depth of the actual integrated seat sling or the wheelchair seat pan mounted to the seat rail. However, in some wheelchair configurations, seat sling depths can be ordered at several sizes without any changes in the depth of the wheelchair seat frame or rail. Although this would not actually change the sitting depth available in the frame, it does affect the amount of support provided by the seat sling or pan underneath the seat cushion. Therefore, because the depth of the seat sling can be different from the depth of the actual frame, it would be useful if different terms were adopted to reflect the potential differences in depth measures of the wheelchair seat rail, the seat pan or sling, and the seat cushion. We propose the terms *seat frame depth, seat sling/pan depth* (measures B and C in Figure 6-14), and *seat depth* to differentiate these measures, respectively. We therefore recommend use of the term *seat frame depth* to describe the depth of the wheelchair frame, independent of the seat pan, sling, or seat cushion.

- *Seat frame depth*: Distance from the front of the back post to the front edge of the seat rail (or the point at which the front frame structure starts to curves downward in a wheelchair with a rigid front end) (Waugh & Crane, 2013b).

Wheelchair seat frame depth is obviously critical in providing appropriate space (not too short or too long) to accommodate the client's buttock/thigh depth as well as the thickness of any after-market back support to be attached to the wheelchair back posts. A wheelchair seat frame depth that is too long may not provide adequate posterior pelvic support through the back support and will frequently cause the client to sit with a posterior pelvic tilt or to slide forward on the seat surface. The seat frame depth is also critical to ensuring that the client's lower legs and feet interface with the foot supports at the desired thigh to lower leg angle.

Front Seat Frame Height, Rear Seat Frame Height, and Seat Surface Height at Front Edge

The term that is commonly used to describe the height of the wheelchair seat from the floor is seat to floor height. However, this term is ambiguous, as evidenced by its use in describing both the vertical height from the floor to the top of the wheelchair seat rail, sling or pan, as well as the height to the top of the seat cushion—two dimensions that are very different. Further, given the angled configuration of many wheelchair seat frames, the seat height at the front and the rear of the wheelchair can also be very different and clinically significant. Therefore, more clarifying terms are needed to distinguish between these dimensions. We propose the three terms *front seat frame height, rear seat frame height,* and *seat surface height at front edge* (measures D, E, and F in Figure 6-14) be used to differentiate these measures.

Many manual wheelchairs are available with either adjustable or configurable differences in height between the front and rear of the seat rail. Therefore, there are two dimensions that can be measured: front seat frame height, and rear seat frame height.

These two measures are proposed and defined in the *Glossary of Terms* as follows:

- *Front seat frame height*: Vertical distance from the floor to the top of the seat rail at its highest point, typically at the end of the seat rail or at the front frame bend (Waugh & Crane, 2013b).
- *Rear seat frame height*: Vertical distance from the floor to the top of the seat rail at the rear, just in front of the back post (Waugh & Crane, 2013b).

When there is a difference in these two heights, it creates a slope in the seat frame. Looking at the wheelchair from the side view, you will note the seat rail is on an angle, typically sloping upward to the front. This type of configuration of a wheelchair frame is commonly referred to as *seat dump* or *squeeze*; although, these terms have not been standardized or defined. The difference in these two descriptors relates to whether there is a concurrent change in the angle between the seat rail and the back post. The term seat dump is typically used to describe a seat frame that is inclined, or sloped such that the rear seat frame height is lower than the front seat frame height. The term squeeze is used to describe a configuration where the seat rail is inclined, and the back posts have remained vertical, creating a smaller, or squeezed angle between the seat rail and back post that is less than 90 degrees. Although most manufacturers measure their front seat frame height to the top of the seat pan or sling, there is currently no uniformity in how or where rear seat frame height is measured. Some manufacturers report the height to the rear-most part of the seat sling or seat pan, others to the rear-most top of the seat rail. It is important to refer to the manufacturer's literature to specify how this measurement is obtained when specifying this dimension.

The term *seat surface height at front edge* is actually a seating dimension (as opposed to wheelchair frame dimension) defined in the ISO and RESNA standards and adapted for clarity in the *Clinical Application Guide*.

- *Seat surface height at front edge*: Vertical distance from the floor to the top of the seat surface at its front edge, in the area intended for distal thigh loading (Waugh & Crane, 2013a, 2013b).

Adding the two dimensions *front seat frame height* plus *seat thickness at front* (see Figure 6-13) will equal the *seat surface height at front edge* (Waugh & Crane, 2013b).

The front seat frame height is important to specify to provide the proper amount of ground clearance needed under a client's foot supports (Waugh & Crane, 2013b), while accommodating lower leg length and lower leg sagittal angles (see next section). This dimension can also significantly affect the wheelchair occupant's ability to transfer in and out of his or her wheelchair, especially when using a stand-pivot transfer technique. It will also affect the occupied wheelchair height (Waugh & Crane, 2013b) from floor to top of occupant's head, which affects access to the client's environment. These wheelchair height dimensions are critical because they either allow or limit sitting under a sink or table, sitting in a van at the correct height to see out the front window or to drive effectively, or clearance entering an adapted van while seated in the wheelchair.

Wheel Axle Horizontal Location

The term commonly used in the industry at this time to describe the fore-aft location of the rear wheel axle in a manual wheelchair with axle adjustability is *center of gravity*. This term is used because changing the location of the rear wheel in a forward-backward direction can alter the stability of the occupied wheelchair system by adjusting the location of the rear wheel relative to the occupant's center of gravity. While the terms center of gravity and center of gravity adjustment are commonly used in the industry, the authors feel that this is an inappropriate label for a linear dimension because the term center of gravity means something completely different in its normal usage.

The term for this dimension defined in the ISO and RESNA wheelchair standards is *horizontal location of the wheel axle* (RESNA, 2009a), which more accurately describes this linear dimension. In the *Glossary of Terms* this was shortened to *wheel axle horizontal location* and defined as the "horizontal distance in the anterior-posterior direction from the front of the wheelchair back post to the center of the drive wheel axle" (Waugh & Crane, 2013b). Specifying the wheel axle horizontal location is typically needed when recommending or making adjustments to a configurable or adjustable manual wheelchair being used for independent propulsion. The location of the rear wheel axle will affect not only the occupant's access to the drive wheels for efficient hand propulsion but also the fore-aft stability of the wheelchair.

Back Post Length

The length of the back post is important as it supports the appropriate back support length and height. If an aftermarket back support is attached to the back posts, they must be long enough to allow attachment of the back support at the proper height but not so long as to interfere with arm movements needed for function. Back post length is also important if a caregiver intends to push the wheelchair using the handgrips. The length of the back posts along with the rear seat frame height will determine the final *handgrip height* from the floor for comfortable pushing.

Seat Sling/Pan to Foot Support

This term is proposed and defined in the *Glossary of Terms* as the distance from the top of the seat sling or seat pan at its front edge to the top back edge of the foot support (Waugh & Crane, 2013b) and is usually adjustable by raising or lowering the foot supports. This distance should be adjusted to support the user's thighs and lower legs at the desired body segment angles, with the seat cushion in place. The *seat surface to foot support* dimension is the distance from the top of the seat cushion to the foot support, and therefore, it is this seating dimension that will more closely match the user's lower leg length. The *seat sling/pan to foot support* dimension plus the *seat cushion thickness at front* will equal the *seat surface to foot support distance*.

Other Wheelchair Frame Linear Dimensions

There are several other potentially relevant wheelchair linear dimensions. These may include the following:

- Ground clearance
- Handgrip height
- Overall wheelchair width
- Overall wheelchair depth
- Overall wheelchair height
- Turning diameter

These six terms are standardized terms defined in ISO and RESNA standards. They are included and referenced in the *Glossary of Terms*, in addition to several other potentially useful, standardized wheelchair-related dimensions, such as wheel diameter, wheelchair footprint, stowage width, depth and height, and camber. The reader can refer to this glossary for a full definition of the terms not described here (Waugh & Crane, 2013b).

Relating Linear Dimensions of the Wheelchair Frame, Seating System and Body

Table 6-1 summarizes the terms for the basic linear dimensions of the wheelchair frame discussed in this section, with their corresponding primary dimension of the seating system and body. (Note that there may be other related body and seating dimensions that need to be considered in making a final determination of the listed wheelchair frame dimension that are not included in this table.)

ANGULAR MEASURES

Angular measures serve to describe or specify the angular orientation of the wheelchair-seated person's body segments and his or her corresponding seating support surfaces. The angular orientation of adjacent and individual body segments defines the position and posture of the person. The angular orientation of the person's seating support surfaces in turn affects the position and posture

TABLE 6-1

RELATED LINEAR MEASURES OF THE WHEELCHAIR FRAME, SEATING, AND BODY

WHEELCHAIR FRAME DIMENSION	RELATED SEATING DIMENSION	RELATED BODY DIMENSION
Seat frame width	Seat width	Hip width, max lower body width
Effective seat frame width	Effective seat width	Hip width, max lower body width
Seat frame depth	Seat depth	Buttock/thigh depth
Front seat frame height	Seat surface height at front edge	Lower leg length
Rear seat frame height	None	None
Seat sling/pan to foot support	Seat surface to foot support	Lower leg length

of the person and is therefore a critical component of the wheelchair seating prescription for many individuals. A few angular measures of the seating system will be familiar to most CRT professionals, such as seat to back support angle; however, there is now a full set of angular measures for both the person's body and a wheelchair's seating support surfaces that have been standardized and defined in international and national standards. As mentioned previously, the *Clinical Application Guide* provides a detailed, but clinically friendly, resource to assist in understanding and applying these measures, providing greater detail than can be included in this chapter (Waugh & Crane, 2013a).

Foundational Principles

The following three foundational concepts apply to all angular measures of the body and seating, and are critical to understanding and applying these measures in practice:

1. The three body reference planes
2. Body segment lines and support surface reference planes
3. Relative vs absolute angles

The Three Body Reference Planes

Body reference planes (Figure 6-15) are imaginary two-dimensional surfaces that pass through the body and are used in the medical field to define joint motion, using the standing anatomical position as the zero reference position to define joint ROM values.

The *sagittal plane* is a vertical plane running from front to back that divides the body or any of its segments into left and right sides. The two basic movements in the sagittal plane are flexion and extension. Hip flexion/extension, knee flexion/extension, and elbow flexion/extension are all defined as movements occurring in this plane.

The *frontal plane* is a vertical plane running from side to side that divides the body or any of its segments into front and back (or anterior and posterior) parts. Most movements that occur in this plane are lateral flexion and abduction.

For example, lateral trunk flexion and shoulder abduction are defined as motions occurring in the frontal plane.

The *transverse plane* is a horizontal plane that divides the body or any of its segments into upper and lower (or superior and inferior) parts. Most movements that occur along this plane involve rotation. For example, pelvic and trunk rotation are defined as motions occurring in the transverse plane.

Postural deviations in the sitting position can also be described as occurring in these same three planes. To analyze seated posture during assessment, it is useful to look at the person in the seated position from three perspectives: the front, side, and top. By looking at the person from the front, you can view postural deviations in the frontal plane, such as a pelvic obliquity. Viewing the person from the side, you can see postural deviations in the sagittal plane, such as a posterior pelvic tilt, spinal kyphosis, or lordosis. Looking down at the person from the top view allows you to note any deviations in the transverse plane, such as trunk rotation or a windswept thigh position. Observation and notation of a person's body alignment in each of the three planes is critical to understanding where and why supports will be needed to achieve and maintain a functional seated posture in a wheelchair.

Similarly for the seating system, we can observe, measure, and/or specify the orientation of any single postural support device in each of the three planes. The new support surface angles defined in the ISO and RESNA standards provide a term and measure for quantifying the orientation in each plane if needed. For example, a head support could be adjusted so that it has a deviation from its typical neutral position in each of these three planes to accommodate a person with fixed neck contractures.

Body Segment Lines and Support Surface Reference Planes

To measure the orientation of a body segment, you have to identify a line on the body segment that will represent its orientation for measurement. For example, if you want to measure the orientation of your client's thigh with respect

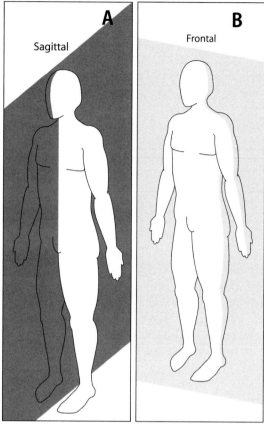

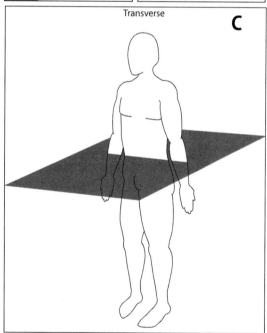

Figure 6-15. The three body reference planes: (A) sagittal plane, (B) frontal plane, and (C) transverse plane.

to the horizontal, how will you line up your goniometer or inclinometer on the thigh to measure an angle? Anatomical landmarks at the end of each body segment define the endpoints of a line on that segment that is used to measure its orientation. These are called body segment lines (Figure

6-16), and you will line up your goniometer or inclinometer along these imaginary lines to measure body segment angles. The *Clinical Application Guide* contains an appendix that lists and defines all body segment lines and their anatomical landmarks (Waugh & Crane, 2013a).

Similarly, to measure the angular orientation of a postural support device, such as a seat or foot support, you have to identify a reference line or plane along the PSD's contact surface, which represents its orientation for measurement. As support surfaces do not have anatomical landmarks like body segments, an imaginary support surface reference plane is used, on which lie imaginary axes and reference lines (Figure 6-17). You will align your goniometer or inclinometer along these planes or lines in order to measure the angular orientation of the PSD. Refer to the *Clinical Application Guide* for more detailed explanation of support surface reference planes, axes, and lines (Waugh & Crane, 2013a).

When a PSD is flat, like a foot support or planar seat, the support surface reference plane coincides with the contact surface, and it is easy to line up your goniometer or inclinometer along the contact surface to measure its angle. However, many seating support surfaces are contoured, and some even have very complex contours. In this situation, you need to identify a flat planar surface somewhere on the PSD that approximates the overall contact surface orientation. Many times this is the noncontact surface side of the support. The accuracy of this measurement will certainly vary depending on how heavily contoured a surface is and the softness of the materials used to create the surface.

Relative Versus Absolute Angles

It is clinically relevant to be able to define the orientation of a body segment or seating support surface in two ways:

1. With respect to an adjacent body segment or support surface, because this reflects joint position and common seating angles

2. With respect to an external, gravitational reference, because this reflects orientation in space and the influence of gravity

Therefore, there are two main types of standardized angular measures:

1. *Relative angles* describe the angle between two adjacent body segments or between two adjacent support surfaces. For example, the angle between the thigh and the trunk is a relative body segment angle called the *thigh to trunk angle*. The angle between the seat and the back support in a seating system is a relative support surface angle called the *seat to back support angle*.

2. *Absolute angles* describe the orientation in space of a single body segment or support surface, with respect to an external, absolute reference, such as the vertical or horizontal. (The term *absolute* refers to the fact that the horizontal or vertical reference is absolute, or not

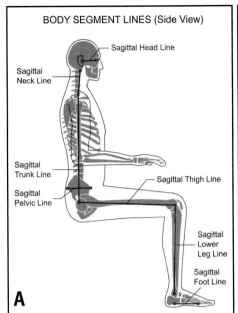

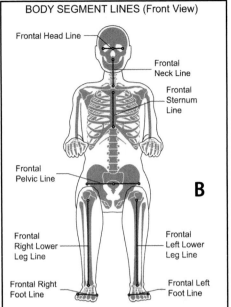

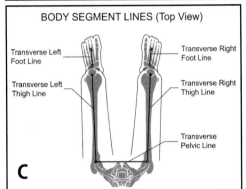

Figure 6-16. Examples of body segment lines: (A) sagittal body segment lines, (B) frontal body segment lines, and (C) transverse body segment lines. *Note*: Not all body segment lines are shown.

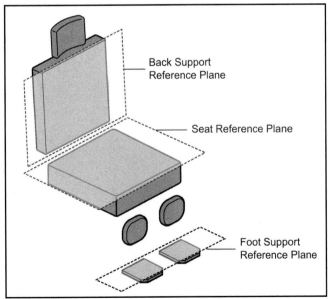

Figure 6-17. Examples of support surface reference planes.

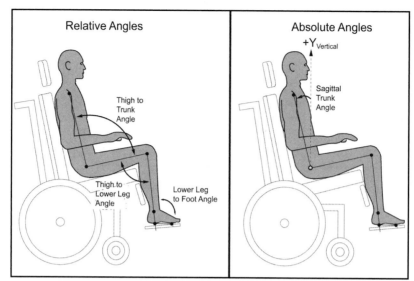

Figure 6-18. Relative vs absolute body segment angles.

changing.) For example, the angle between the thigh and the horizontal is an absolute body segment angle called the *sagittal thigh angle*.

Figure 6-18 shows the difference between relative and absolute body segment angles.

The *thigh to trunk angle* is the angle between the thigh and the trunk, which is a relative angle. This is important to note because it reflects the amount of gross hip flexion the person is sitting in. The *sagittal trunk angle* is the angle between the trunk and a vertical reference; therefore, it is an absolute angle. This is important because this angle may affect the person's trunk and head posture, or functional reach. Note that if you tilted the person in Figure 6-18 posteriorly, such as may occur in a tilt-in-space wheelchair, the thigh to trunk angle would not change, but the sagittal trunk angle would change. Understanding the difference between these types of angles, as well as how they are related, can help with problem solving during assessment and with prescription of corresponding support surface angles and wheelchair features.

Relative Body Segment Angles

There are currently 10 relative body segment angles defined in the ISO (2006) and RESNA (2013) standards; 4 of these more common angles are described in detail in the *Clinical Application Guide* (Waugh & Crane, 2013a). Currently, relative body segment angles are defined in the sagittal plane only.

Basic Measurement Set for Relative Body Segment Angles

The three relative body segment angles shown in Figure 6-19 provide a basic set of measures that can quantify a

person's sitting position from a side view, and help determine the corresponding relative angles of the wheelchair seating system. Documenting these primary angles should become standard practice when assessing any individual with postural support needs for a wheelchair.

- *Thigh to trunk angle*: The relative angle between the thigh and the trunk, viewed from the side. The angle that is above the thigh is measured (Waugh & Crane, 2013b).

- *Thigh to lower leg angle*: The relative angle between the thigh and the lower leg, viewed from the side. The angle that is behind the lower leg is measured (Waugh & Crane, 2013b).

- *Lower leg to foot angle*: The relative angle between the lower leg and the foot, viewed from the side. The angle that is above the foot is measured (Waugh & Crane, 2013b).

Practical Application

Early in a seating assessment, you can measure these three angles with the person sitting in their wheelchair as a way to document their current sitting position. This can help with problem solving during assessment, as you note any discrepancies with the corresponding seating angles or with mat examination measurements.

At the end of the assessment, with the person seated in the desired position and posture (which may be different from their baseline), you can take these measurements again. This is done to document the desired seated position and to help prescribe the corresponding support surface angles, which can then assist with determining the necessary features needed in the wheelchair or seating system hardware. It is the clinician's role to measure these three body segment angles to describe the basic desired resting

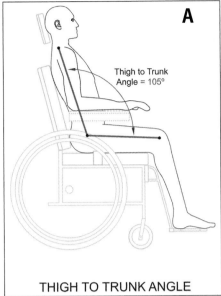

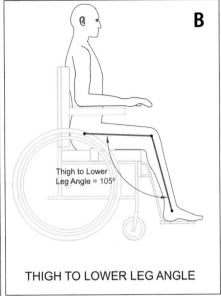

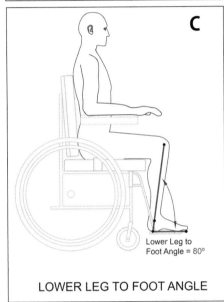

Figure 6-19. Three basic relative body segment angles: (A) thigh to trunk angle, (B) thigh to lower leg angle, and (C) lower leg to foot angle.

sitting position. With these measurements, the clinician and supplier can then have a conversation about product features and recommendations.

Measurement of these angles with the client seated in the desired position and posture will help answer the following (and other) critical questions:

- How will we ensure that the equipment we are recommending will be able to support the client in the desired position?

- What seating system (or wheelchair) components and features are required to achieve the desired relative body segment angles?

- Do we need adjustable angle back posts, or is the hardware on the back support sufficient to support the person with this thigh to trunk angle?

- What type of front frame angle or lower leg support assembly is required to achieve the desired thigh to lower leg angle for accommodation of hamstring tightness?

- Do we need angle adjustable foot supports to achieve the desired lower leg to foot angle?

Translating Mat Examination Measurements Into Relative Body Segment Angles

As a clinician, it is your role and responsibility to be able to translate the information gained from your mat examination and other assessment procedures to help determine the optimal resting seated position for your client. To do this, it is important to understand the difference

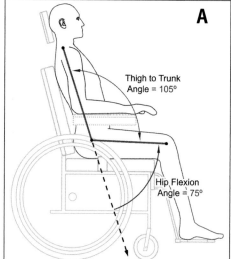
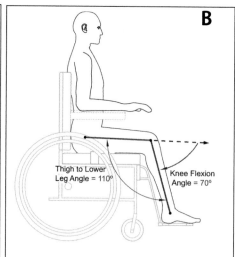

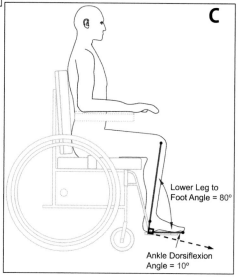

Figure 6-20. Relative body segment angles and corresponding joint angle position: (A) thigh to trunk angle vs hip flexion angle, (B) thigh to lower leg angle vs knee flexion angle, and (C) lower leg to foot angle vs dorsiflexion angle.

between the passive ROM measurements taken during the mat examination and these relative body segment angles. Relative body segment angles describe an angular position—a snapshot in time—as opposed to a range of available joint motion. They are also defined differently, so the values may not be the same. Joint ROM values are based on the standing anatomical position as the zero starting point, whereas relative body segment angles are defined simply as the angle between the two adjacent body segments. For example, you may evaluate a client's passive hip flexion ROM during the mat examination and discover that their range is from 10 to 80 degrees. This means that if you hold the thigh in a position of 80 degrees of hip flexion, the corresponding thigh to trunk angle is 100 degrees. These two measures are related but have different values; they are supplemental angles, meaning they add up to 180 degrees.

Figure 6-20 shows the relationship between these relative body segment angles and the corresponding joint angle position. Figure 6-20A illustrates the relationship between hip flexion and the thigh to trunk angle in the

sitting position. In this diagram, the person is sitting in 75 degrees of hip flexion and with a thigh to trunk angle of 105 degrees. If this is the client's best, most functional sitting position, then it would be important to specify a seat to back support angle of 105 degrees to achieve the desired sitting position.

Figure 6-20B illustrates the relationship between knee flexion and the thigh to lower leg angle. During the mat examination, we typically assess knee extension ROM with the hips flexed to assess hamstring tightness. The resulting popliteal angle is a measure of hamstring tightness, and this equates with the thigh to lower leg angle; however, the knee flexion angle is a different angle—the supplemental angle. In this figure, the person is seated in 70 degrees of knee flexion, creating a thigh to lower leg angle of 110 degrees. If this is the person's desired, resting sitting position, then the prescribed seat to lower leg support angle should be 110 degrees.

Finally, Figure 6-20C illustrates the relationship between ankle dorsiflexion and the lower leg to foot angle. In this

TABLE 6-2		
CORRESPONDING TERMS FOR JOINT RANGE OF MOTION, RELATIVE BODY SEGMENT ANGLES, AND RELATIVE SUPPORT SURFACE ANGLES		
JOINT RANGE OF MOTION	**RELATIVE BODY SEGMENT ANGLE**	**SUPPORT SURFACE ANGLE**
Hip flexion	Thigh to trunk angle	Seat to back support angle
Knee extension with hips flexed (popliteal angle)	Thigh to lower leg angle	Seat to lower leg support angle
Ankle dorsiflexion/plantarflexion	Lower leg to foot angle	Lower leg support to foot support angle

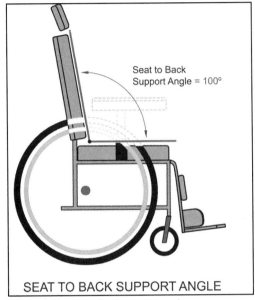

Figure 6-21. Seat to back support angle.

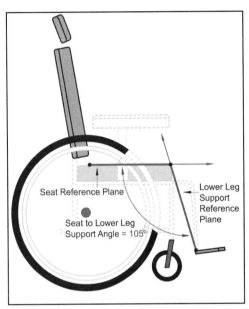

Figure 6-22. Seat to lower leg support angle (with no calf pad).

diagram, the person's ankle is positioned in 10 degrees of dorsiflexion, which creates a lower leg to foot angle of 80 degrees.

Table 6-2 shows the relationship between joint motion assessed during the mat examination, the three primary relative body segment angles, and the corresponding relative support surface angles (discussed in the next session).

It is suggested that the client's desired, resting, sitting position be documented by measuring and recording these three relative body segment angles as part of every wheelchair seating prescription. This will ensure that the appropriate wheelchair/seating components and features necessary to support the client in this position are discussed and included in the final recommendation.

Relative Support Surface Angles

The *Clinical Application Guide* (Waugh & Crane, 2013a) also describes in detail five relative support surface angles based on the three generic definitions provided in the ISO and RESNA standards. As with the relative body segment angles, relative support surface angles are defined in the sagittal plane only.

Basic Measurement Set for Relative Support Surface Angles

The three relative support surface angles described next and shown in Figures 6-21 through 6-23 provide a minimum set of measures to describe the basic angular orientation of the primary support surfaces in a seating system, relative to the adjacent surface. Documenting these three primary seating angles should become standard practice when prescribing a seating system because they can have a significant impact on the wheelchair occupant's posture, comfort, and function.

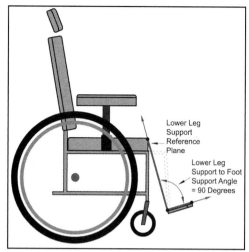

Lower Leg
Support
Reference
Plane

Lower Leg
Support to Foot
Support Angle
= 90 Degrees

Figure 6-23. Lower leg support to foot support angle (with no calf pad).

- *Seat to back support angle* (see Figure 6-21): The relative angle between the seat and the back support reference planes, viewed from the side. The angle above the seat is measured (Waugh & Crane, 2013b).

- *Seat to lower leg support angle* (see Figure 6-22): The relative angle between the seat and the lower leg support reference planes, viewed from the side. The angle that is behind the lower leg support is measured (Waugh & Crane, 2013b).

- *Lower leg support to foot support angle* (see Figure 6-23): The relative angle between the lower leg support and foot support reference planes, viewed from the side. The angle that is above the foot support is measured (Waugh & Crane, 2013b).

It is important to understand that these angles are *seating system* angles not *wheelchair frame* angles. They represent the angles between the support surfaces that are contacting the person's body and, as defined, may not be the same as wheelchair frame angles. For example, the seat to lower leg support angle is defined as the intersection between the seat reference plane and the lower leg support reference plane. In the absence of an actual lower leg support, such as a calf pad, the lower leg support reference plane is an imaginary plane connecting the front edge of the seat with the back edge of the foot support (Waugh & Crane, 2013a). Therefore, this angle is affected by the linear placement of the seat cushion and the foot supports in a forward or backward direction. These types of adjustments can often be done independent of the wheelchair frame configuration. Additionally, the seat to back support angle can be changed with adjustments to a back support's attachment hardware without changing the angle between the wheelchair seat frame and the back posts.

Practical Application

Early in a seating assessment, you can measure these three relative seating angles of the person's wheelchair as a way to document the current seating configuration. This can help with problem solving during assessment because these relative angles can have a significant effect on the person's seated posture and therefore can provide clues as to the cause of a presenting postural deviation or problem, as well as a solution. Here is an example.

CASE EXAMPLE

Mr. Smith presents with a severe posterior pelvic tilt and kyphotic trunk posture. The relative support surface angles of his current wheelchair are as follows: 95 degree seat to back support angle; 120 degree seat to lower leg support angles, and 95 degree lower leg support to foot support angles. Mat examination reveals that he has only 75 degrees of passive hip flexion bilaterally, and mildly tight hamstrings with popliteal angles of 100 degrees bilaterally. He also has mild plantarflexion contractures resulting in passive ankle dorsiflexion of minus 5 degrees bilaterally. His pelvis and spine are flexible to achieve a neutral posture.

From this information, you can hypothesize that a contributing factor to his posterior pelvic tilt and kyphotic trunk posture is that his seat to back support angle and seat to lower leg support angles are not accommodating his limitations in hip flexion and tight hamstrings, resulting in this spinal posture, which you know is flexible. His lower leg support to foot support angle seems appropriate. This information then informs the team as to what to try during seating simulation (test theory by altering seating angles and see if posture improves).

You are able to set up a simulation chair with the following recommended support surface angles, which are based on your mat examination findings: 105-degree seat/back support angle (to accommodate 75 degrees of hip flexion and support a 105-degree thigh to trunk angle); 100-degree seat/lower leg support angles (to accommodate a 100-degree popliteal angle and support a 100-degree thigh to lower leg angle); and 95-degree lower leg support/foot support angles (to accommodate minus 5 degrees of dorsiflexion and support a 95-degree lower leg to foot angle).

At the end of the assessment, with the person's optimal, desired seated posture simulated, you can measure the person's relative body segment angles and from these prescribe the desired seating support surface angles, which may be different from his current setup. As mentioned earlier, the

TABLE 6-3			
SUMMARY OF MEASUREMENTS IN MR. SMITH'S CASE			
JOINT RANGE OF MOTION	**RELATIVE BODY SEGMENT ANGLES**	**RELATIVE SUPPORT SURFACE ANGLES**	**WHEELCHAIR FRAME FEATURE REQUIREMENT**
Maximum hip flexion: 75 degrees	Thigh/trunk angle: 105 degrees	Seat/back support angle: 105 degrees	Adjustable angle back posts or back support hardware
Popliteal angle: 100 degrees	Thigh/lower leg angle: 100 degrees	Seat/LLS support angle: 100 degrees	70-degree swing away LLS assembly with adjustable angle foot supports—slide foot supports rearward to achieve desired seat/LLS angle of 100
Ankle dorsiflexion: -5 degrees	Lower leg/foot angle: 95 degrees	LLS/foot support angle: 95 degrees	Angle adjustable foot supports
LLS=lower leg support			

clinician and supplier can then have a conversation about how the three recommended seating angles will be achieved in the wheelchair prescription. Table 6-3 provides a summary of the preceding clinical example.

It is important to note that the same principles are used to define relative body segment angles and relative support surface angles. Therefore, if the person's body segments are parallel to the support surface reference planes of the back support, seat, lower leg support, and foot supports, then the value of the relative body segment angles will be the same as the values for the relative support surface angles. This helps with prescription.

In summary, these relative seating angles are prescribed specifically to support the wheelchair occupant in the desired sitting position. At the time of any equipment trials, fittings, delivery, or follow-up, these three primary angles are then measured in the desired wheelchair frame and seating system configuration to ensure that the originally prescribed angles have been achieved. This is particularly true with respect to the seat to back support and seat to lower leg support angles, because these angles are affected by the adjustment of the back support hardware, back posts, and placement of the foot supports.

Absolute Body Segment Angles

In addition to the three basic relative body segment angles, you may also wish to quantify additional aspects of a person's wheelchair-seated posture. The new measures for *absolute body segment angles* allow you to quantify the orientation of a single body segment, in any of the three planes. Although these absolute angles are not as commonly measured as the relative body segment angles described earlier, they can be extremely useful when working with individuals with complex postural deviations and complex seating needs.

What if you wanted to measure the orientation in space of a client's trunk because this position is critical to his or her ability to reach with his or her arms due to muscle weakness? Or perhaps you notice that a client's thigh is angling downward and not parallel to the plane of the seat, and you would like to measure the slope of the thigh because this is contributing to complaints of sliding? How would you do it? What if you need to accommodate a client's hip contractures by positioning his or her thighs in a windswept posture, angling to the right? How would you quantify this thigh angle? Or perhaps your client presents with a severe pelvic obliquity and scoliotic posture when viewed from the front, and you would like to quantify this baseline postural deviation. Absolute body segment angle measures allow you to quantify these postural characteristics.

How would you measure the orientation of the relevant body segments in the preceding examples? For each of these examples, you would need to line up a goniometer or inclinometer along the body segment to be measured (using the defined *body segment line*) and measure its angle with respect to a zero reference. It is logical that you would compare the orientation of the person's trunk with the vertical, and you would compare the slope of the thigh with the horizontal. Looking at the person from the front, you would probably compare the angle of the pelvis with the horizontal. But what about the outward angle of the thigh in a windswept posture? What would you use as a reference for that angle? You could compare it to a line going through the seat from back to front, a line that is perpendicular to the wheelchair's rear wheel axle. This line representing the longitudinal centerline of the wheelchair is called the *wheelchair X-axis* (abbreviated X_{WAS}) in the ISO standard

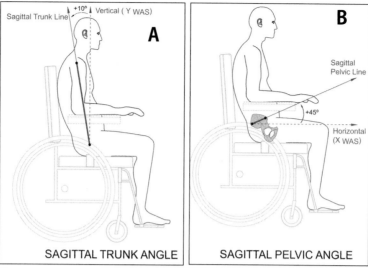

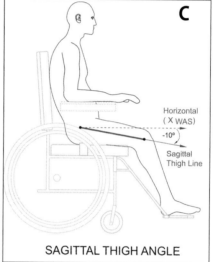

Figure 6-24. Examples of sagittal body segment angles: (A) sagittal trunk angle, (B) sagittal pelvic angle, and (C) sagittal thigh angle.

(ISO, 2006) and *Clinical Application Guide* (Waugh & Crane, 2013a).

Absolute body segment angles are defined for each body segment in at least two of the three planes. For example, the trunk segment of a seated person can deviate away from a neutral position in the:

- Sagittal plane (leaning back or forward from the vertical)
- Frontal plane (leaning to the right or left)
- Transverse plane (rotating to the right or left)

Absolute body segment angles allow you to quantify the position of each body segment relative to a true vertically or horizontally oriented position, which is useful when understanding the impact of gravity on a body segment or the person as a whole. When a body segment deviates from a neutral forward facing position in the transverse plane, its position relative to the vertical or horizontal stays the same; therefore, absolute body segment angles in the transverse plane use a line on the wheelchair as the absolute zero reference.

Remember that you can view, describe, and measure the angular orientation of a body segment in each of the three planes by viewing the person from the side (sagittal), front (frontal), and top (transverse). The convention for labeling the angular measures that define these deviations is consistent and based on the plane, or view, in which the deviation occurs. If you measure the orientation of a body segment in the sagittal plane (side view), it will be called a *sagittal* angle. For example, the degree to which the person's thigh is angled upward or downward compared to the horizontal is called the sagittal thigh angle. Figure 6-24 shows a sample of three sagittal absolute body segment angles. All sagittal absolute body angles are determined by measuring the angle between the body segment (as represented by its body segment line) and either the vertical or the horizontal. In each of the images in Figure 6-24, the body segment line is indicated with a solid line, and the reference axis (either the vertical or horizontal) is indicated with a dashed line. WAS is an abbreviation for the Wheelchair Axis System. The *Clinical Application Guide* (Waugh & Crane, 2013a) is an excellent resource if the reader desires a deeper

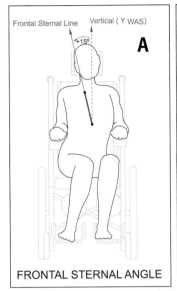

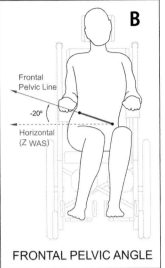

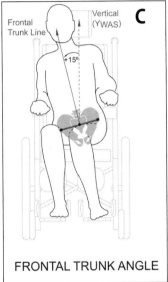

Figure 6-25. Examples of frontal body segment angles: (A) frontal sternal angle, (B) frontal pelvic angle, and (C) frontal trunk angle.

understanding of the coordinate axis system used to accurately define these angles.

If you measure the orientation of a body segment in the frontal plane (front view), it will be called a *frontal angle*. For example, the degree to which a person's sternum is tilted to the right or left is called the frontal sternal angle, and the degree of pelvic obliquity is called the frontal pelvic angle. All frontal absolute body angles are determined by measuring the angle between the body segment (as represented by the body segment line) and either the vertical or the horizontal. Figure 6-25 shows a sample of three frontal absolute body segment angles.

If you measure the orientation of a body segment in the transverse plane (top view), it will be called a *transverse angle*. For example, the degree to which a person's thigh is angled to the right or left with respect to the wheelchair longitudinal axis is called the transverse thigh angle. All transverse absolute angles are determined by measuring the angle between the body segment (as represented by its body segment line) and a specified reference axis of the wheelchair. Figure 6-26 shows a sample of three transverse absolute body segment angles.

You may have noticed in the figures illustrating absolute body segment angles that the value of an absolute angle can be either positive or negative. This is necessary to indicate which direction the body segment has deviated away from the zero reference position. For example, a person's thigh may be angled up or down relative to the horizontal reference, and a convention must be used to indicate this direction. The ISO and RESNA standards use positive and negative numbers to indicate this direction using an engineering principle called the *right handgrip rule*. This is explained in detail in the *Clinical Application Guide* (Waugh & Crane, 2013a). As an alternative while you learn this notation methodology, you can add a descriptive word to the angle value to indicate the direction. For example, right sagittal

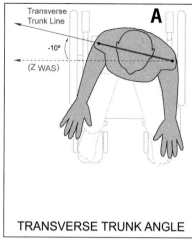

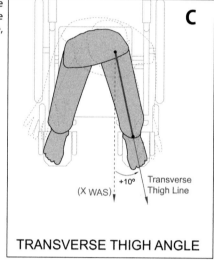

Figure 6-26. Examples of transverse body segment angles: (A) transverse trunk angle, (B) transverse pelvic angle, and (C) transverse thigh angle

thigh angle = 10 degrees (down), or frontal pelvic angle = 15 degrees (right low).

Basic Measurement Set of Absolute Body Segment Angles (Complex Seating)

There are 29 absolute body segment angles defined in the ISO and RESNA standards; 20 of these are described in detail in the *Clinical Application Guide* (Waugh & Crane, 2013a). Although there are many absolute body segment angles available, one would commonly only take a very small set of measures and typically only when managing a client with moderate to severe postural deviations.

The following are the most common absolute body segment angles to measure for documenting existing postural deviations or to set postural objectives:

- Sagittal trunk angle
- Sagittal pelvic angle
- Sagittal thigh angle
- Frontal pelvic angle
- Frontal sternal angle
- Frontal trunk angle
- Frontal head angle
- Transverse pelvic angle
- Transverse thigh angle
- Transverse trunk angle

Practical Application

When a client presents with significant postural deviations and improving seated posture is an identified goal, it can be useful to measure one to three absolute body segment angles to quantify the severity of the postural problem and to establish a baseline. You do not need to measure all of the preceding 10 angles; choose angles that characterize the primary postural problem that the person presents with, and measure him or her sitting in his or her existing wheelchair seating. For example, if the primary postural problem is asymmetry in the frontal plane because of a collapsing spinal scoliosis, then you could measure and document the *frontal pelvic angle* and *frontal sternal angle* because these provide a good measure of the degree of functional asymmetry. If the trunk is leaning to one side or there is a lateral shift of the upper trunk relative to the pelvis, the *frontal trunk angle* provides a measure of this imbalance in the frontal plane. After an assessment of spinal flexibility during the mat examination, and subsequent seating simulation to determine the person's optimal sitting posture, these same three angles could be measured again and documented as the desired sitting posture. This establishes quantifiable postural objectives that can be measured again after the seating intervention to document outcomes.

When the planned seating intervention includes custom contoured seating for an individual with joint limitations and fixed asymmetries, it is recommended that a postural alignment plan be developed and documented before the shape capture. This should include the three relative body segment angles described previously (right and left sides, if different), as well as one to four absolute body segment angles that reflect your primary postural objectives for the individual. This helps not only with setup of the shape capture equipment, but it also guides you during the shape capture to ensure that you have positioned the person in the desired alignment while the body shape is being captured. Angles can be documented again during that session if you were unable to achieve the desired alignment and need to modify your objectives. This is useful so that you can again measure the same angles during the fitting or delivery, to ensure that postural objectives have been met.

Finally, these absolute body segment angle measures can also help monitor postural changes that occur over time if measured and documented carefully, which may be essential in monitoring a progressive condition or the effects of abnormalities in muscle tone or development of secondary complications, such as contractures in joints.

Absolute Support Surface Angles

In addition to the three basic relative support surface angles described earlier in this chapter, there may be times when it is useful to specify and document an *absolute support surface angle*. Similar to absolute body segment angles, these measures allow you to quantify the orientation of a single PSD in any of the three planes. This would only be useful if a PSD needs to be adjusted or oriented at an angle that is not in line with the vertical, horizontal, or wheelchair axes. Similar to the Seated Reference Position, the ISO and RESNA standards define a *support surface reference position* in which all postural support devices in a seating system are aligned with the vertical and horizontal and in a neutral orientation relative to the forward-facing wheelchair frame (Waugh & Crane, 2013a). This is a hypothetical zero reference position in which all absolute angles of support surfaces are zero.

As any PSD in a seating system could technically be intentionally (or unintentionally) adjusted away from its neutral reference position in any of the three planes, absolute support surface angles have been defined and can be measured for any support surface in at least two of the three planes. For example, the head support of a seating system could be adjusted away from a neutral position in the:

- Sagittal plane (angled back or forward from the vertical)
- Frontal plane (tilted to the right or left)
- Transverse plane (rotated to the right or left)

The convention for labeling the angular measures that define these deviations is consistent and based on the plane, or view, in which the deviation occurs. If a support surface is angled away from the horizontal or vertical when viewed from the side (deviation in sagittal plane), it will be called a *sagittal angle*. For example, the degree to which a back support is angled forward or backward from the vertical is called the *back support sagittal angle* (Figure 6-27A). The back support sagittal angle is a standardized measure of the degree of recline or procline of a back support. If a support surface is angled away from the horizontal or vertical when viewed from the front (deviation in frontal plane), it will be called a *frontal angle*. For example, the degree to which a head support is tilted to the right or left is called the *head support frontal angle* (Figure 6-27B). If a support surface is rotated inward or outward, or to the left or right, when viewed from the top (deviation in transverse plane), it will be called a *transverse angle*. For example, the degree to which a lateral knee support is rotated outward or inward is called the *lateral knee support transverse angle* (Figure 6-27C).

Practical Application

Purposeful adjustment of primary support surfaces away from a vertical or horizontal position in the sagittal plane are common, and noting their absolute angle in addition to the relative angles can at times be useful clinically.

CASE EXAMPLE

A client with limited hip flexion of 75 degrees needs to sit with a 105-degree thigh to trunk angle for optimal spinal alignment. This requires the seat to back support angle to be 105 degrees. But she also needs to be able to sit at certain times with a sagittal trunk angle of +5 degrees (reclined 5 degrees from the vertical) to reach forward with her arms due to muscle weakness. Therefore, the back support sagittal angle needs to be able to be adjusted to +5 degrees to bring the client more upright in space for function, while maintaining a 105-degree seat to back support angle if possible. In this more upright position, the seat (and the client's thigh) would be angled downward 10 degrees, a seat sagittal angle of –10 degrees. One solution would be to seat her in a wheelchair with adjustable tilt, configured so that the seat and/or seat frame slopes downward 10 degrees when the wheelchair is in its most upright position. Another solution

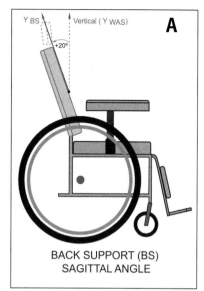

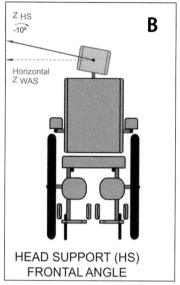

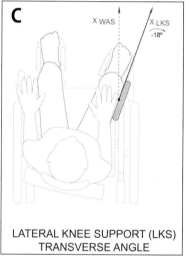

Figure 6-27. Examples of absolute support surface angles: (A) back support sagittal angle, (B) head support frontal angle, and (C) lateral knee support transverse angle.

would be to provide her with adjustable recline in addition to adjustable tilt, so that she can close up her seat to back support angle from 105 to 95 degrees. This would allow her to achieve a sagittal back support angle of +5 degrees (as long as the seat sagittal angle is 0) to facilitate forward reaching. Her posture would most likely be compromised during the reach, and she would need to be educated in the importance of opening her seat to back support angle back up to 105 degrees for improved spinal alignment during rest.

The preceding example shows how describing and measuring both absolute and relative angles can improve the accuracy of communication and prescription, resulting in effective solutions and better clinical outcomes.

Purposeful deviations of a postural support device in the frontal and transverse planes is not common; however, such an adjustment may be necessary to support the person's body in a nonneutral position when there are joint limitations or contractures or to accommodate unique body shapes. For example, a lateral trunk support may need to be angled slightly in the frontal plane (tilted in or out viewed from front) to match the shape and angle of the client's trunk. Measuring the required angle, called the *lateral trunk support frontal angle*, would help in specifying the type of hardware needed to achieve the angle. If the angle was documented in the setup instructions, the lateral trunk support could also be adjusted or set up at this angle before the client fitting or delivery, improving efficiency and accuracy in service delivery. This would also be helpful if the client returned for a follow-up or is seen in the repair shop, with the lateral trunk support out of adjustment causing discomfort or leaning. If the original optimal adjustment was documented at the delivery in the form of an absolute angle measure, then the support can be readjusted quickly by a technician, saving time and cost and improving client satisfaction and outcomes.

It is important to note that the same principles are used to define absolute body segment angles and absolute support surface angles. This helps with prescription. For example, if the desired position of the thigh is windswept to the right, the transverse thigh angle can be measured and used to specify the lateral knee support transverse angle and foot support transverse angle required to support the thigh, lower leg, and foot in the desired position. If the thigh is parallel to the lateral knee support contact surface, the value of the transverse thigh angle and lateral knee support transverse angle should be the same.

Angular Measures of the Wheelchair Frame

Several wheelchair frame angles are critical to meeting the postural support and size needs of clients. These frame angles may or may not be the same as the corresponding seating system angles, depending on how the seating system is mounted to the wheelchair frame. In some wheelchair frames, the angles are adjustable, and in others, they are non-adjustable. In individually configured manual wheelchairs, most of these angles are welded into the frame of the wheelchair and are therefore non-adjustable. These wheelchairs are most frequently recommended for a person who has a long history of wheelchair use and knows exactly the frame geometry and configuration that works best for him or her.

Basic Measurement Set for Wheelchair Frame Angles

The following angular measures of the wheelchair frame should be considered and specified, if necessary, as part of a wheelchair recommendation. The need to specify these angles will depend on the type of wheelchair being recommended and whether there are any options other than a standard configuration to consider. Regardless of whether there is a need to specify the angle on an order form, it is important to understand what these angles represent and how they relate to corresponding seating system and body segment angles. Unfortunately, standardized terminology for all of these angles has not been developed or standardized through the ISO or RESNA process. To aid in discussion of these wheelchair dimensions, we have proposed the following angular measurement terms (Figure 6-28) based on terms used for the relevant wheelchair frame components and following the principles used in the seating standards:

- *Seat frame to back post angle*: The angle between the wheelchair seat frame/rail and the back posts. The angle above the seat frame is measured.
- *Seat frame to front frame angle*: The angle between the wheelchair seat frame/rail and the front frame structure. The angle behind the front frame structure is measured.

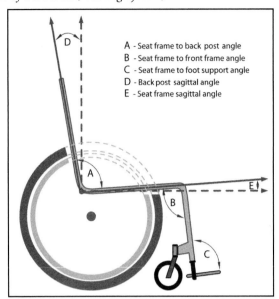

A - Seat frame to back post angle
B - Seat frame to front frame angle
C - Seat frame to foot support angle
D - Back post sagittal angle
E - Seat frame sagittal angle

Figure 6-28. Basic angular measures of the wheelchair frame: (A) seat frame to back post angle, (B) seat frame to front frame angle, (C) front frame to foot support angle, (D) back post sagittal angle, and (E) seat frame sagittal angle.

- *Front frame to foot support angle*: The angle between the wheelchair front frame structure and the foot support. The angle above the foot support is measured.
- *Seat frame sagittal angle*: The orientation of the wheelchair seat frame/rail with respect to the horizontal, viewed from the side.
- *Back post sagittal angle*: The orientation of the wheelchair back posts with respect to the vertical, viewed from the side.

Seat Frame to Back Post Angle

The angle between the seat frame and the back posts is clinically important because it impacts the corresponding seat to back support angle, which can significantly affect the client's seated posture, comfort and function. However, there is currently no standardized term for quantifying this angular measure. We propose the term *seat frame to back post angle*. The seat frame to back post angle may or may not be exactly the same as the corresponding *seat to back support angle*, depending on how the seat and back support are mounted to or integrated into the wheelchair frame. If the back post is attached to the seat frame with angle adjustable hardware, the wheelchair's seat frame to back post angle can be altered by angling the back canes. Achieving the desired seat to back support angle is typically done either through an adjustment of the seat frame to back post angle as described earlier, or through an adjustment of the back support sagittal angle via angle-adjustable hardware attaching the back support to the back posts.

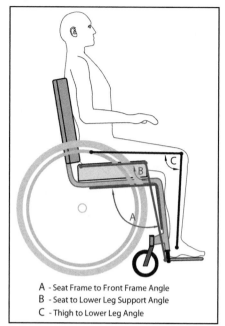

Figure 6-29. Seat frame to front frame angle with corresponding seating and body angles: (A) seat frame to front frame angle, (B) seat to lower leg support angle, and (C) thigh to lower leg angle.

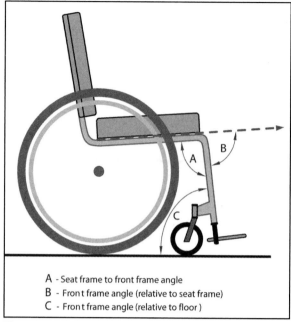

Figure 6-30. Comparing different wheelchair front frame angles: (A) seat frame to front frame angle, (B) front frame angle measured relative to the seat frame, and (C) front frame angle measured relative to the floor.

Seat Frame to Front Frame Angle

The angle between the seat frame and the front frame structure that supports the foot supports is clinically important because it affects the thigh to lower leg angle of the person, and can consequently influence postural alignment, especially when the person has tight hamstrings. This term is sometimes called the *front frame angle*; however, there is no standardized term or definition for this angular frame measure. We propose the term seat frame to front frame angle, measuring the angle behind the front frame structure so that it can be correlated to the seat to lower leg support angle and thigh to lower leg angle (Figure 6-29).

The term front frame angle is commonly used to describe the bend or angle between the seat rail and the front frame structure in a rigid manual wheelchair. However, it is measured in different ways by manufacturers, creating confusion (Figure 6-30). Some manufacturers measure the angle between the front frame structure and the floor, behind the vertically oriented front frame structure (Figure 6-30, C). Others measure the angle between a forward projection of the seat rail and the front frame structure, measured in front of the vertically oriented front frame component (Figure 6-30, B). If the front frame angle is measured relative to the floor, this angle will change if the slope of the seat frame is altered. Therefore, in the manufacturing process this front frame bend is created based on a specified seat frame slope, and the front frame angle measured in this way (relative to the floor) helps to align the caster housing vertically. If the front frame angle is measured relative to the

forward projection of the seat rail, it will not change with changes in seat slope. Both the proposed seat frame to front frame angle (see Figure 6-30A) and a front frame angle measured relative to the seat rail projection represent the true degree of bend between the seat frame and front frame structure, which is not altered by an adjustment of the seat frame slope. The true degree of bend between the seat rail and the front frame is clinically relevant when considering the desired thigh to lower leg angle of the wheelchair occupant, and it will also affect the overall depth of the wheelchair frame.

Many manual wheelchairs have swing-away or removable lower leg support assemblies (RESNA, 2009b), commonly referred to as *legrest hangers*. These are typically available in several angular styles, including 60-, 70-, 85-, or 90-degree options. These angular values represent the angle between a forward projection of the seat rail and the vertical hanger tube, measured in front of the lower leg support assembly. In this way, they are the same as a front frame angle measured relative to the seat rail projection in a rigid manual wheelchair. As use of the term *front frame angle* has not been standardized and is currently used to describe two very different angles on a rigid welded frame, we propose the term *lower leg support assembly angle* (Figure 6-31) to refer to this angle on a wheelchair with a non-fixed, swing away front end. Note that the seat frame to front frame angle and the lower leg support assembly angle are supplemental angles, meaning that the sum of their values equals 180 degrees.

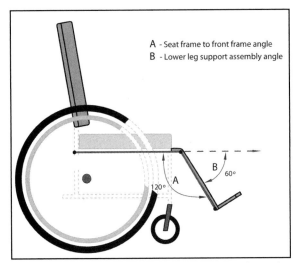

Figure 6-31. Seat frame to front frame angle vs lower leg support assembly angle in a wheelchair with swing-away foot supports

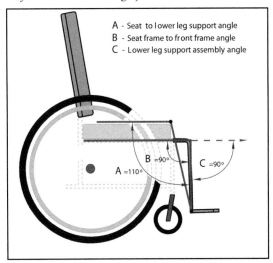

Figure 6-32. Seat to lower leg support angle vs wheelchair frame angles: (A) seat to lower leg support angle, (B) seat frame to front frame angle, (C) lower leg support assembly angle.

The terms front frame angle when measured from the seat frame (see Figure 6-30B) and lower leg support assembly angle represent the same angle (measured in front of the front frame component and relative to the seat rail) but are used with two different frame styles, the term front frame angle being more commonly used for rigid manual wheelchairs with welded front frames. Front frame angle, when measured from the floor, is used exclusively by some manufacturers of rigid frame manual wheelchairs, but it is dependent on a specified seat slope. These terms all represent a different angular measure than the proposed seat frame to front frame angle, which can be used to describe the angle between the seat rail and the front frame structure in a wheelchair with either a fixed or a swing away front end, but it is measured behind the front frame structure so as to better align with the corresponding body segment and support surface angles. It is important to remember that all of the angles described in this section are wheelchair frame angles that are related to, but not necessarily the same as, the seat to lower leg support angle (see Figures 6-22 and 6-32). The seat to lower leg support angle is a seating angle that can be altered by the forward or backward placement of the seat cushion or the foot supports, independent of the wheelchair frame geometry. Figure 6-32 shows the relationship between the seat to lower leg support and the corresponding wheelchair frame angles.

In summary, there is a lot of variation in terms used to describe the angle at the front of a wheelchair seat frame. The proposed term *seat frame to front frame angle* would provide a wheelchair frame angular measure that is defined in the same manner as the corresponding seat to lower leg support angle and thigh to lower leg angle, reducing communication errors, and helping with accurate prescription. This term would help differentiate it from the term *front frame angle*, which is currently used and measured

in varying ways by manufacturers. Using these three corresponding angles—*thigh to lower leg angle* (body), *seat to lower leg support angle* (seating), and the proposed *seat frame to front frame angle* (wheelchair)—would help with translation and prescription. The values for these three corresponding angular measures may or may not be exactly the same, depending on how the body is positioned with respect to the seat and depending on how the seat and foot supports are positioned in a forward-backward position relative to the frame.

Front Frame to Foot Support Angle

The angle between the front frame structure that supports the foot supports and the foot support itself is an important feature because it can affect the degree of ankle dorsiflexion that the client rests in; however, there is no standardized term for quantifying this angular frame measure. We propose the term *front frame to foot support angle* (see Figure 6-28) to differentiate it from the corresponding lower leg support to foot support angle. These two angles may or may not be the same, depending on whether the lower leg support reference plane (on which the seating angle is defined) is parallel to the vertically oriented front frame structure. The front frame to foot support angle may be fixed or adjustable. Adjustability typically comes from angling the foot supports at their attachment to the front frame structure when this feature is available.

Seat Frame Sagittal Angle

The orientation, or angle, of the seat frame with respect to the horizontal is an important feature affecting a client's postural stability, comfort, and function; however, there is currently no standardized term for quantifying this orientation. When the seat frame orientation is adjustable it is typically part of a wheelchair with an adjustable tilt

	TABLE 6-4	
RELATED WHEELCHAIR, SEATING, AND BODY SEGMENT ANGLES		
WHEELCHAIR FRAME ANGLE	**RELATED SEATING ANGLE**	**RELATED BODY ANGLE**
Seat frame to back post angle	Seat to back support angle	Thigh to trunk angle
Seat frame to front frame angle	Seat to lower leg support angle	Thigh to lower leg angle
Front frame to foot support angle	Lower leg support to foot support angle	Lower leg to foot angle
Seat frame sagittal angle	Seat sagittal angle	Sagittal thigh angle
Back post sagittal angle	Back support sagittal angle	Sagittal trunk angle

feature, either power or manual. As discussed earlier in the section on rear and front seat frame height, when the seat frame is inclined (higher in the front than the rear), this is commonly referred to as dump in a standard (nonvariable positioning) wheelchair.

We propose the term *seat frame sagittal angle* (see Figure 6-28) to quantify the degree of seat incline or decline to correlate this measure with the corresponding seat sagittal angle. The seat frame sagittal angle and the seat sagittal angle would be the same when the seat support surface reference plane lies parallel to the wheelchair seat frame. The values for these angles would be different if the seat support is mounted to the seat frame at an angle or if the seat-cushion shape is wedged.

Back Post Sagittal Angle

The orientation of the wheelchair back posts is an important feature because it affects the client's trunk balance and function, and it can also affect the seat to back support angle. However, there is currently no standardized term for quantifying this frame angle. The corresponding support surface angle to this frame angle is the back support sagittal angle, which measures the angle of the back support with respect to the vertical. Accordingly, we propose the term *back post sagittal angle* (see Figure 6-28) to describe the angle of the back posts compared with the vertical. These two angles would be the same if the back support reference plane is parallel to the back posts. However, they are frequently different because many off-the-shelf back supports are mounted to the back posts using angle adjustable hardware, allowing the back support sagittal angle to be altered without a change in the back post angle.

Relating Angular Dimensions of the Wheelchair Frame, Seating System, and Body

As a summary of this section on wheelchair frame angular dimensions, Table 6-4 lists the terms for the basic angular measures of the wheelchair frame, with their corresponding primary angular measure of the seating system and body.

TOOLS FOR MEASURING

Measurement tools will certainly vary based on the setting in which they are used, but it is important to understand the impact of tools on the reliability and accuracy of the measures. The use of any measurement tool requires practice for measures to be reliable (or repeatable). When greater accuracy is desired, it is often useful to take a measurement two or three times to check repeatability. All parties involved in the measurement aspects should be familiar with the available tools and practice their use, as this will only improve accuracy overall.

Accuracy of measures is more critical when prescribing wheelchairs with non-adjustable seating or frame dimensions vs those that have some adjustability in their linear or angular features. In addition, some client diagnoses and clinical presentations will demand higher degrees of measurement accuracy to achieve optimal outcomes. Muscular dystrophy is one example of a diagnostic group characterized by demands for very specific postural support device requirements with respect to dimensions, placement and angular orientation of support surfaces. The *Clinical Application Guide* (Waugh & Crane, 2013a) contains detailed sample measurement methodologies using inexpensive tools for all linear and angular measures defined in the guide and described in this chapter.

Tools for Measuring Linear Dimensions

Linear measures of the body and seating support surfaces are typically taken using a tape measure or caliper system, but a metal ruler or yardstick could also be used for some measures. When using a tape measure, a 1/2-inch or larger metal tape measure that won't easily bend is recommended for greater accuracy. Measuring linear dimensions of the body and the seating system components may be quite challenging at times. The body and many postural support devices have multiple contours and are made of materials with varying degrees of compliance (i.e., softness) that may make them difficult to accurately measure. For some linear measures of the body, it can be helpful to use a firm flat surface, such as a clipboard, to hold lightly against the soft, contoured tissue of the body for greater accuracy. As mentioned previously in this chapter, it is important to understand how the compliance of materials in a PSD may affect its linear dimensions when loaded and in use by the person.

Tools for Measuring Angles

Tools available for measuring the body, support surface, and wheelchair angles vary, depending on the angular measure of interest, the accuracy required, and the setting (clinical vs research). Tools range from simple and inexpensive goniometers to sophisticated (and costly) three-dimensional digitizers used in research labs.

Measuring Relative Angles

All relative angles of the body, seating system, or wheelchair frame can be measured using a standard goniometer. Any of the goniometers available for measuring joint ROM can be used. To measure a relative angle, each arm of the goniometer is aligned with one of the two adjacent body segments, support surfaces, or wheelchair frame components that comprise the angle. For relative body angles, the goniometer arm is aligned with a defined body segment line connecting two body landmarks. For relative support surface angles, the goniometer arms are aligned parallel to the adjacent and intersecting support surface reference planes.

Measuring Absolute Angles

All absolute angles can be measured using either an inclinometer or a goniometer. Unlike relative angle measures, absolute angles cannot be as easily measured using a standard goniometer. For this reason, an inclinometer is preferable for taking sagittal and frontal angles. However, transverse angles cannot be measured using an inclinometer.

Using a goniometer to measure absolute angles is challenging because absolute angles are measured by comparing the line on the body segment or support surface to an external reference—the vertical, horizontal, or axis of the wheelchair. Therefore, you must sight to this external reference when aligning one arm of the goniometer. To measure a sagittal or frontal angle, you must be able to identify a vertical or horizontal line to which you can align one arm of the goniometer. Some goniometers have built-in or add-on bubble levels mounted at the distal end of the stationary arm. This device will convert the stationary arm to a vertical or horizontal reference; however, it must be held steady, which is difficult.

Sagittal and Frontal Angles

It is recommended that for all vertically or horizontally referenced absolute angles of either the client's body or the postural support devices (i.e., all sagittal and frontal angles), an inclinometer, either analog or digital, is a more useful tool to use. Inclinometers will display the angular deviation from either a horizontal or a vertical reference automatically. Analog inclinometers are commonly available at hardware stores and report the deviation of any line or plane from a gravitational vertical line. Some have the capacity to provide measures that are deviations from either a vertical or from a horizontal reference. Digital inclinometers are a bit more costly, but they may provide improved precision over an analog tool, and may be more useful in a research or design setting where higher levels of precision are necessary.

Transverse Angles

Transverse body segment or seating system angles pose different challenges. Inclinometers cannot be used to measure absolute angles in the transverse plane because these angles do not reference the horizontal or vertical, and thus are not gravitationally affected. Measuring these angles requires sighting to a reference line that is based on the wheelchair geometry, a line either parallel to or perpendicular to the rear wheel axle. Using a goniometer, one arm of the goniometer is aligned with the body segment line or support surface reference line, and the other is aligned parallel to the designated wheelchair axis.

New Tools for Measuring Angles

Development of new tools for measuring relative and absolute angles has been occurring in parallel with the development of the ISO seating standard. Additionally, there are many commercially available apps for tablets and smart phones that may be useful in measuring body, seating system, or wheelchair angles.

Two of the new tools developed in Japan are the Horizon tool and Rysis software. The Horizon is a device similar to a digital inclinometer, but it can measure absolute angles in the transverse plane as well as angles in the sagittal and frontal plane. The Horizon is not yet available in the United States; although, plans to bring it to market are underway. Additionally, the capabilities in the Horizon tool are now available in a Horizon app (the i-Horizon) that can be purchased through the iTunes store. This app is available for iPad and iPhone (Apple) hardware devices.

The Rysis software was also developed in Japan, and is specifically used to quantify seated posture by measuring body segment angles. It is available to download at no cost; however, it requires additional setup of cameras and landmark location probes for use. Using this software, clinicians mark body landmarks of interest using 1/2-inch diameter adhesive markers, point to these markers with probes, and then capture a digital image. This digital image is then analyzed using computer-based image analysis software, resulting in a report of sagittal, frontal, and transverse absolute body segment angle values that describe the person's posture.

SUMMARY

Although taking linear measurements of the client's body to prescribe a wheelchair that fits is basic common practice, the use of angular measures in seating assessment is not yet commonplace. We hope that the information in this chapter will encourage readers to incorporate more of these angular measures into practice. Matching the body segment angles and body dimensions to the seating support system for optimal fit and function enhances prescription quality. Use of specific and unique terms for angular measures of the body, the seating system, and the wheelchair helps focus the attention of the clinician and the supplier on the critical impact that angular dimensions have on the client's sitting posture and function. This will help CRT professionals recommend the appropriate wheelchair and seating features needed, facilitate efficient communication of seating system parameters to shop technicians for setup, and ultimately maximize efficiency and quality at the time of delivery.

With such an assortment of measures available, how is a clinician to decide what to measure and when to measure it? It is recommended that the basic set of linear measures, the three relative body segment angles, and the three relative support surface angles described in this chapter be measured and recorded with most every client as a part of best clinical practice in the area of wheelchair seating. However, the set of measures to take will always be situation-dependent, based on the complexity of the presenting problems and the type of wheeled mobility equipment being recommended. Certainly, specific measures that are appropriate for clinical decision-making regarding feature selection will be critical to measure and record. Some clinicians may develop a routine practice of measuring a core set of absolute and relative body segment angles for their clients that they find most useful for making decisions regarding seating strategies and product recommendations or for monitoring their effectiveness. This core set of measures may be determined on the basis of client diagnoses, clinical presentation, type of wheeled mobility device, or other factors involved in the clinic's routine practice. Decisions about what should be measured are not always easy to make, but the power of having the ability to quantify these critical measures is undeniable, and it is likely that many clinicians will expand their basic set of measures as they develop a greater understanding of the measures, as well as confidence and skill in measurement methodologies. We also hope that you will begin to see the benefits of quantifying postural objectives as a way to elevate the quality of your practice as a CRT professional, with positive outcomes for your clients.

As emphasized throughout this chapter, it is vital to use accurate terminology when recording all linear and angular measures. Measures of the seating system and wheelchair must be easily differentiated from the relevant body measures so that it is clear what is being measured. Ultimately, all these measures are interrelated, but during the evaluation and documentation process, it is necessary to be very clear as to what is being recorded—a body measure, a seating system measure, or the associated wheelchair frame measure. Being clear in the use of terms for different measurements supports efficient and accurate communication regarding key parameters of the wheelchair system.

The Need for Standardization of Wheelchair Frame Measures

Although some of the terms for wheelchair frame linear and angular dimensions described in this chapter are defined in international and national standards, there is still significant variation in the terms used for these measures and how they are defined across manufacturers. Until a standard method of labeling, measuring, and reporting the linear and angular dimensions of a wheelchair frame is agreed on and used by all manufacturers, the responsibility of interpreting the manufacturer's literature and order forms falls on the clinician and supplier. Prescribing or choosing the correct wheelchair frame angles or configuration to ensure that the client's optimal seated posture and function can be achieved is a critical final step in the wheelchair evaluation and prescription process. Fortunately, most manufacturers do supply graphic information in their brochures indicating how a dimension is measured. Product literature frequently contains diagrams and descriptions produced by the manufacturer's themselves. Obtaining product demos for specific wheelchair bases is another good method for determining optimal fit and configuration, although this is not always possible, particularly with highly configurable wheelchairs. Close relationships among the client, clinician, supplier, and manufacturer's representative will also help with understanding the plethora of sizes and configurations of manual and power wheelchairs. As the international and national standards development work continues to evolve, efforts will be made to standardize some of these more critical measures and make them consistent with the body and seating system measures.

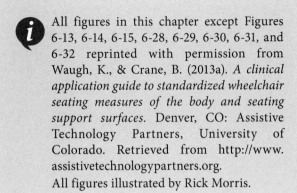

All figures in this chapter except Figures 6-13, 6-14, 6-15, 6-28, 6-29, 6-30, 6-31, and 6-32 reprinted with permission from Waugh, K., & Crane, B. (2013a). *A clinical application guide to standardized wheelchair seating measures of the body and seating support surfaces.* Denver, CO: Assistive Technology Partners, University of Colorado. Retrieved from http://www.assistivetechnologypartners.org.

All figures illustrated by Rick Morris.

REFERENCES

International Organization for Standardization. (1998). *ISO 7176-7: Wheelchairs—Part 7: Measurement of seating and wheel dimensions.* Geneva, Switzerland: International Organization for Standardization.

International Organization for Standardization. (2006). *ISO 16840: Wheelchair Seating, Part 1—Vocabulary, reference axis convention and measures for body posture and postural support surfaces.* Geneva, Switzerland: Author.

Rehabilitation Engineering and Assistive Technology Society of North America. (2009a). *ANSI/RESNA WC 1 Section 7: Measurement of seating and wheel dimensions.* Arlington, VA: Author.

Rehabilitation Engineering and Assistive Technology Society of North America. (2009b). *ANSI/RESNA WC 1 Section 26: Vocabulary,* Arlington, VA: Author.

Rehabilitation Engineering and Assistive Technology Society of North America. (2013). *ANSI/RESNA WC 3 Section 1: Wheelchair Seating—Vocabulary, reference axis convention and measures for body posture and postural support surfaces.* Arlington, VA: Author.

Waugh, K., & Crane, B. (2013a). *A clinical application guide to standardized wheelchair seating measures of the body and seating support surfaces.* Denver, CO: Assistive Technology Partners, University of Colorado. Retrieved from http://www.assistivetechnologypartners.org

Waugh, K., & Crane, B. (2013b). *Glossary of wheelchair terms and definitions, Version 1.0.* Denver, CO: Assistive Technology Partners, University of Colorado. Retrieved from http://www.assistivetechnologypartners.org

Posture Management 24/7

Atli Ágústsson, PT, MSc Bioeng and Guðný Jónsdóttir, PT, MSc

More people are living with a disability now than in the past because we're living longer and improved medical treatments are enabling more people, children and adults, to manage complex health problems (World Health Organization [WHO], 2011). Population aging is a reality in nearly all the countries of the world, and will have a major impact on the organization and delivery of health and long-term care with relatively fewer people to provide the services that disabled people need. It is therefore important to choose well the strategies needed to maintain, support, and improve outcomes for health and quality of life. For people with severe and complex physical disabilities, one of the most important health interventions is 24-hour posture management (PM).

According to WHO (2015), the highest attainable standard of health is a fundamental part of our human rights and our understanding of a life in dignity. Violating the right to health may impair the enjoyment of other human rights. PM is basically a public health intervention and empowerment aimed at the client's health and future possibilities. It empowers parents and caregivers as they gain knowledge and information on what they can do to protect and enhance the individual's health and well-being. PM emphasizes advising, training, and supporting clients, caregivers, clinicians, doctors, and others.

PM recognizes that postural stability is a fundamental necessity for effective functional performance. The effect of poor PM on clients' health and quality of life can be both complex and devastating, as many, or even most, of our vital functions are affected by the ability to control posture.

PM includes positioning using special seating, nighttime support, and standing supports, as well as orthotics, individual therapy sessions, and active exercise, such as horseback riding and swimming. PM interventions may be used in combination with tone reducing medicine (i.e., intrathecal baclofen and botulinum injections) and orthopedic surgery. Medication and orthopedic surgery without PM are not likely to result in improved outcomes.

Clients who will benefit from 24-hour PM are children and adults who, through disease, accident, metabolic malfunction, or congenital abnormalities, have lost or have minimal ability to independently alter their position, maintain an erect sitting position, stand, or walk (Pope, 2007b). This includes clients with cerebral palsy (CP), acquired brain injury, spinal cord injury, multiple sclerosis, amyotrophic lateral sclerosis, and even the elderly. Unmanaged postures will deteriorate due to the crushing effects of gravity, neuromuscular impairment, and the plasticity of body structures.

The underlying assumption of PM is that by preventing secondary complications, clients will have better function, experience less pain and fatigue, and maintain health-related quality of life. They should also need to undergo fewer and less complicated surgeries and enjoy greater participation in society. The need for PM is ongoing and should be incorporated into the client's lifestyle. The situation needs to be monitored with changes made when necessary. Reviews need to be, at a minimum, annually for children and annually or every other year for adults.

Lange, M. L., & Minkel, J. L.
Seating and Wheeled Mobility: A Clinical Resource Guide
(pp. 121-136). © 2018 SLACK Incorporated.

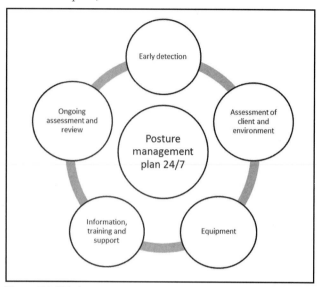

Figure 7-1. PM plan.

PLANNING FOR 24-HOUR POSTURE MANAGEMENT

PM should commence as soon as a motor problem has been identified that is known to lead to postural asymmetry if not managed. As a prerequisite to any PM plan (Figure 7-1), it is necessary to conduct physical, medical and social assessment. The key is an individually tailored PM program.

The Gross Motor Functioning Classification System (GMFCS) is a five-level clinical classification system that describes the gross motor function of people with CP on the basis of self-initiated movement abilities (Palisano et al., 1997). GMFCS can be used to guide and predict the need and nature of PM intervention while remaining dependent on individual circumstances. Children in GMFCS groups IV and V should start 24-hour PM programs in lying as soon as appropriate after birth, in sitting from 6 months of age, and in standing from 12 months of age (Gericke, 2006).

According to the results of the evaluation of the Posture and Postural Ability Scale (PPAS), postural asymmetries and deviations were detected at all GMFCS levels (Rodby-Bousquet et al., 2014; Rodby-Bousquet, Persson-Bunke, & Czuba, 2015). Prevention of secondary complication through PM and physical activity, like swimming, horseback riding and other sports, from an early age is therefore vital for individuals with a motor disorder at GMFCS level I through III.

Assessment of needs includes the client's abilities, critical measures, and need for support, availability of equipment, and caregiver assistance available. It is vital to gather information on health problems, such as pain, risk of pressure injuries, respiratory problems, seizures, gastroesophageal reflux, incontinence, osteoporosis, surgeries,

and medications. Sleep studies may be needed before and after the introduction of the equipment to ensure safety (Hill, Parker, Allen, Paul, & Padoa, 2009).

Other valuable information includes information on daily routines, time spent in different positions over a 24-hour period, what has been tried, and how it has worked. It is necessary to know how the client is handled and if that requires assistance of one person or two. Note the use of orthotics and results of recent x-rays of spine and hips, if they are available.

Parents and paid assistants become the key to successful provision of PM, and so education, information, training, and ongoing support are extremely important.

Posture Management Plan: Key Factors for Consideration

- Assessment of the client and client needs
- Family dynamics and opinions of the client and caregivers
- Lifestyle of the client and family
- Aesthetics and ease of use of the PM equipment
- Risk assessment for nighttime PM equipment
- Team process
- Importance of education, training, and support

SECONDARY COMPLICATIONS

People with lifelong disability may have subtle or no musculoskeletal distortion as newborns, but contractures and asymmetries tend to develop early on. Therefore, in people with ongoing disability, the focus should be on minimizing secondary complications that are not a direct result of the impairment itself. These complications are largely the result of the inability to move effectively, stabilize posture, and change position (Fulford & Brown, 1976; Pope, 2007b).

For the client with motor impairment, the asymmetric habitual posture increases the risk of tissue adaptation and will eventually lead to musculoskeletal distortions. Whenever the body deviates from midline, a gravitational torque is produced, and compounds the deviation (Pope, 2007b). Musculoskeletal complications, such as contractures of muscles and joints, scoliosis, pelvic obliquity, hip dislocations, and windswept distortion, will result in problems with sitting, standing, and walking; risk of fractures; pressure injuries; and increased difficulty with perineal care.

Contractures are a critical secondary complication that affects posture and positioning. These can be defined as a loss of joint mobility due to structural changes of muscles, tendons, ligaments, and other arthrogenic structures. A normal range in the movement of a joint is maintained by repeated movements of the body part each day by a nondisabled person. According to Tardieu, Lespargot, Tabary, and Bret (1988), a muscle must be in a stretched position more than 6 hours daily simply to maintain its length. Evidence suggests that conservative management using 24-hour positioning before the development of hip displacement can reduce hip dislocation in children with bilateral cerebral palsy (Pountney, Mandy, Green, & Gard, 2002).

Upper extremities have not been regarded as a matter of urgency for therapists, although they do need to be addressed. To stress this, Rodby-Bousquet, Czuba, Hagglund, and Westbom (2013) found that limited elbow extension increased the odds ratio for postural asymmetries. Orthopedic distortions in the upper extremities lead to impaired hand function, decreased ability to perform activities of daily living, and increased dependency.

Pain due to progressive musculoskeletal complications is another serious secondary complication and is associated with higher levels of mental health problems and decreases in self-mobility, functional activities, and health-related quality of life (Ramstad, Jahnsen, Skjeldal, & Diseth, 2012). According to a systematic review on comorbidities and functional limitations associated with CP, 75% of the subjects experienced pain in a typical week (Novak, Hines, Goldsmith, & Barclay, 2012).

WHEN SHOULD POSTURE MANAGEMENT START?

PM should ideally be started before muscular and orthopedic changes occur. The following case study illustrates what can happen in as little as 6 months without intervention and should encourage all clinicians to implement PM in all circumstances, regardless of the setting. This child (Figure 7-2) suffered an anoxic brain injury at age 11 years after complications during an appendectomy ended in cardiopulmonary arrest. Before this, he was a healthy and typically developing child who loved to play football and write poems. He survived, but over the next 6 months he developed irreversible asymmetries, including scoliosis and pelvic obliquity, as well as contractures in his neck, arms, hands, hips, knees, and feet.

Distortive positions along with increased tone led to high stress accummulation areas within his body. The tissue adaption rate was high because of his young age, and the resultant stress accummulation (see the later section, "Biomechanics") resulted in severe secondary impairments. The importance of protecting body structures and preventing such outcomes from day one is clear.

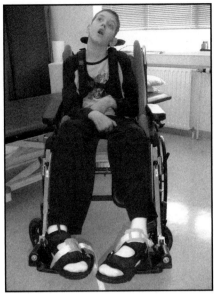

Figure 7-2. Consequences of a lack of posture management for a child with traumatic brain injury.

POSTURE MANAGEMENT FOR EMPOWERMENT

Poor PM compounds secondary complications and affects vital functions, such as respiration, digestion, and swallowing, and will also increase the risk for urinary tract and fungal infections. The inability to stabilize body segments can lead to increased spasticity and excessive muscle work, have an impact on environmental interaction for communication and learning, and affect body image and self-confidence. Last but not least, poor PM can negatively affect self-mobility, functional ability, and overall independence, and lead to an increased need for further intervention, medication, and orthopedic surgery.

Implementation of PM should therefore be considered as empowerment, both for the client and the caregivers who, with knowledge and support, can help minimize or prevent secondary complications for protection of the client's health and function.

Poor Positioning Affects the Client's Functional Potential

- Even though positioned in a custom-molded seating system, the client's posture compounds any distortion of the spine (Figure 7-3).

- Communication potential is restricted and the client is locked in a limited world. The internal organs are compressed and posture has a negative effect on swallowing and breathing—two vital functions. Posture also affects appearance and body image.

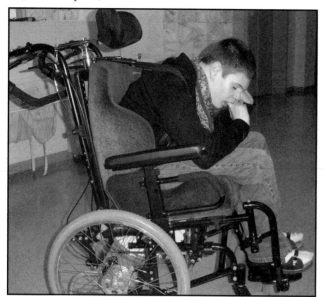

Figure 7-3. The effect of gravity on an unsupported seated position.

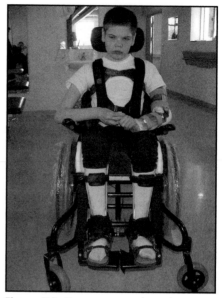

Figure 7-4. Empowerment through posture management.

Empowerment for Health, Communication, and Participation Through Proper Positioning

- Trunk, head, and lower limbs are now well-supported, and the arms are free for functional tasks. Improved comfort and posture result in increased arousal level for communication, learning, and participation (Figure 7-4).

- Pressure on internal organs is reduced, swallowing is easier, and danger of respiratory problems is decreased. This posture does not compound body distortion in the way it did before.

- An adequate lumbar lordosis is necessary to create postural forces that optimize thoracic spine and scapular positioning in upright. Without that structural support, other interventions are unlikely to work. This can be addressed in supine in a hook-lying position with a T-roll or pillow under the knees and a towel roll or soft foam half-roll along the spine or across the lumbar spine as appropriate for thoracic extension.

POSTURE AND POSTURAL ABILITY

Posture is an actively stabilized orientation of the body and its segments in space and in relation to each other. A person's posture is his or her frame of reference with respect to the external world. The frame of reference for a person standing upright differs from that of a person sitting in a wheelchair. The central nervous system regulates the control of posture (Hadders-Algra, 2008; Pope, 2007b).

Good posture is defined as:

[T]he body attitude (position) that helps create maximum performance for minimal energy consumption and does so without causing damage to the body. (Pope, 2007b)

Postural ability is the ability to stabilize the body segments relative to each other and to the supporting surface, as well as to get into the most appropriate body configuration for the performance of the particular task and environment. This means control of the center of gravity relative to the base of support during both static and dynamic conditions (Rodby-Bousquet et al., 2014).

The Posture and Postural Ability Scale

It is clinically relevant to detect asymmetric posture early to apply the appropriate intervention to minimize progressive distortions. The PPAS is sensitive to detect small postural asymmetries and deviations at an early stage at all levels of motor function and provides information relevant to postural support solutions in order to prevent musculoskeletal distortions and improve function. The PPAS can also be used to evaluate effectiveness of therapeutic interventions designed to increase functional ability and to prevent secondary complications (Pope, 2007b; Rodby-Bousquet et al., 2014).

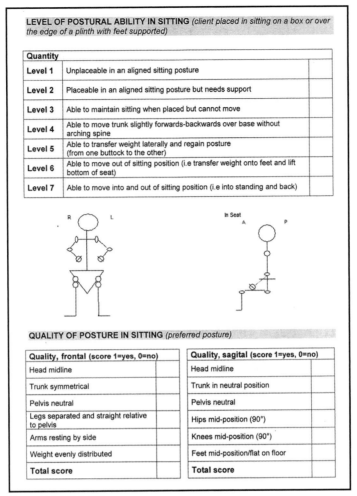

LEVEL OF POSTURAL ABILITY IN SITTING *(client placed in sitting on a box or over the edge of a plinth with feet supported)*

Quantity		
Level 1	Unplaceable in an aligned sitting posture	
Level 2	Placeable in an aligned sitting posture but needs support	
Level 3	Able to maintain sitting when placed but cannot move	
Level 4	Able to move trunk slightly forwards-backwards over base without arching spine	
Level 5	Able to transfer weight laterally and regain posture (from one buttock to the other)	
Level 6	Able to move out of sitting position (i.e transfer weight onto feet and lift bottom of seat)	
Level 7	Able to move into and out of sitting position (i.e into standing and back)	

QUALITY OF POSTURE IN SITTING *(preferred posture)*

Quality, frontal (score 1=yes, 0=no)		Quality, sagital (score 1=yes, 0=no)	
Head midline		Head midline	
Trunk symmetrical		Trunk in neutral position	
Pelvis neutral		Pelvis neutral	
Legs separated and straight relative to pelvis		Hips mid-position (90°)	
Arms resting by side		Knees mid-position (90°)	
Weight evenly distributed		Feet mid-position/flat on floor	
Total score		**Total score**	

Figure 7-5. PPAS sitting.

The PPAS includes a seven-point ordinal scale for postural ability in supine, prone, sitting, and standing conditions, as well as six items for assessment of posture (Figures 7-5 and 7-6). The assessment does not require special equipment, is easy to use in a clinical setting, and takes about 10 minutes to complete. This assessment tool allows postural ability and posture to be assessed separately, but it has no grading and cannot differentiate between a mild, moderate, or severe deviation.

BIOMECHANICS

Basic understanding of biomechanics is vital when practicing PM. Biomechanics applies the laws of physics on living objects. In PM, the biomechanical focus is in two areas: tissue biomechanics and the effects of gravity on posture and positioning.

Plasticity, or tissue adaptation, occurs when the human body as a whole, or individual body parts, remodel in adapting to a new environment. This can be a normal process, such as when a child grows, or a destructive process, as when hip displacement evolves into a hip dislocation. Throughout life, the human body is constantly remodeling itself; mature tissue is removed from the body, and new tissue is formed in its place, thus regenerating the human body. Typically, newborn babies regenerate 100% of their body/year, but adults only regenerate 10%/year. To complicate matters, localized high stress accumulation increases the local regeneration rate, resulting in tissue adaptation.

Tissue biomechanics both explain and predict the consequences on musculoskeletal tissue of staying too long in a harmful position. Biomechanical properties of musculoskeletal tissue have been known for decades and give a solid theoretical foundation for posture management.

Tissue Biomechanics

The main cause of distortion of the human body is the inability to stabilize body parts (Pope, 2007b). Although there are a number of medical explanations for this instability, the distortion is due to the biomechanical effect of staying too long in a harmful position. Plasticity and

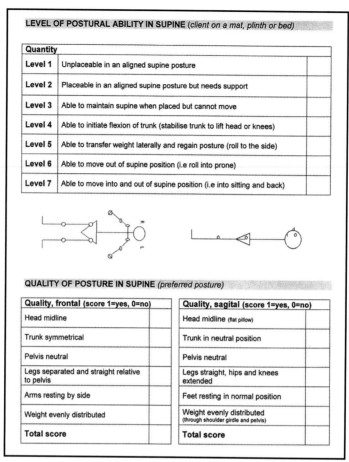

Figure 7-6. PPAS supine.

viscoelastic behavior of the musculoskeletal tissue explains the mechanics behind the formation of distorted body parts.

Windswept hips are a classic example of distortion due to instability and are therefore used here to demonstrate the formation of a functional distortion. This process will happen anywhere in the human body if it is placed in a harmful posture for too long.

When lying on the back with flexed hips, knees, and feet on the mattress, muscle activity is needed to stabilize the knees in a vertical position. Many clients are unable to lay on their back with the legs fully extended due to lack of hip and knee extension. If the client cannot stabilize the knees, the legs will fall to one side (Figure 7-7). When the knees start to fall to the side from a vertical orientation, the effect of gravity acts on the knees and takes them into a downward arc directed to the mattress.

As the knees fall to the side, the slack in arthrogenic and myogenic structures (AMS) (Trudel & Uhthoff, 2000) at the contralateral side in the hips is taken up and becomes stretched. This starts a chain reaction. The stretched AMS pull the pelvis, which starts to rotate and pulls the fifth lumbar vertebrae. This chain reaction continues up the spinal column until the body as a whole is stable (Figure 7-8).

Even though the body is stable, in the sense that it is not moving, gravity is still pushing the body down and the knees over to the side. The AMS on the contralateral side are now fully stretched and will show viscoelastic behavior, which is demonstrated first by a spontaneous elastic and then a slow viscous elongation of the AMS during the time while the knees are under the influence of gravity.

The AMS can elongate only so far before reaching their elastic limit, which is the limit to which a structure can be stretched before it starts to fail. However, gravity does not stop and, when the AMS cannot elongate any further, failure and microruptures occur. This causes permanent damage, and the AMS will not return to their original length; hence, these structures have become permanently elongated.

Tissue remodeling will repair the microruptures of the stretched structures by laying down newly synthesized collagen fibers in the line of the stress. But if one side of a joint is stretched, then the other side will be slackened. This is vital when discussing posture management and 24-hour positioning. Tissue adaptation is occurring on the slack side as well, and because there is no stress on the slack side, the newly synthesized collagen fibers are laid down in all directions, in a hay-like manner.

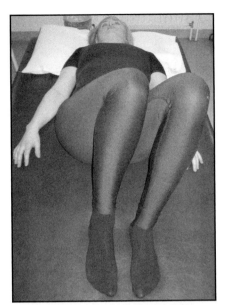

Figure 7-7. Unstable lower extremities in an unsupported supine position.

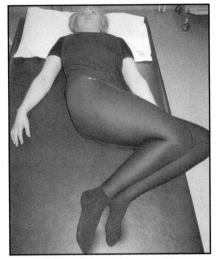

Figure 7-8. Lower extremities have fallen down to the mattress due to effects of gravity.

Staying in this posture repeatedly for long periods of time causes tissues to adapt to the new environment. On one side, all structures shorten, while on the contralateral side, lengthening occurs. This plasticity of tissues will lead to contracture, which will increase with time.

Biomechanical Effects of Gravity on Posture and Positioning

The human sandwich effect (Hare, 1987) is the combined effect of gravity and the ground reaction force on the body. Gravity comes from above, pushing physical objects such as the human body down, and ground reaction force comes from below, pushing the human body up, thus the human body is squeezed in between them like a human sandwich.

Supine

When an able-bodied person lies symmetrically on his or her back, the base of support of the trunk is wide and stable (Figure 7-9). With time, the human sandwich effect will, when lying repeatedly for a long time in supine, give the body a flattened appearance. The back of the skull and the rib cage flatten out and the upper and lower extremities are taken into external rotation with some abduction in the shoulders and the hip joints. The feet go into plantarflexion.

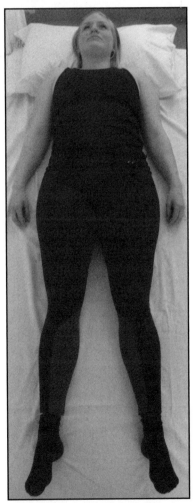

Figure 7-9. Symmetrical supine lying.

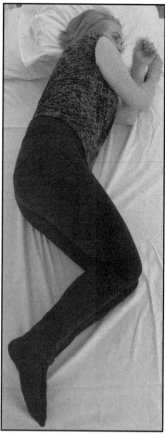

Figure 7-10. Symmetrical side lying.

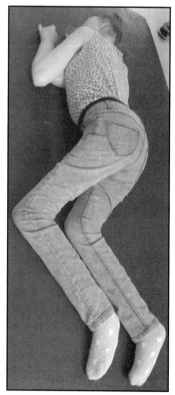

Figure 7-12. An individual lying on the concave side.

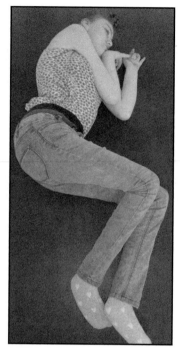

Figure 7-11. Individual with severe scoliosis lying on the convex side of the scoliosis.

Side Lying

When an able-bodied person lies symmetrically with hips and knees in flexion on his or her side, the base of support of the trunk is narrow and small (Figure 7-10). The human sandwich effect of side lying results in the following: the head becomes narrow, the width of the trunk gets narrower, the anterior posterior diameter increases, the sternum goes forward, the shoulders go up, the back becomes kyphotic, and the pelvis assumes a posterior tilt.

Scoliosis and Side Lying

The comfortable posture for side lying for individuals with scoliosis on the convex side is accomplished by rotating the thorax into a supine direction (Figure 7-11). The comfortable posture for side lying on the concave side is accomplished by rotating the thorax into a prone direction (Figure 7-12) (Fulford & Brown, 1976). In both of these side-lying positions, the human sandwich effect will compound scoliosis by enhancing its rotational aspect. This was described by Fulford and Brown (1976) more than 4 decades ago. Even so, large numbers of individuals with scoliosis still sleep in these positions.

Lying Prone

When an able-bodied person lies on his or her abdomen, the base of support of the trunk appears to be wide and stable (Figure 7-13). However, the head is turned to the side, creating internal instability within the trunk. The human sandwich effect squeezes the rib cage even more than in the supine position because the spinal column is the highest and heaviest part of the trunk. Due to the lack of bony support over the abdominal area, the spinal column sinks even further down, exaggerating the lordosis in the lumbar spine and dragging the pelvis into an excessive anterior tilt. The orientation of the legs in prone lying can be classified in three categories: adduction, abduction, or windswept posture (Hill & Goldsmith, 2010). The feet in all three scenarios go into plantarflexion, and the upper extremities will inevitably flex at the elbows.

Whether supine, prone, or side lying, the feet will always go into plantarflexion. As was demonstrated in the tissue biomechanics section, if the AMS of a joint are in a shortened position repeatedly for long periods, they will shorten. Therefore, short calf muscles should not come as a surprise.

HABITUAL POSTURE

The work of Porter, Michael, and Kirkwood (2010) supports the suggestion put forward by Fulford and Brown (1976) that disabled infants may already have a preferred pattern of asymmetrical posture and that there is an association between asymmetrical lying posture adopted in the first year of life and the direction of the subsequent pattern of postural distortion. Rotation of the head to the right during supine lying therefore makes it more likely that the scoliosis will be convex to the left, pelvic obliquity will be lower on the left, the windswept hip pattern will be to the right, and hip subluxation or dislocation will occur on the left. The likelihood of the distortion occurring in the same direction is also increased if consistent lying on the right side is preferred. Limited hip and knee extension are highly associated with postural asymmetries.

Adults with later onset of low level of postural ability, who lie in an asymmetrical habitual posture due to incorrect positioning, will eventually develop musculoskeletal distortions. It is the biomechanical effect of being in the same position over a long period of time.

CASE EXAMPLE

Case Study 7-1: A 4-month-old boy started to show postural asymmetry with deviation over to the right. The mat examination demonstrated that the rotational symmetry of the body was altered because the knees, in hook-lying,

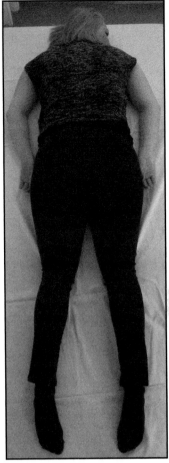

Figure 7-13. Prone lying.

did not rotate as far to the left as to the right. The PPAS qualitative score while supine was 2. All findings indicated postural asymmetry (Figure 7-14).

More than 95% of newborns have no functional distortions, but even so, many will show some sign of postural asymmetry before they begin to sit. This is due to habitual posture.

During the last 10 weeks of pregnancy, the unborn baby spends more and more time in the same position and, at the end, usually stays in that position. The baby carried in a left occipital-anterior/lateral position is more likely to adopt a supine head right-lying posture and vice versa. If the head is turned over to the right, arms and legs go over to the right and the trunk has lateral flexion to the right (Porter et al., 2010).

After the baby is born, he will conveniently fall asleep faster and sleep longer while in this position over to right. In the first 3 months, a newborn sleeps up to 18 hours daily. Lying supine in bed, the baby looks over to the right and the asymmetrical tonic neck reflex enhances that position. Due to the effect of plasticity, postural asymmetry has begun as the baby's body starts to adapt to that position.

When a typically developing baby with postural asymmetries begins to sit up, the postural asymmetry disappears.

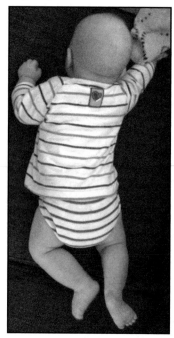

Figure 7-14. Postural asymmetry in an otherwise typically developing infant.

The reason for this is probably that the baby is moving on his or her own and changing positions, exploring the world, and tearing every minor restriction in his or her musculoskeletal system while doing so. The postural asymmetry in the baby in Case Study 7-1 disappeared in less than a week when the mother actively and passively encouraged her son to look over to his left side in supine lying.

The Effect of Habitual Posture in Lying on Positioning in Sitting and Standing

For adults with CP, up to 22 to 24 hours/day are spent in asymmetric positions in lying and sitting (Rodby-Bousquet et al., 2013). Time spent in different positions has a significant impact on the development of contractures and asymmetries.

An individual who is turned two times during the night is in a stretched posture for 3 hours if not properly supported. Up to 50% of adults who cannot independently change their position in bed lie in just one position throughout the night (Rodby-Bousquet et al., 2013). They are stretching for up to 10 hours or more if not properly supported in lying. As explained in the biomechanical section, this extended time in one position will lead to contracture in the slack AMS due to a tissue adaptation.

We have already discussed the implication of a habitual position and the effect on posture in the biomechanical section of this chapter. Evidence suggests that people adopt the same position in sitting and standing as they do in lying (Figures 7-15 through 7-17), indicating that the tissues have adapted physiologically to a lesser or greater degree (Pope, 2007b).

CASE EXAMPLE

Case Study 7-2: A man in his 40s with CP, GMFCS level V, was originally functioning well at a GMFCS level II with minor postural asymmetries. A minor stroke resulted in loss of walking ability. Since then, his asymmetries have increased, and it is clear that he adopts the same position in lying, sitting, and standing. His PPAS level in all positions in the frontal plane is a 2 (see Figures 7-15 through 7-17).

CASE EXAMPLE

Case Study 7-3: This woman is in her 30s with spastic bilateral CP, GMFCS level V, and a PPAS of 0 (Figure 7-18). She has a right hip subluxation (Reimer's Index is 55%). In supine, her head is laterally flexed and rotated over to left and moderate scoliosis, convex to right, and excessive windswept distortion, over to left, are present. The mat examination found a lack of flexion in both hips (right hip 80 degrees of flexion, left hip 30 degrees of flexion), with a lack of abduction and external rotation in the right and lack of adduction and internal rotation of the left. A neutral position cannot be reached in either hip. The knees lack full extension. The lateral scoliosis is fixed but her head can be placed in midline and slightly beyond to the right side.

The client had been in an unsupported supine posture, both for rest and sleep, for the majority of her childhood and adolescent years, leading to severe distortion. Because she did not sit at the age of 6 to 8 months, as a typical baby would, she spent more time lying in supine. Her habitual position has probably been more to her left side, with the head turned and flexed, knees falling over to that side. This individual has the classic footprint of a person with scoliosis and windswept distortion to the concave side. On the convex side, weight is taken through the posterior prominence of the ribs and the right foot. On the concave side, weight is taken through the left shoulder, arm, pelvis, and leg. These are the areas that are prone to pressure injuries for this unstable posture and uneven weight distribution (Figure 7-19).

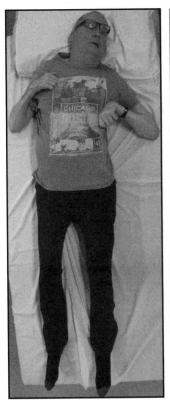

Figure 7-15. A man with spastic bilateral CP, originally GMFCS level II. Asymmetric habitual supine lying posture.

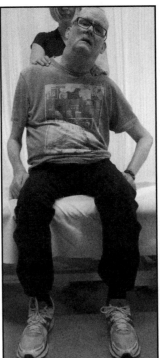

Figure 7-16. He adopts the same posture in sitting as in lying, only compounded by gravity.

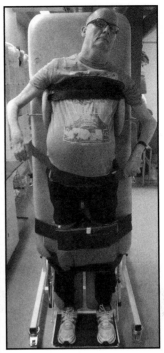

Figure 7-17. The same posture again, but due to postural support the deviation is a little less in standing than in unsupported sitting.

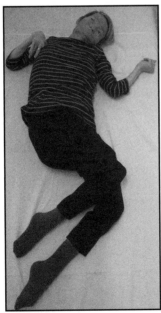

Figure 7-18. An asymmetric habitual lying position is mirrored in seating and vice versa.

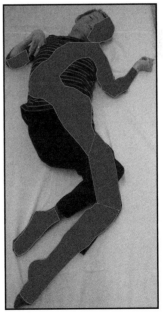

Figure 7-19. Footprint in an unsupported supine-lying position.

What started as a postural asymmetry due to habitual posture evolved with time into contractures due to tissue adaptation, creating a windswept distortion and scoliosis. The excessive windswept position increased the stress within the AMS of the hip joints resulting in tissue adaptation. The tissue adaptation minimized stress over time by reconstructing architecture of the hip joints, leading to restricted movement in the hips and subluxation in the right hip. Being in a harmful position for too long led to a distortion of her body shape.

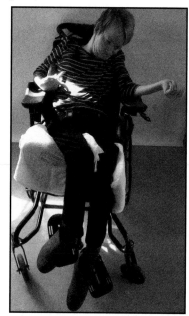

Figure 7-20. An asymmetric habitual lying position is mirrored in seating, and vice versa.

Asymmetric habitual lying posture will be reinforced by asymmetric habitual posture in sitting and vice versa (see Figures 7-18 and 7-20).

POSITIONING FOR REST AND SLEEP

Positioning in lying is essential to the management of the client who is unable to change position without help and aims at maintaining a stable, symmetrical, and comfortable lying or sleeping position. The body is less influenced by muscle tone during the night and gravity can be used in a beneficial way. For the client with motor impairments and complex support needs, at least 3650 of the 8760 hours of the year are spent in bed for rest and sleep. The risk of developing an asymmetric posture, which can lead to musculoskeletal complications, is therefore particularly high in lying.

When the many hours spent in lying are considered, the 24-hour approach is logical. Daytime intervention, such as wheelchair seating, is likely to be less successful if the client is allowed to adopt poor, asymmetrical postures during time spent in bed.

Sleep is an important function in its own right, and, as for anyone else, restorative sleep is essential for people with physical disabilities to maximize cognitive and physical performance during the day. One in five people with CP has a sleep disorder, a rate five times worse than the typical population (Novak et al., 2013). This can be due to an inability to change position, discomfort or pain, respiratory difficulties, or gastroesophageal reflux—all of which can lead to poor sleep quality and duration.

Caregivers in families of children with physical disabilities experience an increased prevalence of sleep issues (Hemmingsson, Stenhammar, & Paulsson, 2009). Although regular change of position throughout the night is important, it is also a source of caregiver burden. Therefore, safety and ease of use of equipment used for rest and sleep are important. Positioning for rest and sleep has two main goals:

1. To prevent or delay the development of musculoskeletal distortion

2. To improve quality and duration of sleep

On the basis of our discussion on biomechanics, effects of gravity, and plasticity of body structures, the most effective position to control posture lying is in supine. On the other hand, a well-supported side-lying position might be a second choice when changing sleep positions and in some cases is better suited for spasticity control. A controlled prone position is a good choice for resting periods during the day rather than for nighttime positioning.

Clients with scoliosis should be encouraged to sleep in supported symmetrical supine lying instead of side lying or in prone.

No matter what sleeping position is chosen for the client, it needs to be correctly and symmetrically supported and be counteracted during the day. In other words, if the client's position in bed is supine or side lying with flexed hips and knees, the client needs to be put into a standing or prone position during the day to stretch the AMS that have been in a shortened position for several hours.

Different solutions are available to support a symmetrical posture during rest and sleep. These vary as much as the clients who need support. Low-tech solutions, such as wedges, rolls, pillows, and T-rolls, can go a long way, and even a teddy bear can come in handy for a infant or a young child. For other clients, these low-tech solutions might not provide enough control and support.

Sleep-positioning systems are commercially available, individualized, lying support systems that may contain one or more component parts, which are held in position by a base layer or sheet (Polak, Clift, & Clift, 2009). These sleep systems are available in different sizes and are made from a variety of materials that conform to body shape or a series of straps that are aimed at holding the body in a neutral and symmetrical position. Some clients find a sleep positioning system useful, while others find this unfriendly, difficult to manage, or unavailable due to funding limitations because these systems are expensive.

Building a Stable Posture in Lying

In general, start with a simple, less restrictive lying support before choosing something more sophisticated

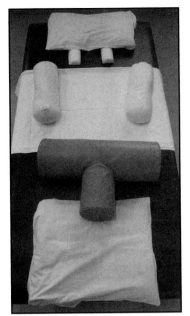

Figure 7-21. Examples of low-tech supports for supine lying.

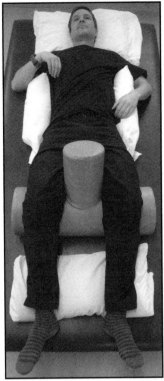

Figure 7-22. Supported supine lying.

because if the less restrictive support is not accepted, the more sophisticated will not be either. Pope (2007a, 2007b) described a simple and inexpensive method in building a stable posture.

Align the body by placing a T-roll under the knees, rotating the central roll upwards and positioning it between the thighs, securing the pelvis in alignment with the thorax. Support the trunk laterally by tucking a roll pillow under a crosswise sheet on each side. Two anchors (small half roll or a towel) are placed under the pillow to guide the head (Figure 7-21). Raise the heels off the mattress by placing a small pillow under the legs (Figure 7-22). The base of a stable posture is a neutral pelvis.

The same applies in side lying. A pillow is tucked behind the back under a crosswise sheet, and the trunk is leaned slightly back against the pillow to take the weight off the shoulder. A roll is placed between the thighs, securing the pelvis in alignment with the thorax and securing abduction in the hip joints; a small pillow is put between the feet for pressure relief. An anchor is placed under the pillow to support the head (Figures 7-23 and 7-24).

When building a stable posture for the client in Case Study 7-3 (Figure 7-25), the adage "correct what is correctable, adapt for the rest" applies. The basis is a neutral pelvis in the transverse plane.

The first step is to secure a stable neutral pelvis in alignment with the thorax, which is done by custom molding a support for the legs in a position that allows the pelvis to be neutral. A T-roll cannot be used due to lack of movement in the hips. The leg support both relieves the stretch on the AMS and improves weight distribution through the pelvis and legs. Weight needs to be off of the heels.

The second step is to support the trunk by tucking a roll pillow under a crosswise sheet on each side. A small wedge is put under the sheet at the thoracic area on the left side to rotate the trunk over to the right, using gravity to counteract the postural asymmetry of the thorax. Support the arms down by the side if possible.

The third step is to secure the head. The goal is to keep the head straight relative to the shoulders. A small anchor on the right side stops the head from sliding over to the right. A wedge on the left side supports the head in a neutral position.

The simplest way to evaluate the new posture is to do the footprint examination again to see whether the weight distribution increases with fewer high-pressure areas (Figures 7-26 and 7-27).

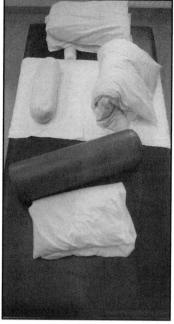

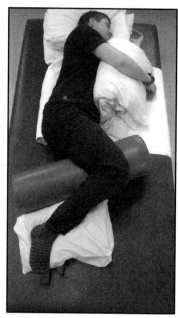

Figure 7-23. Low-tech supports for side lying.

Figure 7-24. Supported side lying.

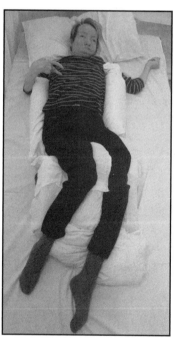

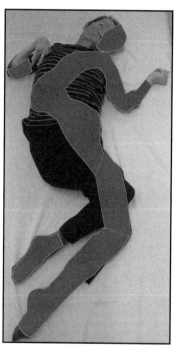

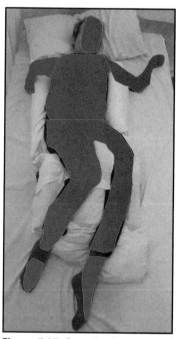

Figure 7-25. Supported supine lying.

Figure 7-26. Footprint in unsupported supine lying.

Figure 7-27. Footprint in supported supine lying.

HEALTH AND SAFETY ISSUES

Many individuals with neurological impairment may have significant health problems, and basic physiological mechanisms, such as breathing and swallowing are influenced by body posture. It is therefore imperative to be aware of the risks that have been associated with nighttime positioning equipment, because it may either aggravate or alleviate these issues. Little research has been done on the effects of sleep positioning systems and their impact on respiratory function and sleep quality. As the clients typically prescribed sleep positioning systems (GMFCS Level IV or V) are often unable to express feelings of discomfort or pain (Gough, 2009), careful consideration should be given to how to assess these effects for each individual.

The most common risk factors are overheating, which may cause epileptic seizures and respiratory issues. Respiratory distress and oxygen desaturation in flat supine lying can be caused by internal organs pushing on the diaphragm and lungs. This can also be due to weakness of the muscles of the chest wall, the diaphragm, or both. Scoliosis also contributes to poor lung function by causing a further reduction in vital capacity and ventilation-perfusion mismatch (Noble-Jamieson, Heckmatt, Dubowitz, & Silverman, 1986). Medications that are taken for pain, sleeping, anxiousness, or muscle stiffness may depress the breathing centers in the brain.

If respiratory distress and gastroesophageal reflux are a problem, the bed may need to be tilted (reverse Trendelenburg position) but kept as minimal as possible; 15 degrees is usually sufficient to minimize the reflux without the client slipping down in the bed. Some children who have seizures at night may need to sleep on their sides with good support to be safe from choking and aspiration.

Other factors to consider are pressure and correct use of the equipment. The risk of pressure injuries due to incorrect positioning or staying too long in the same position must be considered. Incorrect use of the equipment can lead to intolerance of the sleep system. The question of compliance or "will the system be used?" is also a factor not to be overlooked. Some individuals are at risk of becoming entangled in bedcovers or pillows because of uncontrolled movement patterns, leading to possible asphyxia without appropriate sleep positioning (Lange, 2009). The lifestyle of the individual and his or her family and the views of caregivers are critical when using sleeping systems, as is knowledge of therapists and other health care personnel.

SUMMARY

PM, or 24-hour positioning, is an important intervention, aimed at preventing secondary complications and improving health, functional ability, and quality of life for people with neurological impairments and complex support needs. The necessity of posture management in lying is clear when effects of biomechanical forces are considered.

In a world with an aging population, increasing numbers of people with disabilities, and relatively fewer people to assist those clients, it is important to choose strategies carefully to ensure the client's well-being and quality of life. By protecting health and supporting functional abilities and self-mobility, we aim to reduce dependency caused by severe secondary complications as well as lower health care costs.

REFERENCES

Fulford, F. E., & Brown, J. K. (1976). Position as a cause of deformity in children with cerebral palsy. *Developmental Medicine and Child Neurology, 18,* 305-314.

Gericke, T. (2006). Postural management for children with cerebral palsy: Consensus statement. *Developmental Medicine and Child Neurology, 48,* 244. doi:10.1017/S0012162206000685

Gough, M. (2009). Continuous postural management and the prevention of deformity in children with cerebral palsy: An appraisal. *Developmental Medicine and Child Neurology, 51,* 105-110. doi:10.1111/j.1469-8749.2008.03160.x

Hadders-Algra, M. (2008). Why bother about postural control? In M. Hadders-Algra & E. B. Carlberg (Eds.), *Postural control: A key issue in developmental disorders.* London, England: Mac Keith Press.

Hare, N. (1987). *The human sandwich factor.* Presented at the Chartered society of physiotherapy, Oxford, England.

Hemmingsson, H., Stenhammar, A. M., & Paulsson, K. (2009). Sleep problems and the need for parental night-time attention in children with physical disabilities. *Child: Care, Health, and Development, 35,* 89-95. doi:10.1111/j.1365-2214.2008.00907.x

Hill, C. M., Parker, R. C., Allen, P., Paul, A., & Padoa, K. A. (2009). Sleep quality and respiratory function in children with severe cerebral palsy using night-time postural equipment: A pilot study. *Acta Paediatrica, 98,* 1809-1814. doi:10.1111/j.1651-2227.2009.01441.x

Hill, S., & Goldsmith, J. (2010). Biomechanics and prevention of body shape distortion. *Tizard Learning Disability Review, 15,* 15-32

Lange, M. L. (2009). *Sleep positioning. Positioning isn't just for wheelchairs anymore.* Retrieved from http://occupational-therapy.advanceweb.com/Article/Sleep-Positioning.aspx,25,3:34

Noble-Jamieson, C. M., Heckmatt, J. Z., Dubowitz, V., & Silverman, M. (1986). Effects of posture and spinal bracing on respiratory function in neuromuscular disease. *Archives of Disease in Childhood, 61,* 178-181.

Novak, I., Hines, M., Goldsmith, S., & Barclay, R. (2012). Clinical prognostic messages from a systematic review on cerebral palsy. *Pediatrics, 130,* e1285-e1312. doi:10.1542/peds.2012-0924

Palisano, R., Rosenbaum, P., Walter, S., Russell, D., Wood, E., & Galuppi, B. (1997). Development and reliability of a system to classify gross motor function in children with cerebral palsy. *Developmental Medicine and Child Neurology, 39,* 214-223.

Polak, F., Clift M., & Clift L. (2009). *Buyers' guide: Night time postural management equipment for children.* London, England: Department of Health. Retrieved from https://dspace.lboro.ac.uk/dspace-jspui/handle/2134/7368

Pope, P. M. (2007a). Night-time postural support for people with multiple sclerosis. *Way Ahead, 11,* 6-8

Pope, P. M. (2007b). *Severe and complex neurological disability: Management of the physical condition.* Edinburgh, Scotland: Butterworth-Heinemann/Elsevier.

Porter, D., Michael, S., & Kirkwood, C. (2010). Is there a relationship between foetal position and both preferred lying posture after birth and pattern of subsequent postural deformity in non-ambulant people with cerebral palsy? *Child: Care, Health, and Development, 36*(5), 742-747. doi:10.1111/j.1365-2214.2009.01035.x

Pountney, T. E., Mandy, A., Green, E. M., & Gard, P. (2002). Management of hip dislocation with postural management. *Child: Care, Health, and Development, 28,* 179-185.

Ramstad, K., Jahnsen, R., Skjeldal, O. H., & Diseth, T. H. (2011). Characteristics of recurrent musculoskeletal pain in children with cerebral palsy aged 8 to 18 years. *Developmental Medicine and Child Neurology, 53*(11), 1013-1018. doi:10.1111/j.1469-8749.2011.04070.x

Ramstad, K., Jahnsen, R., Skjeldal, O. H., & Diseth, T. H. (2012). Mental health, health related quality of life and recurrent musculoskeletal pain in children with cerebral palsy 8-18 years old. *Disability and Rehabilitation, 34,* 1589-1595. doi: 10.3109/09638288.2012.656794

Rodby-Bousquet, E., Agustsson, A., Jonsdottir, G., Czuba, T., Johansson, A. C., & Hagglund, G. (2014). Interrater reliability and construct validity of the Posture and Postural Ability Scale in adults with cerebral palsy in supine, prone, sitting and standing positions. *Clinical Rehabilitation, 28,* 82-90. doi: 10.1177/0269215512465423

Rodby-Bousquet, E., Czuba, T., Hagglund, G., & Westbom, L. (2013). Postural asymmetries in young adults with cerebral palsy. *Developmental Medicine and Child Neurology, 55*(11), 1009-1015. doi:10.1111/dmcn.12199

Rodby-Bousquet, E., Persson-Bunke, M., & Czuba, T. (2015). Psychometric evaluation of the Posture and Postural Ability Scale for children with cerebral palsy. *Clinical Rehabilitation, 30,* 697-704. doi: 10.1177/0269215515593612

Tardieu, C., Lespargot, A., Tabary, C., & Bret, M. D. (1988). For how long must the soleus muscle be stretched each day to prevent contracture? *Developmental Medicine and Child Neurology, 30,* 3-10.

Trudel, G., & Uhthoff, H. K. (2000). Contractures secondary to immobility: Is the restriction articular or muscular? An experimental longitudinal study in the rat knee. *Archives of Physical Medicine and Rehabilitation, 81,* 6-13.

World Health Organization. (2011). *Global health and aging.* Retrieved from http://www.who.int/ageing/publications/global_health.pdf

World Health Organization. (2015). *Health and human rights* (Fact Sheet No. 323). Retrieved from http://www.who.int/mediacentre/factsheets/fs323/en/

SUGGESTED READING

Nordin, M., & Frankel, V. (2012). *Basic biomechanics of the musculoskeletal system* (4th ed.). Philadelphia, PA: Lippincott Williams & Wilkins.

Please see video on the accompanying website at

www.healio.com/books/mobility

III

Wheeled Mobility
Foundational Information

8

Mobility Assessment
The Mobility Algorithm

Elizabeth Cole, MSPT, ATP

Choosing the appropriate mobility device for each client can be a daunting task considering the variety of choices and options that are available today. Advances in technology, electronics, and materials used in these products, along with sophistication in designs, configurations, and adjustments, provide seemingly endless possibilities. The degree of independence, function, and quality of life provided by the right choice of equipment is immeasurable for the client. So how do you make the right decision? How do you match the most appropriate mobility device to the specific person?

The initial goal in the process is to identify what category of mobility device will provide the client with maximum function. This is determined through a systematic elimination of those devices that will not meet the client's limitations and capabilities. There are two key steps to this process. The first is a critical analysis of the results of the clinical evaluation and technology assessment. The second is to consider the different categories of device in a hierarchy from simplest to most complex. Applying this algorithmic thought process will help you choose the most appropriate and simplest device that will meet each client's needs.

This chapter discusses the algorithm for choosing a category of mobility device. How to choose the specific type of device within each category is discussed in later chapters.

THE EVALUATION FOR A MOBILITY DEVICE

Whether to provide a mobility device and choosing the category of device begins with a thorough clinical evaluation of the client's medical history, social situation, environment(s) of typical use, and physical and functional status. This is true no matter who is being evaluated, whether the mobility needs are basic or complex, who is performing the evaluation, or what the final recommendations might be. It is also true whether the potential device is an ambulatory aid, manual wheelchair, scooter, or power wheelchair. Although the evaluation will be more detailed and involved for someone with complex needs, the fundamental steps will be the same as for someone with basic needs. Implementing all of the appropriate steps to at least some degree for any client ensures that the most appropriate, safe, and efficacious equipment is provided to meet the person's specific needs.

Client Interview

When choosing a mobility device for an individual, it is important to determine the person's capacities, limitations, lifestyle, environments, and, of course, goals and expectations. This begins with information gathering during the

Lange, M. L., & Minkel, J. L.
Seating and Wheeled Mobility: A Clinical Resource Guide
(pp. 139-145). © 2018 SLACK Incorporated.

client interview at the beginning of the clinic visit. Some of this information might also be obtained during a prescreen call or survey.

Medical History

The first step in the interview process is typically the identification of the primary diagnosis that has necessitated the mobility evaluation and the history of this condition, including the date of onset (or date when the symptoms first began) and the nature of the specific symptoms. If the condition or disease has been one of progressive decline, it should be noted whether the progression was sudden and rapid or whether changes occurred slowly over time. Any patterns to the progression such as in the timing of the changes, the severity of the changes, or any regularity in exacerbations and remissions, should be identified. If the condition was caused by a traumatic injury or event, any patterns of recovery should be noted along with the results.

All of this information is a first step in identifying if a mobility device is appropriate for the first-time user or if a different type of mobility device is needed in place of current equipment. It will also identify the need for modularity and adjustability in the mobility interventions to continue to meet potential changes in the individual's function.

The evaluation should also identify any secondary diagnoses or comorbidities and document the date(s) of onset, symptoms, and severity. The identification of these secondary issues is often an essential factor in choosing and justifying the most appropriate base product, as well as any options and accessories. It is especially important to consider secondary conditions that result in cardiac or pulmonary compromise, joint dysfunction, orthopedic issues, seizures, or any conditions causing significant discomfort, pain, abnormal tone, impaired balance, or decreased strength and endurance.

Medications and Surgeries

Any plans to make changes to current medications should be noted, because these can often have an effect on the person's muscle tone, postural stability, medical health, pain level, or body weight. These functional changes could significantly affect the selection of the appropriate mobility device and components. Of particular interest would be medications to manage, prevent or treat spasticity, cardiopulmonary conditions, seizure activity, heterotopic ossification, body weight, pain, psychological conditions, bowel and bladder function, or infection.

The evaluator should also gather information regarding all pertinent past or future surgeries or medical interventions that were in any way related to or will affect the need for mobility equipment. This would include spinal stabilizations or other orthopedic surgeries, surgeries to manage spasticity, or even insertion of a gastrostomy tube. These and other medical procedures could cause changes in the individual's postural stability and balance, muscle and joint

flexibility, skin integrity, functional use of the extremities, pain level, overall function, and body size. In the case of future surgeries, it is sometimes wise to wait until after the procedure is done and the client has stabilized before evaluation and selection of the appropriate mobility device.

Other Considerations

Another important piece of information is the person's body weight and whether there have been any recent or ongoing changes, or if there is the potential for changes. This can help to identify the required weight capacity for certain mobility devices. It can also determine how much adjustability and modularity might be needed in order to continue to appropriately fit the individual. Identifying any changes in size is particularly important when working with children, people with progressive conditions, or those with new traumatic injuries.

Details regarding the client's skin integrity are a must when choosing the appropriate mobility equipment. This includes the current status of the skin as well as the location, stage (or description), cause, and treatment of any past pressure injuries or other forms of skin or soft tissue breakdown. This information can affect the type, features, and materials of the seating components that are required, which can, in turn, affect the type of mobility frame needed to accommodate this seating.

Activity Level and Activities of Daily Living

Many individuals will be using their mobility devices on a daily basis, often throughout the day or for a majority of the day. It is critical to identify all basic activities of daily living (BADL) and instrumental activities of daily living (IADL) that the person performs, needs to perform or participates in on a regular basis in all usual environments, such as home, school, work, or community. BADL might include, but are not limited to, bathing and personal hygiene, dressing, toileting, meal preparation, cooking, eating, child or elder care, personal financial management, home management, house cleaning, laundry, and so forth. IADL might include, but are not limited to, any type of shopping; going to the bank or post office; voting; attending religious services, medical appointments, community, leisure, recreational, and/or family events; activities at work, school, or day care; volunteer work; or any other activities that the individual performs or participates in on a regular basis. Identifying these activities will help to ensure that the mobility device prescribed will allow the individual to continue the most active lifestyle possible (and desired) for maximum fulfillment and quality of life.

It is also important to indicate the activity level of the individual during her daily activities and within her usual environments. Whether the person is mildly, moderately, or highly active can have a significant impact on the most appropriate type of ambulatory aid or wheelchair and its options and accessories, as well as the performance and durability of the device. If the prescribed equipment is not appropriate for the individual's lifestyle, one of two consequences will result. In some cases, the person will be unable to complete all required activities on a day-to-day basis because the equipment is not adequate. In other cases, the equipment will be used to perform all daily activities and will subsequently break down or malfunction, necessitating repairs and time periods when it cannot be used. Either scenario will result in dissatisfaction, decreased quality of life, and potential equipment abandonment.

It is important to identify the expected length of need for the mobility device(s). For most individuals with permanent disabilities, the need will be long-term or lifetime. It is also important to determine whether the mobility intervention will be used for (1) all mobility needs, (2) just for short time periods each day, (3) primarily for long distances and/or outdoor use, or (4) as a backup mobility device.

Environments

Before selecting the appropriate mobility device, information should be gathered regarding the types, features, and characteristics of the environments that the client encounters in daily activities, both indoors and outdoors. This can include indoor surfaces at home, school, work, and/or other environments, such as linoleum, tile, hardwood, low- or high-pile carpet, stone, or a combination. Outdoor terrains might include pavement, gravel, grass, dirt, brick, stone, or other surfaces. The surfaces could be smooth and level, mildly or moderately uneven, or rough. Environments of typical use could also include curbs of various heights and/or inclines of various degrees of steepness.

The accessibility within these environments (especially the home) should be determined with regard to ease of maneuverability. If wheeled mobility is being considered, it is necessary to identify the doorway width and required turning radius for any room or area that the person needs to access. It might also be necessary to know the heights of countertops, sinks, and other work surfaces, as well as beds, toilets, and other transfer surfaces. These dimensions are needed to determine the maximum overall length and width required for a wheeled mobility device, as well as the appropriate seat to floor height.

Goals and Expectations

Most important, the client's goals and expectations should be identified. What would this person like to be able to do that he or she cannot accomplish in the current equipment or at the current functional level? What are his or her satisfactions/dissatisfactions with any current equipment? What are the expected outcomes of the evaluation and equipment prescription? It is critical to consider these first and foremost. Choosing equipment that does not meet the client's goals and needs typically results in dissatisfaction and equipment abandonment.

In the same regard, it is important to make sure that the expectations of the client, caregiver, family members, and all other team members are realistic. Too often, there are hopes or beliefs that a piece of equipment will compensate for a physical or cognitive deficit or ameliorate a limitation in a way that is not possible. It is important to be open and honest about what is and is not realistic.

The Physical Evaluation

Physical and functional capabilities and limitations of the individual must be assessed before identifying the most appropriate category of mobility device. The information that should be obtained from the physical evaluation includes the following:

- Muscle strength
- Coordination and motor control
- Range of motion (ROM) of all pertinent joints
- Presence, type, and severity of any abnormal tone or primitive reflexes
- Static and dynamic sitting and standing balance
- Postural asymmetries, their causes, and whether they are fixed or reducible
- Current skin condition including presence, location, status, stage and cause of any skin/soft tissue injury.

THE CLINICAL THOUGHT PROCESS FOR CHOOSING A MOBILITY DEVICE

In most cases, once the evaluation is complete and the mobility limitation has been identified, you can begin the selection process for an appropriate mobility device. However, in some situations, you might first need to consider whether the physical and/or functional problem(s) could be ameliorated with rehabilitative treatment or other interventions. If there is a good possibility that other treatments could help, it might make sense to delay the equipment selection until the client's physical status and/or function has reached a plateau. However, this is a fine line, because there is certainly the risk that the additional treatment is ineffective in reducing the limitation. If this is the case, then deferring the provision of a mobility device only serves to delay the client's achievement of his or her mobility goals. It is certainly one of the many times when we might wish for the proverbial crystal ball.

If it is determined that a mobility device is the best choice for the client, it is important to view the different categories of devices in a hierarchy, starting with a cane and progressing to a walker, a manual wheelchair, a scooter (power-operated vehicle [POV]), and finally a power wheelchair. The selection process should begin by considering the simplest device and determining whether it would meet the person's needs and accomplish the desired goals on the basis of the results of the clinical evaluation. If this category of device is ruled out as a viable solution, then the next simplest device should be assessed, and it too should be either chosen or ruled out.

This process or algorithm is a clinical thought process that starts with the simplest device (a cane) and systematically rules out each device in the hierarchy until the appropriate one is identified. This is the device that allows the person to complete his or her daily activities safely (without injury, physical or medical compromise, or other adverse effects), in a timely manner, and to his or her fullest capacities. Some considerations as you move through the algorithmic thought process and device selection are discussed in the following sections.

FUNCTIONAL MOBILITY

It is important to keep in mind that functional mobility will be different for each person depending on his or her lifestyle, daily activities, environment, and so forth. For example, consider the client who has a very low activity level and functions in a relatively small environment that is primarily indoors on level surfaces. He or she only needs to walk or propel short distances at a relatively slow speed to complete his or her daily activities of eating, dressing, grooming, bathing, toileting, simple meal preparation, and reading or watching television.

This is very different from the client who is highly active, functions in multiple indoor and outdoor environments of varying sizes and terrains, and has varied responsibilities throughout each day. She needs to travel longer distances at higher speeds to complete all daily activities in a timely manner. If her current mode of ambulation or propulsion only allows her to go short distances before experiencing harmful effects, then she will be unable to complete all necessary activities, or she will suffer consequences if she attempts to do so. Similarly, if her current mode of walking or propelling significantly limits her speed, she will be unable to complete her activities in a timely manner. The same speeds and distances that are fine for the first client are inadequate for the second. If too much time or effort is required, mobility is no longer functional.

IS AMBULATION A FUNCTIONAL MEANS OF MOBILITY?

If the client has any ability to ambulate, this function should be physically assessed with and without ambulatory aids, unless there is an obvious reason why he or she would be unable to do so. There are certainly cases in which it is apparent that ambulation would be impossible or unsafe because of the person's diagnosis and physical limitations, and with these clients, you can move on to the next device in the hierarchy, which is a manual wheelchair. However, there must be clear-cut evidence in the documentation to support this inability to ambulate. This could include objective measurements or descriptions of muscle strength, ROM, tone, balance, motor control, and so forth.

Which Category of Ambulation Is Functional?

If the client has some ability to walk, his or her ambulation should be assessed without an ambulatory aid. If this is not physically possible or safe, or if this is tried and shown to be nonfunctional, then trials with all appropriate ambulatory devices should be conducted beginning with a cane or crutches and progressing through a hierarchy of different types of walkers and gait trainers, as appropriate for that client. Each device should be ruled out as to the person's ability to use it (1) at all, (2) safely in all daily activities and environments, and (3) functionally to complete all daily activities in a timely manner.

The same questions should be posed during each of the trials with the different means of mobility (ambulating without a device, ambulating with a cane, ambulating with a walker). These questions include the following:

- Is the client able to walk with this means of mobility (no device/cane/walker)?

- Are there significant gait abnormalities present with this means of mobility, and do these affect safety, distance, time, or effort of ambulation?

- How much, if any, assistance is needed (supervision; contact guard; minimal, moderate, or maximum assist)?

- Is the speed and distance that the person is able to walk with this means of mobility sufficient to allow him or her to complete all necessary daily activities in all typical environments?

- Does this means of mobility allow the individual to perform these daily activities safely and without harmful effects?

- Does walking with this means of mobility require so much energy and effort that the client is unable to complete his or her daily activities?

- Do attempts to ambulate throughout the day with this means of mobility for all activities cause adverse effects, such as risk of falls or other injury, functionally limiting stress or damage to the upper and/or lower extremity joints, functionally limiting fatigue or pain, cardiopulmonary compromise, or other adverse effects?

- Would the person be able to use this method of mobility throughout the day, every day, day after day?

- If a cane is determined to be appropriate, what type of cane can the client use (straight cane, quad cane, hemi cane)?

- If a walker is determined to be appropriate, what type of walker can the client use (standard walker, rolling walker)?

The evaluations with and without an ambulatory device should identify not only what the limitations in ambulation are, but also the causes of these limitations (e.g., decreased strength, poor standing balance, increased tone, poor endurance, pain, cardiopulmonary compromise, joint instability or degeneration). It is also important to identify how these limitations affect the ability to ambulate safely and in a timely manner.

If the limitations are due to cardiac or pulmonary issues, there should be a record of pertinent quantitative measurements *after* the attempts to ambulate. This could include O_2 saturation, heart rate (HR), blood pressure (BP), respiratory rate (RR), quality of breathing (shortness of breath), and so forth. These test results can then be compared with baseline (at rest) results. Similarly, if limitations are due to pain, there should be documentation of the specific location of the pain and the level of pain before and after ambulation. In all cases, the time needed to recover should also be recorded.

Other Considerations

There are individuals who do have some ability to safely ambulate with or without an ambulatory aid; however, this ability is limited to short distances, short time periods, and certain times of the day or specific environments. In these cases, ambulation is not sufficient or safe for all mobility needs. Most funding sources, including Medicare, recognize this and do not rule out coverage of a wheeled mobility device for the person who is partially ambulatory, as long as the lack of functional ambulation is well-documented. This could include those individuals (non-Medicare) who are able to ambulate within their homes without a device or using a cane or walker but need wheeled mobility to function outdoors and in other environments.

IS PROPULSION OF A MANUAL WHEELCHAIR A FUNCTIONAL MEANS OF MOBILITY?

If ambulation with a walker is not functional, the individual's ability to use an appropriate manual wheelchair should be assessed. Actual propulsion trials should be conducted, unless there is an obvious reason why the client would be unable to physically or safely do so due to his or her diagnosis and physical limitations. In these cases, it is appropriate to move on to the next device in the hierarchy, power mobility. However, there must be clear evidence in the documentation to support his or her inability to participate in propulsion trials. This could include objective measurements or descriptions of muscle strength, ROM, tone, balance, motor control, and so forth.

As with ambulation, objective examination results should be obtained during propulsion trials with a manual wheelchair. These measurements could include the maximum distance the individual was able to functionally propel, and the time required to propel this distance. When the limiting factors involve cardiopulmonary issues or pain, it is important to obtain after measurements of O_2 saturation, HR, BP, RR, shortness of breath, location and level of pain, the time needed to recover, and any other pertinent quantitative measurements. These can then be compared with the client's baseline measurements.

Questions similar to those posed regarding ambulation should be asked. This will help to identify if manual mobility (in general) is appropriate for the client (more information about choosing the specific type of manual wheelchair is found in Chapter 9). Pertinent questions might include the following:

- Is the person able to propel a manual wheelchair?

- What method of propulsion is used (both upper extremities, one upper and one lower extremity, both lower extremities, both upper and both lower extremities, or one upper extremity)?

- Is propelling with a manual wheelchair a functional means of mobility?

- Is the speed and distance achieved while propelling the most optimal type of manual wheelchair sufficient to allow the person to complete all necessary daily activities in all typical environments?

- Does propulsion in this type of manual wheelchair allow the individual to perform these daily activities safely and without risk of injury, physical or medical compromise, or other harmful effects?

- Does propelling any type of manual wheelchair require so much energy that the client is unable to complete his or her daily activities?

- Does propulsion throughout the day cause adverse effects, such as functionally limiting stress or damage to the upper and/or lower extremity joints, functionally limiting fatigue or pain, cardiopulmonary compromise, or other adverse effects?

- Does propulsion cause muscle tone to increase to the point that it significantly affects function, posture, or balance?

- Would the person be able to use this method of mobility throughout the day, every day, day after day?

- Would long-term manual wheelchair propulsion contribute to or increase the risk of repetitive strain injuries of the upper extremities due to compromised joint stability and integrity?

Other Considerations

As with clients who are ambulatory, there are individuals who do have some ability to safely propel a manual wheelchair; however, this is limited to short distances, short time periods, certain times of the day or specific environments. For these individuals, manual mobility might be insufficient or unsafe for all mobility needs. Again, most funding sources recognize this and do not rule out coverage of a power mobility device, as long as the lack of functional propulsion is well-documented. This could include those individuals (non-Medicare) who are able to propel within their homes but need power mobility to function outdoors and in other environments.

We must also consider manual mobility for clients who are unable to ambulate and are unable to independently propel a manual wheelchair, but are also unable to operate any power mobility device. Although they are dependent for mobility, they still need to move from place to place. In these cases, a manual wheelchair is typically the most appropriate category of mobility device, although the specific type of manual wheelchair will most likely be different from that which is appropriate for a self-propeller. This is addressed further in Chapter 14.

Finally, it is important to consider that throughout the evaluation for manual wheelchair propulsion, the individual should be positioned in his or her most optimal posture. This is the posture that was identified during the mat evaluation component of the physical evaluation. All appropriate supports that are needed to maintain stability of the trunk and pelvis and facilitate functional use of the extremities should be provided or simulated. In addition, the evaluation should take place using the most appropriate type of manual wheelchair or a close facsimile (standard, lightweight, high-strength lightweight, ultralightweight, or heavy duty). The mobility device should be adjusted a closely as possible to the optimal configuration for that specific person.

Is Operation of a Scooter a Functional Means of Mobility?

If the individual is unable to functionally ambulate or propel a manual wheelchair, we must evaluate if he or she is safe and able to operate a POV. This should involve an actual trial with a scooter unless, as with ambulation and manual wheelchair propulsion, it is obviously impossible or unsafe. Again, there should be clear evidence of the person's physical limitations in the documentation to support this. Some questions to consider when ruling out a scooter include the following:

- Is a scooter a functional means of mobility?

- Does the individual have the balance and strength to safely transfer on and off a scooter?

- Is the individual's upper extremity strength, ROM, tone, and coordination sufficient to operate the tiller controls?

- Is the person's balance and stability sufficient to maintain an upright posture on the scooter seat?

- Does the person's environment offer sufficient space and accessibility to allow maneuverability of the scooter?

- Are the speed, distance, and power provided by the scooter sufficient to allow the person to complete all necessary daily activities in all typical environments?

- Does the use of a scooter allow the individual to perform these daily activities safely and without risk of injury, physical or medical compromise, or other harmful effects?

- Would the person be able to use this method of mobility throughout the day, every day, day after day?

- Does the client have the cognitive function, behavior, judgment, and perception required for safe operation of a scooter?

Is Operation of a Power Wheelchair a Functional Means of Mobility?

For some clients, a scooter is not appropriate because of physical and/or environmental limitations. He or she might be unable to operate the tiller due to upper extremity compromise, his or her balance might be insufficient to sit on a scooter seat, or he or she might be unable to transfer safely on and off the device. In many cases, a scooter is just not maneuverable within the client's typical environments. If this category of device will not meet the individual's needs, we must determine whether he or she is able to safely operate a power wheelchair. Questions to pose in considering these types of devices include the following:

- What type of base will best meet the individual's activity level, environmental needs, and functional needs?

- How will he or she be able to operate the wheelchair? Is use of a standard joystick possible, or will an alternative drive control be necessary?

- Are power seat functions, such as tilt and/or recline required?

- Would the decrease in energy and time that is achieved with a power wheelchair allow this individual to complete daily activities safely, in a timely manner, and without functionally limiting fatigue, pain, and stress (assuming that a different mobility device does not)?

- Does the person's environment offer sufficient space and accessibility to allow maneuverability of the power wheelchair?

- Are the speed, distance, and power provided by the power wheelchair sufficient to allow the individual to complete all necessary daily activities in all typical environments?

- Does the use of a power wheelchair allow this person to perform these daily activities safely and without risk of injury, physical or medical compromise, or other harmful effects?

- Would the person be able to use this method of mobility throughout the day, every day, day after day?

- Does the client have the cognitive function, behavior, judgment, and perception required for safe operation of a power wheelchair?

This information is critical when determining the most appropriate category of power wheelchair for each individual client, what type of seating support will be required, what types of accommodations are required for postural support or orthopedic asymmetries, what type of drive control device is most appropriate, and what level of electronics is needed (consumer or complex rehab). All of this will influence which type of frame and which options and accessories are appropriate, as well as what degree and type of adjustability is required. This is addressed further in Chapter 10.

Summary

Choosing the most appropriate mobility equipment for any individual requires detailed knowledge of the individual's medical history and a thorough physical and functional evaluation. Once it is determined that the individual needs a mobility device, the various types of devices should be considered and chosen or ruled out in a hierarchy starting with the simplest device, which is a cane. If there is potential that an individual could use this type of device to complete daily activities in a safe, timely, and functional manner, then an assessment with this device should be completed. If mobility with a cane is completely unfeasible or if the evaluation with a cane shows it is insufficient, then the same process should occur with a walker, followed by a manual wheelchair, scooter, and finally power wheelchair. Each type of device must be evaluated and ruled out before going on to the next device in the hierarchy. This ensures that the individual is provided with the most appropriate device to meet his or her specific and unique needs.

Bibliography

Arledge, S., Armstrong, W., Babinec, M., Dicianno, B. E., Digiovine, C., Dyson-Hudson, T.,...& Schmeler, M. (2011). *RESNA wheelchair service provision guide.* Arlington, VA: Rehabilitation Engineering & Assistive Technology Society of North America. Retrieved from https://www.resna.org/sites/default/files/legacy/resources/position-papers/RESNAWheelchairServiceProvisionGuide.pdf

Cook, A. M., & Polgar, J. M. (2008). *Assistive technologies: Principles and practice.* St. Louis, MO: Elsevier Health Sciences.

Isaacson, M. (2011). Best practices by occupational and physical therapists performing seating and mobility evaluations. *Assistive Technology, 23,* 13-21.

Lange, M. (Ed.). (2008). *Fundamentals in assistive technology* (4th ed.). Arlington, VA: RESNA Press.

Petito, C. (2010). Customizing power. A holistic approach to complex power wheelchair and seating evaluations. *Rehab Management, 23*(6), 10.

Schmeler, M. (2010). The need for an outcomes management system in complex rehabilitation equipment. *Directions Magazine, 6,* 26-32.

Sprigle, S., Lenker, J., & Searcy, K. (2012). Activities of suppliers and technicians during the provision of complex and standard wheeled mobility devices. *Disability and Rehabilitation: Assistive Technology, 7,* 219-225.

Walls, G. (2010). Reaching for best practice. A focus on power wheelchair seating and mobility protocols. *Rehab Management, 24,* 14-16.

IV

Wheeled Mobility
Clinical Applications

Manual Mobility Applications for the Person Able to Self-Propel

Lauren E. Rosen, PT, MPT, MSMS, ATP/SMS

Many types of manual wheelchairs available. Some are designed for individuals to propel them full time, whereas others are designed more for people who will use them short term or be pushed by others. Chairs designed for short-term use are not well-designed for efficient, independent propulsion. Generally, they are designed for the ease of pushing for an assistant or for increased stability of the wheelchair. They are usually referred to as *transport chairs* or *standard wheelchairs*. Transport chairs are designed to be lightweight and easy to transport, in an automobile, for example. Standard wheelchairs generally weigh more than 50 pounds and are designed to be stable and durable in multiuser environments, like hospitals and airports (Figures 9-1 and 9-2).

Lightweight manual wheelchairs are, by definition, lighter than standard wheelchairs. They generally weigh more than 30 pounds. They have some limited adjustability of the wheelchair axle, which allows for a small amount of adjustment of the axle up and down. However, they do not have enough axle adjustability for most individuals to be successful, long-term, independent wheelchair hand-propellers at home and in the community. The ability to adjust the axle position to lower the overall sitting height can be helpful to individuals who foot propel because it allows for their feet to make full contact with the floor (Figure 9-3).

Ultralight wheelchairs are generally the best style of wheelchair for individuals who propel full-time. These chairs are the lightest in weight and have the greatest amount of adjustability to customize the wheelchair properly for the individual. In addition to the X-frame-style

chair shown in Figure 9-4, this category of wheelchair also contains rigid frame wheelchairs (Figure 9-5).

Note two possible axle positions:

1. Current position—standard height

2. Top position: lowers seat height to a hemi height for foot propulsion. Need to move both the rear wheel and the front caster position.

Rigid wheelchairs are generally lighter than folding wheelchairs. As they have fewer moving parts, they provide for more efficient propulsion, because the energy is transferred into the ground rather than a moving frame. The cross braces on a folding frame can twist and move in response to rolling across uneven surfaces, which results in energy loss during propulsion. More recent models of ultralight folding wheelchairs have attempted to lessen this motion by adding a second seat rail or a saddle to secure the cross brace when the chair is open and in use, but some movement remains. For some less active wheelchair users, the ease of a folding frame for loading into a vehicle may initially be preferred. However, a detailed conversation about the individual's needs and how to fold a rigid frame frequently results in the provision of rigid frames rather than folding frames.

Ultralightweight wheelchairs require the least amount of force to propel, compared with standard or lightweight chairs, because of lighter weight construction and, more important, the amount of adjustability in their axles. Proper setup of the rear wheels and the frame design lowers rolling resistance, which decreases the forces necessary to propel the wheelchairs. Ultralight wheelchairs have been shown to

Lange, M. L., & Minkel, J. L.
Seating and Wheeled Mobility: A Clinical Resource Guide
(pp. 149-163). © 2018 SLACK Incorporated.

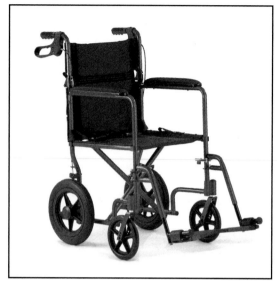

Figure 9-1. Standard transport wheelchair.

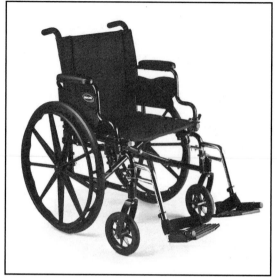

Figure 9-2. Standard wheelchair. (Reprinted with permission from Invacare.)

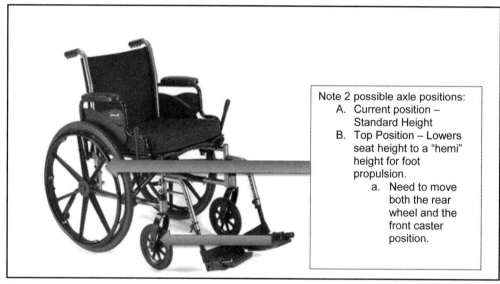

Note 2 possible axle positions:
- A. Current position – Standard Height
- B. Top Position – Lowers seat height to a "hemi" height for foot propulsion.
  - a. Need to move both the rear wheel and the front caster position.

Figure 9-3. Lightweight manual wheelchair. (Reprinted with permission from Invacare.)

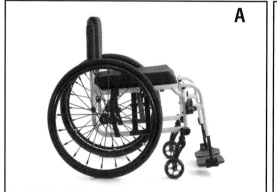

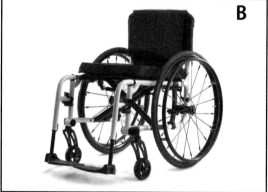

Figure 9-4. Front and side views of two ultralight folding manual wheelchairs. (Reprinted with permission from TiLite and Sunrise Medical.)

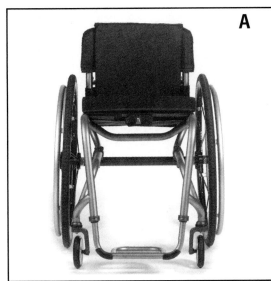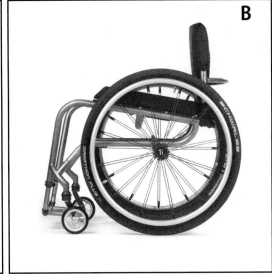

Figure 9-5. Front and side view of an ultralight rigid wheelchair. (Reprinted with permission from TiLite.)

improve push speeds, distance of propulsion, and decrease energy expenditure compared with standard wheelchairs (Beekman, Miller-Porter, & Schoneberger, 1999).

Ultralight wheelchairs have the most adjustability of the axle. As discussed subsequently, this adjustment is important to maximize function and decrease injury risk in individuals who propel. A properly designed ultralight wheelchair functions like a prosthetic in that it is an extension of the individual rather than simply a device that he or she uses. Adjustability of the axle and casters allows for decreased force and reduced frequency of push stroke to achieve and maintain a functional propelling speed.

PAIN IN MANUAL WHEELCHAIR USERS

Individuals who propel manual wheelchairs are at high risk of developing repetitive stress injuries in their upper extremities: 49% to 73% of individuals who use wheelchairs develop carpal tunnel syndrome, and 59% develop pain in their upper extremities including rotator cuff tears (Berner et al., 2010; Boninger et al., 2005; Yang et al., 2009). These injuries result in a decline in function and a decreased quality of life along with increased cost of medical care (Alm, Saraste, & Norrbrink, 2008; Boninger, Impink, Cooper, & Koontz, 2004). The pain affects all aspects of the individual's life and can result in lost days at work or increased need for assistance with personal care.

WHEELCHAIR DESIGN

After selecting the correct type of manual wheelchair for an individual, the appropriate design and setup of the wheelchair is important to maximize function and to lessen the risk of developing upper extremity injuries.

The Rehabilitation, Engineering, and Assistive Technology Society of North America (RESNA) (2012) has a position paper on the proper design and setup of manual wheelchairs. This document can be a helpful addition to this chapter to assist in determining proper wheelchair setup for an individual.

Seat Width

The first measurement that should be determined is seat width. Ensuring that the seat width is as narrow as possible is recommended for most individuals. This is usually accomplished by setting the seat width at or only slight larger than the person's measured hip width (Figure 9-6). A chair that is too wide causes increased shoulder abduction and wrist flexion. This upper extremity positioning, along with decreased sitting stability, can make the chair more difficult to propel and can cause upper extremity injury (Figure 9-7). Additionally, when the chair is made too wide, it can affect the individual's ability to navigate through doorways.

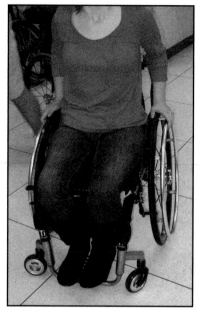

Figure 9-6. Properly selected hip width places the wheels in an easily accessible position.

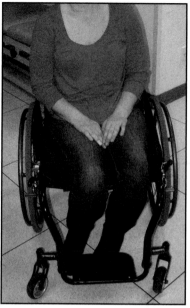

Figure 9-7. A seat width that is too wide makes wheel access difficult and decreases sitting stability.

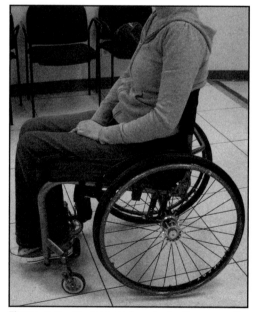

Figure 9-8. An increased seat depth causes the individual to sit with a posterior pelvic tilt.

Seat Depth

Seat depth is important for a proper sitting position (RESNA, 2012). A seat that is too short can increase the load on the buttocks, resulting in the risk of pressure ulcer development at the ischial tuberosity. A short seat depth also shortens the frame length. This increases the amount of weight on the casters, which can make the chair more difficult to propel.

A seat that is too long can put pressure behind the knees and frequently causes people to slide forward in the chair to relieve the pressure on the back of the knees (Figure 9-8). If the person slides forward, the pelvis will often tilt back into posterior pelvic tilt, which puts an increase amount of pressure on the sacrum, which can result in a pressure ulcer. Longer seat depths, also limit the person's ability to tuck his or her feet underneath him or her, resulting in the chair being longer and can limit maneuverability in tight environments.

When determining the correct seat depth, the goal is to maximize the weight on the rear wheels to increase propulsion efficiency and maneuverability. For many self-propellers, an ideal seat depth is at least 2 inches shorter than the person's measured sitting depth to assure proper support (Figure 9-9).

Seat to Footrest Length

Selecting the appropriate distance from the seat support to the footrest is important for sitting stability and positioning. This measurement must include the cushion being chosen because this will affect the height the person will sit relative to the footplate. If the footplate is too high, the individual will have increased pressure under his or her ischial tuberosities, and this could increase the risk of pressure ulcers (Figure 9-10). A properly adjusted footplate will support the thighs and buttocks fully while supporting the feet (Figure 9-11). If the footplate is too low, the individual will have decreased foot support and will be less stable. Additionally, a footplate that is too low can contact the ground and increase risk of injury from falling out of

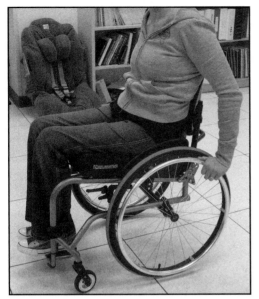

Figure 9-9. A properly adjusted seat depth allows an individual to sit upright without pressure behind his or her knees.

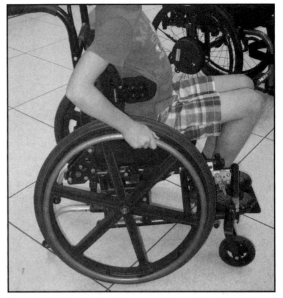

Figure 9-10. Footrests that are positioned too high increase pressure on the ischial tuberosities and can result in pressure ulcers.

the wheelchair. This can happen going down ramps or curb cuts when the footplate catches the ground if it is too low. This sudden stop from footplate contact can cause the individual to fall forward out of the chair, or with the chair if he or she is wearing a pelvic belt.

Front Frame Bend

The front frame bend of the wheelchair frame places the footrest in a position relative to the seat. In Figures 9-12 and 9-13, the front frame bend is measured as the angle that the front frame makes relative to the floor. As you can see, the larger the angle between the ground and the seat, the tighter the position of the footrest is relative to the seat. A tighter fit between the seat and the footrest makes the chair shorter, which improves maneuverability, and also better accommodates tight hamstrings, allowing a person to sit upright and propel. A more extended position of the footrests relative to the seat makes the chair longer and can result in a posterior pelvic tilt if the individual who is sitting in a chair with an extended front end has tight hamstrings. Generally, the tighter the front frame angle a person can tolerate, the easier it is for her to function throughout the day (Figures 9-14 and 9-15).

Seat Height and Vertical Wheel Position

The desired sitting height needs to be discussed when deciding the seat height of the wheelchair. Front seat height

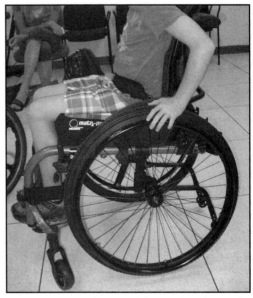

Figure 9-11. Properly adjusted footrest length provides good support under the thighs and buttocks.

is usually determined by the length of the lower legs. The footplates need to be positioned at a length to support the feet while ensuring that the thighs and buttocks are properly supported. It is important that the legs be supported and the footplates are far enough off the ground for safe propulsion to prevent the footplate from contacting the ground, ideally at least 2 inches off the ground.

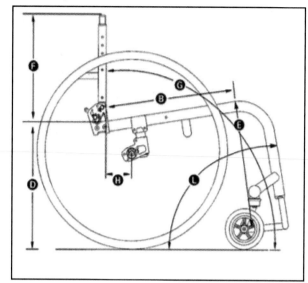

Figure 9-12. Front frame bend: measurement L. Angle of frame to ground.

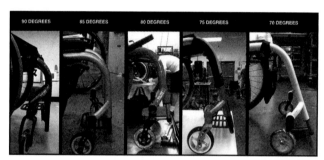

Figure 9-13. Front frame angle. (Reprinted with permission from TiLite.)

There is an important relationship among the lower leg length, cushion thickness, footrest length, and the front seat height. See the following example:

Lower leg length = 12 inches

Cushion thickness = 3 inches

Footrest length should be set at
(12 – 3 inches) = 9 inches

Clearance under footrest = 2 inches

Front seat height needs to be at least
(9 + 2 inches) = 11 inches

The seat height of the wheelchair affects access to tables and desks. When a person has a longer lower leg, the front seat height may need to be positioned so that the individual's knees may be in a position higher than clearance height under standard tables and desks. This should be thoroughly discussed with the individual so that proper modifications can be made to the environment as needed.

The rear sitting height also affects the vertical position of the rear wheel. If the person who is hand propelling sits too low in the wheelchair, he or she will have to flex his or her

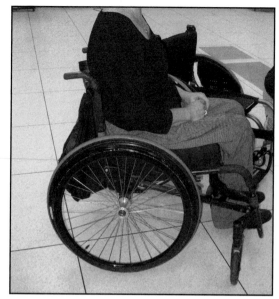

Figure 9-14. An extended front frame bend makes the chair longer and can result in a posterior pelvic tilt in individual with tight hamstrings.

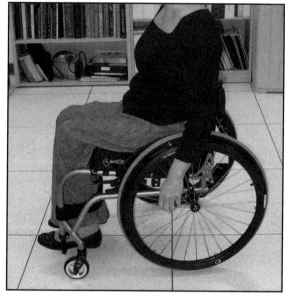

Figure 9-15. A tight front frame bend shortens the overall chair length and allows the individual to sit upright.

elbows and abduct his or her shoulders to access the wheel, which increases the risk of shoulder impingement. If the person sits too high in the chair, he or she will have to fully extend his or her elbows to just reach the wheel, limiting the arc of hand contact on the rim and decreasing push length; this results in very ineffective propulsion

The ideal rear seat height relative to the handrim is when the rider's elbow is in a position of between 100 and 120 degrees of elbow flexion when the hand is on top of the handrim as is shown in Figure 9-16 (Boninger, Baldwin, Cooper, Koontz, & Chan, 2000; van der Woude et al., 2009).

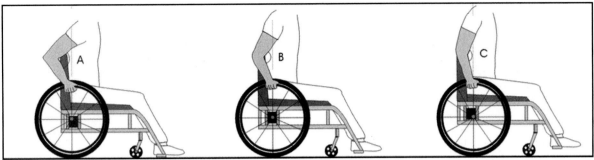

Figure 9-16. (A) Seat height is too low. (B) Adjusting the rear seat height so that it most closely matches this configuration is recommended. (Reprinted with permission from Paralyzed Veterans of America Consortium for Spinal Cord Medicine. (2005). Preservation of upper limb function following spinal cord injury: A clinical practice guideline for health-care professionals. *Journal of Spinal Cord Medicine, 28*, 434-470.)

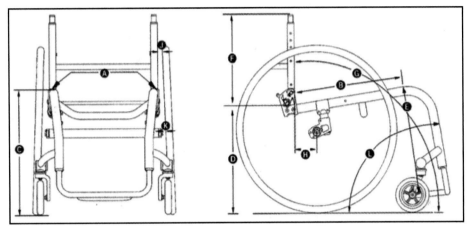

Figure 9-17. Seat slope is the difference between measurement C and D.

In Figure 9-16, part A illustrates when the seat height is too low. When the rider reaches down to the top of the wheel, his or her elbow is flexed more than 120 degrees. To propel the chair, the rider risks impingement at the shoulder due to the increased elbow and shoulder flexion to position the arm on the wheel. Part B of Figure 9-16 is the ideal, with the elbow at a 120-degree angle when the hand is resting on the top of the wheel. In part C, the rider is sitting too high relative to the wheel, requiring almost full extension of the arm to reach the wheel. In this position, the push stroke will be inefficient because of a very short push arc, resulting in increased number of strokes to move the chair.

Seat Slope

Seat slope is the difference between the front seat height and the rear seat height (Figure 9-17). Finding the perfect amount of seat slope for each person is important because it affects sitting balance, transfers, and wheel access. People with less trunk control may need larger seat slopes to maintain their balance (Figures 9-18 and 9-19). However, if the slope is too large and the upper extremities are weak, the person may not be able to transfer out of the chair because he or she has to slide uphill. Additionally, if the slope is large, the person may sit too low relative to the wheels and

have difficulty propelling. In most cases, a minimum of 2 inches of seat slope is used.

Many tall individuals use wheelchairs, and for these individuals, creativity is necessary to design a wheelchair that supports and positions them properly. Usually this requires a combination of an increased seat slope and a tight or increased front frame bend. For example, the gentleman in Figure 9-20 is 6 feet 9 inches tall; seat slope and an appropriate front frame bend allow him to fit under tables and desks.

Backrest Height and Angle

Selecting the correct backrest height can significantly affect propulsion. Higher backrest heights provide more trunk stability. However, if the backrest is too tall, it interferes with propulsion. Generally, lower backrest heights allow the scapula to move during propulsion, which allows for greater shoulder motion (Yang, Koontz, Yeh, & Chang, 2012). This improved motion of the shoulder and scapula decreases push frequency.

When selecting the back height, the individual's trunk control must be considered (Cherubini & Melchiorri, 2012). For individuals with limited trunk control, when possible, placing the back 20 mm below the scapula is recommended.

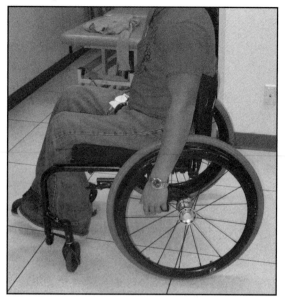

Figure 9-18. A flat seat slope decreases stability.

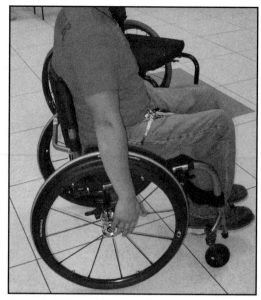

Figure 9-19. A small seat slope improves sitting balance and stability for many individuals.

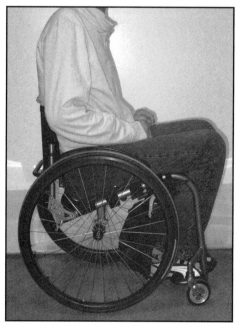

Figure 9-20. Seat slope and an appropriate front frame bend allow this tall client to fit under tables and desks.

When an individual has an intact trunk control, placing the back in the lumbar region provides the rider with the correct support in the low back, while preventing interference with propulsion.

Seat to back angle can affect sitting balance and position. A tighter seat to back angle positions the pelvis in an anterior pelvic tilt, which can assist with propulsion. With a seat to back angle that is too open, the rider may assume a posterior pelvic tilt and slide forward in the wheelchair. Finding the rider's preferred balance is important to give him or her sitting stability and the best position for propulsion.

Center of Gravity—Adjustment of the Rear Wheel

The position of the rear wheels forward or rearward is important and affects a person's ability to propel a wheelchair (Boninger et al., 2000). Moving the rear wheel forward or backward affects the center of gravity of the rider and the chair. By moving the rear wheel forward, you move the center of gravity forward, putting more weight on the rear wheels as compared to a more stable, rearward position, with the weight balanced on the rear wheels and the casters.

For the most efficient self-propelling position, the center of gravity should be as far forward as possible without compromising stability to improve function in many individuals (Paralyzed Veterans of America, 2005). For most individuals, this places the axle of the rear wheel under their middle finger when they hang their hand straight down (Figure 9-21). This is usually 2 to 3 inches in front of the backrest. To test the balance between forward wheel position and compromise of stability, it is suggested to move the wheel forward of the back posts and ask the rider to push from a stand-still position. Stand behind the person when he or she initiates the push to spot the rider and prevent a backward fall. If the chair is "too tippy" (the wheel is too far forward to the rider), when the rider initiates a push from a stand-still position, the front casters will pop up off the ground. The desired forward position of the rear wheel is when the person can easily pop the chair into a wheelie (front caster off the ground) but does not pop into a wheelie with every initial push stroke. More experienced riders will want or need a very tippy chair, whereas someone new to self-propelling will need to learn wheelchair mobility skills

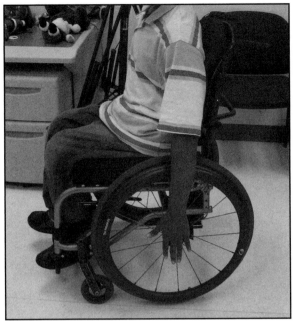

Figure 9-21. A properly adjusted center of gravity improves propulsion ability and decreases injury risk. Note the position of the wheel axle forward of the back posts of the chair.

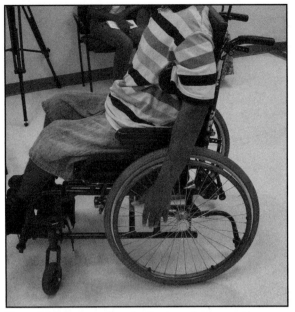

Figure 9-22. A center of gravity that is too far rearward increases rolling resistance and makes wheel access difficult, which decreases propulsion efficiency.

before feeling comfortable with a very forward rear wheel position.

This forward position can reduce rolling resistance and make it easier for the person to perform wheelies. It also positions the wheels for improved general propulsion and minimizes the risks of developing repetitive stress injuries. Each individual is different as to where his or her perfect location rests. Consequently, finding the perfect spot for each individual is important, as a center of gravity that is too far forward will cause the chair to be too tippy and may result in falls. A rear wheel position that is too far back makes the chair hard to propel because wheel contact is limited and can decrease a person's function (Figure 9-22).

Rear Wheel Camber

Increased camber brings the top of the wheel closer to the individual, which can improve propulsion ability because the wheel is easier to access. Increasing camber also increases the lateral stability of the chair (Perdios, Sawatzky, & Sheel, 2007). It is used in sports wheelchairs to improve stability while increasing maneuverability (Figure 9-23). However, increased camber makes the overall width of the chair wider, so access through doors can be difficult if too much camber is used. For most individuals, 2 to 5 degrees of camber works well because they can navigate through doorways with it.

On many rigid frame wheelchairs, this measurement is determined thorough a factory-made axle bar, built with a specific amount of camber. The camber angle cannot be adjusted on this style of wheel axle, so it must be carefully

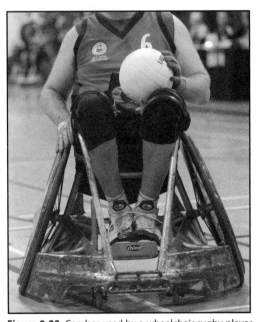

Figure 9-23. Camber used by a wheelchair rugby player to improve stability and maneuverability.

considered before ordering the wheelchair. Asking your supplier if the camber on a wheel chair can be adjusted or altered is an important wheelchair feature to be understood as part of the wheelchair ordering process.

Rear Wheels and Tires

Selecting the correct type and size of the rear wheel and tire is important to assist with effective propulsion. Generally, wheel sizes run from 18 to 22 inches for pediatric

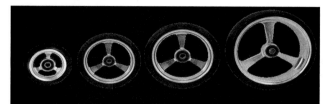

Figure 9-24. Size of caster affects rolling resistance and maneuverability.

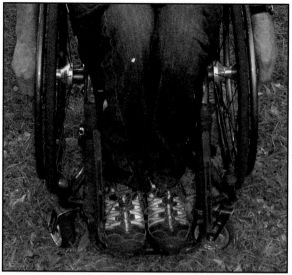

Figure 9-25. Casters that are positioned close to the rear wheel and the footplates provide less rolling resistance.

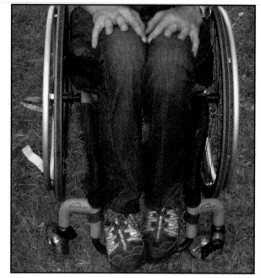

Figure 9-26. Casters that are positioned too wide next to the footplate limit maneuverability.

wheelchairs to 24 to 26 inches for adult wheelchairs. Most adults use a 24-inch rear wheel. However, using the diagram in Figure 9-16 can assist in determining the correct rear wheel size for each individual to assure correct propulsion method. Persons with shorter arms or of shorter stature may find using a small wheel, a 22-inch wheel rather than a 24-inch wheel, allows the rider to position the elbow at the desired, 120 degrees of flexion. When trying out a new chair, it is helpful to have demo chairs with quick release axles to allow them the chance to try a chair with different wheel size configurations.

Heavier rear wheels make it more difficult to start propelling from a stopped position (Hughes, Sawatzky, & Hol, 2005). Lighter weight wheels and those made out of materials like carbon fiber can decrease vibration for a more comfortable ride and less fatigue during propulsion (DiGiovine, Koontz, & Boninger, 2006).

Pneumatic tires generally have a more comfortable ride than solid tires. However, solid tires are frequently used due to ease of care and the lack of risk of punctures to the tire. Air tires have been shown to lessen rolling resistance compared with solid tires (Sawatzky & Denison, 2006). This remains true even when the air tires are poorly inflated.

Casters

There are many sizes and possible positions for casters (Figure 9-24). Smaller casters that are 3 to 4 inches in size turn better, and improve maneuverability compared with 8-inch casters often found on standard chairs (DiGiovine et al., 2006). However, smaller casters increase rolling resistance and get caught more easily on obstacles than larger casters. Newer, wider casters can improve rolling resistance and decrease catching in the smaller casters while maintaining good maneuverability. Many individuals will still require a larger 5- to 6-inch caster to propel safely around their environment if they live in rural areas and cannot effectively perform a wheelie to maneuver over obstacles.

The position of the casters affects propulsion and maneuverability. The caster should be positioned as close to the footplate and rear wheel without interfering with either. The shorter the distance between the rear wheel and the caster, the less rolling resistance there is when propelling the wheelchair (DiGiovine et al., 2006) (Figure 9-25). When the casters are positioned too far lateral to the footplate, the individual has difficulty maneuvering in tight spaces because the front of the chair is too wide (Figure 9-26).

Handrims

The size and design of the handrim affects propulsion. Standard handrims can be slippery and hard to hold, which can reduce their efficiency. Plastic coated handrims can improve propulsion in individuals with limited hand function. Many of these handrims create friction to improve control, and this can result in abrasions to the hands when going down ramps or uneven surfaces. Some of the newer

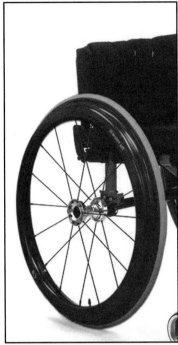

Figure 9-27. Natural Fit Ergonomic Handrim. (Reprinted with permission from Out-Front.)

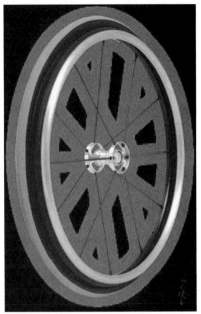

Figure 9-28. Flexrim Handrim; an example of an ergonomic pushrim. (Reprinted with permission from Spinery.)

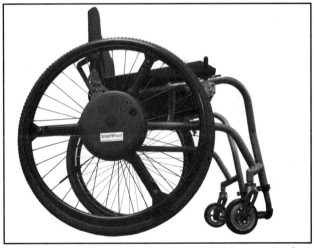

Figure 9-29. Instrumented handrim. (Reprinted with permission from Out-Front.)

coated handrims have decreased this friction, but many wheelchair users also use gloves to lessen the risk of injury.

The use of ergonomic handrims has been shown to decrease pain in wrists and hands during propulsion (Koontz et al., 2006) (Figure 9-27). These handrims use oval rims and provide a contoured surface for the individual's thumb during propulsion. These handrims position the hand more naturally and result in less extreme positions of the wrist and hand. Individuals surveyed stated that it requires less work to propel using this style of handrim. A flexible rubber handrim has been shown to decrease perceived effort and power generation during propulsion (Richter, Rodriguez, Woods, Karpinski, & Axelson, 2006) (Figure 9-28). This style of rim has a standard handrim, but the material that connects it to the wheel allows for movement, which lessens the impact on the wrist and hand from propulsion.

Evaluating propulsion with different styles of handrims is an important part of the process to determine the best equipment for an individual, especially for users who report upper extremity pain at either the shoulder of wrist after years of self-propulsion.

PROPULSION ASSESSMENT

There are both high- and low-tech methods of assessing propulsion. Both are designed to be done in clinical settings and should be completed during evaluation, delivery, and training. This assessment will ensure proper wheelchair setup so that the client has the least risk of developing upper extremity injuries from propulsion, including repetitive motion injuries due to the high frequency of push strokes, combined with the increased force needed to propel a chair that has not been optimally configured.

High Tech

Instrumented handrims provide objective data about propulsion (manufactured by Out-Front) (Figure 9-29). These devices provide kinetic and temporal spatial data about propulsion. The devices provide graphical data that shows propulsion in real time or throughout a trial

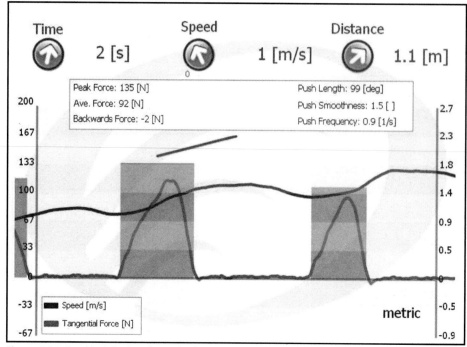

Figure 9-30. Graphical display of an individual's propulsion. (Reprinted with permission from Out-Front.)

(Figure 9-30). There is a database of wheelchair users propelling with one of these devices, and these data can easily be used to compare an individual's propulsion with others with similar diagnoses (Figure 9-31).

The data can be used to show a client his or her current efficiency and to teach him or her more efficient push mechanics—long, smooth strokes, using less force to maintain an effective propulsion speed. The data, including the graphical display, can also be sent to payer sources to justify why a certain wheelchair setup or style is necessary for an individual.

Low Tech

Many clinics do not have access to instrumented handrims. However, much information can be obtained with the use of items that most clinics possess. A stopwatch can be used to assess how long it takes an individual to propel a fixed distance. Most people use 10 meters for this test, but the distance can vary based on the size of the testing space available. The use of a video camera can allow for assessment of push frequency. These data can also be used to document an individual's propulsion ability and help to improve it or justify necessary equipment. As a functional baseline for minimally effective manual mobility propulsion, a person should be able to self-propel at least at the same speed as a person walking. A great functional test, if you are in an urban environment, is to test if the person can get across a street while the walk sign is still flashing. If the person is unable to self-propel at least at walking speed, due

to decreased upper extremity strength, coordination, pain, or shortness of breath, then power mobility, including the use of scooter, may be considered, especially for community mobility needs.

PROPULSION TRAINING

Time should be spent at delivery and during follow-up appointments to teach the individual the best, most efficient propulsion technique for him or her. Video and kinetic data can help to provide feedback to the client to teach him or her the best pattern.

Hand Propulsion

The most common technique selected by wheelchair users is a single-looping method where the client recovers with his or her hand above the handrim (Boninger et al., 2002). However, the best technique is the semicircular pattern in which the hand remains below the handrim during the recovery phase of propulsion. This method results in a lower push frequency and decreased forces generated for propulsion for most individuals.

Figure 9-32A illustrates the goal of a long smooth stroke: recovery below the rim. Figure 9-32B illustrates inefficient stroke mechanics. The rider needs to contact the rim too frequently using this technique, again resulting in risk of overuse injury.

Key Data From Client Session and Comparison to Database Averages

(These key parameters are calculated from all pushes except for the first 3. Database average may not be available depending upon protocol chosen.)

	CLIENT SESSION 1	CLIENT SESSION 2	CLIENT SESSION 3	CLIENT SESSION 4	DATABASE AVERAGE[†]	DATABASE TOP 25%[‡]
SPEED (M/S)	1.35	0.90	1.17	0.79	1.20	1.50
PUSH FREQUENCY (L/S)	0.80	1.08	1.26	0.45	1.00	1.14
PUSH LENGTH (DEGREE)	77.93	43.54	39.99	70.34	100.6	107.12
FORCE (WEIGHT NORMALIZED) %	9.32	5.59	10.99	6.78	9.70	11.34

[†] Database averages cited are from *Archives of Physical Medicine and Rehabilitation*. 2008;89:260-268 and is for informational purposes only.

[‡] Speed, frequency, push length, and force data are drawn from the database population that fell within the top 25% of speed (upper quartile).

AVERAGE SPEED VS WEIGHT NORMALIZED PUSH FORCE ON TILE

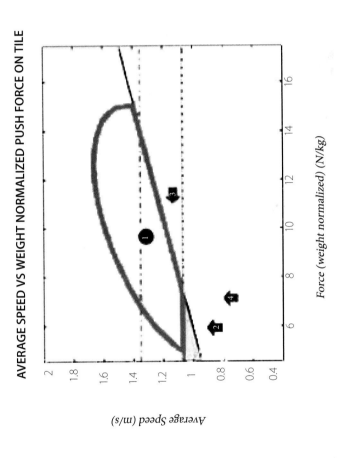

Figure 9-31. Comparison of an individual's propulsion to the SmartWheel Database. (Reprinted with permission from Out-Front.) *To see this image in color, please visit the companion website at www. healio.com/books/mobility.*

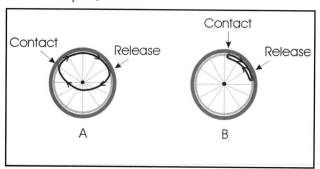

Figure 9-32. (A) A single-loop pattern for propulsion, which is the preferred method to preserve shoulder function. (B) An arc pattern, which is a less efficient stroke mechanics. (Reprinted with permission from Paralyzed Veterans of America Consortium for Spinal Cord Medicine. (2005). Preservation of upper limb function following spinal cord injury: A clinical practice guideline for health-care professionals. *Journal of Spinal Cord Medicine, 28,* 434-470.)

Alternative Propulsion Techniques

Some people cannot effectively self-propel a manual wheelchair using their hands alone. For these individuals, foot propulsion, or a combination of hand and foot propulsion, can be used. At delivery, training for these individuals to ensure an effective technique is important. Unlike hand propulsion, there is no gold standard method, so observation should be used to determine the most effective technique for each client.

Advanced Skills

When working with a wheelchair rider, a discussion of and training on advanced skills is important to ensure that an individual reaches his or her highest level of function. The ability to perform a wheelie (lifting the casters off the ground and holding rear-wheel balance is important skill for navigating uneven surfaces). Learning and using advanced mobility skills allows the rider to experience the highest level of independence in manual wheelchair propulsion. To safely and effectively perform a wheelie, the individual must have the appropriate chair setup. A forward center of gravity (rear wheel moved as far forward as possible) greatly decreases the effort needed to pop a wheelie. The more forward the person's weight is in the chair, the easier it is to move the center of gravity behind the rear wheel, causing the chair to tip backward and raising the front caster off the ground. The advance mobility skill of rear-wheel balancing is the learned skill of controlling the rearward tip of the chair and being able to push the chair while balancing only on the rear wheels. Learning these skills is the result of a progression of learned tasks, including being able to:

- Hold the rear-wheel balance, once positioned in the rear wheel balance position

- Pop into the rear-wheel balance position from a stand-still position

- Lift the casters off the ground, in a controlled fashion while moving forward

- Coordinate the lifting of the casters off the ground, maintain forward propulsion, and pop a wheelie to go over a 2- to 3-inch curb

Professionals involved in the setup and recommendation of an ultralight, high adjustable manual chair should also be skilled in training riders on how to use the chair, especially teaching the advanced mobility skills needed to maximize independent mobility. An informative website, designed to assist the clinician to learn and teach these skills, is found at www.wheelchairskillsprogram.ca/eng/index.php

With plastic-coated or ergonomic handrims, many individuals with limited hand function can effectively perform wheelies with the correct equipment and chair setup. Additionally, depending on the individual's trunk balance and upper extremity function, a properly designed seat slope is needed to ensure the necessary trunk balance while performing a wheelie.

Many individuals also need to learn how to upright their wheelchair if they fall or to go up or down steps and escalators. Without a therapist to teach them these skills, many people do not know that these activities are possible and their function is consequently limited.

SUMMARY

When working with clients, clinicians have a large range of wheelchairs and seating components available to them so that they can best meet the needs of each client. Equipment selection and design can change a person's life in both positive and negative ways. The prescribing of manual wheelchairs is complex and requires a thorough understanding of the client, his or her needs, and the equipment options to achieve best outcomes. Follow-up and adjustments made over time can help to ensure optimal function

REFERENCES

Alm, M., Saraste, H., & Norrbrink, C. (2008). Shoulder pain in persons with thoracic spinal cord injury: Prevalence and characteristics. *Journal of Rehabilitation Medicine, 40,* 277-283.

Beekman, C. E., Miller-Porter, L., & Schoneberger, M. (1999). Energy cost of propulsion in standard and ultralight wheelchairs in people with spinal cord injuries. *Physical Therapy, 79,* 146-158.

Berner, T. F., DiGiovine, C. P., & Roesler, T. L. (2010). Manual Wheelchair Configuration and Training: An Update on the Evidence. 26th International Seating Symposium. Vancouver, British Columbia.

Boninger, M. L., Baldwin, M., Cooper, R. A., Koontz, A., & Chan, L. (2000). Manual wheelchair pushrim biomechanics and axle position. *Archives of Physical Medicine and Rehabilitation, 81,* 608-613.

Boninger, M. L., Impink, B. G., Cooper, R. A., & Koontz, A. M. (2004). Relation between median and ulnar nerve function and wrist kinematics during wheelchair propulsion. *Archives of Physical Medicine and Rehabilitation, 85,* 1141-1145.

Boninger, M. L., Koontz, A. M., Sisto, S. A., Dyson-Hudson, T. A., Chang, M., Price, R., & Cooper, R. A. (2005). Pushrim biomechanics and injury prevention in spinal cord injury: Recommendations based on CULP-SCI investigations. *Journal of Rehabilitation Research & Development, 42*(3 Suppl 1), 9-20.

Boninger, M. L., Souza, A. L., Cooper, R. A., Fitzgerald, S. G., Koontz, A. M., & Fay, B. T. (2002). Propulsion patterns and pushrim biomechanics in manual wheelchair propulsion. *Archives of Physical Medicine and Rehabilitation, 83,* 718-723.

Cherubini, M., & Melchiorri, G. (2012). Descriptive study about congruence in wheelchair prescription. *European Journal of Physical Rehabilitation Medicine, 48,* 217-22.

DiGiovine, C., Koontz, A., & Boninger, M. (2006). Advances in manual wheelchair technology. *Topics in Spinal Cord Injury Rehabilitation, 11*(4), 1-14.

Hughes, B., Sawatzky, B. J., & Hol, A. T. (2005). A comparison of spinergy versus standard steel-spoke wheelchair wheels. *Archives of Physical Medicine and Rehabilitation, 86,* 596-601.

Koontz, A. M., Yang, Y., Boninger, D. S., Kanaly, J., Cooper, R. A., Boninger, M. L.,...& Ewer, L. (2006). Investigation of the performance of an ergonomic handrim as a pain-relieving intervention for manual wheelchair users. *Assistive Technology, 18,* 123-145.

Paralyzed Veterans of America Consortium for Spinal Cord Medicine. (2005). Preservation of upper limb function following spinal cord injury: A clinical practice guideline for health-care professionals. *Journal of Spinal Cord Medicine, 28,* 434-470.

Perdios, A., Sawatzky, B. J., & Sheel, A. W. (2007). Effects of camber on wheeling efficiency in the experienced and inexperienced wheelchair user. *Journal of Rehabilitation Research and Development, 44,* 459-466.

Rehabilitation Engineering & Assistive Technology Society of North America. (2012). *RESNA position on the application of ultralight wheelchairs.* Retrieved from https://www.resna.org/sites/default/files/legacy/resources/position-papers/UltraLightweightManualWheelchairs.pdf

Richter, W. M., Rodriguez, R., Woods, K. R., Karpinski, A. P., & Axelson, P. W. (2006). Reduced finger and wrist flexor activity during propulsion with a new flexible handrim. *Archives of Physical Medicine and Rehabilitation, 87,* 1643-1647.

Sawatzky, B. J., & Denison, I. (2006). Wheeling efficiency: The effects of varying tyre pressure with children and adolescents. *Pediatric Rehabilitation, 9,* 122-126.

van der Woude, L. H., Bouw, A., van Wegen, J., van As, H., Veeger, D., & de Groot, S. (2009). Seat height: Effects on submaximal hand rim wheelchair performance during spinal cord injury rehabilitation. *Journal of Rehabilitation Medicine, 41,* 143-149.

Yang, J., Boninger, M. L., Leath, J. D., Fitzgerald, S. G., Dyson-Hudson, T. A., & Chang, M. W. (2009). Carpal tunnel syndrome in manual wheelchair users with spinal cord injury: a cross-sectional multicenter study. *American Journal of Physical Medicine & Rehabilitation, 88*(12), 1007-1016.

Yang, Y. S., Koontz, A. M., Yeh, S. J., & Chang, J. J. (2012). Effect of backrest height on wheelchair propulsion biomechanics for level and uphill conditions. *Archives of Physical Medicine and Rehabilitation, 93,* 654-659.

10

Power Mobility Applications
Mobility Categories and Clinical Indicators

Michael Babinec, OTR/L, ABDA, ATP

The number of individuals requiring a power mobility device (PMD) for participation in activities of daily mobility in the United States continues to grow each year. In 2011, there were estimated to be 3.3 million wheelchair users in the United States (Disabled World, 2011). The growth rate for additional wheelchair users is estimated to be from 5% to 8% (Flagg, 2009). Although statistics indicating the number of replacement power wheelchairs prescribed each year are difficult to compile, this represents a large volume of PMDs, most noticeably in the complex rehabilitation technology (CRT) segments to be discussed later. Many current PMD users in the United States receive a recommendation for a new or replacement power wheelchair on an average of every 5 years after receiving a previous system. This 5-year benchmark is not a universal rule but is based on one U.S. reimbursement policy guideline regarding eligibility for coverage of a replacement power chair only after it is 5 years old, unless there are additional or extenuating circumstances. For example, the beneficiary has a new diagnosis or the equipment was irreparably damaged (NHIC Corp., 2007). Some third-party funding agencies will reimburse for a new power chair earlier than the 5-year benchmark with appropriate justification. Some, however, will authorize replacement only if documentation can be provided stating why the original needs to be replaced, regardless of the age of the current system.

In any case, new or replacement, the recommendation for a power wheelchair needs to match the technology of the power wheelchair (and accessories) to the user's clinical, functional, and environmental needs and preferences.

This chapter examines various power wheelchair categories and the clinical indicators for each.

POWER MOBILITY: SYSTEMS DEFINED

Power wheelchairs for mobility are complete systems. Primary components include the base, seating, driver control(s), motors, and batteries. Additional components include positioning accessories, electronic accessories, and even integrated electronic aids to daily living. Poorly prescribed power mobility systems can be dangerous and cause harm. Critical when recommending an appropriate power mobility system is the seating and positioning system. Not all power wheelchairs can accept all seating systems. Inappropriate seating, at its worst, can cause pressure injuries, pain, discomfort, and loss of function. At its best, seating will contribute to stability, comfort, and function. The best programming, driver control selection, and mounting, and latest software upgrades for a power mobility control system cannot substitute for incorrect seating and positioning. Power mobility systems are intended to provide function and mobility. Without stability there can be no function. Stability within any powered seating device—whether a simple van/captain's seat or a complex powered tilt/recline system with custom seating—is essential to function.

Lange, M. L., & Minkel, J. L.
Seating and Wheeled Mobility: A Clinical Resource Guide
(pp. 165-177). © 2018 SLACK Incorporated.

POWER MOBILITY:
USER CATEGORIES

Age Segments

Who is appropriate for powered mobility? A better question to ask may be "Who would benefit from powered mobility?" Independent (and sometimes least assisted) mobility is essential for participation in many instrumental activities of daily living (IADL). Few can argue the functional gains from use of powered mobility. For some, powered mobility is medically necessary to prevent pain/overuse syndromes or manage positioning for those at risk for pressure injuries. Powered mobility has applications from pediatric through adult to geriatric users.

Pediatric users are generally considered those up to 18 years of age. The age a child should get his first power chair is changing, however, and rapidly becoming younger (Jones, McEwen, & Neas, 2012). Some advocate for early intervention with supervised power mobility use beginning at 18 months and earlier. Normal development requires mobility, specifically vestibular stimulation and interaction with the environment (Livingstone & Paleg, 2014). Mobility even plays a key role in the development of vision and visual perceptual skills (Jones et al., 2012). Common attributes of pediatric power chairs include the ability to accommodate growth, accommodation of both standard and alternative driver controls, and the ability to accommodate transportation requirements. Common diagnoses requiring pediatric powered mobility include but are not limited to cerebral palsy, spinal muscular atrophy, spina bifida, spinal cord injury, muscular dystrophy, juvenile rheumatoid arthritis, and osteogenesis imperfecta. More information on pediatric mobility can be found in Chapter 17.

Power mobility for adults needs to meet the widest range of needs from very basic to the most challenging. Adults use powered mobility in the widest range of environments—home, community, social, educational, recreational, and vocational settings. Powered mobility may not only be required for a client's own independence and participation but also to provide for those who are dependent on him or her.

Power mobility for geriatric users may be required for participation in activities of daily mobility but also be necessary for managing the aging process. Indoor safety, accessibility, and maneuverability are key factors in power mobility for the elderly. These individuals are often unable to tolerate the bumps and jolts associated with some outdoor terrains. Elderly individuals often present with multiple disease processes. Some studies estimate the prevalence of chronic shoulder pain in the elderly population to range from 28.9% to 59.3% (McCarthy, Bigal, Katz, Derby, & Lipton, 2009)—a factor certainly not compatible with manual wheelchair propulsion for independent mobility.

More information on geriatric mobility can be found in Chapter 18.

Basic Criteria for Use of Powered Mobility

If an individual meets one or more of the following criteria, a PMD may be indicated:

- The individual has a mobility impairment that cannot be safely mitigated through use of a cane or walker.
- The individual demonstrates insufficient strength, range of motion (ROM), coordination, or endurance for manual wheelchair propulsion (mobility-related ADL).
- The individual presents with cardiorespiratory endurance deficiencies that impair participation in activities of daily mobility.
- Manual mobility is painful; propulsion method is not functional.
- Manual mobility places the individual at risk for development of overuse/pain syndromes.
- The individual is at risk for pressure injury development and requires power positioning to mitigate these risks.
- The individual has a progressive disability where use of power mobility or powered seating systems are anticipated.
- Manual propulsion method increases muscle tone and/or postural asymmetry.
- The weight of the individual negates independent manual or caregiver assisted mobility.

Not even 20 years ago, it was not unusual for some to recommend a manual wheelchair for mobility needs with the assumption that if an individual did not use his or her upper extremities with daily mobility, he or she would lose the strength and endurance required to do so. Fortunately, this "use it or lose it" mentality is being replaced with "conserve to preserve." If the goal is mobility, many recommend the correct device to meet not only today's needs but also those anticipated in the future. For more information on aging with a disability, please refer to Chapter 22.

User Segments with Clinical Indicators

Power mobility users can be broadly classified into three segments:

1. Intermittent in-home user/community user (light duty)
2. Active user—not at risk for pressure injuries (active duty)
3. Active user—at risk for pressure injuries or requiring CRT

Intermittent In-Home User/ Community User

This individual can be described as only requiring power mobility in the home for limited periods of the day or managing outdoor/community mobility. Most all who require power mobility in the home will also require assistance in the community, even if only on a limited basis. Power-operated vehicles (POVs), sometimes referred to as scooters, often accommodate those able to navigate indoors without a PMD but who require assistance for mobility in the community due to either mobility or endurance limitations. Some three-wheel POVs are able to be used in many home environments but are not as maneuverable as indoor power wheelchairs.

Clinical indicators for power wheelchair use in this segment include the following:

- Unable to mitigate mobility limitations through use of a cane, walker, or manual wheelchair
- Insufficient endurance to safely manage required mobility distances
- Able to operate a standard proportional joystick or Tiller control
- Not at risk for pressure injuries (able to maintain skin integrity through posture changes and weight shifts)
- Requires seating only for comfort and support
- Able to manage standard indoor obstacles and limited outdoor obstacles
- Needs are not anticipated to change for the expected life of the equipment
- May need a portable power wheelchair or scooter for community use

Active User—Not at Risk for Pressure Injuries

This individual requires a PMD for all activities of daily mobility and is active in a variety of home and community environments. POVs generally do not meet needs for indoor accessibility while also accommodating varied outdoor environments. Many active users will require CRT due to postural requirements, programming to accommodate multiple environments, or fitting/fabrication of accessories for positioning.

Clinical indicators for power wheelchair use in this segment include the following:

- Able to operate a standard proportional joystick with multiple drive profiles, but may require an alternative drive control input
- Requires seating for comfort and stability
- Does not require power seating to manage positioning needs/pressure redistribution

- May require seating to accommodate postural asymmetries
- Requires the features of an indoor/outdoor, or outdoor power wheelchair as described to meet daily mobility needs
- Able to manage outdoor terrain including inclines/declines, curb cuts, obstacles greater than 2 inches in height, and uneven grades/terrain

Active User—At Risk for Pressure Injuries or Requiring Complex Rehabilitation Technology

This segment describes a unique population of power wheelchair users with needs that require the skills of a team of health care professionals. The majority, but not all, will have a diagnosis classified as a neurologic condition, myopathy, or congenital orthopedic conditions. Neurologic conditions include diagnoses such as spinal cord injury, paraplegia and tetraplegia, cerebral palsy, multiple sclerosis, postpolio syndrome, cerebral vascular accident (stroke), traumatic brain injury, and amyotrophic lateral sclerosis (ALS). Myopathies include many muscular dystrophies. Congenital orthopedic conditions (present since birth) may result from one of the preceding diagnoses or from conditions such as arthrogryposis or juvenile rheumatoid arthritis. Some of these conditions/diagnoses, such as multiple sclerosis, ALS, and certain muscular dystrophies, are progressive and result in diminishing function over time.

Clinical indicators requiring CRT may include the following:

- Limitations in upper extremity function, such as diminished ROM, decreased strength or endurance, impaired sensation, impaired coordination and/or dexterity, or fixed orthopedic asymmetries/joint limitations that impair function. These users will require a driver control input other than a standard proportional joystick and custom programming to meet operational needs.
- Absent upper extremity or hand function requiring other means to operate the power wheelchair, such as head, chin, or pneumatic controls
- Muscle tone in the trunk and all or some extremities that ranges from absent, low or high, requiring full positioning and support. Some clients may even exhibit spasms and/or abnormal reflexive responses that need to be accommodated.
- Some clients will have full trunk control, whereas others will have either impaired or absent trunk balance that requires accommodation.
- Some clients will lack the physical ability/skills to perform a weight shift for pressure redistribution and require powered seating for pressure redistribution, positioning, and repositioning.

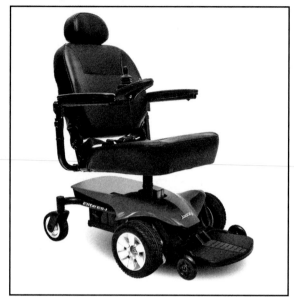

Figure 10-1. Pride Mobility Jazzy Elite ES.

- Some clients will have limited head control or ROM requiring support and positioning, whereas other clients will exhibit full head control without support.

POWER MOBILITY: ENVIRONMENTAL CATEGORIES

In terms of intended use environments, power wheelchairs fall into one of three basic categories: indoor, indoor/outdoor, and outdoor.

Indoor

Power mobility devices intended primarily for indoor use are often considered light-duty systems. This segment includes both power wheelchairs and POVs. Power wheelchairs in this segment include all three-drive wheel configurations: rear-, center-, and front-wheel drive (for more information on drive wheel configurations, refer to Chapter 12). The small turning radius of the center wheel configuration dominates this arena (Figure 10-1). The POVs in this segment are compact scooters (Figure 10-2).

Indoor PMD features include the following:

- Smaller drive wheels (10 to 12 inches)
- Slower driving speeds
- Standard proportional joysticks with speed control (no alternative driver controls)
- Comfort seating with only mild postural support (van-style seats)

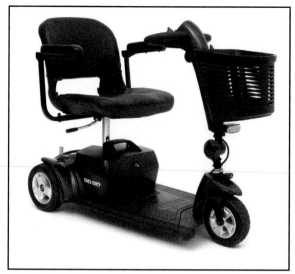

Figure 10-2. Pride Mobility GoGo Scooter.

- Obstacle-climbing capabilities of 2 inches (Centers for Medicare & Medicaid Services [CMS] Healthcare Common Procedure Coding System [HCPCS] Group 2) or less (CMS HCPCS Group 1) (National Government Services, 2013)
- Battery range of 7 miles (CMS HCPCS Group 2) or less (CMS HCPCS Group 1) (National Government Services, 2013)

Although intended primarily for indoor use, many of these devices do perform adequately in some outdoor environments that include minimal obstacles and firm, paved surfaces.

Indoor/Outdoor

Many PMDs are designed to have both indoor and outdoor capabilities. This category is often considered moderate-duty power wheelchairs (Figures 10-3 through 10-5). This is the largest segment of power chairs designed to meet the widest range of needs and includes all three drive wheel configurations (rear-, center-, and front-wheel drive). These are often included in the CRT segment. CRT includes products that are medically necessary and individually determined that require evaluation, fabrication, configuration, fitting, adjustment, and/or programming.

Indoor/outdoor power wheelchair features include the following:

- Larger drive wheels (12 to 14 inches)
- Faster driving speeds (>5 mph)
- Standard and alternative driver control options
- Van, rehab, and power positioning seating options and compatibility with custom seating
- Obstacle climbing capabilities of up to 3 inches
- Tracking (veer compensation) driving technologies

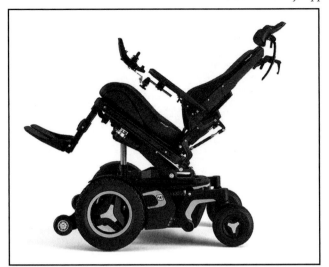

Figure 10-3. Permobil F3 Corpus.

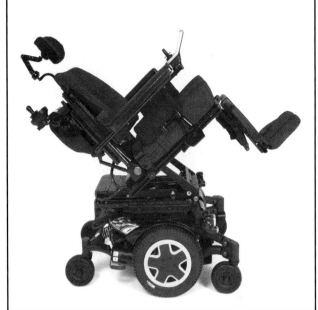

Figure 10-4. Invacare TDX SP.

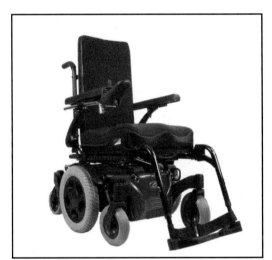

Figure 10-5. Sunrise Medical Pulse.

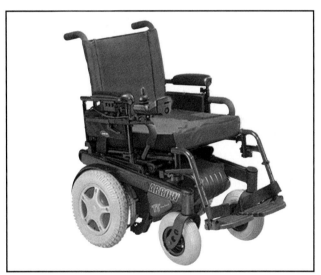

Figure 10-6. Invacare 3G Storm Arrow.

- Suspension
- Transport tie-down compatibilities
- Battery range ≥ 12 miles
- Compatibility with positioning accessories
- Compatibility with ventilator trays

Outdoor

Some PMDs are primarily intended for outdoor use and are considered active-duty devices (Figure 10-6). These include both four-wheel POVs and power wheelchairs. Power wheelchairs in this segment include many of the features of indoor/outdoor systems, and may also include the following:

- Faster driving speeds (> 6 mph)
- Large drive wheels (≥ 14 inches)

- Suspension
- Battery range ≥ 16 miles
- Obstacle-climbing capabilities of at least 3 inches

POWERED MOBILITY TYPES

Power-Operated Vehicles

A scooter is also known as a *power-operated vehicle*. Scooters come in all types and sizes, although the typical configuration is either three-wheel (Figure 10-7) or

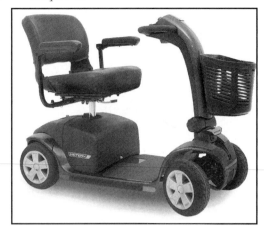

Figure 10-7. Pride Mobility Victory 10.

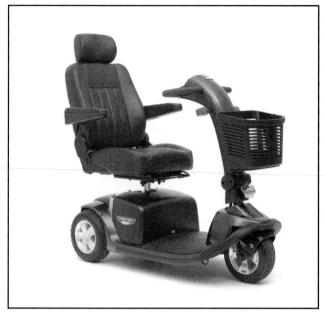

Figure 10-8. Pride Mobility Victory Sport.

four-wheel (Figure 10-8). Scooters are often more accepted and sought after by first time power mobility users. These are generally lower profile than a power wheelchair and more socially acceptable to some. POVs are intended to provide for only basic mobility needs for individuals with at least limited ambulatory skills and are not intended for the mobility-dependent user without ambulatory skills.

The greatest strength of a POV is its ability to provide mobility. A weakness of a POV is its limited maneuverability, especially in tight spaces. Scooters with three wheels (two rear, one front) generally have a smaller turning radius (required for indoor mobility) than scooters with four wheels, but can be less stable. Not all indoor environments, however, provide the space necessary to allow a user to maneuver even with a three-wheeled base. Four-wheel scooters have a larger turning radius, accommodating outdoor mobility more readily, and can be more stable at faster speeds and when traversing outdoor, unleveled terrain.

Most all scooters have some style of padded seat similar to the captain's seat of some power wheelchairs. The captain's seat on some POVs has a back angle adjustment, which is critical for accommodating sitting postures with a kyphotic trunk or posteriorly tilted pelvis.

Many seat types swivel and lock into position 90 degrees left or right of the standard position. This can be useful in performing some ADL from the scooter seat, such as sitting sideways at a table for meals or even for meal preparation, as well as facilitating transfers into and out of the seat.

Some armrests on scooter seats adjust, and others are fixed. Adjustments include width, height, and angle:

- Width: Required to accommodate torso size if different than hip width
- Height: Required for arm support for stability
- Angle: Required for support while matching back angle

- Flip back: Required by some to allow independent transfers into/out of the chair

Although many scooters have head- and taillights, these are more useful to enable the scooter driver to be seen rather than lighting the road or path for safe driving. Although intended for outdoor use, POVs are not intended for mobility on streets, roads, or highways.

Clinical Indicators for Use of Power-Operated Vehicles

Scooters are appropriate for users who are considered *partial ambulators*—users who have limited ambulation skills but can negotiate tight indoor spaces with or without an assistive device. In addition, the following are clinical indicators required for safe and independent POV operation.

Limited Ambulation Skills

- Lower extremity strength, endurance, or coordination required to manage the distances needed by activities of daily mobility is insufficient.
- Cardiorespiratory endurance to manage the distances required by activities of daily mobility is insufficient.

Adequate Transfer Skills

- User is able to safely transfer into *and* out of the POV with or without caregiver assistance.
- User has the ability to swivel and lock the seat at a 90-degree position to enable safe transfer to surfaces and participation in ADL.

Sufficient Upper Extremity Function for Tiller Operation

- Shoulder strength and ROM are appropriate to allow the user to reach and sustain hand placement on the tiller handles to operate the POV in all required environments.
- Upper extremity strength and coordination are appropriate for steering and controlling the POV using tiller control in all required environments.

At Least Limited Hand Function

- Hand function must be sufficient to grasp and sustain hold on the tiller grip.
- Thumb dexterity must be sufficient to allow for operating and controlling speed.
- Pinch dexterity must be appropriate to operate the on-off key for power.
- Finger dexterity appropriate for operation of the lights and horn.

Functional Trunk Balance

- Positioning needs when seated are mild and for support only.
- Stability in a seated position when driving is adequate for safety and control.
- Balance is sufficient for safe transfers and for stability when driving.
- Head control is good without support.

Sensory Function

- The user is not at risk for pressure injuries.
- The user has the awareness and ability to redistribute seated pressure.
- Visual acuity is adequate for safe mobility and POV operation.
- Visual perceptual skills are adequate for safe and efficient POV operation.

Cognitive Skills

- The user has the cognitive and judgment skills required for safe and efficient POV operation in all required environments.

Care of a Power-Operated Vehicle Mobility Device

As with all PMDs, a POV requires either the user or the caregiver to charge the batteries. POVs that are driven only intermittently indoors may not need the batteries charged daily.

In these instances, it may be acceptable to wait until the battery gauge shows half full. POVs that are driven daily or driven outdoors should have the batteries charged daily. A battery is essentially the gas tank for a PMD. Running "out of gas" at the wrong time can be more than just inconvenient. Although POVs have a brake release to put them in a free wheel mode and enable pushing, this is primarily for maneuverability or for transportation purposes and is not intended to allow manual mobility through a caregiver's assistance.

Who May Not Be Appropriate for Power-Operated Vehicles

Although preferred by some, there are individuals for whom a POV may not be appropriate. These include the following.

Individuals With a Progressive Disability

Although a POV may be appropriate for some clients in the early stages of certain progressive disabilities, as physical function or positioning needs progress, the individual may need a power wheelchair but lack the resources to obtain one because a scooter was already funded. Many third-party funding agencies will not reimburse for a new powered mobility device before 5 years, even if a disability has progressed.

Individuals With Postural-Positioning Needs

POVs are not capable of accepting after-market wheelchair backs for positioning or postural control or accepting seat cushions used for skin protection or positioning.

Individuals With Poor Trunk Balance

POVs require the user to be capable of sitting only with the support of a standard scooter seat and maintain her trunk control when maneuvering the scooter.

Individuals With Impaired Upper Extremity Function

The individual must be able to control the speed and direction of the scooter using only the standard tiller controls.

Individuals With Insufficient Environmental Space/Accessibility

Some living environments are too small to allow a POV to maneuver. Those who require the POV for mobility outdoors must either have the ability to get the POV outdoors or the means to store it outdoors.

Individuals Who Are Unwilling or Unable to Accept or Maintain the Power-Operated Vehicle

If the user is unable, arrangements must be made for a caregiver to charge the batteries and follow the manufacturers recommended maintenance schedule. If the user is unwilling to accept the POV, technology abandonment will occur sooner rather than later.

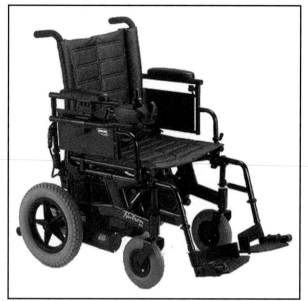

Figure 10-9. Invacare Nutron LX.

Power Wheelchairs

There are many types and configurations of power wheelchairs, with a large variety of seating systems and driver controls available. These can be categorized many ways. One method is by drive wheel configuration (rear-, center-, and front-wheel drive; see Chapter 12). Another method is by construction. Power chair construction falls into two basic design categories, power wheelchair frames and power wheelchair bases. Both categories are available in all three drive wheel configurations.

Frame-Style Power Chairs

Strengths

A folding design allows the chair to fold if needed for transportability (Figure 10-9). Although transportability is an option, it is often used intermittently rather than every day. When disassembled, the heaviest component can still weigh more than 70 pounds. To be considered truly portable, some reimbursement agencies require the heaviest component of the disassembled power chair to weigh no more the 55 pounds.

The cross-brace construction does allow for some flexibility of the left and right sides of the frame as the chair traverses outdoor terrain, providing a basic level of suspension.

Challenges

A disadvantage to this style of design is the inability to add powered seating systems or driver controls beyond a standard proportional joystick. This style of power chair is limited in seat geometries available (width, depth, seat to floor height, and back height). Options are often limited as well (arm styles, legrest options, positioning accessories). Terrain capability is dependent on the configuration of the

gear and motor package. Driving range is often limited by the smaller battery size. Folding-style power wheelchairs are not considered robust enough to meet the requirements of American National Standards Institute-Rehabilitation Engineering & Assistive Technology Society of North America WC-19 and are not available with integrated tie-down brackets (see Chapter 24 for further information).

Clinical Indicators

The user will primarily be operating the power chair indoors and on firm, paved surfaces with minimal obstacles outdoors. The following are clinical indicators:

- There is no present or anticipated requirement for powered seating systems.
- The user can operate a standard proportional joystick.
- There are no current or anticipated needs for alternative driver controls.
- Seating and positioning needs are able to be met through standard after-market options.
- The user does not have a progressive disability.
- There is a need for transportability met through use of a folding power wheelchair.

Base-Style Power Chairs

Strengths

Base style power chairs are available in many configurations including light duty for primarily indoor use, moderate duty for indoor and outdoor use, and active duty for the highly active community user (Figures 10-10 through 10-12). These chairs are available with the largest range of arm and legrest options and styles, drive wheel/motor packages, seating accessory options, and driver control alternative choices. More information on alternative drive controls can be found in Chapter 11.

Many base configurations include integrated tie-down accommodations for transportation needs.

Very often, one model will offer more than one type of seating. Seating types available include van seats, rehab seats, and powered seating systems.

Challenges

Suspension: Some base configurations manage suspension better than others. Rear-wheel drive configurations are currently the best at managing suspension through spring shock absorbers, pneumatic wheels, front caster suspension, and even center of gravity adjustment, which can aid in avoiding front-loading the casters (excessive weight over the front casters), a contributor to rough rides. Benefits of suspension include management of pain and fatigue associated with whole body vibration, comfort, reduced muscle tone, and fewer abnormal reflexive responses. Technology is changing. Look for future power chairs to better address

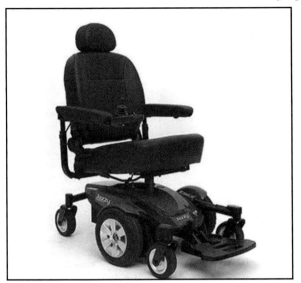

Figure 10-10. Pride Mobility Jazzy J6.

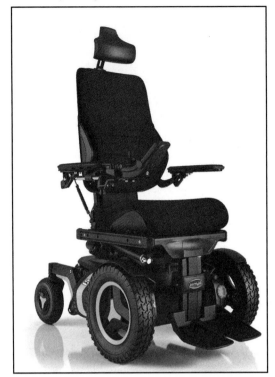

Figure 10-11. Permobil F3 Corpus.

the benefits of suspension, including center and front wheel configurations.

Center-of-gravity distribution: Eliminating or reducing front loading is important to optimize driving. Some base-type systems allow the seating system to be moved fore or aft more readily. Reducing front loading makes the chair easier to drive and turn by reducing caster rolling and turning resistance, generally reduces overall length for a smaller turning radius, reduces wear and tear on the front caster assembly and motors, and can even increase driving range.

POWER WHEELCHAIR SEATING WITH CLINICAL INDICATORS

Van-Style Seating

Van seats are often viewed as comfort seats (see Figure 10-10). Most van seats include the ability to partially recline the back (open the seat to back angle). This may be required to accommodate posture or may be a convenient way to change position in the course of a day for comfort. Some van seats are available with a solid seat pan for use with after-market wheelchair cushions for positioning or skin protection. Some models have manual reclining van seats.

Drawbacks to van seats include limited size configurations, armrest options, and seat to floor height options.

Rehab Seating

Rehab seats accommodate a wide range of needs and are available in the largest range of geometries (Figure 10-13). Widths and depths generally range from 10 to 24 inches or greater. Some allow for adjustment of width and depth

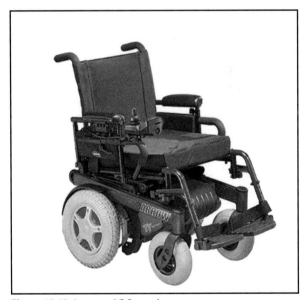

Figure 10-12. Invacare 3G Storm Arrow.

without using additional parts. Most include a solid seat pan for support of a wide range of wheelchair cushions. Most all arm styles flip back out of the way for transfers while staying attached to the frame for easy return to start position. Back canes are available in a variety of heights to accommodate positioning needs as well as support a wide variety of after-market positioning backs.

Key to rehab seating is the ability to adjust the seat to back angle to accommodate fixed postural asymmetries.

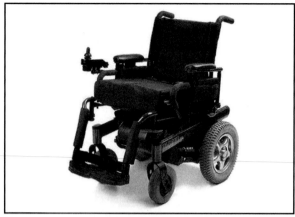

Figure 10-13. Invacare 3G Torque SP.

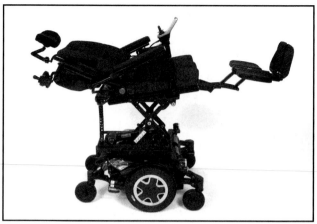

Figure 10-14. Invacare Tilt with recline and power elevating legrests.

Power Seating

Power seating systems use an actuator to move or change the position of the seat or a component of the seat. The actuator is operated either through an external switch or through the driver control. Power seating systems include tilt, recline, elevate, standing, individual power elevating legrests, or power-elevating center-mount legrest. Some recline systems also include an actuator to move the back up and down the back canes to reduce shear displacement while others use a mechanical linkage for this function. Some elevating legrest systems also articulate, lengthening during extension to prevent pushing the legs back toward the client.

Although a primary benefit for powered tilt and/or recline systems is pressure redistribution to manage the risk for pressure injury development, there are many more benefits or clinical indicators (Dicianno et al., 2009). Certain clinical benefits are unique to tilt systems and others unique to recline systems. The combination of tilt and recline together can incorporate the benefits of each while eliminating or reducing any disadvantage to either. The use of tilt to meet one or several objectives while also using powered recline to accommodate different requirements can be beneficial for many clients (Figure 10-14).

Benefits of standing are well-documented in the literature. Additional benefits of using a standing feature as a part of a power wheelchair include improved compliance with a standing program, increased functional reach, and pressure relief/redistribution (Arva, Paleg, et al., 2009).

The following section includes a list of some of the clinical benefits/applications for each system.

Clinical Indicators/Functional Benefits: Power Tilt Systems (Posterior Tilt)

Tilt changes the position of the seating system in space without changing the seated angles at the hips, knees and ankles. Posterior tilt moves the client posterior of an upright position. Benefits include the following:

- Pressure relief/redistribution
- Independent performance of weight shifts
- Decreased fatigue associated with high muscle tone
- Increased sitting tolerance in the course of the day
- Improved postural/proximal stability
- Improved upper extremity function through increased postural stability
- Improved head control through increased postural stability
- Increased power wheelchair driving capabilities through increased head control and upper extremity functioning
- Reduced caregiver or attendant hours required due to the ability to independently perform weight shifts with resulting increased sitting tolerance
- Effective shear displacement management during position changes (shear displacement can result in sliding out of position)
- Absent to minimal triggering of abnormal muscle tone or reflexes triggered by hip extension (*Note*: a supine tonic labyrinthine reflex can be triggered for some by tilting back)
- Gravity-assisted caregiver repositioning of the user in the chair

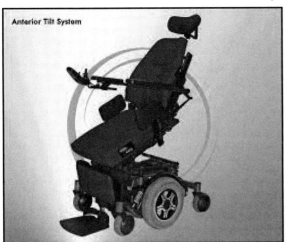

Figure 10-15. Motion Concepts anterior tilt systems.

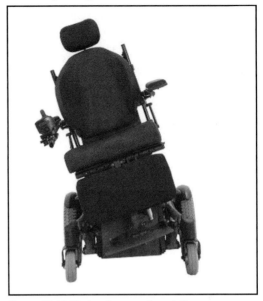

Figure 10-16. Motion Concepts lateral tilt.

- Gravity-assisted postural support (by holding the individual to the seating contours)

- Improved line of sight (visual field)

- Easiest accommodation of lower extremity contractures during position change

- Easiest accommodation of trunk or postural asymmetries during position change

- Muscle tone management
  - Positioning for relaxation of high muscle tone
  - Positioning for stability with low muscle tone
  - Positioning for feeding and improved swallowing due to relaxed muscle tone in the neck region

- Lower extremity edema management (limited unless combined with elevating legs to get feet above the level of the heart)

- Reduced respiratory difficulty through reducing pressure on the diaphragm by facilitating extension of the spine and trunk

- Independent initial management of hypertensive episodes, including autonomic hyperreflexia, through independence with return to an upright position

- Effective use for position change with limited hip ROM

- Postural and balance accommodation when traversing challenging terrain

- Comfort

- Pain relief

Clinical Indicators/Functional Benefits: Anterior (Forward) Tilt Systems

Anterior tilt moves the client anterior of an upright position (Figure 10-15). It is often used in conjunction with a posterior tilt. Benefits include the following:

- Positioning for function
  - Assist with transfers
  - Positioning with recline to facilitate trunk extensor tone

Clinical Indicators/Functional Benefits: Lateral Tilt Systems

Lateral tilt moves the client lateral to an upright position (Figure 10-16). Lateral tilt is sometimes uses to provide weight shifts for a client who cannot tolerate a posterior tilt because of a reflexive response. Benefits include the following:

- Pressure redistribution

- Comfort

- Reduced rain

- Increased gastric emptying

- Facilitates oral secretions to drain

- Counteracts effects of scoliosis

- Improves head balance

- Decreases need for repositioning

- Reduces abnormal muscle tone

- Reduces reflux

- Increases sitting tolerance

Clinical Indicators/Functional Benefits: Power Recline Systems

Recline dynamically opens the seat to back angle and is sometimes used with a height adjustable back to reduce shear forces. Recline is often used in conjunction with elevating legrests. Benefits include the following:

- Pressure relief and redistribution (allowing the largest available surface area to distribute pressure)
- Passive ROM of the hip joints (and knees, with power or mechanical elevating legrests) during recline (helpful with pain management for some clients)
- Decreased fatigue
- Increased sitting tolerance
- Positioning for bladder management
- Positioning for toileting hygiene
- Lower extremity edema management (limited unless combined with elevating legrests)
- Positioning for respiratory care
- Muscle tone management
- Improved blood flow to the lower extremities reducing incidents of venous stasis and concomitant vascular problems
- Positioning for safe supine transfers
- Independent performance of weight shifts
- Armrests and lap trays stay perpendicular to the floor during recline (unless mounted to the back canes)
- Pressure relief/redistribution performance without moving away from a table or desk
- Reduced respiratory effort through decreasing pressure on the diaphragm and increasing extension of the trunk
- Improved line of sight
- Independent initial management of hypertensive episodes, including autonomic hyperreflexia/dysreflexia, through independence with return to an upright position
- Independent initial management of orthostatic/postural hypotension by laying back
- Improved postural and proximal stability
- Improved upper extremity function through increased postural stability
- Improved head control
- Increased power wheelchair driving capabilities through increased head control and upper extremity functioning
- Reduced caregiver or attendant hours required due to the ability to independently perform weight shifts with resulting increased sitting tolerance
- Reduced pain
- Comfort with increased sitting tolerance

Clinical Indicators/Functional Benefits: Power Tilt-and-Recline Systems

Tilt-and-recline systems allow for each of these functions to be used separately or in combination with one another. Benefits include the following:

- Allows combination of benefits and applications of each tilt and recline (e.g., tilt for pressure relief with recline for bladder management; recline for pressure management with tilt to abate swallowing difficulties)
- Most effective means of managing lower extremity edema, particularly when combined with elevating legrests
- Most effective means of reducing respiratory distress through increased trunk extension in the supine position and by facilitating respiratory therapy interventions
- Allows end-user to choose and manage pressure relief options and combinations thus reducing reliance on caregivers
- Most effectively manages shear displacement during repositioning by first tilting to initiate a position change, then recline. This also assists in maintaining the client's posture during the weight shift cycle.

Clinical Indicators/Functional Benefits: Seat Elevation

Seat elevation maintains all seated angles and raises the seat from the starting seat to floor height (Arva, Schmeler, Lange, Lipka, & Rosen, 2009). Benefits include the following:

- Allows independent or less-assisted safe wheelchair transfers by changing the seat height in relation to the transfer surface (always moving from a higher surface to a lower one or to a same level surface)
- Allows independent safe meal preparation by allowing access to multiple surfaces and avoiding unsafe reaching
- Allows independent home ADL (e.g., dressing, hygiene, feeding) and IADL by extending a user's functional reach capabilities
- Allows independence and participation in a variety of activities
- Allows independent community ADL (e.g., shopping)

- Meets vocational and educational access requirements to safely reach multiple surfaces
- Facilitates social interactions
- Improves line of sight in crowded environments

Clinical Indicators/Functional Benefits: Independent Power Elevating Legrests/ Power Center Mount

Elevating legrests extend the knee beyond its starting position. Benefits include the following:

- Works simultaneously with recline to prevent sliding out of the chair during position changes
- Comfort
- Management of lower extremity edema (when combined with power tilt)
- Management of lower extremity pain associated with edema
- Management of hypotensive episodes
- When used with power tilt and or recline, management of episodes of autonomic hyperreflexia/ dysreflexia
- May be indicated for the treatment and management of lower extremity pressure injuries
- Allows an individual to raise the feet in response to terrain requirements (i.e., transitioning from a steep decline to a level surface)

SUMMARY

There are many types of and configurations for powered mobility devices. Technology within this segment is evolving rapidly. A large number of PMDs introduced less than 10 years ago have already been made obsolete by the manufacturer and replaced with new technology. Inappropriate matching of a prescribed PMD can have dire consequences for the user and, in some cases, cause harm. In contrast, matching the correct PMD to the user's needs can mean the difference between success and failure and improve quality of life.

REFERENCES

Arva, J., Paleg, G., Lange, M., Lieberman, J., Schmeler, M., Dicianno, B.,...& Rosen, L. (2009). RESNA position on the application of wheelchair standing devices. *Assistive Technology, 21,* 161-168.

Arva, J., Schmeler, M. R., Lange, M. L., Lipka, D. D., & Rosen, L. E. (2009). RESNA position on the application of seat-elevating devices for wheelchair users. *Assistive Technology, 21,* 69-72.

Dicianno, B. E., Arva, J., Lieberman, J. M., Schmeler, M. R., Souza, A., Phillips, K.,...& Betz, K. L. (2009). RESNA position on the application of tilt, recline, and elevating legrests for wheelchairs. *Assistive Technology, 21,* 13-22.

Disabled World. (2011). Disability in America infographic. Retrieved from http://www.disabled-world.com/disability/statistics/american-disability.php

Flagg, J. (2009). Wheeled mobility demographics. In *Industry Profile on Wheeled Mobility.* Buffalo, NY: RERC on Technology Transfer, University of Buffalo. Retrieved from http://t2rerc.buffalo.edu/pubs/ip/MT/2009%20IP%20on%20Wheeled%20Mobility%20v2.0.pdf

Jones, M. A., McEwen, I. R., & Neas, B. R. (2012). Effects of power wheelchairs on the development and function of young children with severe motor impairments. *Pediatric Physical Therapy, 24,* 131-140.

Livingstone, R., & Paleg, G. (2014). Practice considerations for the introduction and use of power mobility for children. *Developmental Medicine & Child Neurology, 56,* 210-221.

McCarthy, L. H., Bigal, M. E., Katz, M., Derby, C., & Lipton, R. B. (2009). Chronic pain and obesity in elderly people: Results from the Einstein aging study. *Journal of the American Geriatrics Society, 57*(1), 115-119.

National Government Services, Medical Policy Center. (2013,). *Power mobility devices* (Policy Article A47122).

NHIC, Corp. (2007). *Reminder of the reasonable useful lifetime guidelines.*

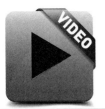

11

Power Mobility
Alternative Access Methods

Michelle L. Lange, OTR/L, ABDA, ATP/SMS

Mobility is so much more than getting from Point A to Point B. We move for many reasons: to get a better look at something, to reach and acquire an object, to approach someone for social interaction, to increase our alertness or decrease our boredom, to provide a bit of vestibular stimulation and to get to specific destinations for a variety of purposes (Cullen, 2012). Mobility bases, whether an adaptive stroller or a complex rehab power wheelchair, can provide movement to clients who otherwise are limited in their mobility. Ideally, our goal is to provide a means of independent mobility for the clients with whom we work.

As Elizabeth Cole pointed out in Chapter 8, mobility bases fall into a hierarchy of choices. It is critical to evaluate a client's abilities to determine the optimal mobility category required. At the end of the mobility product spectrum (from walkers to wheelchairs) are complex rehab power wheelchairs. Even if a client has limited ambulation or is able to self-propel a manual wheelchair, a power wheelchair may still be indicated and can still be successfully covered by funding sources. Mobility is all about efficiency. If a client is inefficient in a particular environment using one type of mobility device, a more efficient mobility category may be indicated. For example, if a client is an effective self-propeller in the home, is the same client efficient self-propelling in a community environment?

What is efficiency? *Efficiency* is a combination of time and energy (Merriam-Webster.com, n.d.). If getting from math class to history class in high school is taking too much time (i.e., the student is late for class) or energy (i.e., the student is too tired to pay attention), the client may require a more efficient means of getting around in this environment.

Various power mobility options are available, as discussed by Michael Babinec in Chapter 10. The majority of power wheelchair drivers use a joystick (Dicianno, Cooper, & Coltellaro, 2010). For those power wheelchair riders with the motor control to safely operate a joystick, this driving method provides an effective means to control speed and direction in one input device—an ideal combination.

This chapter, however, primarily examines alternative access methods to provide a means of power wheelchair control for clients unable to use a standard joystick. Power wheelchair access methods include proportional (analog) and digital access methods. Standard joysticks, as well as some alternative access methods, provide proportional control. Proportional control generally provides full directional control within a 360-degree circle. Proportional control also provides control of speed. The farther a joystick is deflected from its center, the faster the wheelchair will move. Stopping is generally achieved by returning the control to its center or letting go. Digital access uses switches. Each switch controls a specific direction: forward, reverse, left, and right. When the switch is activated, only one speed is available. Power wheelchairs, which support alternative access methods, fall into the complex rehabilitation category of mobility products. The power chair must include expanded electronics required to support these driver controls. The expanded electronics feature is one of the characteristics of power chairs categorized under complex rehabilitation technology.

Lange, M. L., & Minkel, J. L.
Seating and Wheeled Mobility: A Clinical Resource Guide
(pp. 179-198). © 2018 SLACK Incorporated.

The mobility evaluator must determine the optimal power wheelchair access method for an individual client to provide the intended, successful outcome: independent mobility. If the optimal access method is not determined, the client may be inefficient, or even unsuccessful, in using a power wheelchair. Positioning is critical. The client must be positioned optimally with adequate stability to facilitate access. This cannot be overstated: Many of the clients I have evaluated for power mobility are unsuccessful because of inadequate postural support and stability.

Once the client is evaluated for power mobility and an access method is determined, other factors must be considered to optimize driving a power wheelchair. In Chapter 12, Amy Morgan describes how drive wheel configuration, tracking, and programming are essential to achieving a successful outcome. A power wheelchair can be customized to meet an individual's needs but can also be configured in such a way as to be unsafe or even unusable. Recommendations must include the best drive wheel configuration for a client and tracking technologies, as appropriate. Delivery must include programming the wheelchair to support the access method and to meet that individual's needs.

Power wheelchairs and their electronics packages vary widely, around the world. As of 2017 in the United States, three main electronic packages are available. The Mk6i package is used on Invacare power wheelchairs. Q-Logic is used on Quantum power wheelchairs (the rehab division of Pride Mobility). The R-Net package is used on Permobil, Quickie, Rovi, and some other power wheelchairs, produced by smaller manufacturers. These electronic packages are updated frequently, mainly by software upgrades. Each system is programmed differently and similar programmable parameters may have different labels across electronic packages. In addition to the wheelchair manufacturers' electronics, after-market alternative control packages are available, such as the Stealth Products iDrive and Movis products. iDrive and Movis products can be programmed through the power wheelchair electronics package or through the iDrive or Movis software that offers additional programming options.

ASSESSMENT

Before evaluating a client for the best access method, optimal seating must be provided. This can be challenging if the optimal seating happens to be in a manual wheelchair and cannot easily be transferred to a power wheelchair for mobility assessment. If possible, the current seating system should be transferred to an assessment chair or seating mocked up in a power wheelchair as ideally as possible. In a clinic at the Children's Hospital of Denver, we mounted a seating simulator, which included highly adjustable postural supports, to a power wheelchair base to provide the needed postural support during mobility assessments. Another option would be using a temporary positioning pillow that can be placed in the mobility base to support the client as optimally as possible (i.e., Versaform).

The next step of mobility assessment is to determine whether this client can use a power wheelchair. In general, using a power wheelchair requires adequate motor control, mobility concepts, and vision. In this chapter, I focus on motor control and how this determines the access method. Mobility concepts include cause and effect, stop and go, directional concepts, problem-solving, and judgment (Livingstone, 2010). Competence in each of these areas is not required before a power wheelchair is recommended; rather potential is identified. Readiness is discussed in more detail by Jan Furumasu in Chapter 17.

Specific assessment strategies are discussed as we move through each access method.

THE ACCESS METHODS

Power wheelchair access methods fall into a hierarchy. For clients with the required motor control, the access method of choice is a standard joystick. As client abilities dictate, the evaluator will move further down the hierarchy (Table 11-1).

The first power wheelchairs offered only one access method: a joystick (Smith, 2013). Over time, alternative access methods were introduced. Early examples of alternative access methods include sip-and-puff (a pneumatic switch housed in a straw at the mouth controlling multiple directions of movement by varying air pressure) and simple switch arrays (each switch moving the wheelchair in a discreet direction when pressed). In the 1980s, Adaptive Switch Labs introduced the Head Array (Figure 11-1). Many more access options followed to provide a means of independent mobility to clients who were previously unable to use a power wheelchair.

Proportional Access Methods

As noted earlier, a proportional controller, which combines control of speed and direction in one input device, is the preferred input method whenever possible.

Clinical Indicators

Joysticks seem fairly intuitive and easy to use, especially for a generation that has grown up with video games. Using a joystick is more difficult than it looks, however, both from a motor and cognitive standpoint. Moving forward requires forward deflection of the joystick. To make a turn from forward, the driver must pull back a bit on the joystick and push it to the side. This requires voluntary motor control for the grading of force and distance. People with abnormal muscle tone, common in conditions such as

TABLE 11-1
HIERARCHY OF ACCESS METHODS FOR EFFICIENT MOBILITY
PROPORTIONAL METHODS
• Standard joystick
• Joystick modifications: handles, programming, placement
• Alternative joysticks
• Alternative proportional controls (i.e., touch pad)
DIGITAL METHODS
• Three-to five-switch array (any combination of mechanical or electrical switches at any location)
○ Head array
○ Proximity array under tray
○ Fiberoptic array
• Pneumatic array (sip-and-puff)
• Two-switch array
• Single-switch scanning
• Eye gaze

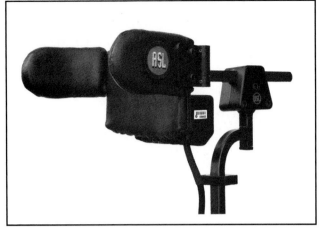

Figure 11-1. Adaptive Switch Labs electronic head array.

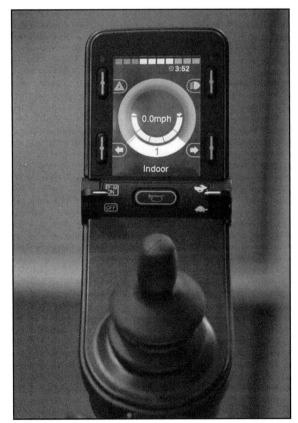

Figure 11-2. Permobil joystick module.

cerebral palsy and traumatic brain injury, have difficulty with cocontraction of the muscle groups and, in turn, with grading a movement pattern. These clients may be able to move a power wheelchair with a joystick, particularly in a forward direction, with only poor motor control. Standard joysticks have an initial stiffness that must be overcome to move the joystick away from center and then a degree of resistance that must be countered to sustain the position of the joystick and the movement of the chair. This requires muscle strength. Some clients do not have adequate strength to move or maintain the joystick away from center. In these cases, specialized joysticks are available that require less force.

A joystick moves in a 360-degree circle. This joystick movement then translates into direction of movement of the power wheelchair. The driver must understand that the relative position of the joystick in relation to center determines the direction of movement of the chair. How far the stick is moved away from the center will determine the speed of the chair. This is often difficult for young children and clients with cognitive limitations. In these cases, a joystick may not be the input device of choice.

Standard Joystick

As previously mentioned, the most common power wheelchair access method is a joystick and the most common placement is by a hand. Standard joysticks comprise a box, vertical rod, joystick handle, and sometimes a flexible hood between the handle and box to prevent moisture and debris from entering the box where vulnerable electronics are located (Figure 11-2).

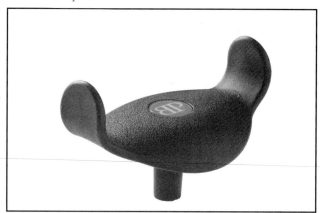

Figure 11-3. Body Point goalpost-style joystick handle.

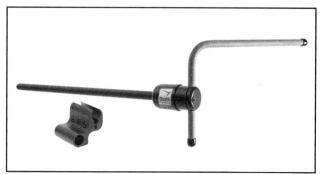

Figure 11-5. Swing-away joystick mount for midline placement (Stealth Products).

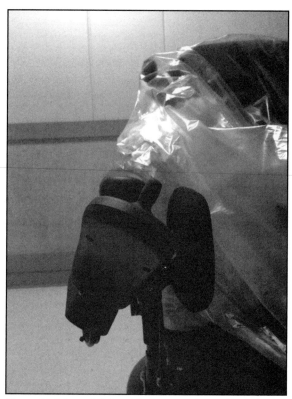

Figure 11-4. Lateral tilt joystick placement (viewed from beneath the joystick box).

Handles

Various handles are available. Standard handles are typically grasped between the first two fingers and thumb when the forearm is pronated, and in a palmer grasp when the forearm is neutral. Some clients grasp the joystick too firmly due to increased muscle tone and this limits driving control. Using a large round handle may reduce tone in the hand and improve success in driving the chair. Some clients use a palmer grasp with the forearm pronated. A T-shaped handle accommodates this type of grasp. Finally, some clients have limited hand grasp, but do have good motor control of the shoulder and elbow. These clients sometimes benefit from a goalpost-style handle (Figure 11-3). Clients with a high level spinal cord injury (SCI) who still have limited upper extremity control frequently use goalpost-style handles (C5 level). The mushroom joystick has an integrated handle shaped like a dome. This design is so clients with a poor grasp can control a joystick using their palm, which rests on the dome-shaped surface. However, the joystick is rather stiff and hard to hang onto with the palm. A separate dome-shaped handle is also available that is textured for better grip.

Placement

Joystick placement is typically by the hand, in line with an arm pad and parallel with the floor; however, this placement is not always optimal. For a client whose forward arm movement veers toward midline, a mounting angle with the distal end of the joystick facing midline may be helpful. Some clients' high muscle tone pulls the forearm into extreme pronation during forward movement. In these cases, laterally tilting the joystick box, so that the medial side is lower, matches this pattern (Figure 11-4). Midline placement is often useful. In this case, a swing away mount is required for transfers (Figure 11-5). If the client can transfer independently, a power joystick mount is available because midline joystick mounts are usually too difficult for the client to swing away independently. Clients who frequently benefit from a midline placement include those with short arms and those with muscle weakness. People with muscle weakness often have better control in midline and close to the body, particularly clients with Duchenne muscular dystrophy. A standard joystick can be difficult to place close to the body as it is bulky. In this case, a smaller joystick, sometimes called a *compact* or *remote joystick,* can be used or even a mini joystick.

Mini Proportional Joystick

Not everyone can use a standard joystick due to lack of strength or range of motion of the hand or upper extremity. Specialized joysticks require less force and less range of motion to control the operation of the chair. Clients with muscular dystrophy commonly lack sufficient strength to move the standard joystick. A great alternative control for these clients is a mini proportional joystick.

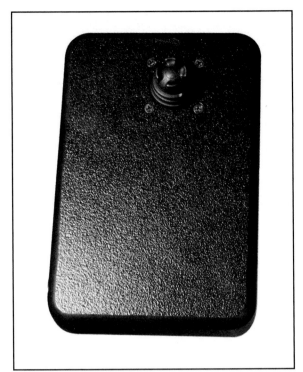

Figure 11-6. Mini proportional joystick in hand platform (Stealth Products).

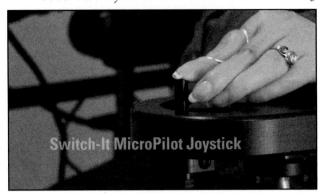

Figure 11-7. Isometric joystick mounted in handpad (Switch It).

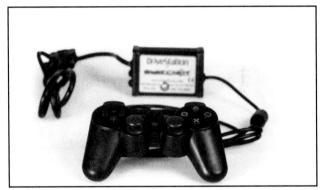

Figure 11-8. Drive Station adapted video game controller (Switch It).

Mini proportional joysticks are small joysticks that require significantly less force and travel distance than a standard joystick. A standard joystick requires between 180 and 220 grams of force while mini proportional joysticks requires 10 to 50 grams of force. These are often fragile and do not hold up to standard forces. If a caregiver needs to drive the power wheelchair, a standard attendant control joystick is required as the mini joystick is too sensitive and fragile for the attendant to use functionally. Mini proportional joysticks are ideal for clients with very limited strength, including clients with spinal muscular atrophy (SMA), muscular dystrophy, and amyotrophic lateral sclerosis (ALS). Midline placement is often required because many clients with muscle weakness have the most control at midline and close to the body. Support of the hand, wrist, and forearm may be required as well. A special rectangular hand platform is available that allows placement of the joystick at a specific height in relation to the support surface (Figure 11-6).

Various styles of mini proportional joysticks are available. One style includes a reset switch activated by pushing down on the joystick top. Reset places the power wheelchair into another mode of operation, such as power seating.

One style of specialized joystick, an isometric mini proportional joystick, responds to force, rather than movement. The force required is still minimal (Figure 11-7). Eliminating the movement required may allow the client to stabilize against the joystick. Also, an isometric joystick is less likely to move in response to movement of the wheelchair. This may reduce extraneous movement of the wheelchair when an isometric joystick is used. Finally, because some clients have better control with the fingers flexed (i.e., over the edge of a tray), an isometric joystick can be placed parallel to the floor without sinking downward.

CASE EXAMPLE

Michael is a 32-year-old man with the diagnosis of SMA. He has significant muscle weakness but good fine motor control at midline. He does not have adequate strength to use a standard or compact joystick, but he is able to use a mini proportional joystick mounted midline and low. He rests his arms on his lap and uses the joystick between his knees. He can also activate a small mechanical switch by the joystick as a reset to access other features such as power seating.

ADAPTED GAME CONTROLLER

Two companies have adapted video game controllers to access a power wheelchair (Figure 11-8). These game controllers already incorporate one or two mini joysticks that require 40 to 50 grams of pressure (still significantly less than the force needed for a standard wheelchair joystick). These joysticks are then used to control the power

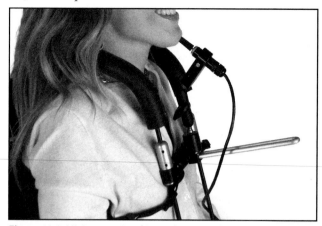

Figure 11-9. Mini proportional joystick mounted at chin (Switch It).

wheelchair. If two mini joysticks are present, one can be programmed to control movement of the wheelchair and the other can be used to control other features. It is even possible to control movement using both joysticks; for example, the first joystick can be programmed for forward and reverse, and the second joystick for left and right. Besides looking cool and fun, these joysticks are fairly robust, being designed for hours of rough-and-tumble video game play. The game controller buttons can be designated for various functions as well, such as power seating. This is not programmable in the field, but can be custom ordered to meet an individual client's needs.

CASE EXAMPLE

Brad is a 16-year-old young man with the diagnosis of Duchenne muscular dystrophy. He was driving with a standard joystick until a respiratory incident placed him in the hospital. By the time he was back in his power wheelchair, he had lost the ability to use his joystick. He was, however, still able to play his video games. The game controller joysticks were much more sensitive, and he could hold this controller in his lap, close to his body and at midline where he had more control. Brad trialed a Drive Station and did quite well. Brad was initially reluctant to change access methods but was excited to find this as an option.

Chin Joystick

Chin joysticks are mounted on a swing-away arm or on a bib worn against the chest (Figure 11-9). Standard compact proportional joysticks are stiff and can lead to repetitive stress injuries of the jaw or cervical area. Mini proportional joysticks require significantly less force and so reduce this risk. Before the development of many alternative controls, persons who sustained a high-level SCI developed skill in using a joystick under the chin to be able to control both direction and speed of the chair. Other options for these

clients now include the Head Array Mini proportional joysticks are so sensitive that these can be challenging to operate with one's chin, particularly outdoors. The bumps in the road translate into client movement, which may result in extraneous movement of the joystick and erratic driving.

CASE EXAMPLE

Doug is a 24-year-old man who sustained a high-level SCI. He has no control over his extremities but is able to move his neck. He will use his power wheelchair primarily indoors and at slower speeds. A mini proportional joystick was mounted at his chin on a power swing away mount. This allowed Doug to use a switch mounted by his head to move the joystick in and out of position for driving so that he did not have this directly in front of him at all times. An isometric joystick was selected because this was less sensitive to movement from the wheelchair.

Proportional Head Control

The proportional head control (sometimes referred to as *RIM—Rehabilitation Institute of Montreal* control) is a head pad mounted to a compact (proportional) joystick. This type of controller operates on a 180-degree arc, not the full 360 degrees of the standard joystick. The chair moves forward when the head presses against this head pad, moving the joystick to which it is attached. When the head turns to the side (maintaining pressure against the rear pad), the chair turns to the side. To go into reverse, a separate mode switch toggles the forward function to reverse. Once toggled, the same head movement will result in the chair being driven in the reverse direction. The primary drawback of the proportional head control is that pressure is required against the head pad to sustain movement. This may lead to neck pain and headaches but is primarily a safety concern. Sustained force against the rear pad tends to lead to increased muscle tone, making stopping (by bringing the head forward) difficult for people with abnormal muscle tone. This head pad is also hard to rest against when the client is not driving because it moves, even when the wheelchair is powered down (Figure 11-10).

CASE EXAMPLE

Carly is a 20-year-old woman who sustained a high-level SCI. She has no control of her extremities, although she demonstrates good head control. Carly trialed a proportional head control in a clinic setting and drove with good control. She was able to direct the power wheelchair accurately and stop without difficulty. Carly was also able

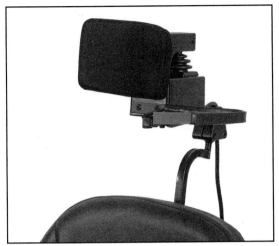

Figure 11-10. Proportional head control (Adaptive Switch Labs).

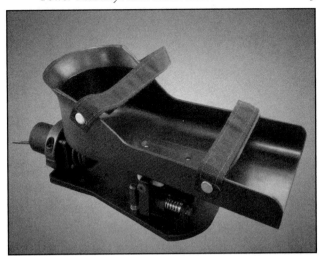

Figure 11-11. Foot control mounting adaptor (Adaptive Switch Labs).

to drive using a chin joystick, as well as a sip-and-puff control. She preferred the proportional head control as this remained behind her, rather than having a joystick or straw in front of her chin.

Foot Joystick

Attaching a compact joystick to a special footplate allows control using the foot (Figure 11-11). Some clients may have little motor control in other areas of the body and yet have isolated control of a foot. This is sometimes seen in people with athetoid-type cerebral palsy. Pressing down on the forward portion of the footplate moves the power wheelchair forward. Lifting the forward portion of the footplate results in rearward movement of the chair. Laterally turning the foot to the left or right turns the chair. Often a shoe-holder is required to keep the foot on the footplate while these movements are made.

An alternative to this specialty controller and footplate is to mount the standard joystick in front of the footplate, eliminating the need to order a specialized foot joystick. In this case, the client must hover the foot above the joystick for driving, rather than resting on a footplate.

CASE EXAMPLE

Juan is a 17-year-old male with a diagnosis of athetoid cerebral palsy. Juan had a power wheelchair, but it was difficult for him to control using the joystick mounted by his right hand. He had little postural support or stability in his seating system, and his team tied his forearm to the arm pad to facilitate his driving. Juan was evaluated to determine the optimal seating system for his needs, and with additional support and stability, he was much more functional. We determined that Juan needed to stabilize

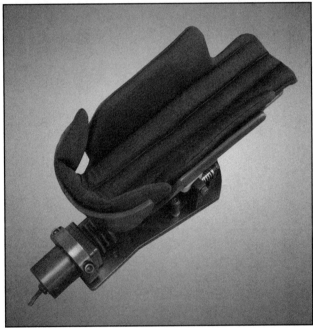

Figure 11-12. Arm drive (Switch It). *Note:* Joystick is mounted below the armrest trough.

with his arms to isolate control in his left foot. He was able to tuck his arms under a padded tray to provide this stability and could then drive with a joystick mounted by his left foot with good control and minimal effort. If his arms were not stabilized, he was unable to drive.

Arm Joystick

Attaching a joystick to a special arm trough allows control using the forearm (Figure 11-12). This type of controller is operated largely by shoulder motion. By dropping the hand lower than the elbow, the chair will move forward, conversely raising the hand higher than the elbow will result in driving in reverse. To turn, moving the forearm to the left or right drives the wheelchair in that direction.

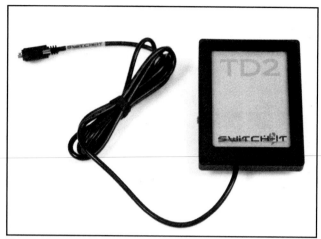

Figure 11-13. Touch Drive 2 (Switch It).

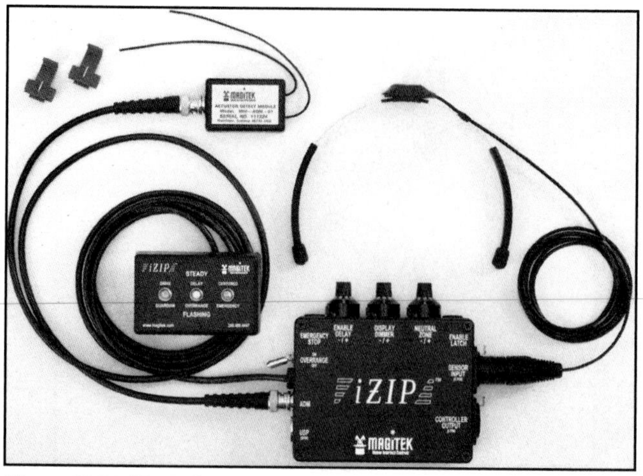

Figure 11-14. Magitek Drive Control.

No wrist or hand control is required because the joystick is attached to the arm trough. This is appropriate for a client with shoulder and upper arm control but limited forearm, wrist, or finger control (i.e., high-level SCI). This client may also use mobile arm supports but lack adequate control to use a hand-controlled joystick.

CASE EXAMPLE

Manuel is a 12-year-old boy with the diagnosis of congenital myopathy. He has significant muscle weakness throughout his body but is able to move his arms with the use of mobile arm supports. He trialed the Arm Drive, which provided similar support to his mobile arm supports and capitalized on his shoulder strength. Manuel was able to use this successfully and the increased leverage of this system allowed him to overcome the resistance in the attached compact joystick.

Touch Pads

Various graphic pads are available that are activated by a finger touch (Figure 11-13). The chair moves in the direction the finger drags and moves faster the farther the finger is moved from center. These range from small (3 x 3 inches) to large (8 x 10 inches). The larger version is no longer available in the United States. Some versions incorporate buttons that can control other features, such as a power tilt. The Switch-It touch pads include two modes of operation.

In Absolute Mode, the client must start in the center of the pad. In Relative Mode, center is wherever the client starts on the surface of the pad. The smaller pads accommodate clients with limited active movement and force whereas the larger pad can accommodate a fisted hand and larger movements.

CASE EXAMPLE

Ruth Anne is a 39-year-old woman who sustained a traumatic brain injury in the past. She does not have adequate motor control to use a standard joystick but is motivated to use her hands. Her movements are large, and she has difficulty grasping. She trialed a large touch pad and was able to accurately move her fisted hand around the surface and drive a power wheelchair.

Magitek Drive Control

Magitek is a unique access method (Figure 11-14). A sensor placed on a metal band sits directly on top of the head. Head movement translates into chair movement. The farther the head moves in a direction, the faster the chair moves. The chair stops when the client's head enters the neutral zone, generally when the head centers upright. If the neutral zone is programmed to be large, the chair is easier to stop but requires more head movement for activation. This access method is appropriate for clients with very good head control and little or no extremity control.

CASE EXAMPLE

Marjorie has a high-level SCI that prevents her from moving her extremities, yet spares head movement. Marjorie has very good head control and would be able to use a Magitek, chin joystick, proportional head control, head array, or sip-and-puff. Although she could operate a chin joystick or proportional head control, Marjorie tended to fatigue. She prefers the proportional control of the Magitek over the more limited directional and speed control of the head array or sip-and-puff.

Peachtree

Peachtree is another proportional head control (Figure 11-15). The client moves his or her head in front of the pad without any contact with the pad itself. Movement is sensed and translated into movement of the wheelchair. Moving further away from the pad increases speed. Tilting the head to the left or right (neck lateral flexion) provides directional control.

Proportional Programming

Power wheelchairs offer many programming options to customize driving performance to a particular client's needs and abilities. Programming is discussed at length in Chapter 12. In this chapter, I touch on programming for specific access methods. Proportional control programming parameters include short throw, sensitivity, changing axes, three direction, deadband, and switch joystick. The specific name of each programming parameter may vary from manufacturer to manufacturer.

Short Throw

This parameter reduces the amount of travel the proportional control must move before reaching maximum speed. This is useful for clients with muscle diseases who are still using a standard joystick. By adjusting the short throw parameter, the client must move the joystick only a portion of the distance typically required when using a standard joystick to achieve the same speed. Shorter distances to achieve the same level of speed does require a greater about of motor control when driving the chair. Using shorter distances to achieve the same level of speed requires a greater amount of motor control when driving.

Sensitivity

This parameter adjusts how quickly the power wheelchair responds to the access method. If the wheelchair drives jerky, the sensitivity is probably too high. If the wheelchair seems unresponsive, the sensitivity is probably too low. Sensitivity can be turned down so that tremors are ignored and only intentional movements are translated into

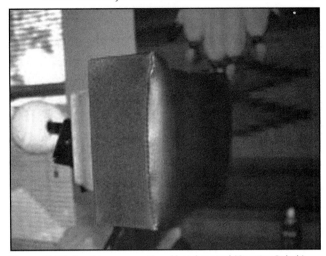

Figure 11-15. Peachtree proportional head control (Creative Rehab).

chair movement. Sensitivity may be increased for a client with muscle weakness. This setting does not change the force required to move the joystick but only the responsiveness of the chair once the controller has been engaged.

Changing Axes

The changing axes parameter allows the programmer to map forward, reverse, right, and left to different directions of movement. Pushing the joystick forward is often difficult for clients with abnormal muscle tone, while pulling back may be easier. The electronics can be programmed to swap one direction for another (i.e., pulling back on joystick will result in the chair moving forward) or to assign a specific directional movement for each direction the joystick is moved.

Three Direction

The three-direction parameter allows programming the joystick in a 180-degree arc, as opposed to the standard 360-degree circle. A reset switch toggles forward and reverse commands. This may be helpful for a client who can move the joystick in three directions but cannot manage a fourth.

Deadband

Deadband draws an imaginary line around the joystick. The client must move the joystick past this boundary to initiate movement of the wheelchair. This is specifically designed for people using a goalpost handle. When someone rests a hand on a goalpost handle, gravity tends to pull the joystick to one side, and the wheelchair motors may attempt to engage. Deadband prevents unexpected movement by requiring a great degree of joystick deflection before the chair responds with movement.

Switch Joystick

This parameter turns the proportional joystick into four switches. Some clients have the general ability to use

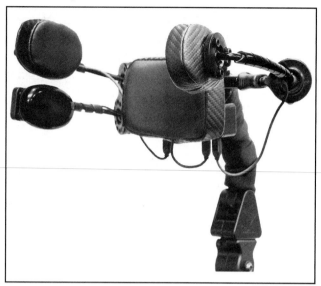

Figure 11-16. Head array in a Stealth Products Head Support.

a joystick but perhaps tend to veer to one side if unable to hold the joystick in an absolute forward position. Switch joysticks accept any general forward movement as true forward.

Digital Access Methods

The primary advantage of digital access is provision of power wheelchair control for the client who does not have adequate motor skills or strength to use any proportional access method. For some clients, digital access is also easier from a cognitive standpoint because it is more concrete. As such, many young drivers begin with switches rather than a joystick, even if they have adequate motor control to use proportional control.

As mentioned previously, standard proportional control combines direction and speed control: 360 degrees of directional control and the farther the joystick moves from center, the faster the wheelchair moves. In nonproportional control, speed is static. Once the switch is activated, the chair will move at one set speed. Direction of movement is limited to four primary directions (forward, left, right, and reverse). Some digital access methods provide diagonal movement when the forward and left or right switches are activated simultaneously. Switches are nonproportional access methods, meaning the chair will respond at one preset speed, when the switch is activated though one manufacturer uses switches that increase speed in response to increased force. Any type of individual or switch array can be placed in any location to provide discrete directional control of the chair. So the evaluator must determine individual switch sites where the client can activate a switch, sustain contact, and release quickly for stopping. The client needs to be able to do so repeatedly for continued driving.

The appendix at the end of this chapter provides a decision-making tree for these digital access methods.

Head Array

One of the most common alternative access methods is the head array (Figure 11-16). The head support pads contain electrical proximity switches. A proximity switch is a capacitive switch and does not require any force. If the head approaches the switch, it activates. Touching the rear pad moves the wheelchair forward, touching the left pad moves the wheelchair to the left and touching the right pad moves the wheelchair to the right. Touching the rear pad and a side pad simultaneously results in diagonal movement. The chair is stopped by bringing the head forward and away from the switches. Specific manufacturer electronics packages offer several methods to place the chair in reverse. Often a reset or mode switch toggles the forward and reverse functions. Head arrays always have at least three switches. Some styles include a reset and reverse switch, one at the distal end of each side pad. These switches can be placed at other locations as well.

Newer versions of the head array allow mechanical and electrical switches to be combined and include more programming options. A wide range of head supports can be used to incorporate the switches. Providing increased support, particularly at the base of the neck through the use of a suboccipital support, can provide increased control of the head, optimizing driving.

The head array works best for clients who cannot use proportional control and have fair to good head control. The head support pads provide a surface to stabilize against, which can be helpful for clients with only fair head control. The client cannot rest against the head support, however, unless the chair is off or in a nondriving mode, because head support contact results in chair movement. Clients with strong reflexive movement of the head, referred to as an *asymmetrical tonic neck reflex*, may have difficulty releasing the side pads. Clients with strong extensor tone may have difficulty stopping, particularly under stress, because quick forward movement of the head and neck is required to stop movement of the chair.

CASE EXAMPLE

Taylor is an 8-year-old boy with the diagnosis of cerebral palsy (Figure 11-17). He demonstrates significant extensor tone throughout his body and has little control of his extremities. His head control is fair. He often drops his head forward and has some difficulty returning to upright. Taylor trialed a head array and, with some mobility training, was able to drive with this access method. He does have a suboccipital support, which provides stability and gives

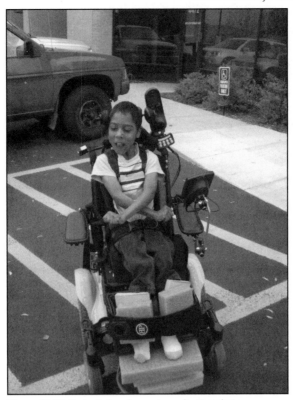

Figure 11-17. Taylor in head array in evaluation chair.

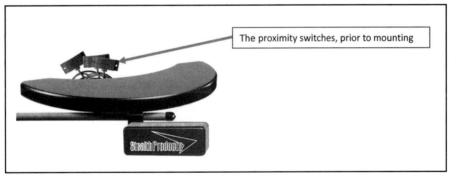

Figure 11-18. Proximity switch array, placed in hollow tray (Stealth Products).

him a consistent starting point for his head movements. Despite his high tone, he does not have difficulty stopping. He does get distracted at school and turns his head to the side to look at things. This leads to the wheelchair moving in that direction, which may be where he would like to go, but this has led to some contact with walls as well. Overall, he is driving quite well for his developmental level.

Proximity Switch Array

The same proximity switches used in the head array are available in a four-switch array (Figure 11-18). These are typically placed under or inside a tray. The client then slides a hand or arm over the switch for activation. As capacitive switches, activation occurs when something capable of conducting electricity passes over them. The tray or a book placed on the wheelchair tray are not able to conduct electricity and thus do not activate the switches. The client's hand, however, does conduct electricity, and thus when the hand passes past the switch, the switch will be activated. If the switches are too close together, they will activate each other. If the switches are under a tray and too close to the client's lap, their legs will activate the switches from below. Each switch has a small dial on the side that turns to adjust the size of the activation field. The switches control forward, left, and right directional control, with the fourth switch acting as reverse or a reset.

Proximity switches provide larger targets than fiberoptic switches and so work better for clients with impaired fine motor control. Placing proximity switches under the tray has several advantages over using mechanical switches (e.g., AbleNet Jellybean switches) on top of the tray. To

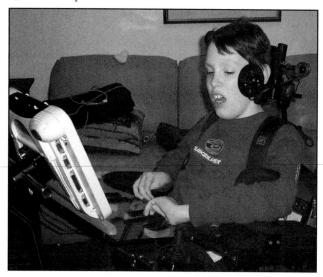

Figure 11-19. Mark and colored proximity switches (Adaptive Switch Labs) under clear tray (joystick is for caregiver, and head switch is for a speech-generating device).

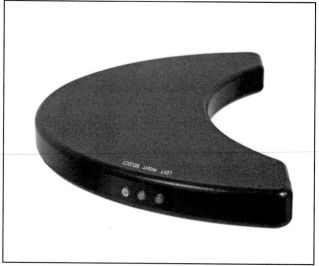

Figure 11-20. Fiberoptic two-switch array in Eclipse Tray (Stealth Products).

access a mechanical switch, the client must move the upper extremity in two planes: vertically to move higher than the surface of the switch and horizontally to move directly over the switch for activation. Placing the switches under the tray eliminates a plane of movement. Now the client needs only to slide a hand over the switch location using back-and-forth or side to side movements. Many clients have difficulty with this vertical movement, particularly clients with abnormal muscle tone. Leaving spaces between the switches allows the client to rest on these areas without moving the wheelchair.

When a switch is under a solid colored tray, it cannot be seen. Stickers can be placed over individual switch locations to cue the client. Velcro (loop side) can be used instead so that the client can feel where the switch is without having to look down. We want the client to be looking where he or she is driving, not at the drive switches. Various colors of Velcro are available for each individual direction. Colors are fairly easy to see peripherally.

Proximity arrays are appropriate for clients with fair upper extremity control who cannot use a proportional access method or mechanical switches.

CASE EXAMPLE

Mark is a 12-year-old boy with the diagnosis of cerebral palsy (Figure 11-19). He does not have adequate motor control to use a joystick or large touch pad, but he wants to use his right hand. He trialed mechanical switches on his tray, but had difficulty with the vertical movement required. We next placed proximity switches under his tray with Velcro prompts above so he could detect whether he was in the

right location. He was able to drive using these switches, but his left hand would sometimes drift over and inadvertently activate some of the switches. He was unable to volitionally control this movement. A cuff was placed facing outward on the left side of his tray. His left arm sat within this cuff to prevent accidental switch activation. Mark was also able to stabilize against this cuff, improving his access with the right arm.

Fiberoptic Switch Array

Fiberoptic switches are very small electronic switches that emit a beam of light (Figure 11-20). When the light encounters an obstacle, such as a finger, it is reflected back and activates the switch. This happens instantaneously. Fiberoptic switches are available in two- and four-switch arrays for power wheelchair access. The switches mount just about anywhere but are most often accessed with very small finger movement. The surface area of the switch is only about 1/8 inch across. The activation range is adjustable. These can be mounted in an arm trough handpad, facing upward. A finger or thumb resting on the handpad moves laterally to cover the beam to activate the switch. Little movement is required and no force. The switches also mount horizontally in the edge of an arm trough or tray (e.g., the Stealth Eclipse tray) so that the client's hand can rest with his or her fingers curled over the edge of the tray (see Figure 11-20). Finger flexion will activate the switch and finger extension will release the switch and the chair will stop. Switches can also be placed on a gooseneck mounts for maximum flexibility of switch placement (Figure 11-21).

In a four-switch array, three of the switches are for forward, left, and right directional control. The fourth switch is a reset switch and can be used to access reverse and other

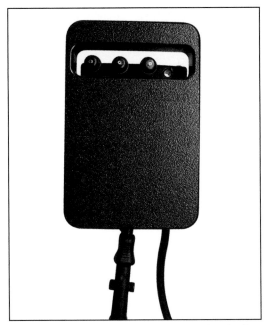

Figure 11-21. Three fiberoptic switches in a handpad on mini gooseneck mounts (Stealth Products).

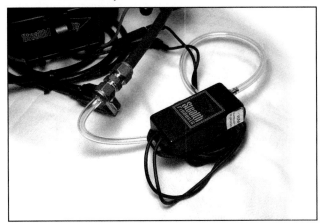

Figure 11-22. Sip-and-puff pneumatic control (Stealth Products).

features. In a two-switch array, one switch executes left movement, one switch executes right movement, and, if both switches are covered, the chair moves forward. If the client is able to activate a third switch, this is designated as reverse or reset.

Fiberoptic switches are appropriate for a client who is unable to use a mini proportional joystick and has very small active movement with little or no force. Clients with ALS, multiple sclerosis, or SMA often use this access method. The cables are fragile and must be protected to prevent damage.

CASE EXAMPLE

Alex is a 42-year-old man with the diagnosis of ALS. His condition has deteriorated to the point that he only has slight finger movements. Fiberoptic switches were trialed in his handpad (an extension to the arm trough), but he had difficulty moving his fingers over the locations of the switches. We next placed the switches along the edge of a tray so that his fingers could drape over the edge, allowing him to use finger flexion for activation. This worked well for him and provided control of driving and power seating.

Sip-and-Puff

Sip-and-puff is one of the oldest alternative access methods (Figure 11-22). Originally designed for use by clients

with high-level SCIs, sip-and-puff is still used with this population. Sip-and-puff is a pneumatic switch activated by changes in air pressure. Specific changes in air pressure result in specific directional commands: hard puff controls forward, soft puff controls right, hard sip controls reverse, and soft sip controls left. It is unreasonable to sustain a hard puff for continued forward motion, so Latch Mode is typically used. When a system is programmed with Latch Mode, one hard puff engages latch and the chair continues forward movement until a hard sip is executed, stopping the chair. With latch engaged, soft puff and soft sip commands correct course (right and left) as the wheelchair moves forward. Pneumatic commands can control speed as well. Once latch engages, subsequent hard puffs increase speed.

Sip-and-puff is appropriate for a client who has little volitional movement, yet good oral motor control. The client must precisely control the air pressure within the mouth, which requires good lip closure and a competent soft palate. If the client can puff out his or her cheeks and suck them in, as demonstrated through drinking through a straw, he or she can probably use this access method. Most clients with abnormal tone have difficulty with lip closure or precisely regulating air pressure within the mouth. Many clients with ALS, once unable to use a joystick, have difficulty with sip-and-puff as the soft palate loses competency and air escapes through the nose.

Programming is essential when using sip-and-puff to customize parameters to meet an individual's needs. The pressure required to execute each pneumatic command is programmable. Hand held programmers have a display that gives the client feedback as they sip or puff while choosing ideal pressures. Some newer electronics include a programmable delay before a pneumatic command is accepted. This is helpful for clients who need time to build up pressure and may unintentionally make a right turn (soft puff) while building air pressure to move forward (hard puff). A more recent option is two-pressure control. With this option

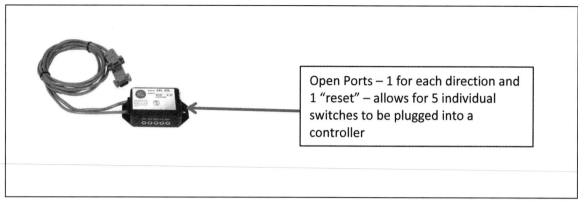

Open Ports – 1 for each direction and 1 "reset" – allows for 5 individual switches to be plugged into a controller

Figure 11-23. Switch interface (Adaptive Switch Labs).

enabled through programming, any two puffs moves the chair forward, a single puff turns the chair to the right, two sips moves the chair in reverse, and a single sip executes a left turn. This was designed for clients who can execute a sip and a puff, but who cannot discriminate between a hard and soft command. The time between double pneumatic commands must also be programmed.

CASE EXAMPLE

Travis is a 15-year-old male with a C2-level SCI secondary to a motor vehicle accident. He is vent-dependent and unable to move his extremities. He has minimal head movement. The only method available to him for independent driving was pneumatic control. Travis, having previous mobility concepts from before his accident, caught on quickly to the controls. He was able to use latch for forward movement and could change his speeds through hard puffs while in latch mode. He drove with excellent control for several years. One day, while driving in his family room, he ran over a bump, and the straw moved out of his mouth. He was unable to retrieve this due to lack of neck movement, and the wheelchair was in latch. The wheelchair drove itself across the room and through a sliding glass door! A fiberoptic switch was placed on the distal end of the straw. This switch detected Travis's chin. If the straw moved out of position, the fiberoptic switch no longer detected his chin and stopped the chair. Travis also used this switch as his reset switch. He would open his mouth wide, activating the switch, changing from driving mode to power seating mode to access his power tilt.

Three- to Five-Switch Control

Any combination of mechanical or electrical switches can be placed where the client can access these to provide control of the power wheelchair. The access methods mentioned earlier are already part of an array, such as four fiberoptic switches. If a combination of mechanical and electrical switches is used, a switch interface is required (Figure 11-23). This interface has five switch ports labeled forward, left, right, reverse, and reset. If the client will use an AbleNet Jellybean switch placed in the center of his or her tray for forward directional control, the switch is plugged into the forward port of the interface.

As mentioned previously, if only one switch site can be identified, the client can use single switch scanning. If two switch sites are identified, the client may be able to use two-switch control. If three switch sites can be identified, then these can be used for forward, left, and right. Reverse does not have to be available immediately and actually can be problematic for new drivers. New drivers often reverse for longer distances than are required, resulting in collisions. Many drivers cannot see behind their wheelchair, also leading to collisions. If the driver learns to rely on forward, left, and right, then when reverse is added in the future, excessive use is minimized. Many of the power wheelchairs available today are so maneuverable that reverse is not as critical as it once was. When using four switches for driving, use the strongest switch site for Forward, as this is used most frequently. Use the weakest switch site for Reset, as this is not a timed or sustained switch activation.

Another means of accessing reverse is by using a reset or mode switch. Reset places the power wheelchair into another mode of operation, allowing the client to access features such as reverse, preprogrammed speed packages, powered seating, infrared transmission, mouse emulation, and interfaced assistive technology devices. This is covered in more detail in Chapter 13.

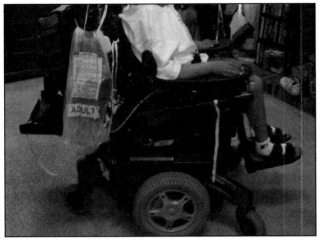

Figure 11-24. Julian and combination of switch types and sites.

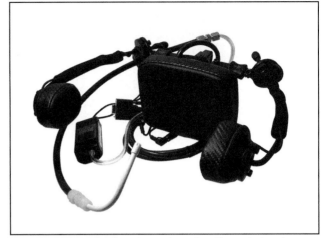

Figure 11-25. Combination sip-and-puff and head array (Stealth Products).

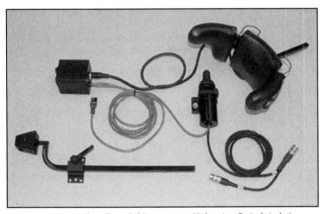

Figure 11-26. Analog digital drive system (Adaptive Switch Labs).

CASE EXAMPLE

Julian is 17 years old and has SMA (Figure 11-24). He uses four switches for driving and to control his power tilt. He uses a fiberoptic switch in his right arm trough for forward, which he activates with his thumb, a proximity switch embedded in the left pad of his headrest for left, an AbleNet Microlite switch by his medial right knee for right, and an AbleNet Specs switch in the right side of his headrest for reset. These are the locations where he has the volitional movement to accurately use switches for driving. Each had to be mounted in a precise location for access, and the knee switch swings out of the way for transfers. Julian is independent in driving and in control of his power tilt.

Hybrid Systems

Several hybrid systems are available that combine features of other access methods. One system combines features of sip-and-puff and the head array (Figure 11-25). Any puff is forward, any sip is reverse and left and right are controlled by the side pads of the headrest. This is appropriate for a client who can execute sip and puff commands, but cannot discriminate between the hard and soft pneumatic commands. The client must have adequate head control. This may also be beneficial for the client who can use a head array, but may have difficulty releasing the rear pad to stop (i.e., due to extension). The client must be able to execute pneumatic commands.

Another hybrid system combines a joystick and head array. The joystick controls forward and reverse and the head array controls left and right (Figure 11-26). This system would meet the needs of a client who perhaps had difficulty with lateral control of the joystick and releasing the rear pad of the head array but was able to control both joystick forward and reverse movement and lateral movement of his or her head.

Two-Switch Control

Another configuration option available on two electronics packages is two-switch control. If the client presses the first switch once, twice, and holds, the chair moves forward. If the client presses the first switch once and holds, the chair moves left. A double click of the first switch is a reset. If the client presses the second switch once, twice, and holds, the chairs moves into reverse. If the client presses the second switch once and holds, the chair moves right. This provides full directional control with only two switches (any mechanical or electrical switches can be used). The client must be able to activate the switches in this manner and discriminate between commands, which may present a significant cognitive load for some individuals.

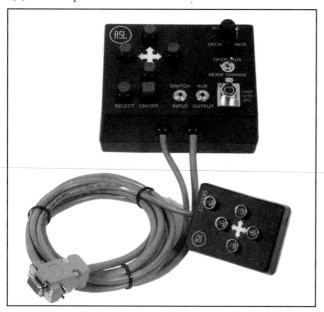

Figure 11-27. Single-switch scanner (Adaptive Switch Labs).

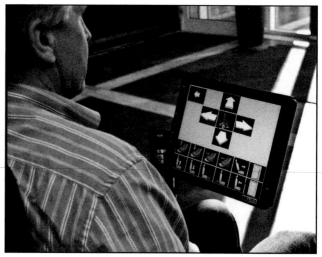

Figure 11-28. Roll Talk eye gaze system (Adaptive Switch Labs).

Single-Switch Scanning

Finding switch sites can be challenging. If only one switch site is identified, it is possible to drive by using switch scanning (Figure 11-27). A single switch activation starts a scan on the wheelchair display or on an external display. Directional options are scanned (a mode option can be scanned as well). When the desired selection is highlighted, the client activates and holds the switch for as long as movement in that direction is needed.

Depending on the wheelchair electronics, the scan can be programmed for four, eight, or even more directions. The scan speed can be adjusted. The pattern of the scan can also be programmed; for example, reverse can be scanned half as often as forward, left, and right. All of these strategies are designed to increase efficiency of a rather inefficient means of driving.

Scanning is a slow and laborious means of driving a power wheelchair but does provide mobility for clients with extremely limited motor control. The client must be able to accurately use a single switch site and visually monitor the display. If the client has the ability to use just one other switch, this can be designated for reset. Single switch scanning is a last resort access method that is inherently inefficient, so all other possible access methods should be explored before this is selected.

CASE EXAMPLE

Paul is a 46-year-old man with the diagnosis of cerebral palsy. He has significant extensor tone and little volitional movement. He is able to access a switch by the left side of his head. No other volitional switch sites were identified. He uses this one switch to drive via scanning. His driving is slow, but he can generally get where he needs to. He is also able to control his power tilt by scanning and selecting mode.

Eye Gaze

Roll Talk is an eye gaze operated system (Figure 11-28). It is a combination system that is also a speech-generating device and electronic aid to daily living. The back of the device has four small cameras. In driving mode, the client sees four quadrants on the screen. To drive the wheelchair, the client looks at the desired quadrant, and the chair moves in that direction, subsequently displaying four new quadrants. The system does require an initial switch activation to wake up. The client can use eye gaze to operate power seating functions as well. This system is specifically designed for clients with advanced ALS and is not available in the United States.

FUTURE

Researchers are working on power wheelchairs that can be operated by brain, voice, and computer. Brain and voice control will most likely not come to market because of safety concerns. Computer-controlled chairs follow special tape laid on the floor to get to specific destinations. Sensors prevent collisions with obstacles. These systems are also unlikely to become available commercially due to funding. Most funding sources are unwilling to purchase a power wheelchair if the client cannot drive it with less external assistance.

Power wheelchair electronics continue to advance. New access methods will continue to come to market, along with new programming options. Careful assessment remains essential to match these products and features to client needs.

REFERENCES

Cullen, K. E. (2012). The vestibular system: Multimodal integration and encoding of self-motion for motor control. *Trends in Neurosciences, 35,* 185-196.

Dicianno, B. E., Cooper, R. A., & Coltellaro, J. (2010). Joystick control for powered mobility: Current state of technology and future directions. *Physical Medicine and Rehabilitation Clinics of North America, 21,* 79.

Livingstone, R. (2010). A critical review of powered mobility assessment and training for children. *Disability & Rehabilitation: Assistive Technology, 5*(6), 392-400.

Merriam-Webster. (n.d.). Efficiency. Retrieved from www.merriam-webster.com/dictionary/efficiency

Smith, M. (2013). *Wheels of change: The story behind how complex rehab technology was born, evolved, and fosters the independence of Americans with disabilities.* CreateSpace Independent Publishing Platform.

SUGGESTED RESOURCES

Access to Independence, Inc. Complex Rehab Power Wheelchair Electronics Comparison Matrix: www.atilange.com/resources.html

Adaptive Switch Laboratories, Inc.: www.asl-inc.com

Stealth Products, Inc.: www.stealthproducts.com

Switch It, Inc.: www.switchit.com

Please see video on the accompanying website at

www.healio.com/books/mobility

Appendix

Note. CP = cerebral palsy; MD = muscular dystrophy; RIM = Rehabilitation Institute of Montreal; SMA = spinal muscular atrophy; TBI = traumatic brain injury.

Non-Joystick Driving Methods

Decision-Making Tree

Each client functional category includes a list of diagnoses. These are diagnoses in which this functional level is sometimes seen. Functional levels vary greatly within a diagnosis, and these functional skills may be seen in clients with other diagnoses.

Specific driving methods are also labeled proportional or digital. Proportional typically provides 360 degrees of directional control, as well as speed control, by moving further from a starting point. Digital control uses switches and discreet directional control and does not typically provide speed control via how the switch is activated.

Client cannot use any type of joystick.

Joystick control requires grading of the force and distance of movement. The client must also have adequate movement and motor control to use a joystick.

Client has fair upper extremity control (CP, TBI, MS, MD).

- Individual mechanical switches on a tray surface (digital)
  - Typically four switches: forward, left, right, and reverse or reset.
  - Choose the switch size and force that matches the client's abilities.
  - The client must be able to move his hands horizontally and vertically to move up and over the switch surface.

The client does not have controlled vertical movements (more difficult for clients with increased tone).

- Proximity array under tray (digital)
  - Typically four switches: forward, left, right, and reverse or reset.
  - Place switches at a distance apart and in a pattern that matches the client's abilities.
  - Provide a tactile cue on the tray surface so the client knows where the activation area is located, even when looking forward to drive (i.e., Velcro).

Adjustment of activation area: Activation distance is a bubble around the switch. If the activation area is too large, the switches may activate one another or be activated by the top of the client's thighs.

Proximity switches are capacitive switches and are activated by items that are conductive. The switch can be activated by certain items on the tray within the activation area, including beverages or a cat. The switches will not be activated by other items, such as a book. The switches must be protected from moisture.

Client has good fine motor (finger/hand) control but limited activation travel and force (ALS, SMA, MD).

- Touch pad (proportional; i.e., Switch It Touch Drive 2)
  - The client must have adequate movement of a finger or thumb to move within a 360-degree circle for full available directional control.
  - The farther the finger or thumb moves from center, the faster the wheelchair moves.
  - A client with this control may be able to use a mini proportional joystick.

Note: A larger Touch Pad (HMC International) is no longer available in the United States. This would be used by a client with fair upper extremity control.

- VIC Touchless finger joystick (proportional) is no longer available in the United States.
- Fiberoptic switches (digital)
  - Typically four switches: forward, left, right, and reverse or reset.
  - Place switches at a distance apart and in a pattern that matches the client's abilities.
  - Tactile cue: The client should be able to feel the tip of the fiberoptic switch or mount to determine location.

Adjustment of activation distance: Activation distance is a straight line from the end of the switch. Match this to the client's available movement, which is typically quite small.

Switch placement: Fiberoptics can be placed at the angle required by the client. These can be placed facing directly upward or parallel to the floor, allowing the fingers to be moved while curled over the edge of a handpad or tray in a flexed position.

Switch mounting: Cables are fragile and need to be well-protected. Switches can be mounted in a tray, handpad of arm trough, or in a hollow gooseneck mount.

Upper extremity support: To provide postural support and facilitate a very small movement, support of the forearm, wrist and hand is required.

Client has good head control but little extremity control (high-level SCI, ALS, CP, MS).

- Magitek (proportional)
  - A sensor is typically mounted at the top of the head on a headset. Movement of the head is translated into movement of the power wheelchair.
  - *Precautions:* Client must be able to consistently bring head to upright to stop movement of power wheelchair. Programming required to allow power seating control through left and right directional control only.
- Proportional head control (RIM; proportional)
  - A posterior head pad is attached to a joystick behind the head. Moving the head rearward moves the power wheelchair forward.
  - *Precautions:* Client must sustain pressure against back pad to sustain forward. This can lead to increased tone in some clients or require excessive muscle strength for others. Increased tone can affect the client's ability to stop. Difficult to use with tilt or recline as posterior head pad moves. A reverse strategy is required.
- Head array (digital)
  - Despite not providing proportional control, head arrays may provide better driving control for some clients in this category. Further information follows.

Client has fair head control but little extremity control (CP, TBI, high-level SCI).

- Head array (digital)
  - Typically, three to five proximity switches in a tripad head support. The pad behind the head is for forward directional control. Various style head supports can be used.
  - A reverse strategy is required. This may be accomplished through an external switch to toggle forward/reverse, a quick hit on the rear pad, a reset switch, or standby. Options vary by base electronics.
- Permobil Total Control head array allows a combination of mechanical and proximity switches. It has two proximities in the rear pad to better capture diagonals
- Switch It Dual Pro has three options: (1) proximities only; (2) mechanical only—increased force on switch increases speed; and (3) proximities and mechanical—proximities respond immediately, and mechanicals allow increased speed with increased force. Speed for each switch/direction can be changed on the rear of the head array.

- *Precaution:* Increased force can lead to increased tone and difficulty stopping as well as increased fatigue.
- ASL Atom offers a user switch that plugs into the head array. Pressing the user switch turns off the head array (double beep), allowing the client to rest on the headrest without driving, changing modes or powering off the chair. If the user switch is held down for a longer amount of time (long beep), a directional command from the head array can now send a wireless switch signal to an assistive technology device (no interfacing component or cable required). Can turn on auditory feedback when a directional switch is activated.
- iDrive head array allows mechanical and proximity switches to be combined. Each switch is assigned using iDrive programming, which also provides other programming options.

Client has good oral motor control but little head or extremity control (high-level SCI).

- Sip-and-puff (digital)
  - Requires good intraoral pressure control, which requires good lip closure and a competent soft palate.
  - Latch is used to sustain forward movement without sustaining a hard puff. Typically turned on by a second hard puff and turned off with a hard sip. Consider a fiberoptic stop switch if the client will use latch.
  - Four pressure control: hard puff (forward), soft puff (right), hard sip (reverse), soft sip (left). Various strategies for changing speed which vary by base electronics.
  - Two pressure control (Q-Logic): two puffs (forward), one puff (right), two sips (reverse), one sip (left).
  - Stage control (iDrive): Stage 1 only controls forward and reverse and is not latched. A softer puff moves the chair forward slowly (i.e., creeping up to a table). Stage 2 (entered via a hard puff) provides four pressure controls with latch option.

Client has partial oral motor and head control (MS, TBI, SCI, CP).

- Sip-and-puff head array combo (digital)
  - Any puff is forward, any sip is reverse, and head array controls left and right. This may be appropriate for a client who cannot discriminate between hard and soft pneumatic commands but has some head movement.

Client has adequate motor control at four specific body sites (CP, TBI, ALS, SMA, MD).

- Four mechanical and/or electrical switches for forward, left, right, and reverse or reset (digital)
  - An optimal switch placement is where the client has small, isolated, repeatable, and sustained ability to activate and release a switch. Switches vary in size and force requirements.
  - A few electronic systems allow any mechanical and electrical switches to be combined.

Client has adequate motor control at three specific body sites (CP, TBI, ALS, SMA).

- Three mechanical and/or electrical switches for forward, left, and right (digital).
  - Reverse or reset can be added later or consider standby, as needed.
  - A few electronic systems allow any mechanical and electrical switches to be combined.

Client has adequate motor control at two specific body sites (CP, TBI, ALS, SMA).

- Two mechanical and/or electrical switches used to emulate four directions (digital)
- Q-Logic two switch control
  - Switch 1: Two switch activations, second sustained (forward), one sustained switch activation (left), double click (reset).
  - Switch 2: Two switch activations, second sustained (reverse), one sustained switch activation (right).
- iDrive Link:
  - Sustained activation of both switches simultaneously (forward).
  - Sustained activation of Switch 1 (left)
  - Sustained activation of Switch 2 (right)
  - Double click of Switch 1 (reset)
- ASL 2 switch fiberoptic array (can only be used with fiberoptic switches):
  - Sustained activation of both switches simultaneously (forward).
  - Sustained activation of Switch 1 (left).
  - Sustained activation of Switch 2 (right).
- ASL Single Switch Scanner with Dual Switch Step Scan
  - Switch 1: Each activation moves through driving direction choices (forward, left, right, and reverse).
  - Switch 2: Sustained activation moves the power wheelchair in the selected direction.

Client has adequate motor control at one specific body site (CP, TBI, ALS, SMA).

- Single-switch scanning (digital)
  - Uses an external scanner (ASL) or the base electronics display.
  - Options vary by base electronics.
  - First switch activation starts the scan, and a second sustained activation moves the power wheelchair in the highlighted direction.
  - Directions and reset are scanned.

Client has inadequate motor control to use any of the previous driving methods but has good eye movement control (ALS).

- Roll Talk Nova (digital) (Not available in the United States)
  - A single switch command is required to wake up the system.
  - Also provides communication and electronic aids to daily living functions.

Note: Reset redefines what the forward, left, and right directional switches control by changing the mode of operation of the wheelchair, providing control of reverse, speeds, power seating, infrared transmission, mouse emulation, and interfaced external assistive technology devices.

Power Mobility
Optimizing Driving

Amy M. Morgan, PT, ATP

Many factors go into adjusting how a power wheelchair handles and drives. The drive wheel configuration of the base will change the way a wheelchair performs in various environments. Additionally, how that chair is programmed also has a major impact on overall performance. This chapter discusses how both base characteristics and programming adjustments impact the way a power wheelchair drives. It also reviews various tracking technologies and how these impact power wheelchair driving. Finally, ongoing training strategies and tools are discussed to help clients continue to optimize their driving skills.

OPTIMIZING DRIVING THROUGH DRIVE WHEEL CONFIGURATION

Three main types of drive wheel configurations are available for power wheelchair bases: front-wheel drive (FWD), mid-wheel drive (MWD, or center-wheel drive), and rear-wheel drive (RWD; Figure 12-1). Each configuration has its own pros and cons. It is important to assess the individual client's needs at the power wheelchair evaluation to help determine which drive wheel configuration will best meet the identified functional mobility requirements.

Rear-Wheel Drive

RWD was the first type of power wheelchair base configuration. It is still used and offered as an option today, but more rarely utilized than front or mid-wheel drive due to its larger turning radius. The following pros and cons should be considered when thinking about RWD configuration. Remember, these are general concepts and apply differently to each individual chair model.

Pros of Rear-Wheel Drive

- Typically, RWD power bases offer good suspension, minimizing vibration in the chair and softening the ride for the client.

- Four wheels on the ground minimize the energy and forces that are distributed through the chair, which can potentially create issues with durability.

- RWD bases provide good tracking for successful use at higher speeds.

- The configuration may feel intuitive to clients who are familiar with driving a car because it maneuvers similarly.

Cons of Rear-Wheel Drive

- The smaller front casters on a RWD power wheelchair move during turning tasks, making turns wider. This may compromise maneuverability in tight spaces and during turning tasks.

- These rotating front casters must be straightforward to climb obstacles and may make climbing difficult from the side.

Lange, M. L., & Minkel, J. L.
Seating and Wheeled Mobility: A Clinical Resource Guide
(pp. 199-214). © 2018 SLACK Incorporated.

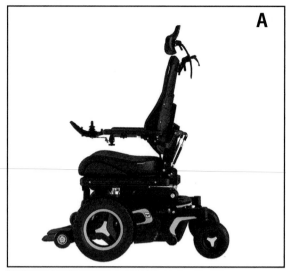

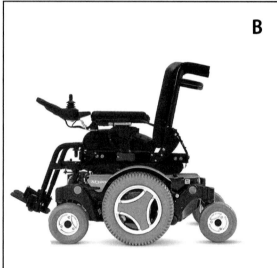

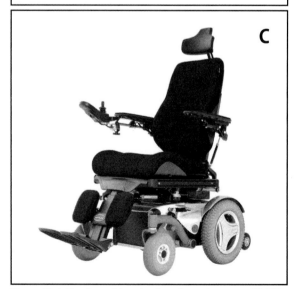

Figure 12-1. The three drive wheel configuration types: (A) FWD; (B) MWD; and (C) RWD.

- The area for proper weight distribution and balance in a RWD wheelchair is small. As most of the weight is in the back, it can be difficult to position the client properly while maintaining stability and balance in the base.

- As the weight is more rearward, the client may have limited access to larger angles of tilt-and-recline, which shift the client's weight posteriorly. This can also cause imbalance in the base. Larger tilt-and-recline angles may be required for medical management and adequate pressure relief.

- Rotating front casters may limit lower extremity positioning options and potentially interfere with stand-pivot transfers.

Front-Wheel Drive

FWD power wheelchair bases typically offer good maneuverability indoors and are optimal for use outdoors. However, because the rear casters move during turning tasks, this creates a difficult learning curve for some users.

Pros of Front-Wheel Drive

- As the front wheels are connected to the drive motors, these pull the casters over obstacles and through various terrains in a more effective way than other configurations where the casters are being pushed. When casters are being pulled, as in FWD, the force generated is forward and upward allowing the chair to get over obstacles and through softer terrains. On the contrary, when the casters are being pushed, the force generated is forward and downward, which can increase the likelihood of becoming stuck in certain situations.

- The drive wheels located in the front allow for climbing obstacles from any direction (the base does not need to be straight on in relation to the obstacle).

- The rear casters turning allows for tight turns and hugging the corner, taking less space to complete 90-degree turns.

- Four wheels on the ground minimize the energy and forces that are distributed through the chair.

- Weight distribution in FWD is forward, providing good balance when utilizing power seat functions that shift a client's weight posteriorly.

- FWD bases offer unlimited options for lower extremity positioning because there are no rotating front casters to avoid. This also allows the feet to be positioned in tighter, improving access to items in front, as well as keeping the overall footprint of the base smaller.

Cons of Front-Wheel Drive

- Some people feel uncomfortable with the rear casters turning in FWD, and there is a learning curve to establish successful driving techniques.

- Historically, FWD bases tracked poorly at higher speeds; however, current tracking technology has eliminated this concern.

- Weight distribution forward creates the possibility for base instability when descending ramps or large inclines, especially at higher speeds with abrupt stopping.

Mid-Wheel Drive

MWD is the most recent technology developed for power wheelchair bases. It attempts to combine the positive aspects of FWD and RWD into a hybrid product. MWD does provide the smallest overall turning radius, but has some limitations in use outdoors and over varied terrains.

Pros of Mid-Wheel Drive

- The smallest turning radius may improve maneuverability in tight spaces.

- MWD driving is intuitive as the client is typically sitting directly over the drive wheel (axis of rotation).

- Six wheels on the ground offer superior stability. The front or rear casters ensure this stability is maintained whether ascending or descending ramps/inclines.

Cons of Mid-Wheel Drive

- With six wheels on the ground, there is a chance for the center drive wheels to lose traction and not be able to move the base in certain situations (commonly known as *high centering*). This is probably the biggest disadvantage of MWD power wheelchair bases. However, newer technologies on complex bases can compensate for this risk.

- Six wheels on the ground allows for more energy transfer from the ground to the chair (and ultimately the client). This can potentially limit ride comfort for the client and possibly elicit pain, abnormal tone, or fatigue.

- Rotating front casters may limit lower extremity positioning options and potentially interfere with stand-pivot transfers. If the revolving front casters collide with optimally positioned footrests, adjustments may be required to compensate for this, such as raising the seat to floor height, or positioning the client more forward on the base (using caution not to impact balance and stability)

Specific Techniques to Optimize Driving

RWD drives most like a car (wider turns, front end moves):

- Keep feet in as close as possible while avoiding front caster interference.

- Wider turns are necessary around corners (Figure 12-2).

- Line up front casters straight on for obstacle climbing.

- Be careful with weight distribution/stability when navigating inclines and rough terrain.

FWD drives like a forklift (back end moves):

- When positioned adjacent to a wall/barrier, turn toward the wall/barrier, then reverse slightly to allow rear caster clearance for turning in the desired direction (away from the wall/barrier).

- Pull all the way in before starting the turn (Figure 12-3).

- Hug the corner (Figure 12-4).

- Obstacle climbing is possible from any direction, but the client must commit and follow through; do not back off.

- Navigate declines slowly without abrupt stopping; it also helps to tilt the chair (if equipped with power tilt) to help distribute weight for improved stability.

MWD turns on its own center (tight turning, quick turns):

- Keep feet in as close as possible while avoiding front caster interference.

- Line up drive wheel with corner for turning around obstacles (Figure 12-5).

- Line up front casters—straight on for obstacle climbing.

- When navigating soft, rounded curbs, go up from the side instead of straight on to avoid high centering.

- On uneven terrains, remember that high centering is a risk with any MWD chair.

In a recent study, various power bases were compared with the following results reported. The study was through the Human Engineering Research Laboratories, Veterans Affairs Pittsburgh Health Care System, Departments of Bio-Engineering, Rehabilitation Science and Technology, University of Pittsburgh, Pittsburgh, PA; and Department of Design and Environmental Analysis, Cornell University, Ithaca, NY.

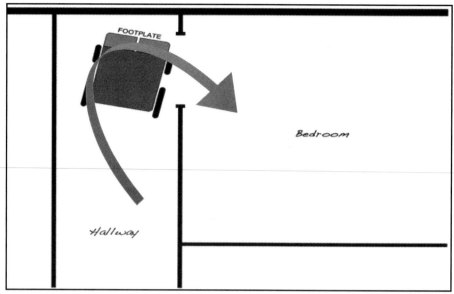

Figure 12-2. RWD 90-degree turn. Need to take a wider turn and may have difficulty clearing the footplates and/or front casters when turning around a corner.

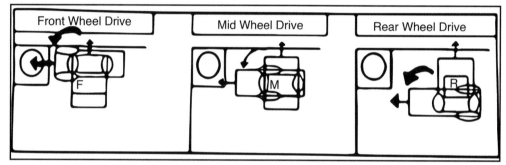

Figure 12-3. Imagine a small bathroom with access required to a sink right next to wall. The only configuration able to get the user correctly to the sink is FWD. Other configurations might work better in alternative situations.

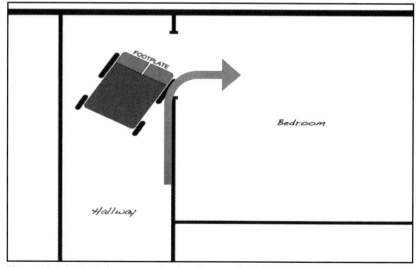

Figure 12-4. FWD 90-degree turn. Staying closer to the side you are turning to and lining up the center axle of the drive wheels allows for a tight turn around the corner. If the chair is not close to the turning side, the rear casters may contact the opposite wall of the hallway.

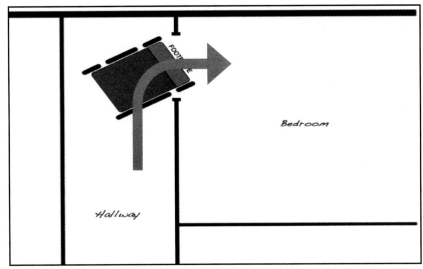

Figure 12-5. MWD 90-degree turn. Staying in the middle of the hallway helps improve this turn. Footplates and front casters may interfere with doorway clearance.

Mid-wheel drive PWCs [power wheelchairs] required the least space for the 360-degree turn in place compared with front-wheel drive and rear-wheel drive PWCs ($P < 0.01$) but performed equally as well as front-wheel drive models on all other turning tasks.

Even though the front-wheel drive models were longer and likely had larger swing angles in the rear compared with mid-wheel drive and rear-wheel drive configurations, users maneuvered these chairs in the least amount of space around the L-turn.

Our PWC findings combined suggest that front-wheel drive and mid-wheel drive wheelchairs are better than rear-wheel drive wheelchairs for maneuvering in confined spaces. Maneuverability of front-wheel drive PWCs may be more intuitive and easier to learn for users who are new to powered mobility or have impaired proprioception because turns can be initiated closer to the bend.

The handling of front-wheel drive PWCs may be more intuitive for some users because the center of rotation is toward the front of wheelchair, enabling the user to initiate a turn at the bend versus having to judge when to begin initiating a turn in order to accommodate a wider front-end swing angle. (Koontz, Brindle, Kankipati, Feathers, & Cooper, 2010)

Regardless of the power wheelchair drive wheel configuration, the size of the drive wheels and casters also has an important bearing on how the wheelchair base performs. The larger the wheel, the larger the obstacle it can negotiate. This is especially important when looking at the size of the drive wheel.

Again, it is important to reiterate that each individual chair model will offer various degrees of the characteristics just listed. This information is generalized information, and when prescribing an actual power wheelchair, one must consider the features of the specific model being recommended.

OPTIMIZING DRIVING THROUGH PROGRAMMING

Programming through the power wheelchair electronics is a beneficial tool to optimize driving for the client. If you are attempting to manipulate the programming setting on a client's power wheelchair, it is critical that you have been trained to do so. Improper adjustment in the programming can do much more harm than good and can even result in unsafe driving situations. Training can be obtained through educational courses, manufacturer in-services, or one-on-one training with qualified professionals.

Is Programming Necessary?

Why is programming necessary? Aren't power wheelchairs set up with standard programs that are adequate? These are common questions, and although it is true that manufacturers do much testing and attempt to create preset or default settings for each power wheelchair, there are times when these parameters need to be modified to optimize driving and safety for individuals. Programming is typically done for the following reasons:

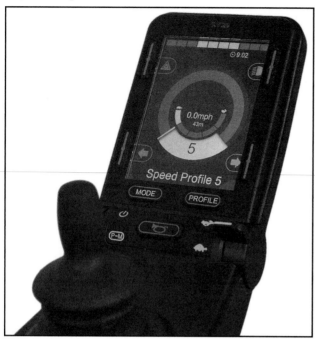

Figure 12-6. This R-Net joystick display shows a driving profile (Profile 5). The amount of battery power is displayed, as well as the speed of the power wheelchair.

- To optimize driving by adjusting performance settings

- To assign specialty input devices (alternative access methods/driver controls) used to drive the chair (see Chapter 11)

- To set up specific power seating features, such as seating angle limits, and memory seat positions, etc. (see Chapter 10)

- To allow the chair to be used in nondriving modes of operation, including control of power seating through the drive method, mouse emulation, infrared transmission (to control devices in the environment such as a TV) and control of interfaced external assistive technology devices (such as a speech generating device; see Chapter 13).

Electronics and Programming

Before getting into the specifics of programming, it is important to understand the difference between expandable and nonexpandable electronics. When thinking about expandable electronics, we are referring to doing more than just driving the wheelchair. With nonexpandable electronics, the joystick plugs directly into the controller. We typically see nonexpandable electronics on more basic power configurations such as scooters (Group 1 products) and consumer power chairs (Group 2 products). Power seat function operation (usually no more than two power options) and basic speed adjustments may be available.

(*Note*: Some manufacturers have more or less capability than what is explained here.) With expandable electronics, advanced features can be added if needed. For example, if a client requires an alternative driver control (input device other than a standard joystick) or needs to access the computer or control devices in the environment through the driving method, expandable electronics must be present. It is important to request the correct type of electronics package at the initial power wheelchair prescription so driving can be optimized effectively for the client. This is particularly important for clients with progressive conditions but also applies to those clients with advanced needs and a more involved clinical presentation.

Additionally, it is important to know some of the terminology that manufacturers use. *Drives* or *Profiles* are sets of driving parameters dictating how the chair performs under various driving conditions. Profile 1 may be programmed to drive indoors (lower speeds, increased responsiveness), and Profile 2 may be programmed to drive outdoors (higher speeds). *Drive Modes* or *Modes* are tasks that the wheelchair can do in each individual Drive/Profile. For example, power seating is a mode that may be accessible in Profiles 1 and 2; mouse emulation (for computer access) is a drive mode that may be programmed to be accessed in Drive 2. Knowing the differences in this terminology will help you communicate more clearly with other members of the team. See Figure 12-6 for an example of the information on a joystick display.

The three major brands of electronics power wheelchair manufacturers used in the United States are PG Drives Technology (R-Net), Dynamic (MK6i), and Curtis (Q-Logic). Each of these electronics packages are constantly improving and evolving. Unfortunately, the rate of programming improvements is not quick enough to keep up with the consumer electronics industry. Some of the differences among the various electronics manufacturers include varying number of drives or profiles, semantics used to describe different programming parameters, the availability of timers/compatibility with apps to monitor seating (e.g., the Virtual Seating Coach), look and feel of display, and how the chair is programmed, to name a few. For the most part, one can obtain similar results through programming in each type of electronics package, but how this is accomplished may be slightly different among manufacturers. Although various manufacturers use different terminology, all electronics packages allow you to manipulate driving parameters, seating, and management of external devices.

How Is Programming Done?

Power wheelchairs can be programmed in several ways. Most people are familiar with the handheld programmer. This is a device that is plugged directly into the wheelchair and changes are made directly on the handheld display and uploaded to the chair. This option is still available for all electronics packages; however, new and improved techniques can also be used. As most power wheelchair controllers have a visual display built in, it is now possible to complete on-board programming (OBP). OBP is not available from all manufacturers, but when it is present, the chair's display becomes the programmer when a special programming key is connected. Finally, there is programming through a computer or memory card. In this case, the programming is done on a computer and saved to the chair either by direct upload or through the insertion of a memory card that has the data stored on it. This method of programming allows the supplier or manufacturer to save drives or profiles, and even share them with others when the settings might be beneficial for another client. Some manufacturers have even developed various presets or subset files for common scenarios. The saved set of programming parameters can be emailed to a clinician or supplier to upload to a client's chair. The rehab team can then complete fine-tuning of the settings while assessing the client's driving performance.

When adjusting programming parameters, it is sometimes possible to adjust global settings instead of individual parameters. These global adjustments incorporate several parameters that affect the overall responsiveness and speed of the wheelchair. For example, response of the chair incorporates adjustments to acceleration, deceleration, braking, and tremor dampening, all of which are discussed in the following sections.

Specific Programming Parameters and Adjustments

Speeds and Rates (Responsiveness)

Speed

Speed is how fast a chair moves (higher number = faster). Often, clients will begin using slower speeds, but as they get more comfortable with driving the power wheelchair, these values can be adjusted to provide increased speed for more efficient mobility.

Each direction (forward/reverse/turning) can be independently adjusted.

Acceleration

Acceleration is how quickly the chair achieves its top speed (higher number = accelerates more quickly). If the acceleration is too high, the chair may be over-responsive or drive jerky. If the acceleration is too low, the client may not realize the chair is moving or will not be able to get the chair moving as quickly as necessary.

Each direction (forward/reverse/turning) can be independently adjusted.

Deceleration (Braking)

Deceleration is how quickly the chair slows to a stop (higher number = brakes more severely). If the deceleration is too high, the chair will stop very abruptly and can possibly cause postural instability with the client feeling like he or she is falling forward. If the deceleration is too low, the chair will coast to a stop and may overshoot the intended stopping point.

Each direction (forward/reverse/turning) can be independently adjusted.

CASE EXAMPLE

Sarah is an 11-year-old girl with undiagnosed neurodegenerative disorder. She obtained her first power wheelchair (RWD) when she was 7 years old and now requires a new one because she has grown. The team wanted to see whether Sarah was able to use a MWD power wheelchair and standard joystick. She and her family, along with the rehabilitation team, chose a MWD power base with 8-inch (larger) front casters to allow her to navigate obstacles and varying terrains more successfully. Sarah uses a standard joystick on the right with a modified joystick knob (combination stick with ball) (Figure 12-7). This modification was necessary due to her abnormal tone and improved driving in full extension (at end range). However, even with these hardware modifications, Sarah continued to veer to the right when driving. When she attempted to correct her path deviation, she would overcorrect and seemed to constantly be adjusting her path, unable to maintain forward consistently (see Video 12-1 on the companion site).

Programming

Sarah's school therapist contacted the manufacturer's representative, who came to the school and helped make the following adjustments to her programming: reduced turning speed to 9% and reduced turning acceleration to 10%. This was done to keep Sarah from getting off course and overcorrecting by increasing time for her to respond. They also modified the tremor dampening setting to 20 and increased the neutral (deadband) zone to 25 (these programming parameters are described in detail later in the chapter).

Hardware

The team also discussed the possibility of potential hardware changes if the programming adjustments were not successful. These included potentially changing to smaller 6-inch casters to improve maneuverability (although this wasn't preferred because it might limit her access on varied terrains), as well as adding gyroscopic tracking technology to improve forward tracking (see Tracking Technology later in the chapter). Tracking was not the preferred first response because of the additional cost of adding this unit.

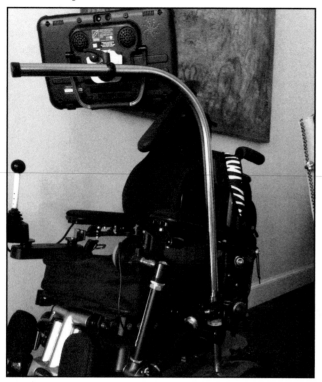

Figure 12-7. Sarah's wheelchair includes a special joystick knob to help her control her power wheelchair.

After the programming, adjustments were made and then fine-tuned, Sarah was able to maintain a forward path while driving her chair with much fewer corrections required. At that time, she did not need to pursue any of the hardware changes that had been considered (see Video 12-2 on the companion site).

CASE EXAMPLE

Brooklyn is a 5-year-old girl with arthrogryposis. She had been trialing power mobility using a FWD power base with a standard joystick mounted for use with her right foot. The joystick used a modified handle (dome-shaped) to allow her foot to rest on and manipulate this successfully. As it was her first time using powered mobility, the programming was adjusted globally to reduce the speeds (forward, reverse, and turning), which allowed her to be more successful with driving because she had more time to react and change her direction. She did well with the trial and demonstrated good safety awareness. Her speeds were quickly increased to default settings.

CASE EXAMPLE

Jin is a 14-year-old female with spastic cerebral palsy. She had been dependent for mobility her entire life with the exception of minimal indoor manual wheelchair propulsion using both her upper and lower extremities. This mobility was nonfunctional for her, and her school therapist and family wanted to trial power mobility using a standard joystick. Although Jin could move the joystick independently, she was easily distracted and seemed to not realize that she was moving herself.

Programming

The team decided to temporarily increase the forward acceleration and deceleration to accentuate her going and stopping in the chair. This helped improve her attention and allowed her to feel and know that she was in control of the chair. (*Note:* This adjustment would be a precaution or contraindication for any client with an uncontrolled startle reflex or who had significant weakness and severely limited postural control.)

Occasionally, Jin would also rest in a position that moved the joystick into reverse (out of neutral). To avoid her moving in a direction she could not see, the team turned down the reverse speed to 5% during the training period. The goal was to reintroduce reverse when Jin was more confident and aware of her independent mobility and the potential safety hazards in the environment.

Motor Performance

Power

This is the amount of power to the motors; lowering this value reduces collision damage by creating a *stall point*. Use this setting with caution because you do not want to restrict a client's ability to navigate his daily environments (e.g., ramps, thresholds, carpeting).

The power adjustment is typically used with clients newer to power mobility. Reducing this setting can allow the client to practice in the power wheelchair without raising concern for damaging the environment or client safety.

Torque

Torque is increased to overcome obstacles at low speed settings by providing a momentary burst of power. *Note*: This value cannot exceed the setting for overall power.

If a client needs to navigate over obstacles or rough terrain, increasing the torque may be necessary.

Steer Correct

This adjusts the balance of power to each motor. Use this with caution; attempt other strategies first because this adjustment may increase wear and tear on the equipment.

Many factors can cause a chair to not maintain a straight path. The steer correct setting can be used as a Band-Aid to fix the resulting path deviation but may not correct the source of the issue.

CASE EXAMPLE

Remember Jin? One additional adjustment in her programming was to reduce the power setting on her chair to 30%. This was done to allow her to safely interact with obstacles in the environment (bumping things, rather than causing damage to a wall) to help her develop an understanding of three dimensions, depth perception, and safety. This also helped her understand that objects are not always going to move out of the way and allowed her to begin to navigate around stationary obstacles. Since she was training in the school setting and the floor was level and made of tile, the chair would still move at this lowered power setting. If she needed to navigate a threshold, ramp, or thicker carpet, the chair may not have moved consistently due to the power being set too low to overcome this resistance.

With this trial chair, additional drive profiles were set at 100% power in case the chair got into an area where the additional power was necessary to keep the chair moving.

CASE EXAMPLE

Nick is a 40-year-old man with spina bifida at the T2 level who works in the home construction business. He is constantly encountering obstacles that he must be able to navigate successfully. Upon delivery of his new power wheelchair, an additional drive profile was created to provide the settings he needed for navigating his work sites. The supplier increased the torque settings in this drive profile to allow him to successfully negotiate the obstacles that he encounters daily.

Joystick Adjustments

Tremor Dampening

Also called *sensitivity*, tremor dampening is how quickly the chair responds to joystick movement. Higher values reduce the effect of hand tremoring by reducing responsiveness to smaller hand movements.

Caution: Higher values = larger stopping distance. Sometimes adjusting the "neutral zone" of a joystick can accomplish the same goal without compromising the braking speed.

Joystick Throw

Joystick throw is how far from center the joystick must move to achieve full speed. Various joysticks have different maximum values, and this will affect drive performance. The type of joystick chosen for a client depends on his or her capabilities, strength, tone, range of motion, and so on. For example, ultralight types of joysticks have maximum throw ranging from 0 to 6 mm, light joystick throw ranges from 13 to 17 mm, and standard joysticks have a throw of approximately 28 mm.

- Within each of these maximum values, the joystick throw can be reprogrammed from 0% to 100% of maximum.
- Joystick throw can be also adjusted individually in each direction of movement (forward, reverse, right, and left).

Note: When equipped with OBP, one can use active orientation to have the client physically move the joystick to his or her individual maximum position. The display will show the percentage of throw used, and the clinician or supplier can adjust the throw from that point to fine-tune the values.

Joystick Force

Various joysticks also have differing levels of force required to move the joystick out of neutral. The force of a joystick is *not* programmable and cannot be changed through programming (see Optimizing Driving Through Hardware later in the chapter).

Joystick Orientation and Axes

These parameters define which movement of the joystick (north, south, east, or west) controls which direction of travel (forward, reverse, right, or left).

- Directions for forward/reverse and left/right are always opposite one another. For example, forward can be defined as south, and reverse will automatically be defined as north.
- The joystick axes are also always 90 degrees apart from one another.
- Inverting axes refers to changing north to south and south to north or east to west and west to east.
- Swapping axes refers to changing north and south to east and west.

Note: When equipped with OBP, one can use active orientation to have the client physically move the joystick to the desired forward direction (reverse will automatically be the opposite movement), and to the desired left direction (right will automatically be the opposite movement).

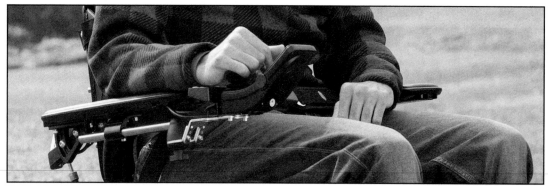

Figure 12-8. Swing-away joystick mount pivots medially and laterally to swing in to a midline position or out of the way.

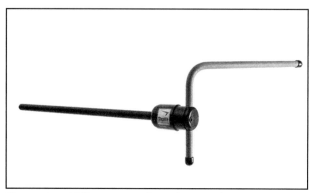

Figure 12-9. Midline mount allows the joystick to be positioned centrally in front of the client. The mounting hardware typically will swing away to allow for transfers in and out of the chair.

CASE EXAMPLE

Mr. X has advanced Parkinson's disease and would like to drive his power wheelchair with a standard joystick. However, the tremoring in his hand consistently causes the chair to move off course. This requires him to constantly move the joystick back and forth to correct his path deviation, contributing to frustration and fatigue. His supplier suggested using the tremor dampening feature in programming to decrease the effect of his hand tremors. The supplier adjusted tremor dampening to 40%. This helped Mr. X maintain a forward course; however, when he needed to turn abruptly, he was unable to do so. As he has several dogs in his home, this was important for him to be able to do. The supplier then lessened the tremor dampening to 20% and also increased the neutral/deadband zone to 25%. Mr. X now needed to move the joystick out of the expanded neutral/deadband zone for the chair to respond. This compensated for his tremoring while also preserving his ability to make quick turns and stops in his chair.

CASE EXAMPLE

James is a right-handed 31-year-old man with C5 tetraplegia (American Spinal Injury Association [ASIA] A). He is able to complete elbow flexion and forearm supination and is weak in shoulder external rotation, abduction, and flexion. He is trialing use of a standard joystick on the right with a modified handle (goalpost-style) to compensate for his lack of hand function. However, James is having some difficulty turning to the right due to his weak shoulder external rotators. The therapist asked if there was anything that could be done to help with this issue. The team manufacturer's representative was present and offered to reduce the joystick throw in the right direction and adjusted this value to 50%. This change helped James with his right turns and also helped him maintain his course appropriately.

CASE EXAMPLE

Kendle is a 6-year-old girl with congenital muscular dystrophy. She can sit with support but is unable to stand or walk on her own. She has extremely limited proximal muscle strength, but has good hand control for joystick operation when her arm is properly supported in midline. Kendle cannot independently move a midline mount to move the joystick out of the way, and it interferes with pulling up to desks and tables. She is able to independently operate a swing-away joystick mount with the tension slightly released. She has poor head control and requires assistance to lift her head if it falls forward. Figures 12-8 and 12-9 show images of some different types of joystick mounting options.

Input Device

Kendle is able to use a standard force joystick, but she does have significant weakness. When the swing-away joystick mount was swung in across her body, the joystick achieved midline position, and she was able to manipulate the joystick and mount independently without requiring specific midline mounting hardware.

Programming

The joystick throw was adjusted globally (all directions) to 50% to compensate for her weakness and manage fatigue. Additionally, the joystick orientation needed to be adjusted when the joystick was swung in (midline position) and swung out (for pulling up to desks). Her power wheelchair used R-Net electronics, and active orientation was utilized to achieve the appropriate directions with joystick movements in these positions. Additionally, a drive profile was created to allow her caregivers to drive the chair in the standard orientation. Each of these profiles were specifically named using PC programming (through a computer) such as "Kendle," "Desk," and "Mom" to clarify how the joystick would operate in each profile and letting everyone know which position the joystick should be in while driving.

Special Situations

Latched Driving

When a command is given for the chair to move, it will continue moving until a different command is given to stop the chair. This is typically only used for forward, and is most commonly used with sip-and-puff controls. However, any input device can be programmed to drive in latch. There are several latch types; two of the most common include the step latch and cruise latch:

- Step latch—a series of forward commands are given, gradually increasing the chair speed with each step.
- Cruise latch—a continuous forward command is given until the desired speed is reached.

Caution: Latched driving should only be used with clients who are able to easily and consistently execute a stop command. If the client is unable to execute the stop command reliably, latched driving would be unsafe to implement and is therefore contraindicated.

Standby

After a programmable amount of inactivity, the chair enters standby. From standby, the client can choose the function of the chair by which directional command is given. The chair can also be programmed to enter standby by activating a separate switch. When the client enters standby, several scenarios can be programmed:

- The input device becomes totally inactive, and movements do not result in any action from the chair.
- Each direction of the input device selects a specific function (e.g., forward—return to drive; right—enter seating mode; reverse—enter computer/mouse emulation). These directions can be individually programmed using a computer (OBP will use default features). When specifically programming

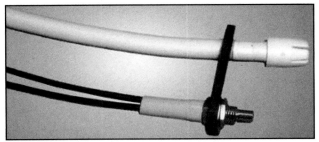
Figure 12-10. Switch-It Sip N' Puff with Opti-Stop.

features, be sure to assign a direction to return to driving so the client can exit standby.

- A specified direction will allow the client to cycle through all available modes and profiles for that chair. The client selects the desired function with a different command, typically forward.

Note: Standby options and terminology vary by manufacturer and these are examples of common standby options available.

CASE EXAMPLE

John is a 26-year-old man with an incomplete spinal cord injury (C4 ASIA B). John uses sip-and-puff to drive his power wheelchair.

Programming

To keep John from having to maintain the intraoral pressure required to sustain a hard puff, the rehabilitation team programmed the chair to drive in latch for forward. This also allowed John to more efficiently navigate through his environment (veering) by using soft sips and/or puffs while the chair continued to move forward. John executes one hard puff to enter latch. The chair continues forward movement until he executes a hard sip to stop. While the chair is moving forward, he is able to execute soft puffs (for right directional control) and soft sips (for left directional control) to change course.

Hardware

One additional component provided with the sip-and-puff drive control was a fiberoptic switch used as an optical emergency stop (Figure 12-10). This switch was programmed to be normally closed, which allowed the chair to move as long as the switch was in proximity to John's lip (detecting that the sip-and-puff straw was in his mouth). If the straw were ever removed from John's mouth, (causing him to lose control of chair operation) the fiberoptic switch would automatically stop the chair from moving. This is particularly important when the chair is driven in latch because the chair would continue to drive if the straw moved away from the client's mouth.

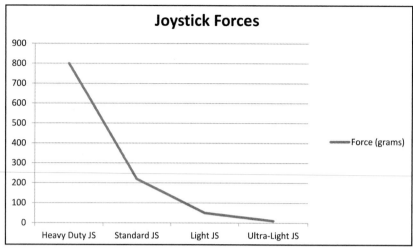

Figure 12-11. Common force requirements for various JS categories. (JS = joystick.)

CASE EXAMPLE

Mary is a 32-year-old woman who uses a standard joystick with a goalpost handle to drive her power wheelchair. It is difficult for Mary to access the buttons on her joystick to change speeds or control her power seating through the joystick. Every time she tries to push the buttons, the chair ends up turning or moving into reverse because she bumps the joystick unintentionally. This has gotten her into some difficult situations. When Mary tries to take her hand off the joystick, she is unable to get it back on successfully, especially when she is fatigued at the end of her day. Her therapist considered changing her input device to an alternative drive control, such as a head array or sip-and-puff, to help with this issue. Mary's supplier suggested that they attempt to program the chair to use standby before making changes to the input device to see if that solved the problem. The supplier attached a mechanical switch on a swing-away mount to Mary's headrest.

Programming

Standby was set up to engage with switch activation. Through computer programming, each direction of her joystick was individually programmed to enter a specific mode. When Mary pressed the switch at her head, her joystick movements then allowed her to access the following features (modes) of her chair: right/left allowed her to change drive profiles (essentially changing her speed); forward allowed her to return to driving (exiting standby); and reverse selected the seating mode (operating power seat functions of the chair).

This was successful for Mary, and she was able to continue driving her power wheelchair with the proportional control of her standard joystick and avoiding the unnecessary purchase of an additional input device.

OPTIMIZING DRIVING THROUGH HARDWARE

Options are also available to improve driving through hardware or physical characteristics of the power wheelchair itself. Changing or adding components on the power wheelchair base creates additional costs. Therefore, it is best to attempt to solve issues through programming whenever possible. Programming adjustments should be done before making equipment changes or purchasing additional components for the power wheelchair. Occasionally, the issue cannot be resolved through programming alone, and hardware changes are necessary. The following items are potential ways to improve driving performance through hardware.

Input Device

The type of input device a client uses to drive the power wheelchair can have a significant impact on his or her successful driving. Most power wheelchair users will drive using a standard joystick. There are many types of joysticks. One of the distinguishing characteristics among joysticks is the amount of force the client must generate to move the joystick out of neutral. This is a mechanical characteristic of the joystick and any changes to manipulate the amount of force required would need to be made physically to the mechanics/structure of the joystick itself. This is not commonly done. If the force of a joystick is more than the client can exert, a different joystick is typically chosen. Joysticks can be classified into four categories: standard, light, ultralight, and heavy duty. Forces required with these various joysticks can range from 8.5 to 800 g (Figure 12-11).

Common Force Requirements for Joysticks

Standard joystick: approximately 220 g

Light joystick: range from 18 to 50 g

Ultralight joystick: range from 8.5 to 13 g

Heavy-duty joystick: up to 800 g

Additionally, there are times when a joystick or other proportional input is not appropriate for the client. Other input devices may make driving more successful for that individual. These alternative drive controls and applications for use are discussed at length in Chapter 11.

Front Caster Size

Rotating front casters (for MWD/RWD bases) result in an initial shift in the direction of the wheelchair after a forward command is executed if they are not properly aligned (straight in a trailing position) for forward movement. The size of these casters directly correlates to the magnitude of that initial shift (larger casters will shift more than smaller casters). If this shift is problematic for the client and he or she is unable to correct the pattern of movement and get the chair on proper course, changing to a smaller front caster may be a possible solution.

Tracking Technology

Tracking technology has significantly improved over the years. This has allowed power wheelchairs, especially FWD models, to travel at higher speeds without losing course or fishtailing. Tracking has a strong application when the client is using a digital (switched) input device. In these cases, tracking technology allows the chair to remain on course, even if traveling on varied terrain, therefore requiring fewer corrections (switch hits) by the client. Additionally, tracking may be necessary when the power wheelchair has additional weight attached, such as a ventilator tray. This additional weight alters the chair balance and may result in a loss of forward course. Finally, when a chair encounters an obstacle, this can also cause the chair to lose course and veer to one side. Tracking technology helps manage this and ideally keeps the chair on proper course. If the power wheelchair remains on course, the client has to make less compensatory joystick movements or switch activations, reducing effort and time.

Three main types of tracking technologies are used in power wheelchairs today: gyroscopes (ESP/G-Trac), tachometers (Tru-Trac), and encoders (Accu-Trac). Gyroscopes directly measure the actual position of the power wheelchair base and offer more accurate management of tracking. Tachometers and encoders indirectly measure wheel revolutions per minute to detect whether the chair is moving off course. For tachometers and encoders to work accurately, traction on the wheels must be maintained.

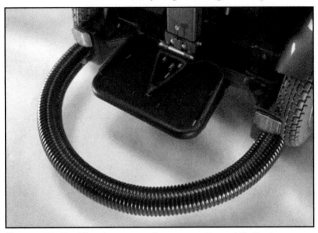

Figure 12-12. The bumper, shown on Permobil Koala power wheelchair, is sometimes used during training to minimize damage to the environment when a child is initially learning to use the power wheelchair.

In a *Mobility Management* article from June 2013, results from an informal study examining tracking technology were reported. Both MWD and FWD models were used with either three switches on a tray or a three-switch head array. The results showed that when equipped with tracking technology, the wheelchair user required significantly fewer switch hits (57% to 76% less). Also, the subject was able to complete the course in significantly less time (38% to 52%), indicating improved efficiency and energy conservation when using tracking technology. According to the authors, "This efficiency is critical for consumers, as driving efficiency reduces motor effort, energy expenditure and can prevent fatigue, loss of function and increased muscle tone" (Brown & Lange, 2013).

Bumpers and Safety Switches

Special circumstances may warrant the addition of hardware to promote safe driving for clients. These are most commonly used for clients who are new to power mobility or are still in training, as well as those clients with visual impairments.

Some wheelchair models offer front bumpers that attach to the wheelchair base to provide tactile feedback to protect the client's feet as well as alert him or her to obstacles in the environment. These are often used on a temporary basis and can be removed once the client is able to safely navigate his or her environment (Figure 12-12).

Special switches can be attached to the base of the wheelchair to detect obstacles in the path of the power wheelchair (Figure 12-13). These switches can provide either an auditory input or, in some cases, physically stop the wheelchair from moving. When working with a client who has a visual impairment, these safety switches may be necessary. While the switches will detect obstacles up to approximately 20 inches away from the wheelchair base. It is important to

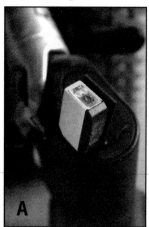

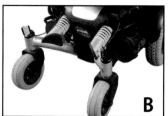

Figure 12-13. ASL 405 Two Sensor Alert with One Tone.

note that the switches do not detect any drop off (e.g., curbs, steps). If the switches are adjusted at maximum range, these may be inadvertently activated by simply moving through a room.

ONGOING TRAINING TO OPTIMIZE DRIVING

Every power wheelchair user will become more and more proficient at driving over time through everyday experiences in the chair. For some, it may be beneficial to have several ongoing training sessions to help maximize driving performance and gain confidence in using the new power wheelchair. These training sessions begin with more basic use (e.g., driving straight, incorporating turning tasks in open, noncluttered environments) and progress to more complex tasks (e.g., crowded environments, static and dynamic obstacles, loading/unloading in vehicles). It is not uncommon for clinicians to dedicate therapy sessions to work on improving driving and maneuverability. However, for some clients, this training is best done in the natural environments where the chair is being used (e.g., home, school, grocery store, church/temple). Generally, it is more beneficial to conduct training sessions more frequently at shorter durations (e.g., 30 minutes/day, 5 days/week) than longer sessions done less frequently.

In the clinic, a clinician may choose to use specific outcome measures to quantify performance and progress, such as the Wheelchair Skills Test developed at Dalhousie University, Halifax, Nova Scotia, Canada (Kirby, Swuste, Dupuis, MacLeod, & Monroe, 2002). Both manual and power wheelchair versions of this tool are available, as well as a Wheelchair Skills Training Program Manual (www. wheelchairskillsprogram.ca). These outcome measures, along with other tools, can assist with wheelchair training or serve as a resource for clients to help improve efficiency and mobility skills (Rushton, Kirby, Routhier, & Smith,

2016). The Suggested Reading section lists some of these resources. Additionally, typical daily tasks can be simulated, and the clinician can help the client learn strategies for maneuvering in difficult situations, such as getting on/off an elevator, navigating through and accessing items in the kitchen, using a small restroom or accessible stall in public restrooms, and so on. During training, it is imperative that consideration be taken for the type of drive wheel configuration being used by the client (see specific maneuverability tips in the Drive Wheel Configuration section of this chapter). Once a client has completed training sessions with supervision by a clinician, it is beneficial to train a caregiver or attendant to continue instruction in the natural environment. This is typically done with the client and trainer during the therapy visits. Many times, in the school setting, this ongoing training is provided by a one-on-one aide or paraprofessional and not directly by the treating therapist.

Approaching wheelchair skills training for pediatric clients compared with adults requires differentiation between the two groups. For example, a child may not understand the need to perform skills well to be successful, whereas an adult realizes the importance of completing daily skills effectively. Therefore, motivational strategies tend to require much more creativity when working with the pediatric population. In both cases, daily activities and interests should be incorporated into the training program.

CASE EXAMPLE

Pediatric Training

Luke is a 5-year-old boy with cerebral palsy who loves to read and play basketball. He received his first power wheelchair one week before his first outpatient physical therapy visit for advanced mobility training. The main goals identified for these treatment sessions were to:

- Maximize independence with self-care and activities of daily living mobility skills

- Improve accuracy and efficiency with power mobility driving in tight and crowded spaces

- Provide client and caregiver education regarding high-level mobility skills using the power wheelchair in the home and community environments

Initially training included a review of Luke's chair features and basic driving instruction (e.g., turning chair on and off, using power seat functions, driving a straight path). Several activities that incorporated Luke's interests were initiated to help him with higher level driving skills. For example, a story was created for Luke to read. Each page of the story was placed along the walls in an area where both right and left turns were required. As Luke was using a

FWD power wheelchair, the pages were posted on the side of the wall that he was turning toward (to help him get used to hugging the corner). Also, a basketball net was set up with some obstacles (e.g., cones, foam cubes, therapy balls) scattered around. Luke was required to scan his environment and navigate to the basketball hoop, and then also use his seat elevator to make a slam-dunk.

After playing basketball, Luke needed to wash his hands, so the session then proceeded to the restroom where hygiene skills could be practiced. Finally, Luke, his mother, and therapist went outside to the family vehicle (navigating an elevator—allowing Luke to push the buttons) and ended the session working on getting in and out of the vehicle safely and efficiently. Traveling to the outdoor parking lot also allowed education regarding safety with curbs, crossing streets, and other skills.

After a few training sessions and some slight modifications to the programming parameters in his power wheelchair electronics, Luke and his mother were ready to continue working on refining his skills in their daily environments. He was discharged from physical therapy for power mobility training.

Case Example

Adult Training

Beth is a 55-year-old woman who has multiple sclerosis. She began using a power wheelchair recently because of her decline in function. Her occupational therapist determined that it was necessary for her to receive services on a short-term basis for additional mobility training. Beth's goals were very specific and included the following:

- Maximize independence with cooking and meal preparation
- Independently navigate her small bathroom for basic hygiene activities
- Improve safety and accuracy in crowded areas and busy environments in the community

During Beth's first session, her therapist reviewed the power chair features including powering the chair on and off, using power seat functions effectively to manage her medical needs, and basic operation, including speed adjustment. Beth successfully used an application on her mobile device to help her remember to perform power seat functions, and this worked particularly well for her because she had some difficulty with her memory.

Next, the therapist set up several cones with yardsticks in them and created a boundary with caution tape to simulate a small bathroom as well as her kitchen. This was an ideal place to begin training Beth in the techniques to get her out of difficult situations in tight spaces. After Beth successfully completed the simulation, it was time to proceed to an actual bathroom and kitchen (the staff kitchen and restroom were used for this training). One session even involved baking cookies (using premade cookie dough). Beth was able to complete all of the steps independently with few modifications to the cooking equipment.

In the final session, Beth and the therapist ventured to a public restroom near the hospital cafeteria at lunchtime and worked on navigation in crowded areas. This task allowed the therapist to help Beth become more comfortable around dynamic obstacles as well as using a public restroom stall.

Beth was discharged from occupational therapy after four sessions (1 session per week). She was much more comfortable using her power wheelchair, and her maneuverability skills continued to improve as time went on.

Summary

Optimizing driving in the power wheelchair can be accomplished in a variety of ways. Many compounding factors must be considered when determining why a client is having difficulty using the power wheelchair successfully. It is beneficial to attack these issues with a team approach. The more people who are thinking about the issues, the more likely a solution will be identified. In each case, more conservative, less costly changes are preferred (i.e. programming), and equipment changes and purchasing new equipment can be pursued as a last resort if more conservative measures are unsuccessful.

References

Brown, L., & Lange, M. (2013). Tracking technologies: A Phase 1 study to validate efficacy. *Mobility Management*. Retrieved from https://mobilitymgmt.com/Articles/2013/06/01/Tracking-Technologies.aspx

Kirby, R. L., Swuste, J., Dupuis, D. J., MacLeod, D. A., & Monroe, R. (2002). The Wheelchair Skills Test: A pilot study of a new outcome measure. *Archives of Physical Medicine and Rehabilitation, 83,* 10-18.

Koontz, A. M., Brindle, E. D., Kankipati, P., Feathers, D., & Cooper, R. A. (2010). Design features that affect the maneuverability of wheelchairs and scooters. *Archives of Physical Medicine and Rehabilitation, 91,* 759-764.

Rushton, P. W., Kirby, R. L., Routhier, F., & Smith, C. (2016). Measurement properties of the Wheelchair Skills Test-Questionnaire for powered wheelchair users. *Disability and Rehabilitation: Assistive Technology, 11*, 400-406.

SUGGESTED READINGS

Minkel, J., Perr, A., & Yamada, D. (2002). *The powered wheelchair training guide.* New York, NY: PAX Press.

Lange, M. (2007). *Mobility training guidelines.* Retrieved from http://www.atilange.com/Resources.html

---

Please see video on the accompanying website at

www.healio.com/books/mobility

Power Mobility
Advanced Applications

Michelle L. Lange, OTR/L, ABDA, ATP/SMS

Power wheelchairs are primarily designed to provide a means of independent mobility to the client. Complex rehabilitation power wheelchairs, using expanded electronics, also include features that can increase independence beyond mobility. These features include control of power seating or interfaced external Assistive Technology devices (e.g., a speech-generating device [SGD]) through the driving method. Infrared (IR) transmission from the power wheelchair to control devices in the environment (e.g., audiovisual equipment) and mouse emulation for access to a computer or SGDs are also available. In addition, power wheelchairs can be used with emerging technologies, such as tablets and smartphones.

Many clients who require a power wheelchair will also require other assistive technologies due to physical, cognitive, or sensory limitations. For example, a client requiring power mobility is more likely to require power seating for weight shifts than a client using manual mobility. A client using alternative driving methods is more likely to require control of that power seating through the access method, rather than a through standard toggle or button control.

These advanced applications can be difficult to fund. Funding sources may be unfamiliar with specific components that are required to access these features. Documentation must justify the necessity of each component as well as detail the functional difference these features will make in the client's level of independence. For example, if a client needs to access his or her SGD through the power wheelchair driving method, an interfacing component and cable will typically be required. Documentation justifying the necessary components may state: "The interfacing component and cable are required for the power wheelchair driving method to be used to access the current SGD." Documentation detailing the functional need may state: "The client's optimal driving method is using a head array. The optimal switch location for the SGD is the left side of the head. For the client to use the optimal access method for both mobility and communication while in the power wheelchair, these two devices must share the same switch."

Just as funding can be challenging, it may be difficult to find clinicians and suppliers who are familiar with these advanced applications. If the team members are not aware of features that may be helpful to a client, these options will not be considered in product recommendations. If team members are aware of these features but do not know how to set up the features, the client may still not benefit from this technology. Seating and mobility professionals need to be competent in these areas to meet client needs.

Before exploring advanced power wheelchair applications, it is of course critical to ensure the client is positioned well, is using the most appropriate driving method (as addressed in Chapter 11) and that the power wheelchair has been configured to optimize driving (as addressed in Chapter 12).

Lange, M. L., & Minkel, J. L.
Seating and Wheeled Mobility: A Clinical Resource Guide
(pp. 215-235). © 2018 SLACK Incorporated.

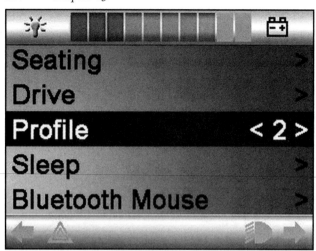

Figure 13-1. Screenshot of user menu.

FEATURE NAVIGATION

A power wheelchair is typically operated in drive mode. Once the wheelchair is powered on, in drive mode, use of the drive method results in movement of the wheelchair. To use the driving method (e.g., a head array) to control other features (e.g., a power tilt), the client must navigate between features, choosing a different mode of operation. Feature navigation varies between manufacturer's electronic systems and sometimes more than one strategy is available within a system. Currently, complex rehabilitation technology uses a variety of electronic packages, including MK6i and LiNX (used on Invacare chairs), R-Net (used on Permobil, Quickie, and Rovi chairs), and Q-Logic (used on Quantum Rehab chairs).

Features that can be accessed through the driving method include the following:

- Driving in reverse: A separate reset switch is commonly used to toggle forward and reverse directional control on three-switch driving methods such as the head array

- Power seating, including tilt, recline, elevating legrests, seat elevation, and stand

- Preprogrammed driving profiles, allowing the client to change which driving profile is active

- IR transmission for control of a compatible device in the environment

- Mouse emulation to replicate the functions of a computer mouse

- Auxiliary, used for interfacing external assistive technology devices, such as a SGD

Feature navigation may not seem very interesting, but it is critical in providing client control of nondriving features. Various navigational strategies are available to meet an individual's motor, cognitive, and visual requirements.

As specific feature navigation varies and changes, this section provides general information. Specific information may be obtained from the manufacturers. Two main strategies used to access features other than mobility are *reset* and *standby*.

Reset/Mode Navigation Methods

The terms *reset* and *mode* are often used interchangeably. A reset/mode switch is usually plugged into a 1/8-inch switch jack on the joystick or display. Any type of switch can be operated by any part of the body that the client has adequate motor control. A reset switch does not require the accuracy of a driving switch, freeing up stronger sites for driving control. Activating the reset/mode switch places the wheelchair into a nondriving mode of operation.

One navigation method moves through a predicable *sequence* of features with each reset switch activation, such as reverse, power seating, and auxiliary. Features can be added or removed from this sequence depending on client need. A primary advantage of a predictable sequence is that the client may be able to memorize this sequence and choose the desired feature without actually needing to see the display. This is helpful for clients who have adequate vision for driving the wheelchair but not enough vision to read the display. This is also helpful for clients who can see the display but who are not literate.

Another navigation option (sometimes called *manual scroll*) shows a feature menu on the display when the reset switch is activated (Figure 13-1). Directional switches are used to move through and select the displayed features. For example, the client activates the reset switch to get to the feature menu (sometimes referred to as *user menu*). The forward directional switch moves up the list of available features, reverse moves down the list, and right selects the desired feature. The left directional command goes back a level in the hierarchy. This navigation method allows the client to move through many options, but does require adequate vision and literacy. If the client is using three switches for driving, a forward directional command would move up the displayed choices and wrap to the bottom of the display because reverse is unavailable for feature navigation.

A third navigation technique available when using a reset switch is an auto scroll. The reset switch begins a scan of the feature menu. The speed is adjustable. The client activates the right directional switch to choose a highlighted feature or the left directional switch to move back in the hierarchy.

Depending on the electronics system, the specific text displayed on the menu can be customized to meet an individual's needs. For example, instead of *auxiliary*, the display can show *talker* if this feature is used to interface an SGD.

Standby Navigation

Standby is the second general feature navigation strategy and is used primarily with clients who are unable to access a reset switch. For example, a client may have adequate head movement to control a three-switch head array, but inadequate motor control to access a separate reset switch. In standby, if the client does not access the driving method for a programmed amount of time (e.g., 30 seconds), the power wheelchair enters standby mode. The next direction chosen (e.g., left) dictates the feature chosen (e.g., power seating). Depending on the driving method, this limits the client to three or four feature choices (as the client drives with three or four directions). Another option is for the chair to go to a feature menu after an elapsed period of time, allowing navigation and selection using only the directional switches.

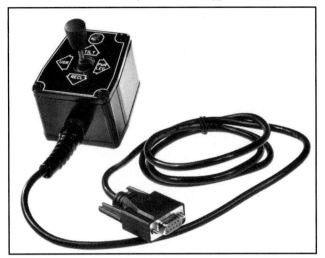

Figure 13-2. Power actuator toggle switches: different methods to directly operate power seating function.

CHANGING DRIVE PROFILES THROUGH MODE SELECTION

Speed is typically controlled by deflecting the joystick to the desired point. If the client desires and has adequate fine motor control, speed can also be changed by pressing buttons or turning a speed dial on the joystick. Most power wheelchairs have several *drives* or *profiles*. Each drive can be programmed separately. For example, Drive 1 may be controlled by a head array and programmed at slower speeds for indoor driving around furniture and through doorways. Drive 2 may also be controlled by head array but may be programmed at a higher degree of speed and responsiveness for outdoor driving. Drive 3 may be controlled by an attendant control (typically a smaller joystick mounted behind the client and operated by a caregiver) and set at a slow speed for getting in and out of the van. The client can change his speed by changing the drive or profile. A joystick driver can accomplish this by pressing buttons or operating a toggle switch on the joystick. If a joystick driver is unable to press a button or use the toggles, a separate switch can be plugged into the joystick and used as a reset. A switch driver can accomplish this by using a reset/mode switch or the standby navigation method.

CASE EXAMPLE

Alyssa is driving inside her home using a head array. She is in Drive 1, which is set at a slow speed and degree of responsiveness. However, she is going outside to play with her friends and wants to drive faster and needs her chair to be more responsive. She presses her reset switch located by her right knee, once, toggling the rear pad of the headrest to reverse directional control. She presses her reset switch again, placing her in a mode to select her drive. By activating her right headrest pad, she changes from Drive 1 to Drive 2. Pressing her reset switch again returns her to driving mode, and she can now keep up with her friends. If she doesn't have a fourth switch for reset, she can access drives through standby. After waiting for the programmed amount of time to pass, a directional command will place the chair in drives mode from which she can choose the desired drive.

CONTROL OF POWER SEATING THROUGH THE DRIVING METHOD

Power seating, or actuators, allows a client to independently change her position in space. Actuators include tilt, recline, elevating legrests, seat elevators, and standers. Changing position in space is important for redistributing pressure to reduce risk of pressure injuries, improving comfort, increasing sitting tolerance, postural management, fatigue management, and more (Dicianno et al., 2009; this is addressed in Chapter 10). Typically, a client controls power actuators through a toggle switch, separate from the drive control (Figure 13-2).

Various styles of toggles and buttons are available for power seating control, but these generally require fairly precise finger control. A single switch can be used for direct control of a seating actuator, allowing the switch to be placed in another location, such as by the side of the client's head. If one switch is used, this is often programmed to toggle movement of a single power actuator in one direction and back. For example, the first switch activation moves the power tilt anteriorly, and the second switch activation moves the power tilt posteriorly. If more than one seating actuator is being controlled or if the client cannot easily

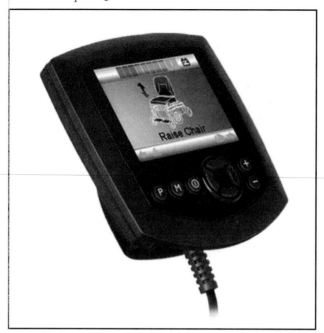

Figure 13-3. Screenshot of power seating mode on display.

control an additional switch site, the driving method can be used to also control the power seat functions. The client places the power wheelchair in a mode of operation other than drive mode. So instead of driving mode, the power wheelchair is now in power seating mode. Terminology varies depending on the electronics package used.

Once in power seating mode, the client uses a reset switch and/or directional switches to choose which power actuator to control. This requires the client to visually monitor the display where text and/or graphics show these options (Figure 13-3). The directional switches are then used to choose the direction and duration of movement. One directional switch may be used for a discreet direction of movement (e.g., the left directional switch used to control anterior tilt movement and the right directional switch used to control posterior tilt movement) or a single directional switch can toggle two actuator movements (e.g., initial activation of the left directional switch controls anterior tilt movement and a second activation of the left directional switch controls posterior tilt movement).

CASE EXAMPLE

Alyssa has been playing with her friends for a while and is getting tired. She wants to tilt posteriorly to help with neck and trunk control. She doesn't have the dexterity to operate a toggle switch. Alyssa drives with a head array. She presses a reset switch by her right knee to move through features on her display sequentially. The first reset activation toggles forward and reverse directional control.

The second reset activation allows her to change her drive/profile. The third reset activation places her in tilt mode. Activating the left head array pad now allows her to tilt posteriorly and activating the right head array pad allows her to tilt anteriorly. Now a fourth reset switch activation puts her back in driving mode.

If Alyssa used a feature menu, she could activate her reset switch once to toggle forward and reverse and activate her reset switch again to display other feature choices. When tilt is highlighted, she could select this option with a right switch activation. The power tilt is then controlled by left and right switch activations, unless programmed otherwise. The display lists all the actuators that are included on the chair to provide control of each through the drive controls.

If Alyssa couldn't activate a separate mode switch, she could use standby. However, she only has three switches to choose her mode of operation from standby (forward, left, and right on the head array), and she has four features she wants to access (drive, reverse, speed, and power tilt). Standby can be programmed to go to feature navigation, which is seen on the display. These choices can be navigated and chosen directly with drive switch selections, or the choices can be automatically scanned and selected with a right switch activation when highlighted.

INTERFACING

Interfacing has traditionally referred to connecting two assistive technology devices (e.g., a power wheelchair and an SGD) so that the same access method (e.g., a head array) can be used to control each device (Lange, 2015). A power wheelchair can be interfaced with an SGD, computer, or electronic aid to daily living (EADL). The main advantage of interfacing is streamlining access so that multiple access methods are not required for a client who uses more than one assistive technology device. Many assistive technology devices used for one primary purpose (e.g., speech output) include built-in features for secondary purposes (e.g., electronic aids to daily living). Less actual physical interfacing is required as a result; however, these features must still be enabled and programmed and the client trained.

CASE EXAMPLE

Ben is a 17-year-old male with a traumatic brain injury. He has a power wheelchair and an SGD. He drives using three individually mounted switches. Left hip abduction activates the switch by his left lateral knee for forward directional control. Left upper extremity abduction activates a switch for left directional control. Right hip

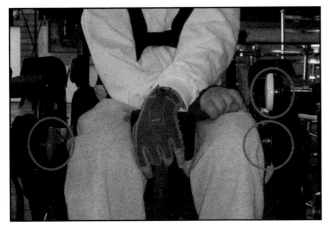

Figure 13-4. Ben and three-switch driving method.

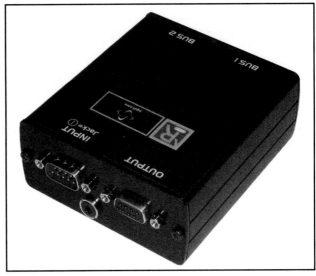

Figure 13-5. Interfacing component.

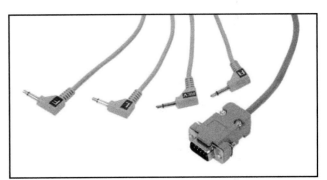

Figure 13-6. Interfacing cable.

abduction activates the switch by his right lateral knee for right directional control (Figure 13-4). Ben also uses an SGD with single switch scanning. His strongest switch site is by his left knee; so, he has a potential problem. If he uses this switch site for driving, then he can't stop and talk to people along the way unless he uses another switch site for the SGD. He doesn't have adequate control of scanning using another switch site, which would compromise his communication with others. If he only used the left knee switch for the SGD, then he couldn't drive forward because he doesn't have another strong switch site for forward directional control. Typically, the client's strongest switch site is used for forward because this switch is activated most frequently and for the longest distances. So the SGD was interfaced with the power wheelchair, enabling Ben to access both devices and share the left knee switch.

An interfacing component and cable are required that allow the joystick or switches used for driving to send a signal to the interfaced assistive technology device. So in Ben's case, his Invacare TDX power wheelchair has an AUX12M6 interfacing component (Figure 13-5) and Adaptive Switch Labs 802-1F interfacing cable (Figure 13-6), which plugs into the standard switch jack on his Dynavox SGD. He activates a reset switch with his left hand, which places the power wheelchair in AUX mode (an auxiliary mode). Now when he presses his forward switch by his left knee, a switch output is sent to the interfaced Dynavox SGD. Some electronic systems require the auxiliary port to be activated by the programmer before use.

Pros and Cons of Interfacing

Like anything else, interfacing has its advantages and disadvantages.

Advantages of Interfacing

- Streamlined access: The main advantage of interfacing is using several switches to control multiple assistive technology devices and features, rather than requiring a separate means of access for each device and feature. Clients with significant physical limitations simply cannot access that many switches.

- Cost savings: A separate access method is not required for each device and feature, which may be a cost savings.

- Increased functional independence: Interfacing may provide access to devices and features that could not be accessed otherwise because of lack of motor control. Specifically, interfacing allows strong switch sites to be used for more than one function.

Disadvantages of Interfacing

- Increased cost: The client may require a backup access method or methods, which could increase cost. For example, a client who interfaces a SGD with the power wheelchair may also require access to the SGD from a manual wheelchair and from bed. Also, interfacing requires additional power wheelchair components.

- Interdependent system: Interdependency means that if one part breaks, everything breaks. So if a

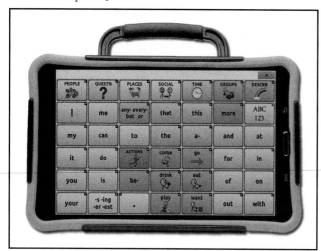

Figure 13-7. Speech-generating device.

client interfaces an SGD to the power wheelchair and the power wheelchair needs repair, the SGD can no longer be accessed through the drive control. This is another reason backup access is important.

- Complexity for the consumer and team: When technology works together, the level of complexity goes up. The team working with the client now has to be familiar with not only the power wheelchair and the SGD, but how the two work together as well. Many suppliers or clinicians do not have the knowledge or experience to determine whether a client can benefit from interfacing and to help with setup, programming, and training.

- Cognitive requirements: Interfacing can add to the cognitive load. Specifically, memory and sequencing are required to recall and execute the specific steps required to change from driving to control of the interfaced device. Memory and sequencing are often impaired in clients who have brain injuries. Training and cognitive reminders (e.g., a written list of steps) may be required.

- Visual requirements: Interfacing can be difficult visually, or for those who do not read, because the client typically must monitor the display to move between modes of operation. If a sequence method is used for feature navigation, visual monitoring of the display may not be required if the client can remember the feature choices and what order they are in.

- Access requirements
  - Interfacing may add to the access requirements, rather than streamlining access. If only one item is being interfaced, adding a reset switch may be no different from adding another control switch, as long as the client has adequate control of that switch for optimal access of the interfaced device.

  - Interfacing allows a switch to control both driving and an interfaced device. However, the same switch is used in a very different manner. Sustained contact and quick release is required for driving, whereas momentary contact is required for scanning (commonly used with switch access on interfaced devices) with accurate and timely activation. Additional switch training may be required for the client to develop these disparate switch skills.

  - It is also critical to determine whether the interfaced method is the optimal access method. For example, if a client can access an alternative mouse, such as a trackball, switch control of the mouse (through interfacing) is less efficient. Just because interfacing is technically possible doesn't mean it is always optimal.

Interfacing Speech-Generating Devices

When interfacing an SGD with a power wheelchair, teamwork is required. A speech-language pathologist working with augmentative communication generally recommends the SGD (Figure 13-7). An occupational therapist or other team member may determine the optimal power wheelchair and SGD access method and mounting and assist with interfacing. The supplier often determines the necessary components, connections, and programming.

As with interfacing in general, interfacing an SGD streamlines access, allows a client to share a strong access method between devices, and the access method does not need to be moved to the power wheelchair. It is imperative to ensure that if a switch is shared, the client can use it not only for driving but also for scanning. If the client ever uses the SGD outside of the power wheelchair, a backup access method is required. A reset switch is required when interfacing an SGD. This allows the client to change from driving mode to auxiliary mode. Although standby can be used to select auxiliary mode, this is not recommended when interfacing an SGD. While the client is using the SGD for communication (particularly in scanning, while waiting for the desired selection to be highlighted), the power wheelchair will enter standby, and a switch activation will choose a mode of operation rather than the desired vocabulary. It is possible to deactivate standby while in auxiliary mode. However, the only way to return to driving mode is to use a reset switch, which negates the need for standby.

If a client is able to directly access an SGD (i.e., finger to display location), then interfacing is not required. The exception would be if the direct access is less efficient then another access method that can be interfaced. Seth is an adult with cerebral palsy. He is able to directly access his SGD, but his increased muscle tone causes him to retract his arm after each selection. This slows him down and increases effort. Seth was able to use a joystick to access his SGD with more efficiency as he could sustain his grasp on the joystick while navigating vocabulary choices on the SGD display.

If the client is using single-switch scanning to access his or her SGD, then an interfacing component and interfacing cable are required. The cable terminates in a switch jack that corresponds to the directional switch on the wheelchair. For example, if the client uses his or her left directional switch to control the SGD, then the interfacing cable switch jack needs to be designated as left. The cable is ordered with the required directional jacks. The interfacing cable is connected to the interfacing component and the switch port on the SGD, typically labeled switch Port 1.

If the client uses two-switch scanning, then the interfacing cable needs to include two switch jacks, designated for the two directional switches used to control the interfaced SGD. For example, if the client uses the left and right pads of a head array to control the SGD, the interfacing cable would terminate in two switch jacks labeled L and R. These would then plug into the SGD switch Ports 1 and 2.

Some clients, like Seth, will access their SGD through a joystick. This requires the SGD to have a joystick input option, which is different from mouse input. Mouse input controls movement of a cursor or a highlight in unlimited directions. Joystick input typically moves a highlight over potential selections in horizontal or vertical directions only. For joystick input, a nine-pin to nine-pin interfacing cable is required. The SGD will have a nine-pin port if joystick input is an option. Some SGDs also accept diagonal movement through the joystick. On some power wheelchair electronic systems, this requires specific programming. This programming feature can be found under transmission methods, communication, to provide this diagonal movement for joystick input.

Joysticks and other access methods, such as the head array, can be used to emulate a mouse. Many SGDs accept mouse input. This requires either an external mouse emulator (in addition to the interfacing component) or mouse emulation, which is a standard or optional feature on complex rehabilitation power wheelchairs. Mouse emulation is discussed later in this chapter.

CASE EXAMPLE

Mark is a 16-year-old male with a diagnosis of cerebral palsy. He is nonverbal and uses an SGD to communicate with others. He also drives a power wheelchair for mobility. Mark uses a single switch by the left side of his head to access the SGD via scanning. He also uses individually mounted switches for driving his power wheelchair. The forward directional switch is on his tray, and he accesses

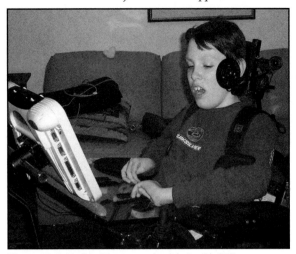

Figure 13-8. Mark in his power wheelchair with SGD.

this using his right hand; the right directional switch is mounted by the right side of his head on his headrest; and the left directional switch is mounted by the left side of his head, also on the headrest. He has to share the left head switch to access the SGD and for left directional control of the wheelchair (Figure 13-8).

Mark can change his modes using a reset switch that is mounted by his right knee on the lateral side. The first reset activation takes him out of drive mode and places the power wheelchair into reverse. Mark only has three driving switches, so he needs to activate reset, which toggles the forward switch on the tray to act as reverse. The next reset activation places the chair in tilt mode. Now Mark can use the switches on either side of his head to control his position in space. The left head switch tilts the chair posteriorly, and the right head switch tilts the chair anteriorly. The third reset switch activation places the chair into auxiliary mode. This is the mode that allows Mark to send a switch signal from his left head switch to the SGD.

The interfacing component has one to nine-pin ports on it. The interfacing cable attaches to this nine-pin port and the SGD switch port. These cables have a female nine-pin connector on one side (that connects to the interfacing component on the power wheelchair) and one or more switch plugs (1/8-inch male) on the other. Mark uses his left directional control switch to send a signal to the SGD, so he needs a cable that has a single switch jack that sends a signal from the left directional switch.

Mark's caregivers put him in the wheelchair, make sure he is positioned well, and turn on the power wheelchair. They then place his SGD on a mount attached to the wheelchair. Finally, they take the interfacing cable, which is hanging on the back of his chair, and plug the single switch jack into the switch port on the SGD. When Mark enters auxiliary mode, he sends switch signals to the SGD by pressing his left directional switch. To return to driving, he presses reset again.

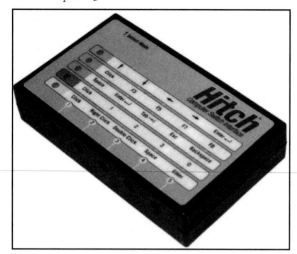

Figure 13-9. Computer switch interface.

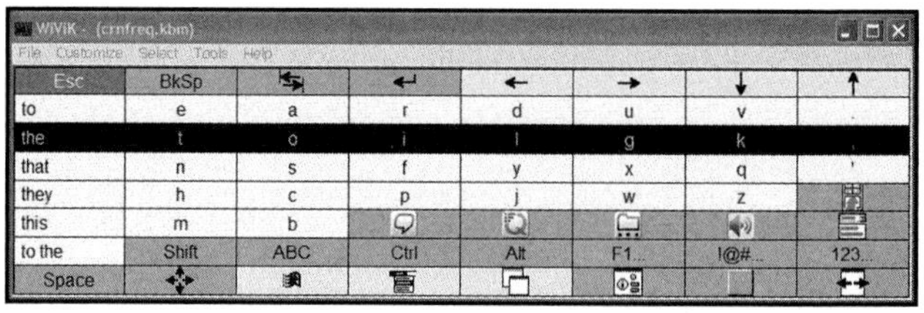

Interfacing Computers

As with SGDs, teamwork is needed when interfacing computers, particularly in determining the optimal computer access method. Often, more efficient access methods are available for computer access than what is possible through interfacing. If the driving method provides the optimal access method, then interfacing can streamline access for the client. A laptop can be mounted on the power wheelchair, or the client can drive up to a desktop computer. Wireless options are available so that assistance is not required to connect interfacing wires. An exciting advantage of interfacing computers is mouse emulation, available through an external mouse emulator or directly through the power wheelchair electronics. When interfacing computers, keep in mind both keyboard and mouse emulation for the client. As with interfacing SGDs, standby is not recommended.

If the client is using an SGD, that device may also be a computer or be able to interface to a computer. Many SGDs are computer-based, and the client may be able to move back and forth between communication and other computer features using the same SGD access method. In this case, interfacing through the power wheelchair is not necessary or, if the SGD is already interfaced through the power wheelchair, a separate computer does not also have to be interfaced. SGDs can be a very efficient computer access method because individual letters, words, and even entire phrases can be sent to the computer at one time.

Single-Switch Input

Some clients only need to send a single-switch signal through the interfacing component and cable to a computer. Using a switch interface (Figure 13-9), this signal can be designated as a switch signal, specific keyboard character (i.e., space bar), or mouse click. Single-switch software is activated by a switch signal and is often used to develop cause-and-effect concepts and to provide simple

Figure 13-10. Scanning onscreen keyboard.

recreational activities for young children and those with significant cognitive limitations. This single-switch signal can also be used in conjunction with an onscreen scanning keyboard for keyboard emulation (Figure 13-10).

If more than one switch or a joystick is used for computer access, typically mouse emulation is used. Mouse emulation allows the client to open software applications, use the Internet, and access an onscreen keyboard for keyboard input. The cursor is moved over a specific location on the keyboard and a mouse click executed to select. If the client cannot execute a mouse click, the client can dwell over that location for a programmable amount of time until the selection is automatically made. An external mouse emulator or power wheelchair electronics including mouse emulation are required, and are discussed later in this chapter.

Tablets are computers themselves. We will discuss control of tablets under Emerging Technologies later in this chapter.

CASE EXAMPLE

Jessica was diagnosed with amyotrophic lateral sclerosis 6 months ago. She currently uses a power wheelchair with a joystick. She can no longer use a standard keyboard and mouse. Jessica is interested in an alternative way to access the computer. She is quite familiar with computers, having used them in her job for many years. She has, until recently, been able to use the standard keyboard and mouse. As her condition has progressed, she no longer has this fine motor control. She can, however, use the joystick on her power wheelchair. After evaluating the options, Jessica decided to use a combination of voice recognition and alternative cursor control using the joystick on her power wheelchair. She recognizes that eventually she will no longer be able to use voice input as her condition progresses, but this is her most efficient access method at this time. Voice recognition can be used to control the cursor with voice commands, but this can be tedious. Voice recognition can also be used to execute keyboard shortcuts (i.e., Ctrl + P for print), which reduces the need for cursor control, but Jessica preferred direct cursor control. Jessica had a laptop computer that she wanted to keep on her power wheelchair. This eliminated the need for a wireless emulator and the associated higher cost that would be required if she drove up to a desktop

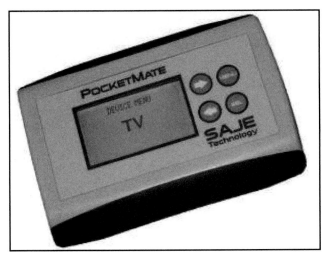

Figure 13-11. Switch-activated EADL system.

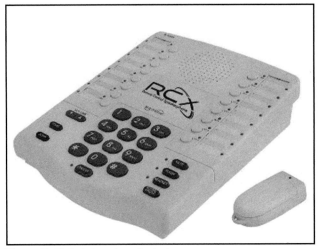

Figure 13-12. Switch-activated telephone.

computer. She chose a standard mouse emulator that was connected to her power wheelchair electronics and to her computer's USB port. With these modifications, Jessica was able to "talk" to her laptop computer, which was mounted to the power wheelchair, and control the computer cursor using the joystick as an alternative mouse. All she had to do was change the operating mode of the power wheelchair from drive to an auxiliary mode. Once in auxiliary mode, joystick movement resulted in direct and corresponding cursor movement on the screen. Joystick buttons were used for mouse clicks.

As her condition progressed, Jessica was no longer able to use her voice to control the computer. She now required a different means of emulating the keyboard. As she was still able to use the joystick as a mouse with her mouse emulator, Jessica began using the mouse with an onscreen keyboard for keyboard control. This particular onscreen keyboard included word prediction and abbreviation expansion features, which increased her speed and efficiency.

As Jessica continued to progress, she was no longer able to use the joystick and began driving her power wheelchair with a head array. This nonproportional access method requires a different mouse emulator for cursor control. Jessica would have been able to use her head movements to control cursor movements on the computer, however, as she used her computer throughout the day, this was too fatiguing. Instead, she used the left switch in the head array to send a single switch signal to the computer. She was no longer able to emulate the mouse, but was able to continue to use an onscreen keyboard through scanning. She also used keyboard shortcuts for commands typically executed by the mouse.

Interfacing Electronic Aids to Daily Living

EADLs provide an alternative means of controlling devices in the environment to facilitate daily living tasks (Figure 13-11). EADLs can be accessed directly (e.g., finger to button), by switch scanning, or by voice. The client can control audiovisual equipment, lights, appliances, hospital beds, door openers, and telephones. EADLs can be simple, such as a remote control with large buttons, or sophisticated, such as a voice-controlled system that controls multiple devices and features throughout the home. EADLs increase safety, independence, and quality of life. If interfacing an EADL through a power wheelchair, the only access method available is switch scanning. If switch use is the optimal access method for the client, then interfacing may be helpful. Single-function EADLs can be interfaced as well, including power door openers and switch-activated telephones (Figure 13-12).

Complex rehabilitation power wheelchairs often include or offer IR transmission, which can be used to control devices in the environment. This is addressed later in the chapter. For now, the discussion considers how and why to interface an external or stand-alone EADL. The main advantage of interfacing is streamlining access. It is important to ensure the client have a backup access method for use from other positions, particularly from bed. If the client will control an electric hospital bed, then access is required from this position. That same client may also want to turn on a light during the night or watch TV from bed. Most EADL systems are portable, so use from a power wheelchair is possible. As with other interfaced devices, use of standby is contraindicated because the wheelchair may revert to

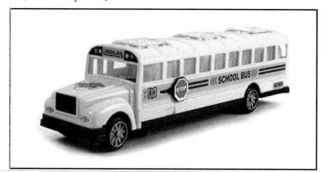

Figure 13-13. Interfacing a remote-controlled toy.

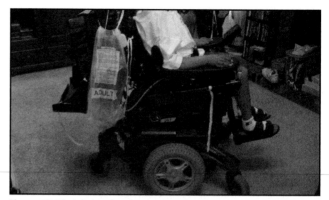

Figure 13-14. Julian.

standby while the client is waiting for the desired EADL feature to be scanned.

As with other interfaced devices, an interfacing component is required. An interfacing cable then connects to the nine-pin port of the interfacing component and the 1/8-inch switch port of the EADL. If the client needs to control an EADL, a switch-activated telephone and a power door opener, this can be accomplished in two ways:

1. First, an interfacing cable can be ordered with three switch jacks. One directional switch (i.e., forward) sends a switch signal to the EADL, another directional switch (i.e., left) sends a signal to the telephone transmitter and the final directional switch (i.e., right) sends a signal to the power door transmitter while in auxiliary mode. The telephone and power door transmitters are available with a switch port.

2. A second option is to use the second nine-pin port on the interfacing component and a second interfacing cable. Port 1 can control the EADL using one directional switch (i.e., left), and Port 2 can control the telephone and door opener using two directional switches (i.e., left and right).

Basic EADLs provide control of battery operated toys and simple appliances. It is possible to interface a switch toy to the power wheelchair. Imagine a child learning to change modes of operation on the power wheelchair by changing between driving the wheelchair and driving a toy car! In this case, the interfacing cable is connected to the battery interrupter or switch port on the battery-operated toy. Wireless options are available as well, so that the interfacing cable connects to a transmitter to control a toy remotely (Figure 13-13).

CASE EXAMPLE

Julian is a 13-year-old boy with the diagnosis of spinal muscular atrophy (Figure 13-14). He has little volitional movement and uses a ventilator. He is verbal, although difficult to understand. He has a very high-pitched voice, as is common with this diagnosis, and a fair amount of secretions because he does not swallow. In combination with the ventilator, which creates background noise and affects rate of speech, he is unable to successfully use voice input to control an EADL.

Julian has driven a power wheelchair since age 3 years. He uses a combination of switches to allow him to drive using the very small movements that he can control. His forward directional switch is a fiberoptic switch under his right thumb. This is embedded in the palm pad of his arm trough. He uses a slight rotational movement of his head to activate a proximity switch embedded in his headrest by the left side of his head for left directional control. For right directional control, Julian activates a Microlite switch mounted by the medial side of his right knee, using hip adduction. Finally, Julian has a proximity switch mounted by the right side of his head for reset.

Julian is able to change modes with his reset switch and control his power tilt using his knee switch. However, Julian has no other control over his environment. He loves to watch TV (especially wrestling) and movies (especially horror movies). Julian also likes to listen to rap music. He would like to control the movement of his bed and make phone calls to his friends in private, not with his nurse holding the receiver by his ear. He needed EADLs to provide independence and quality of life.

Julian could use an EADL to control all of these devices and their features; however, we were out of switch sites. He did not have another switch site on his body that we could use for accessing an EADL system. As mentioned earlier, he was unable to use voice to control an EADL. He certainly didn't have the motor control for a direct access system. We needed to interface the EADL with the power wheelchair so that he could use the drive control switches to send signals to the EADL. We did not choose to use the power wheelchair IR transmission because Julian required control from both the power wheelchair and his bed. A switch accessed EADL was selected. An interfacing component and cable were ordered and connected. The interfacing port was enabled through the power wheelchair programmer (Figure 13-15).

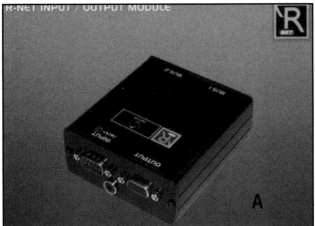
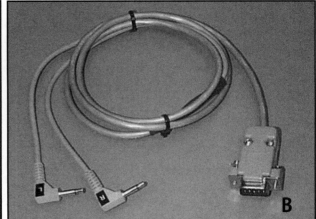

Figure 13-15. (A) Interfacing component. (B) Interfacing cable.

Now, when Julian wants to watch a movie, this is how he does so. It sounds complicated, but he has it down pat. From drive mode, he activates his reset switch. The power wheelchair display shows *reverse*. This allows him to use the forward switch under his right thumb to reverse the power wheelchair, as needed. He activates his reset switch a second time. The display now shows *tilt*. This allows him to use the right directional switch by his knee to control his power tilt. He activates his reset switch a third time. The display now shows *AUX*. The displayed message varies by manufacturer. AUX, in this case, is now set to the EADL system. He then uses his left directional switch mounted by the left side of his head to send switch signals to his EADL system. Julian activates the left directional switch to start a scan on the EADL. When TV is highlighted, he activates the switch again to choose TV. Now, TV features are displayed on the EADL. He waits for and chooses *power* to turn on the TV. He now activates the switch to start the scan on his EADL again and waits for *input* (this is a required signal on his TV to receive input from the DVD player). After choosing Input, Julian chooses *go back* on the EADL to return to his main page. On the main page of the EADL, he selects *DVD* to open DVD features. He then chooses *play* to watch his movie. Julian's family or nurse could certainly start the movie for him, but he prefers to do so himself. He can mute the sound, pause the action, or skip ahead whenever he chooses.

Another advantage of interfacing the EADL, rather than using the built-in IR transmission available on many power wheelchairs, is that Julian can also access the EADL from bed. He spends up to 12 hours a day in his bed and likes to listen to music, watch TV and movies, talk on the phone, and adjust his bed while in it. After all, he is a teenager! The EADL is mounted to his bed rail so that he can see it. While supine, Julian is able to access a fiberoptic switch using right thumb lateral movement. He uses a custom arm trough in bed to keep his arm in a consistent position in relation to the fiberoptic switch that is embedded in the

trough, just like the forward switch is embedded in the power wheelchair arm trough. The fiberoptic switch is an electrical switch that typically draws power from the power wheelchair batteries. While in bed, the switch is plugged into an outlet in the room, using an adaptor available from the manufacturer.

INFRARED TRANSMISSION

Some of the complex rehabilitation power wheelchair electronic packages include standard or optional capabilities to send IR signals to control devices in the environment (Lange, 2014a). The IR signals are sent from diodes in the display or a separate emitter (Figure 13-16). The display now acts as an EADL, eliminating the need to purchase a separate device. It is challenging to get funding for EADLs, despite their importance in providing independence and safety in the home, so having this option on a power wheelchair is very attractive.

The advantages of IR transmission from the power wheelchair are obvious: increased independence, cost savings, and streamlined access. However, onboard IR transmission limits the client's control to the power wheelchair. If the client requires control from bed or a manual wheelchair, an external EADL is still required. Also, the client has to send switch signals or use discreet joystick movements to control these features, so direct or voice control is not supported. Finally, someone has to set up this system to work in the home. This requires a professional who has the required knowledge, funding, and time.

IR signals are light signals and are commonly used to control audiovisual equipment, such as televisions and stereo systems. These signals are line of sight and will not go through walls or ceilings. Other light sources, such as natural light and florescent lighting, can sometimes interfere with the signal. IR signals can be prestored or learned. Prestored signals work just like a universal remote control

Figure 13-16. IR transmission from a display.

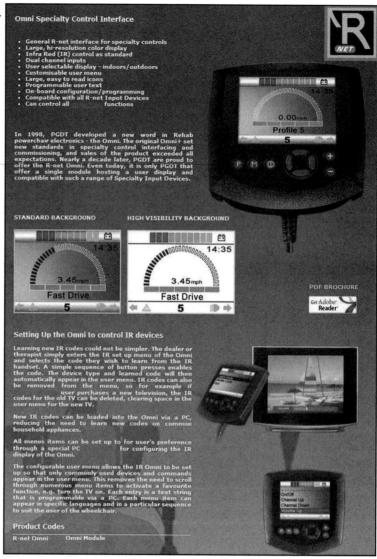

that you may have purchased when your TV remote broke. A booklet lists codes by device and brand (e.g., TV, Sanyo). You look up the code for your device and enter this into the universal remote, and then the remote can control your TV. The power wheelchair electronics may contain preprogrammed codes that are entered in the same way. The ability to learn IR signals is important as well. If an IR controlled device doesn't have a preprogrammed code, this code can be learned by the power wheelchair electronics. The electronics read, learn, store, and transmit any IR signal. How does the power wheelchair learn an IR signal? Typically a remote control (i.e., TV remote) is aimed at the learning window of the power wheelchair electronics (i.e., back of the display). The display is placed in learning mode and lists step-by-step instructions, including when to press a command on the remote control and indicating when that command has been received and learned. If the power wheelchair is not learning the IR signals, try the following:

clean the windows on the power wheelchair emitter and the remote control (over the IR diodes), replace the batteries in the remotes with brand new batteries and use the original remotes. If the client does not have the original remote control and the system is not learning the IR signals from a universal remote, the original remote can often be purchased from Internet sources. Some devices also require a longer IR signal, so you may need to hold down the button longer during the learning process.

Some audiovisual remote controls send more than just IR signals. Many television and cable provider remote controls also send radio signals. Power wheelchair electronics and external EADLs cannot learn radio frequency signals and so cannot transmit these signals. If you can execute a function while covering the IR window on a remote, chances are the signal is really radio frequency and cannot be learned. The only way these devices and features can be controlled without use of the standard remote control is

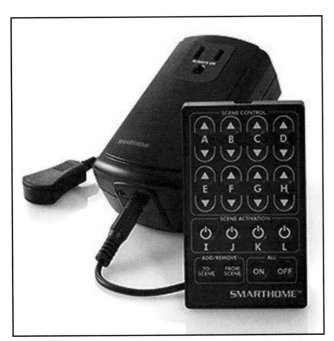

Figure 13-17. Insteon IRLinc receiver.

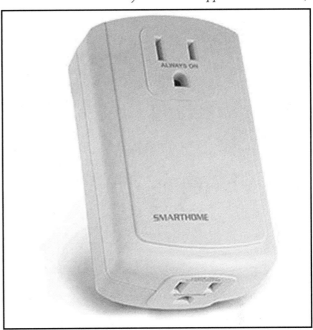

Figure 13-18. Insteon module.

through wireless networks. Apps on tablets and phones can be used to control this audiovisual equipment through a wireless network in the home.

Many clients require access to a telephone. Several IR telephones are available commercially. These include a remote control so that the features can be learned by the power wheelchair electronics. Remember, the client will only be able to use the phone while in the power wheelchair. These IR phones are expensive and typically not covered by funding sources.

IR transmission can also be used to control lights, simple appliances (e.g., a fan), and thermostats. The power wheelchair sends IR signals to a converter (Figure 13-17) that converts the IR to Insteon signals. Insteon technology uses the house wiring to send signals to individual lamp or appliance modules (Figure 13-18). The module is then turned on or off. The desired device, such as a lamp, plugs into the module. Insteon wall switches are available for control of overhead lights. Insteon thermostats are available to control heating and air conditioning. This technology is generally funded by the client, but the cost is reasonable.

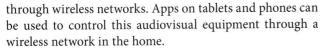

CASE EXAMPLE

Tony has Duchenne muscular dystrophy. He is now 16 years old and a sophomore in high school. Tony has been driving a power wheelchair for a number of years now, and currently drives with a mini proportional joystick. He can drive his power wheelchair well, but he is not as independent as he would like to be. He is unable to control devices in the home environment.

Tony no longer has the active range of motion (ROM) or strength to use a remote control for the TV and his other audiovisual equipment. He cannot use a phone, open the door, or change his position in bed. When he comes home from school, the bus driver opens the unlocked front door and Tony drives in and waits for his parents to get home. He can't turn on the TV or music, and if it gets dark, he can't turn on a light. He knows the door is unlocked, and this makes him nervous, but because he cannot open it independently, it has to stay that way.

Tony could use an EADL to control all of these devices within the home environment. Unfortunately, his state Medicaid will not fund this category of equipment. As a matter of fact, few funding sources will pay for EADLs, even for people who are left unattended and cannot open the door or make a phone call in an emergency. His family is unable to afford the equipment he would need to be safe and independent; however, Tony needs a new power wheelchair. A new power wheelchair that included IR transmission standard was recommended. Tony can now use his mini joystick to drive, tilt, and turn on the TV. A reset switch was mounted next to the mini joystick. When Tony activates the switch, his display now shows the driver's menu, a list of shortcuts to frequently used functions. One of the functions on the list is *infrared control* (the specific wording can usually be changed using a computer programming tool). Using joystick movements, Tony can move down the list until he reaches infrared control and then use a right directional command to choose this option. Now he sees a new list of device options, including his TV, DVD and CD players, and lights. By choosing one of these categories, he can see the corresponding features, such as TV power, and make his selection. Once a feature selection is made,

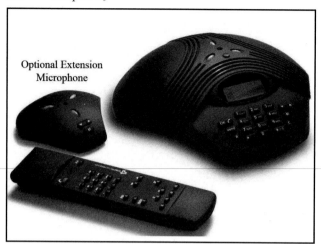

Figure 13-19. IR telephone.

an IR signal is sent out the rear of the display and the TV turns on.

Tony's family was able to purchase an IR/Insteon converter and modules. This converter plugs into the wall and the power wheelchair display sends IR signals to it (see Figure 13-17). Those signals are translated into Insteon signals and are sent over the house wiring until a module is found. A module is a box that a light or simple appliance plugs into and then the module is plugged into the wall outlet (see Figure 13-18). Tony can send a signal, using his joystick, to turn that module on or off.

Tony still needed to open the door. The IR signals could be used to control a door opener, either directly using IR or through a converter to send Insteon signals. The family still had to purchase a door opener, but this was less costly than buying a door opener and a stand-alone EADL system.

Few stand-alone EADLs come with a phone. Several adaptive phones on the market can be controlled with IR, although these are costly. Tony's family did some fundraising and managed to get one of these. We programmed the power wheelchair with these commands and Tony was then able to use this IR receiving speakerphone to answer, hang up, and dial calls (Figure 13-19).

One disadvantage of using the power wheelchair to control devices in the environment is that you need to be in the power wheelchair. Tony did not have the ability to control devices from bed, and that included control of the bed itself. If you are working with a client who requires control from bed, a stand-alone EADL is still a good option, if the family can afford one.

MOUSE EMULATION

The same complex rehabilitation electronics that can send IR signals also include or offer mouse emulation. This

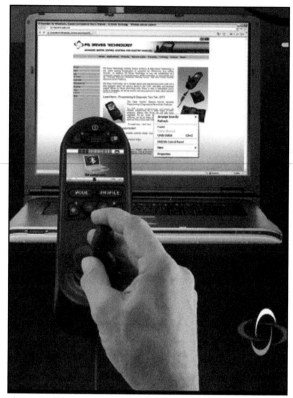

Figure 13-20. Joystick emulating a mouse.

mouse emulation can be used to access a computer or many SGDs (Lange, 2014b). Before considering use of the power wheelchair mouse emulation, it is critical to ensure that this is the optimal access method for the client. Many access options are available for computers and SGDs in addition to mouse control. Many alternative mice are also available and may meet the client's needs more efficiently than using the power wheelchair driving method to emulate a mouse. For clinicians and suppliers primarily working with seating and mobility, additional team members may be required to address computer or SGD specific needs.

If a client is able to drive with good control using a joystick, it is natural to conclude that this same joystick can be used to emulate a mouse. Keep in mind that use of a joystick to move a power wheelchair throughout a room does not require the same precision as using that same joystick to move over an onscreen keyboard on a computer display. Mouse emulation requires more refined control than driving, whether the client is using a joystick or other access method.

Controlling the mouse through the driving method, as with interfacing an external mouse emulator, streamlines access, is wireless (increasing independence for the client), and may save costs. If mouse emulation is standard, then certainly there is a cost savings. If mouse emulation is an option, this may still be less costly than purchasing and interfacing an external mouse emulator, interfacing component, and interfacing cable (Figure 13-20).

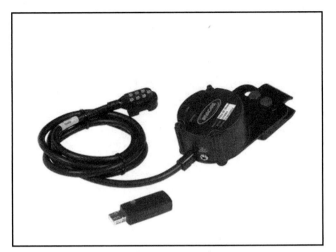

Figure 13-21. Power wheelchair mouse emulator.

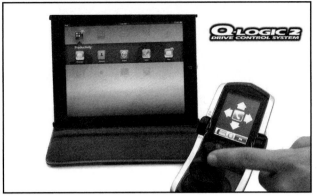

Figure 13-22. Display in mouse emulation mode.

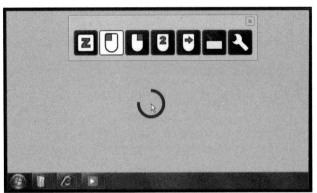

Figure 13-23. Click emulation software.

This area of technology is changing quickly, so it is important to check with the wheelchair manufacturer for the most current options. Mouse emulation requires the power wheelchair electronics to act as a wireless mouse, sending a signal to the controlled device. This signal is typically Bluetooth (BT), like many of the wireless mice used by the general populace. This may be an issue for some clients who have multiple control needs. Currently, the power wheelchair can only pair with one device at a time. If the client needs to use the mouse emulator to access both a computer and a separate SGD, this is a problem. Each power wheelchair electronics system has a different method of pairing with a device. Prentke Romich SGD devices, at the time of this writing, require an external BT dongle and downloadable software to allow the SGD to be "discovered" by the power wheelchair during the pairing process.

Signals are sent from the display or a separate mouse emulator (Figure 13-21). The client must place the power wheelchair into mouse emulation mode. The display will show available options (Figure 13-22). The driving method then moves the cursor on the computer or SGD display.

If the client is using a proportional control, such as a joystick, then directional movement and speed of the cursor will also be proportional. The client will be able to move the cursor in any direction within a 360-degree radius, and the further the joystick is deflected from center, the faster the cursor will move. If the client is using digital (switch) access, the directional switches move the cursor in the corresponding direction. If three-switch access is used (e.g., head array), forward typically moves the cursor up. Once the top of the computer display is reached, the cursor wraps around to the bottom of the screen. Forward/reverse and left/right directional movements can be combined to provide diagonal movement of the cursor. The cursor usually moves at one speed, set within the computer's operating system.

Mouse emulation not only moves the cursor, but must emulate mouse clicks, as well. Common mouse commands include left and right click, double click, drag, and scroll up and down. When using the power wheelchair driving method, strategies are available to emulate or execute a click. In click emulation, software displays various mouse commands and the client hovers or dwells over the desired selection for a preset time to choose that command (e.g., double click) (Figure 13-23). The client then moves the cursor to the appropriate location to execute that command (e.g., over a word processing program to open that application).

To physically choose and execute a mouse command, the client must be able to use an additional switch that represents a specific mouse command or be able to discriminate between quick hits and sustained contact of the driving switches to execute specific mouse commands. One or two switches may be connected to the mouse emulator itself for mouse commands. On some electronics systems, joystick buttons can be programmed to execute mouse clicks.

Mouse emulation uses three- or four-quadrant control. Four-quadrant control is typically used with a joystick and allows all four quadrants of driver control (forward, reverse, left, and right) to operate the mouse in four directions. Three-quadrant control is typically used with a head

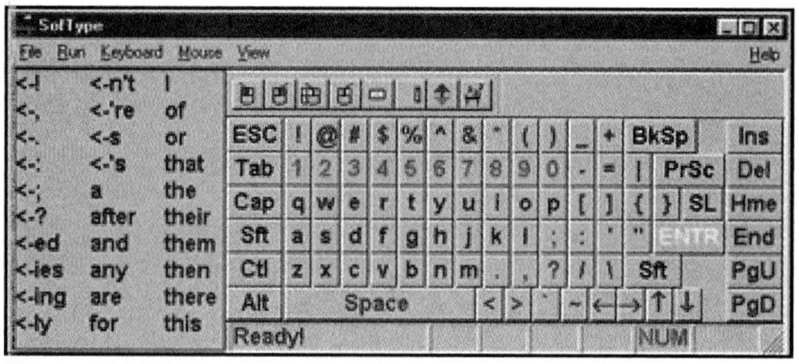

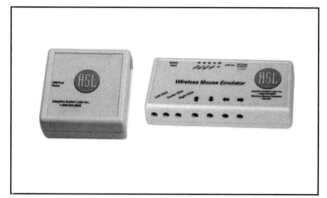

Figure 13-24. Onscreen keyboard.

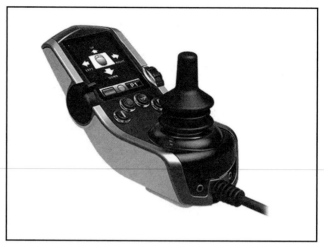

Figure 13-25. Joystick-based mouse emulator.

Figure 13-26. External wireless mouse emulator.

array. Forward either toggles the mouse up and down or is changed to reverse with an external switch.

Keyboard emulation requires an onscreen keyboard (Figure 13-24). This requires very precise cursor control to move over the desired character and either dwell or click to make a selection. Many onscreen keyboards include abbreviation expansion or word prediction for rate enhancement.

When considering mouse emulation, the team must decide whether using the power wheelchair emulator or an external mouse emulator will best meet the client's needs. The power wheelchair emulator is incorporated into the display or requires a separate mouse emulator component. For clients using a joystick, a display is sometimes required if a separate mouse emulation component is not used (for systems with mouse emulation contained within the display). Even for those systems using a separate component, the display is still typically required to monitor mouse movement and commands. An optional mouse emulator and a display used solely for the purposes of mouse emulation will not usually be funded. Some electronics are now incorporating mouse emulation into a joystick that has its own display (Figure 13-25).

External mouse emulators require an interfacing component and cable, which increases cost. These items are also typically difficult to fund. External mouse emulators send radio signals and include three- and five-switch configurations. The five-switch version is for joystick control (Figure 13-26). Wired and wireless versions are available. These are able to pair with more than one device. External mouse emulators often have more features and flexibility than those incorporated into power wheelchairs.

Generally, if cost is the main concern, power wheelchair mouse emulators are least expensive, particularly if included as a standard feature. External mouse emulators, although costly, allow the client to pair with more than one device if needed (e.g., computer and SGD) and have more features.

CASE EXAMPLE

Let's revisit Tony. Recall that Tony has Duchenne's muscular dystrophy. He is now 16 years old and a sophomore in high school. Tony has been unable to use a computer for some time. He used to use a standard keyboard and mouse. After this became too difficult due to lack of active ROM, he used a trackball and an onscreen keyboard. The trackball is now too difficult as well because of the force required. The new power wheelchair Tony is receiving includes mouse emulation features so that Tony can move the cursor on the computer screen using the movements of his mini joystick.

Tony presses the reset switch next to his joystick by his right hand. This brings up the driver's mode on the display. One of the displayed choices is *mouse*. He scrolls down his choices by pulling the joystick back into reverse and selects Mouse with a right joystick movement. Now, another screen displays his mouse movement options. Any direction he moves the joystick results in corresponding cursor movement on the screen.

Tony has resumed using his onscreen keyboard but uses the mini proportional joystick instead of his old trackball. He hovers or dwells over the desired keyboard character to select it. He also uses word prediction and abbreviation expansion to increase his typing speed.

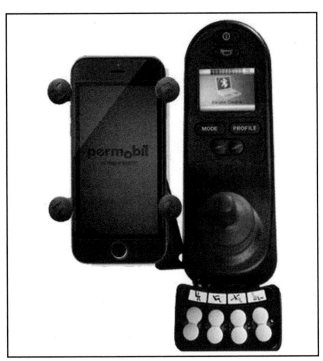

Figure 13-27. R-Net iDevice for iOS access.

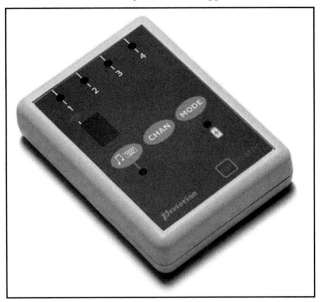

Figure 13-28. iOS switch interface.

Tony can move the cursor on the screen but clicking requires other strategies. He already has a reset switch placed to the left of his mini proportional joystick. A second switch was placed to the right of his mini proportional joystick. One activation sends a left click and two activations a double click.

EMERGING TECHNOLOGIES

Emerging technologies are challenging to address in a book because this area of assistive technology changes so rapidly. Therefore, always check with the power wheelchair manufacturers for the latest information. Emerging technologies in terms of advanced power wheelchair applications include control of tablets and smartphones through the power wheelchair. Other useful advanced applications will also be addressed in this section.

A gap exists between consumer electronics and assistive technology. Assistive technology cannot keep up with the rapid pace of consumer electronic development for several reasons. First, the demand is much smaller for clients wishing to control a smartphone through a power wheelchair joystick than consumers wanting a new and better smartphone. Second, because demand is relatively low, product development is less of a priority. Third, because funding sources generally will not reimburse this technology, as it is not considered medically necessary, product development is also affected. Fourth, many clients are unaware of these applications and so do not request these features. Finally, and arguably most challenging, consumer electronics are

not designed to meet the physical, cognitive, and/or sensory limitations present in clients using assistive technologies and so modifications must be made.

Tablets

A client in a power wheelchair can access a tablet through switch or mouse access (Breaux, 2015). Mouse control provides more control but can only be used to control tablets that are designed for standard mouse access. The BT power wheelchair mouse is able to pair with most tablets. At the time of this writing, iPads (Apple) do not support mouse access. A new product from R-Net does provide an alternative means of mouse emulation to iOS products, including tablets and smartphones (Figure 13-27). The power wheelchair joystick or other access method can access a tablet using mouse emulation (internal or external). An external mouse click is generally required, rather than use of dwell. Tablets incorporate an onscreen keyboard that can be used for character input.

Not all clients have the motor ability to use mouse emulation. Another option is switch access.

iPads can be controlled by any BT switch. Several of these are available. If the client is unable to use the BT switch directly, any ability switch can connect to the BT switch adapter and be placed in a location the client is able to access. Strategies are available to scan and select *apps* on the iPad. Some apps are specifically designed to be switch accessible. Although a switch interface is not required on i-devices (iOS7 and above), interfaces can provide a means to customize switch access for an individual client (Figure 13-28). For example, a switch signal can be programmed to send a *volume down* command. In camera mode, Volume Down takes a picture. Now the client can mount the iPad,

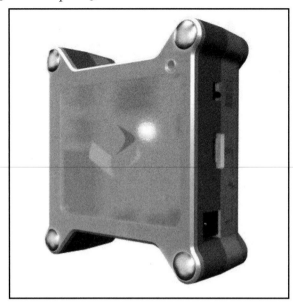

Figure 13-29. Tablet and smartphone switch interface.

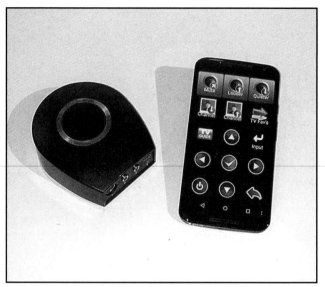

Figure 13-30. Smartphone interfaces.

use his or her driving method to move into position for a nice picture, and access a switch to send the command through the switch interface to take the shot. If the client cannot use a separate switch for iPad control, the switch interface can be interfaced through the power wheelchair using an interfacing component and cable. The switch interface can be controlled by one or two switches.

To provide similar switch access to both iPads and other tablet platforms, a different switch interface is required (i.e., Tecla Shield) (Figure 13-29). This particular switch interface uses BT transmission with one or two switches. When using a head array, the left and right pads move the highlight in a linear pattern on the display and the back pad selects. This interface also allows specific customization to meet a client's individual needs.

Smartphones

Smartphones can also be navigated by switch signal. Some switch interfaces that work with tablets also work with smartphones. As the display is smaller, the client needs to be able to visually monitor this accurately. HouseMate with ClickToPhone software provides joystick or switch access to Android smartphones (Figure 13-30). An interfacing component and cable are required to allow control through the driving method.

Tablets and smartphones are common in our society, and many clients desire control of these emerging technologies. Although control is possible through the power wheelchair driving method, using joystick or switch control, this technology can remain difficult to use for clients who have cognitive or visual limitations. More and more applications are being developed that are meeting these needs. Keep in mind, as with other interfaced technologies, joystick or

switch may not be the client's optimal access method. If the client can touch the screen and use this technology directly, interfacing is not required. Direct access usually refers to touching the screen with a finger. Pointers may not work because the touch screen requires direct skin contact. Some types of stylus are available that do activate these touch screens and can be held in the hand or used as a mouthstick. Some systems are now available that provide voice or eye gaze control of tablets, as well.

Gaming

Other emerging technologies are available to meet individual client needs. Many clients would like to play video games but lack the physical ability to use a standard game system controller. Adaptive Switch Labs has a PlayStation modification to allow video game control through the power wheelchair driving method (Figure 13-31). An interfacing component and cable are required.

Audio Output

Much of these emerging technologies have audio output. However, sharing that audio with those around us is not always appropriate. Most people use earbuds or a headset to listen privately to audio, including music, audio from video files, and audiobooks. These listening options may not work for clients due to intolerance or excessive movement. Instead, speakers can be placed within the headrest and used for private listening of any audio (Figure 13-32). Many clients who use SGDs use auditory scanning to provide an auditory cue as to what is being scanned. Speakers can provide private listening of the cues and the SGD only "speaks" the selected message.

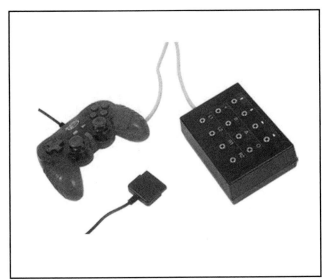

Figure 13-31. Game controllers.

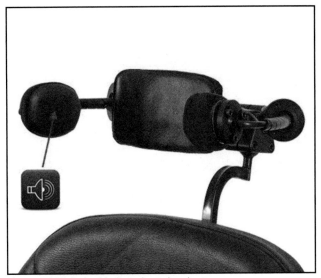

Figure 13-32. Embedded speaker in headrest.

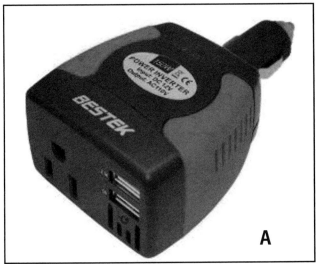

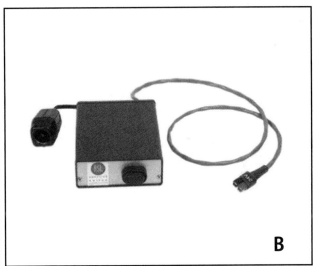

Figure 13-33. (A) Power source. (B) Power invertor.

Power Options

All of this technology requires power. SGDs, notebook computers, tablets, and smartphones do not always last a full day. Convertors are available to provide a power source from the power wheelchair batteries (Figure 13-33). Complex rehabilitation power wheelchairs generally have adequate battery power to support driving, power seating, interfacing, and power to other devices.

Obstacle Detection

Sensors can help clients with low vision, or even poor attention, avoid obstacles. These photoelectric sensors are placed on the front or rear of the wheelchair (or both) and are programmable to beep when an obstacle is detected in an adjustable 4- to 21-inch range (Figure 13-34). If these are set with a large range, the sensors may beep frequently in close quarters. If set with too short a range, the client may not have time to react to the auditory warning.

Remote Emergency Stop Switch

A great mobility-training tool is the remote emergency stop switch (Figure 13-35). This may not be an emerging technology, having been available for some time, but it is definitely a useful and underused mobility option. A trainer or caregiver presses a remote switch to stop the power wheelchair from a distance. This is helpful for clients who are still learning to drive or who may not see or notice

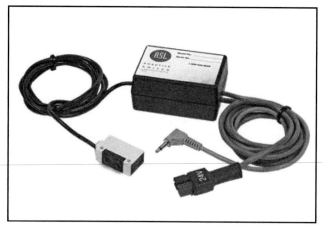

Figure 13-34. Photoelectric sensor switch.

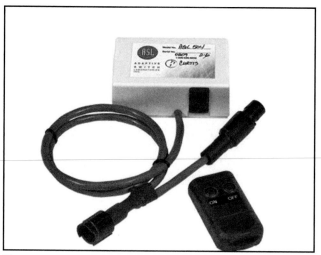

Figure 13-35. Remote stop switch.

a potential obstacle. Apps are available that allow a smartphone to be used as a remote stop and even an attendant control.

Additional Items

Many other devices can be interfaced through the drive control. These include power swing away mounts by the head (for chin joysticks, sip-and-puff, or even hydration), power SGD mounts, power trays, and power leg-bag emptiers. As with any interfaced device, the goal is to provide access through the drive control when another switch site cannot be located. As a result, the client is more independent.

The Future

Many innovations are on the horizon. Research has led to the development of prototype smart wheelchairs. Similar to work being done on driverless cars, smart wheelchairs will use a combination of technologies to assist the driver in navigating his or her environment. Prototype features include auto-stop if the wheelchair gets too close to obstacles, a backup camera that automatically engages when the wheelchair is in reverse and strategies to accurately reach the desired destination.

FUNDING CONSIDERATIONS

What about funding? Is it really possible to fund all of these bells and whistles? First, it is important that we remember and communicate to others the importance of these power wheelchair advanced applications. This technology isn't about fun and games; it provides independent control to clients. Funding is challenging for much of this technology. For example, funding a switch interface for a tablet is quite difficult. Why? Because the funding source does not view tablet use as medically necessary. However, someone bought that tablet and may be willing to pay for the switch interface to provide that access. I believe it is important to inform clients of any technologies that may increase their independence, even if it may not be funded. It is up to the client to decide whether an option is worth pursuing funding for.

SUMMARY

Assistive technology is more interdependent and multifunctional than ever, changing the very definition of interfacing. Assistive technology can improve independence for many clients. This requires professionals to stay current with available assistive technology devices and applications. Although a daunting task at times, this is also an exciting opportunity to take advantage of these advances for the benefit of our clients.

REFERENCES

Breaux, B. (2015, February). *Access to mobile devices through the power wheelchair drive control system.* Presented at the International Seating Symposium, Nashville, TN.

Dicianno, B. E., Arva, J., Lieberman, J. M., Schmeler, M. R., Souza, A., Phillips, K.,...& Betz, K. L. (2009). RESNA position on the application of tilt, recline, and elevating legrests for wheelchairs. *Assistive Technology, 21,* 13-22.

Lange, M. (2014a). *Power wheelchairs and infrared transmission.* Arlington, VA: Rehabilitation Engineering & Assistive Technology Society of North America Webinar.

Lange, M. (2014b). *Power wheelchairs: Mouse emulation.* Arlington, VA: Rehabilitation Engineering & Assistive Technology Society of North America Webinar.

Lange, M. (2015). Power wheelchairs: An overview of advanced features. *PhysicalTherapy.com.* Retrieved from http://www.physicaltherapy.com/articles/power-wheelchairs-overview-advanced-features-2502

SUGGESTED RESOURCES

Complex Rehab Power Wheelchair Electronics Comparison Matrix: http://www.atilange.com/resources.html

Adaptive Switch Labs step-by-step mouse emulation instructions by electronics package: www.asl-inc.com/technical-support/programming-documents.php

Please see video on the accompanying website at

www.healio.com/books/mobility

Manual Mobility Applications for the Dependent User

Sheila N. R. Buck, BSc (OT), OT Reg (Ont), ATP

Clients who are unable to move a manual wheelchair themselves are known as *dependent users*. Although the client may not be able to self-propel, her mobility base must provide him or her with a safe and efficient sitting surface with supportive seating. A full assessment of the client, the caregiver, the environment of use and transport of the client, and mobility base must be completed to provide the best system for desired use. This chapter reviews considerations when choosing a mobility base for a dependent user. There are a variety of mobility bases available and these include transport, folding and rigid, adjustable and non-adjustable, tilt-and-recline wheelchairs, and adaptive strollers. With each dependent mobility base prescription, consideration must be given to variations in frame design to allow for ease of pushing of the mobility base, balance of the client in the chair, and foot-loading required to maintain client seated support. Orientation in space to maintain client safety and upright sitting within client capacity must be considered, as well as the ability to insert a seating system onto or into the mobility base.

When being pushed, does the wheelchair really need to be more than four wheels? Just because a client is dependent on others for mobility, does that mean that the seating and wheelchair setup does not matter? Does the assessment of the client change? What should or shouldn't be considered? All of these questions are important to ask when completing a prescription for a mobility base for a dependent user.

How does one define a dependent user? A dependent user encompasses all age-groups and diagnostic categories. Therefore, this type of user can only be determined by an assessment of his or her specific functional capacity level,

including physical and cognitive aspects. It is important to remember that this functional capacity must be reassessed every time the client is evaluated for a new mobility base. Changes in function, including regression, relapse, or improvement, may have occurred since the last evaluation. To define someone as a dependent user, he or she must be unable to wheel his or her manual wheelchair with two hands, one hand, one hand and one foot, or two feet. If the client cannot self-propel a manual wheelchair in one of these manners, a one-arm drive or lever drive wheelchair, gear reduction or power assist wheels may provide a means of independent manual mobility. This is addressed in more depth in Chapter 9. If no manual option is viable, power mobility can then be assessed. When reviewing a client's capacity to drive a power chair, optimal seating is required to facilitate access to a variety of switches or drive controls for sustained and repetitive movements. It is important to assess not only hand function but alternative body access points that allow for switch access. This is addressed in more depth in Chapter 11. Once the client is seated and access points have been determined, perception and cognitive capacity must also be evaluated with respect to driving capacity. This is also discussed in Chapter 17. At this point, if the client is unable to self-propel a manual wheelchair or drive a power wheelchair, he or she would be determined to be a dependent user.

A person in a seated position must be stable and secure to maximize functional potential, even if that is only achieving a resting posture. Pressure management must also be addressed. When prescribing mobility devices for the dependent user, the seating system design must be

Lange, M. L., & Minkel, J. L.
Seating and Wheeled Mobility: A Clinical Resource Guide
(pp. 237-250). © 2018 SLACK Incorporated.

simulated after the assessment of body range of motion (ROM) and postural balance. Seating can then be determined on the basis of postural control needs, as well as pressure management. This seating design must address physical, perceptual, cognitive, and social needs as well. Seat to back angle and chair orientation in space need to be determined to maintain postural control, balance, pressure relief, and basic physical functions. These functions may include breathing, swallowing, visual gaze, and verbal and assisted communication. A client may still be able to complete activities of daily living (ADL) even though he or she can't mobilize his or her chair. Therefore, all activities done from the mobility base must be reviewed, including transportation of the device. It is important to review the environment of use and ensure that the client can be mobilized over all expected terrains safely and without loss of posture.

Even if a client is not independent in his or her mobility, he or she must still have a secure and comfortable seated position when being pushed or injury can occur. These injuries may occur due to the client becoming agitated, sliding out of the chair, or demonstrating intolerance for being in his chair. This might be better defined as a *do no harm scenario* to maintain the clients' physical and emotional sense of well-being at all times. This well-being often comes from a sense of postural control, balance, comfort, and pressure relief. If postural control does not occur, a client will tend to grab on to her armrests, if possible, or slide out of his or her seating system. He or she will then be at greater risk for injury, as well as skin breakdown due to shearing and pressure issues.

Once the seating system has been determined, the mobility base can be prescribed. The widths, depths, angles, and orientation in space of the wheelchair will have been determined by the assessment and parameters of the seating system. It is important to remember to fit the seating and mobility base to the client, not the client to the equipment, even if he or she cannot wheel the chair him- or herself. Often, clients who are not independently mobile are provided with loaner or standard issue generic wheelchairs. We are not all the same shape and size and, therefore, the seating of the trunk, pelvis, and/or lower extremities, as well as the size of the wheelchair, must address the complexities and differences in human shape. Improperly prescribed wheelchair sizing may result in decreased social interaction or basic bodily functioning due to limited accessibility or sitting tolerances.

ASSESSMENT

The completion of a thorough assessment is critical in determining product design and setup. Incorrect prescriptions can create potential changes in posture and basic functioning due to incorrect forces being applied to the body, insufficient postural support, inadequate pressure relief, or lack of stability. Therefore, a full seating assessment must be completed before prescribing a dependent mobility base. The measurements and parameters of the seating system will then be reflected in the size and design of the mobility base. If the seating is altered midassessment, it is important to reflect on how the change will affect the mobility base, including size and center of gravity.

First, it is important to review what type of base is required for each individual client. This will be based on a number of factors, including wheel size, adjustability, and position or orientation in space. A transportation assessment of the client must include the environments of primary and secondary use. Questions to ask include the following:

- Is the client mainly staying indoors?
- Are there accessibility issues within this space?
  - Consider door and hallway widths, turning radius from hall to door to inner room, washroom space, dining table space and heights, access to computer services, desks, and counter heights. Refer to Chapter 23 for further information.
- Does the client use speech-generating devices (SGDs) mounted on his or her wheelchair, and, if so, how does the mounting system and device affect the overall width of the wheelchair?
- Will the client be moving outdoors and, if so, on what type of terrain? Is vibration an issue to be addressed?
- Will the client be transported in a vehicle in his or her mobility device, or will he or she be transferred to a passenger seat? If he or she is transferred, how will the mobility base be transported? Refer to Chapter 24 for further information.
- Who is doing the pushing, and what is the height and strength of the person pushing the chair?
- Are there multiple caregivers?
- How does the client transfer into the chair?
  - Consider pivot transfer and bed heights, mechanical floor lift vs ceiling lift, location of the ceiling tracks, and space in and around the transfer areas (e.g., bed, toilet).

DEPENDENT MOBILITY OPTIONS

The following frame styles are available but need to be matched to the client with the previous considerations in mind.

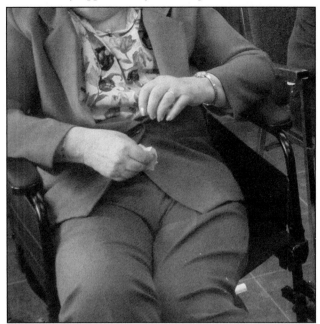

Figure 14-2. Windswept posture.

adjustment of the feet (dorsi/plantarflexion or eversion/inversion). As the name describes, a transport chair should only be used for temporary transportation as opposed to a daily sitting and mobility device due to limitations in support and a small wheel size, which does not bode well in outdoor settings.

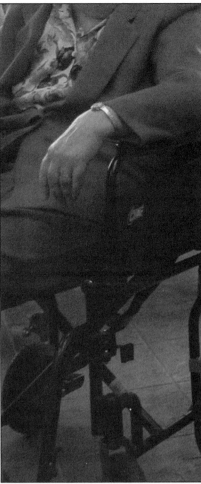

Figure 14-1. Transport chair.

Transport Chair

A transport chair is typically a 16-, 17-, or 18-inch-wide chair with a 16- or 18-inch seat depth, 4 small wheels of 8- or 12-inch diameter, and foot locking or low mount brakes. The back may collapse in half from top to bottom to reduce the size of the chair when folded. This style of chair is used for quick transport of clients who do not have any postural issues and need only be transported between perhaps a car and short time frame appointment. Typically, no additional back support is added due to arm support restrictions (e.g., nonremovable armrests limit mounting options), but a seat cushion can be provided on top of the chair upholstery for pressure reduction and some minimal postural support. It is important that the cushion be provided with a solid seat insert (Applewood or ABS plastic) if the cushion does not have a sling contour base. If a solid base is not applied, the client's body weight will cause the upholstery to stretch. Additionally, the cushion will also take on the sling upholstery shape, creating pelvic obliquity or internal rotation of the hips and lead to client postural instability. This can also lead to increased pressure points. The footrests have a minimal height adjustment but do not allow for angle

CASE EXAMPLE

As seen in (Figure 14-1), a client has been provided with a transport chair to take her from the main floor of her retirement home to a community appointment. She has severe osteoarthritis of her spine, hips, and knees and has had multiple joint replacements. She uses a wheeled walker for ambulating the short distances within the retirement home. The transport chair allows her family to take her to appointments or events beyond the facility. No seating has been provided and the seat depth is short compared with her thigh length. Notice her tendency to slide forward into a posterior pelvic tilt with increased kyphotic curvature of her upper back, pelvic rotation, and windswept legs (Figure 14-2). This chair does not provide support for thigh, hip, and pelvic alignment or trunk support. She is also experiencing shoulder elevation from supporting her arms on the fixed armrests. The client complains of increased pain after sitting in this chair for greater than 15 minutes. This transport chair, therefore, should only be used for short distances, because long-term postural changes will occur if this is used as the sole means of mobility. The use of a contoured cushion with solid insert would assist in increasing

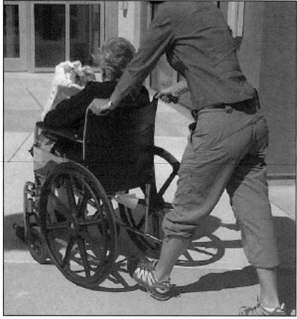

Figure 14-3. Non-adjustable wheelchair.

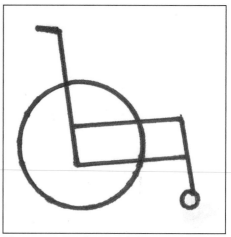

Figure 14-4. Fixed rearward tilt.

her comfort and posture for short outings by leveling her pelvis and gaining a more supportive armrest height.

Non-Adjustable Wheelchair

A non-adjustable wheelchair is typically 16 or 18 inches wide by 16 or 18 inches deep, with limited footrest height adjustment. Some alternative sizing may be available. Arm supports may be fixed and non-adjustable or adjustable in height. This style of chair may be altered to provide an additional seat cushion or alternate adjustable tension or rigid back support. It does not, however, provide any height adjustment of the front caster or rear wheel to change seat to floor heights. Center of gravity adjustments of the rear axle (the ability to move the rear axle forward or back to accommodate client weight or posture) cannot be completed because of a fixed axle position. This style of chair is therefore used for the client who is of average body shape, size, and weight. This chair style is typically heavy, and therefore, due to a lack of center of gravity or frame angle adjustment, is typically more difficult to push. These frames come in standard and bariatric weight capacity. The client who is provided with this type of chair would typically not demonstrate any potential for change in muscle tone, postural control, or body weight. Seldom is this style of chair used in conjunction with seating systems applying forces of gravity to assist in maintaining or gaining an upright posture.

CASE EXAMPLE

The elderly client seen in Figure 14-3 has generalized weakness and dementia, and was provided with a non-adjustable wheelchair to be transported with family on outings. Unfortunately, she is losing overall strength and now requires a wheelchair on a daily basis. The same chair is being used for manual mobility, but the seating has not been adapted or changed to provide greater comfort or postural support. The sling back is starting to hammock, creating increased kyphosis. The lack of seat cushion puts her at high risk for skin breakdown, postural instability, discomfort, and overall postural changes to her pelvis and spine. The inability to adjust the axle position or armrest height will not allow this chair to accommodate changes as she ages. The chair cannot change position in space, and therefore, as her kyphosis progresses, she will have limited postural support, which will affect eye gaze, communication, eating, and overall comfort.

Adjustable-Frame Folding Wheelchair

The adjustable-frame folding wheelchair can be ordered in a variety of seat widths and depths, as well as seat to floor heights. These wheelchairs often include adjustable options, such as height adjustable armrests, various footrest hangar angles, adjustable angle footplates, back cane angle adjustability, and various back cane heights. The front riggings may be fixed with flip-up or swing-away and removable footplates. The rear axle and front casters can be positioned at varying heights and changed as conditions warrant, providing increased seat angle or fixed position in space by altering seat to floor heights differently front to back (Figure 14-4). For example, the front of the chair frame is set higher than the rear. This is often referred to as *chair dump*. The rear axle is placed higher on the frame to lower the rear end of the frame, while the front casters are moved to a lower position to raise the front of the chair. After completing these changes, the front caster housing must be readjusted to vertical alignment to prevent difficulties associated with poor alignment, such as caster flutter or poor caster turning.

These chairs are produced in aluminum, carbon fiber, and titanium frames, decreasing overall weight to ease lifting for transportation and to ease propulsion. The side-folding capacity of this style of chair reduces overall size during nonuse hours and for transportation. Even though a client may be dependent for propulsion, the weight factor may be important to the caregiver who must lift the chair in and out of vehicles or push a client of higher weight. As a result of the adjustability of the axle and caster positions, angles, and position in space, this chair is suitable for clients who have existing or potential changes noted in body stature, spinal curvatures, and postural control. The chair setup can be altered as the client changes to maintain postural control and pressure management. For the client who has decreased trunk control and tends to fall forward without support systems, after seating has been addressed, the chair can be placed in a rear fixed position in space to allow gravity to assist in postural control. When the chair and client are tilted in a fixed rearward position, the line of gravity is in front of the client's head, acting as a force rearward to assist with the gravitational pull of the head and trunk back into the seating system.

The footprint of the chair can also be set up to maximize accessibility (e.g., by decreasing width for doorway clearance). This can be done by changing handrim spacing as well as axle threading (i.e., changing the space between the axle and the wheel). The length of the chair or the depth for turning radius can be adjusted by moving the rear wheel forward or back, as well as by adjusting the caster position from a leading to trailing positioning. Clients who may be agitated and rock or transfer with less controlled movements are at risk of tipping their wheelchair and being injured. Safety can be ensured by increasing stability and reducing tendency to tip through moving the rear wheel back and hence increasing the footprint of the chair. The center of gravity of the chair can also be set up to maximize the ability of the caregiver to easily push the chair. This is done by maximizing the position of the rear wheel under the center of the client mass (i.e., the average center of client body weight measured in a seated position). By having the bulk of the weight of the client over the rear wheel, less force will be required to push the chair. If the client's mass is forward over the front caster, the chair will be difficult both to steer and to push.

Additionally, the seat angle changes set through the vertical and horizontal wheel and axle adjustments can assist with providing increased postural control or pressure reduction by changing the position of the client's center of mass with respect to the forces of gravity. This is done by placing the rear of the chair lower than the front end. The client will then sit in an overall fixed posterior tilted position, which may assist in moving his or her head, shoulders, and trunk (upper body mass) behind the center line of gravity. This will allow gravity to assist the trunk and head to achieve a more upright position. This position may also reduce pressure on bony prominences in the pelvic and thigh areas. It is important, however, to assess the pressure gradients after altering this angle because gravitational forces may increase pressure through the ischial tuberosities. For example, a client who develops an increased forward kyphosis can have the chair adjusted to allow for the rear seat to floor height to be lower than the front seat to floor height. This will allow his or her center of mass to be moved back toward the center of gravity of the chair to make it easier to push. Additionally, his or her line of gaze will be more forward, rather than pointing down to the ground, because his or her head will move upward as the orientation of the whole body moves in a rearward orientation. An added benefit is gained through improved postural control with assisted head and spinal positioning. Adjustable-frame folding wheelchairs are typically used when the client requires customized seating to provide three points of support to correct, modify, or maintain a seated posture in the client's functional midline. Customized seating may include fully molded systems, a modified seat cushion or back support, or just the capacity to change seat to back or seat frame angles to gain better postural control and maintain skin integrity. If an adjustable frame has been prescribed, it is important to adjust it—and keep adjusting it as the client changes.

CASE EXAMPLE

A client living with dementia lives at home with her elderly spouse, who is also her caregiver (Figure 14-5). In this scenario, the family is concerned that the client is sliding and falling out of the wheelchair and that the chair is heavy to push. The client frequently requests to go back to bed. Although an adjustable frame was prescribed, seating was not provided for postural control or pressure management, and therefore sliding occurs, leaving the client at risk for skin breakdown through shearing and pressure issues. The seat depth is too short, putting increased pressure on the ischial tuberosities with minimal posterior trunk support to limit posterior pelvic tilt. Additionally, the available adjustments on the chair have not been used. The footrests have not been adjusted low enough, leaving her thighs unsupported. This adjustable frame chair is not set up to assist with pushing or postural control. The rear wheel is set behind the client's center of mass, resulting in front-loading of the casters. This makes the chair very difficult to push on carpet. The handrims of the chair have been removed, resulting in reduced integrity of wheel rim,

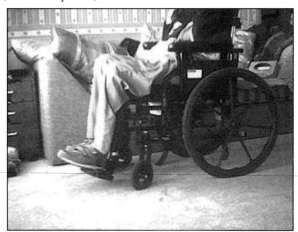

Figure 14-5. Adjustable chair not set up for pushing, postural control, or accessibility.

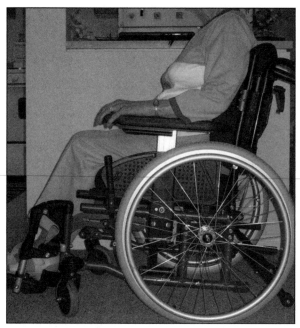

Figure 14-6. Adjustable folding chair with good setup for maneuverability, trunk control, and pressure management.

which will lead to wheel malfunction. The overall footprint of the chair can be reduced by bringing the rear wheel forward. Additionally, beyond proper seating, the seat to floor height could be adjusted with the front higher than the rear to assist with upright posture. After the seating is completed, the footrest height should be set to ensure good thigh-loading.

Once the client is provided a chair with proper seating and setup, she no longer slides out of the chair, she can sit up longer, and her chair is much easier to push (Figure 14-6). The adjustable frame is set up with supportive seating to maximize seat depth, thigh-loading, and trunk and posterior pelvic support. The center of client mass is positioned over the center of gravity of the rear wheel to improve pushing of the chair. The seat angle of the frame is set in fixed posterior tilt for visual stimulation and postural support. The back canes are angled open for shoulder clearance and caregiver access to push handles. The footrests have been adjusted to allow for thigh-loading. Overall, her chair is now providing better support to decrease sliding, improve visual gaze, and ease the work of pushing the chair for her spouse, both inside and outside.

Adjustable-Frame Rigid Wheelchair

This style of chair can also be ordered in a variety of seat widths, depths, and seat to floor heights. It often has adjustable options, such as armrests, front frame angles, footplates, and back cane angle and height adjustability. The front end and front riggings may be fixed with a standard rigid footplate, optional flip-up footplate, or, occasionally, swing-away and removable footrest hangars. Rear axle and front casters can be positioned to provide increased seat angle (fixed posterior tilt) by altering seat to floor heights differently front to back. These chairs are produced in aluminum, carbon fiber, and titanium frames. These lightweight frames ease lifting, transportation, and propulsion.

Even though a client may be dependent for pushing, the weight factor may be important to the caregiver with respect to lifting the frame in and out of vehicles or pushing a client of greater weight. This chair is suitable for clients who have existing or potential changes noted in body stature, spinal curvatures, and postural control because the chair can be adjusted for fixed posterior tilt, center of gravity, and overall stability. The footprint of the chair can be set up either to maximize accessibility (by shortening the frame) or to increase safety for clients who may be agitated and rock or transfer with less controlled movements (by lengthening the frame). The center of gravity of the chair can be set up to maximize the ability of the caregiver to easily push the chair by shifting the rear wheel forward or backward to be positioned under the center of mass of the client. Additionally, the seat angle changes set through the vertical and horizontal wheel/axle adjustments can assist with providing increased postural control or pressure reduction by changing the position of the client's center of mass with respect to the forces of gravity. For example, by moving the rear wheel axle higher on the frame, the rear of the seat will drop. This will result in the client sitting in a fixed posterior tilt position in space, which shifts his or her head and trunk rearwards with respect to a vertical line of gravity (Figure 14-7). Typically this style of chair is used for the client who does not perform a stand-pivot transfer, but would be transferred using a transfer board, or mechanical lift system. The rigidity of the frame allows for improved pushing efficiency when used with heavier clients or those who may have increased tremor or agitated movements in their chair when resting.

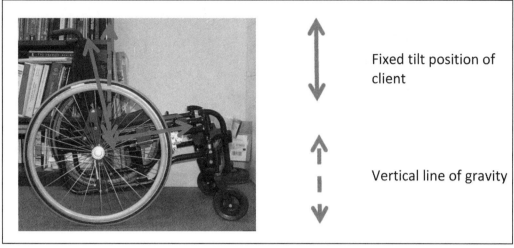

Figure 14-7. Vertical line of gravity compared with fixed tilt rotation in space.

CASE EXAMPLE

In Figure 14-8, we see a client who presents with a spinal cord injury and higher personal weight. The client is no longer able to independently wheel the chair due to a repetitive strain injury of his shoulder. An adjustable-axle rigid frame chair provides good weight distribution of the client's body mass over the center of gravity of the chair by moving the rear wheel forward on the frame. The chair frame is lighter in overall weight. These two factors allow his spouse to easily push the chair, despite the client's larger body size and weight.

Manual Tilt-in-space Wheelchair

This chair is most typically of rigid frame design and aluminum materials. The chair is able to tilt-in-space using a lever action to tilt the chair backward (posteriorly) from 0 to 25, 45, or 60 degrees of tilt. Some frames will allow for an anterior tilt, which may assist in positioning clients to a table for eating or other ADL. A lesser or reduced tilt angle may be used for clients to change the forces of gravity, working in conjunction with their seating to improve posture. Clients with a significant kyphosis may require some tilt to balance the head and gain improved visual gaze; however, an altered tilt position may still be needed for access to the table for eating, either for accessibility or to optimize swallowing. During the assessment, it is important to evaluate feeding and determine whether tilt will assist or interfere with swallowing, gastronomy tube or jejunum tube, or position to the table for self-feeding. A reduced tilt angle may also be good for a client who demonstrates agitation. A slight amount of posterior tilt may assist with reducing the agitated behavior by allowing the client to remain with his or her feet on the ground for stimulation

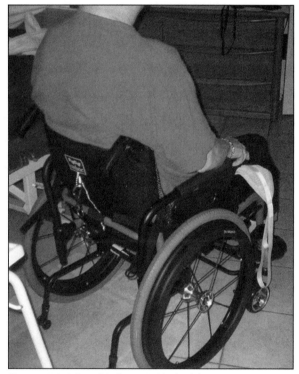

Figure 14-8. Adjustable-frame rigid wheelchair.

or grounding of agitated behaviors, while positioning his or her body into a posterior tilt angle. The seat to floor height must be assessed to still allow for full thigh-loading and the tilt mechanism set to allow for adjustments in tilt angle without the front of the seat frame changing height (i.e., the rear of the seat tilts down with the lever of action occurring at the front of the frame to keep the front seat to floor height consistent for feet to remain on the ground (Figure 14-9).

Larger tilt angles will provide greater off-loading for clients who may have issues with pressure on their buttocks, greater degrees of agitation, or very limited postural control. Additionally, some medical conditions may require a

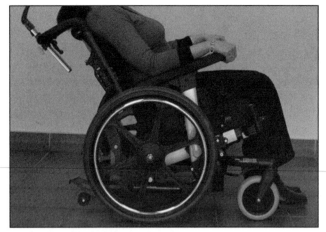

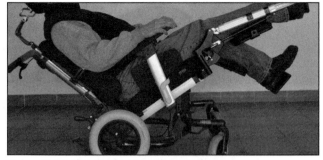

Figure 14-10. Chair in tilt with elevating leg rest.

Figure 14-9. Chair slightly tilted with feet on floor.

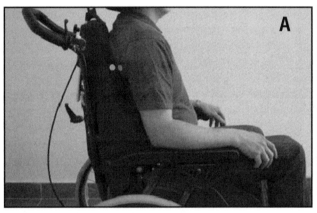

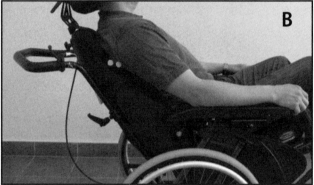

Figure 14-11. (A) Closed seat to back angle. Client mass is in front of rear wheel/axle, loading the front casters. (B) Open seat to back angle. Client center of mass is situated over the rear wheel.

greater tilt angle to enhance respiratory status, circulation, or edema reduction. To reduce edema of the lower extremities, the client's feet need to be in a position above the level of the heart (Figure 14-10). This may require the use of elevating legrests in conjunction with the tilt. If this is the case, it is important to assess whether the client's hamstring ROM will allow the knee to be extended.

When addressing the use of a tilt chair for a client with altered respiratory status, it is beneficial to use pulse oximetry to determine oxygen levels when the client is in varying degrees of tilt. This will provide a guide as to the amount of tilt required for maximal respiratory function. Lastly, larger tilt angles may be used for fatigue management. This may be the case when the client is unable to return to bed for a rest due to limitations in staff or transfer equipment. Altering the tilt angle will reduce trunk and head fatigue and allow the client to rest without returning to bed.

Some frames are non-adjustable and cannot accommodate changes in client center of mass, spinal curvature, or weight changes. Therefore, it is important to consider the client's prognosis for change before prescription. The inability to shift the axle position for center of mass and

center of gravity will also increase resistance of the frame during pushing or result in front-end-loading. This will occur if the rear wheel position cannot be set to accommodate heavier client weights (forward center of mass), forward postural tendencies, or seating that decreases the rear seat depth of the chair. Use of customized seating or some off-the-shelf rigid back supports in tilt chairs often places the client mass forward on the frame. These clients do require adjustability to change the rear axle position to accommodate the center of mass and their seating system combined. It is often critical to use angle adjustable back posts with custom seating to gain the specific seat to back angles required by the client. Changing the seat to back angle also changes the center of mass of the client and will therefore require a change in the center of gravity setup of the rear wheel/axle (Figure 14-11).

Additionally, the style of frame tilt will also affect the client's ability to tolerate abrupt changes in position. Therefore, it is important to review whether the frame tilts from a (1) posterior single pivot-point fulcrum, which may promote a sudden movement backward; (2) midframe multipivot point fulcrum, which reduces the amount of

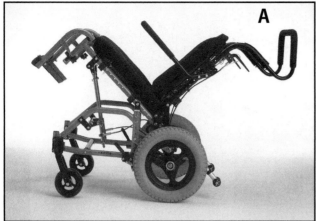
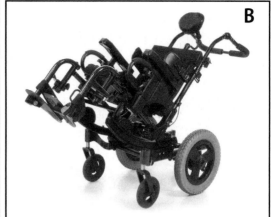

Figure 14-12. (A) Single pivot point tilt chair. (B) Rotation-in-space tilt chair.

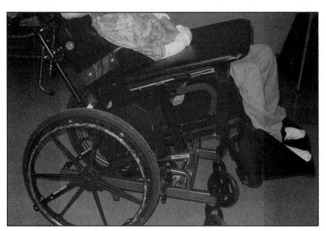

Figure 14-13. Single pivot point tilt chair, non-adjustable center of gravity.

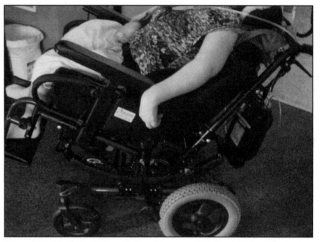

Figure 14-14. Adjustable rotation-in-space tilt wheelchair with oxygen tank.

horizontal movement but still may create sudden movements with tilt; or (3) if it travels through a C-curve or rotation in space tilt, which reduces horizontal head and jerking movements (Figure 14-12). Sudden changes in tilt angle may negatively impact client posture by increasing muscle tone due to elicitation of primitive reflexes, affecting postural control.

These chairs are usually set up for caregiver control of the tilt lever, either by hand or foot function, but some models do provide the opportunity of self-tilt by the client. Self-tilt may be achieved with a manual lever on the armrest or activation of switch for power tilt. This is of benefit for the client who has the cognitive capacity to change his or her tilt angle for pressure reduction, postural support and comfort, or a change in position for ADL. Stroller handles can benefit the caregiver pushing the chair, especially if the client is pushed in a tilted angle. This allows the caregiver to efficiently push the chair without increased back flexion, which can promote back injuries.

In the instance of a client presenting with cerebral palsy, a non-adjustable tilt chair has been set up with custom seating (Figure 14-13). The center of mass is too far forward of the rear wheel and axle due to the depth of the custom seating. The casters are front-loaded, making the chair difficult to push. The front-loading also causes sudden dropping of the upper frame when returning to upright, causing the client to startle and resulting in increased extensor tone of her upper and lower extremities. The front-loading and single pivot point-style of chair also make it difficult for staff to activate the tilt mechanism. Due to the difficulty tilting the chair, this feature is not frequently used by staff, therefore creating postural and pressure difficulties for the client.

CASE EXAMPLE

In Figure 14-14, we see a client with a diagnosis of cerebral palsy and presenting with scoliosis and changes to her rib cage, creating a posterior lateral rib prominence. She was provided with custom seating, which pushes her center of mass forward due to the depth contours of the back support. She requires continuous oxygen, and is therefore

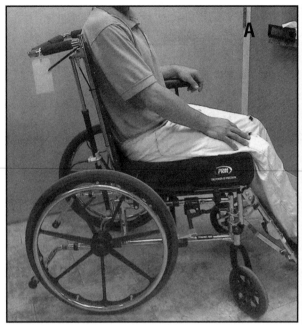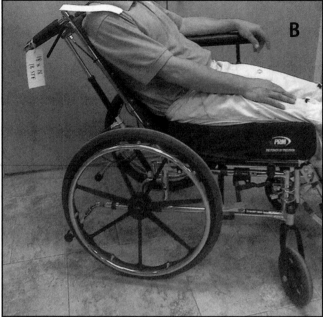

Figure 14-15. (A) Upright position with shoulders above backrest level. (B) Reclined position. Shoulder migrated down backrest by 4 inches.

required to have the oxygen tank with her at all times. By hanging the oxygen tank on the back of the chair, it counter balances her body weight. In this scenario, an adjustable tilt chair is set up with center of mass (including the weight of the oxygen tank) over the center of gravity of chair to maximize ease of pushing. The small rear wheels keep her hands out of danger if they drop to the sides of the chair. Stroller handles on the back of the chair provide an improved height for the pusher when the chair is tilted. If this client's condition were to change and the oxygen is no longer used, then the center of gravity (rear wheel) of the chair will need to shift forward to accommodate the change in weight on the rear of the chair.

Reclining-Back Wheelchair

This style of chair is rarely used for dependent users who also require moderate trunk lateral support. When the back of a chair is moved into recline, shearing of the client's back relative to the back support of the chair occurs due to a difference in position of the fulcrum of the reclining back and the position of the client's hip joint. As these two joints are not in the same alignment, the movement of the wheelchair back causes the client to move out of position relative to any lateral trunk supports, resulting in postural issues for the client, such as the lateral support contacting the axilla. Fixed mounted, rigid back supports with deep laterals can also become hung up under the clients axilla when the back is moved into full recline. The dynamic movement of the back reclining also creates skin shearing against the back

support as the back canes move at a different rate of recline than the client does. Low shear options are not available on manual wheelchairs, although these options are available for power wheelchairs. If a seat to back angle change is required, adjustable back canes may be more appropriate because these can provide the required angle without movement. Reclining backs have historically been used when catheter changes are required during the day and the client is unable to return to bed to do so, or in combination with manual tilt to provide larger surface contact to decrease peak pressure points.

CASE EXAMPLE

In Figure 14-15, we see a reclining wheelchair that is being used to transport a client requiring a change of hip angle due to recent hip surgery. As the hip heals, the back angle can change to allow the client to slowly sit up to a 90-degree angle. No lateral thoracic supports are used due to the shearing, which occurs when the back is in a recline position. Note the change in the client shoulder level compared with the top of the back support when reclined. This change in position is a result of the movement of the backrest relative to the cushion and client height because the cushion thickness raises the client above the low pivot point of the reclining back.

Adaptive Strollers

Adaptive strollers are typically used for young children, although adult sizes are available. Independent propulsion is not an option as the rear wheels are small and placed behind the client. Some of these look like a large umbrella stroller with a fixed tilt and minimal positioning options. Others styles include seating options, tilt-and-recline features, and oxygen and ventilator holders, and allow the seat to be turned on the base so that the caregiver can better monitor a medically fragile young child. Some strollers allow the caregiver to change the height of the seating system so that a young child can sit at peer level but also be raised to kitchen table height for meal times. The seat portion of the frame can sometimes be removed and placed on an indoor base that takes up less space and may offer this hi-low feature.

Adaptive strollers can support clients as small as infants just discharged from the neonatal care unit, as well as the medical equipment these children may require. They can also support young adults of smaller weight and body size for long distance transportation when they are no longer able to walk distances. These bases may also be used as backup to a manual wheelchair because the frame is lightweight and easy to fold, making transport easy. In general, these strollers do not offer as much growth, frame adjustment, or seating options as manual wheelchairs.

In Figure 14-16, we see a young client in a stroller that is set up with customized seating and additional medical equipment (e.g., suction, supplies, intravenous pole, ventilator). It is important that the medical devices are situated low and toward the middle of the frame to keep the stroller balanced and prevent rear tipping. The stroller is easy for the parents to transport and the custom seating is removable to put in a manual wheelchair base.

CONTRIBUTING FACTORS INFLUENCING FRAME STYLE

Critical thinking is required to determine which chair frame design to prescribe and whether or not adjustability is required. The following factors need to be considered.

Ease of Pushing

The footprint (overall outside width and depth of the chair) will determine accessibility of the wheelchair in different environments and spaces. Van lifts, ramps, doorways, and spaces for maneuvering (turning radius), such as hallways and bathrooms, must be measured to determine whether a recommended mobility base will meet these specifications. Floor-based mechanical lifts must clear the overall width of the chair based on the expandable width

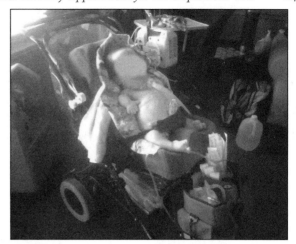

Figure 14-16. Adaptive stroller for transportation.

of the lift floor base. The overall wheelchair width will be determined primarily by the size of the seating system; however, this overall width will also affect maneuvering. Additionally, the overall depth of the wheelchair will be determined by the position of center of mass of the client and seating within the center of gravity of the wheelchair. This must be set up appropriately to ensure that the client mass is not front-loaded over the front casters, making the chair hard to push and less maneuverable due to the longer depth. Keeping the rear wheel position under the center of mass will provide the easiest point for the caregiver to push the chair and decrease the turning radius and depth of the chair. However, moving the rear wheel back from the center of mass can achieve greater safety and stability for agitated clients or for those who complete a transfer landing heavily into the chair causing it to tip backward. A longer depth chair with a more rearward axle can also increase the comfort level of the client who may feel that she is at risk of falling out of the chair if it is "too tippy."

As noted earlier, it is important to monitor the front-loading of the client and seating mass as the rear wheel moves back and ensure a longer front wheel base is provided, if required, to eliminate front-loading. This may be accomplished through a longer frame or by placing the casters in a leading vs trailing position. This is done by mounting the caster housing facing forward on the front frame of the wheelchair (Figure 14-17).

Placing the client's center of mass over the rear wheel also decreases the vibration experienced when being pushed on rough ground. It is important to use antitippers when changing rear axle position to prevent accidental rear tipping of the wheelchair. Unfortunately, antitippers can be a hindrance to the caregiver pushing the chair. Adjustable antitippers provide the pusher the ability to set the position of the antitipper out of their foot space but re-engage it when the client is no longer being pushed.

Seat to floor height adjustability can also alter ease of pushing the client. Adjusting the seat to floor height may

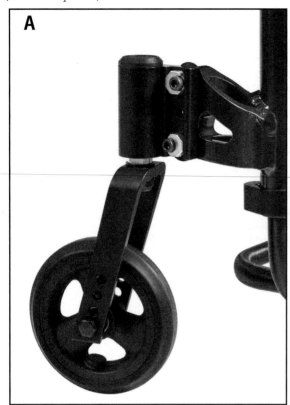

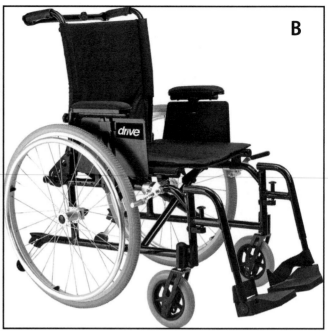

Figure 14-17. (A) Forward leading position. (B) Rear trailing position.

affect the method of transfer in and out of the wheelchair, as well as access to various height tables or alternate heights for ADL. If the frame height is set too high (vertical positioning of the rear axle and front caster), the client completing an assisted standing pivot transfer may not land and then sit all the way back in his or her seat cushion. Alternately, if the frame height is too low, the client may not be able to assist with standing from the wheelchair, or on sitting, he or she is dropped to the low height, causing the chair to tip. Caregiver pushing will also be altered by the overall chair, back support, and push handle height. Therefore, the chair, back support and cane height must be reviewed with the caregiver, client and transfer method in mind before determining the finished seat to floor height.

Ultimately, the best ergonomic position for the caregiver pushing the wheelchair is to have the push handle height set at 45 to 90 degrees of elbow flexion to reduce forward bending while pushing. Unfortunately, with multiple caregivers, this is difficult to achieve for all involved. Therefore, an average push height should be determined but only after the wheelchair and back cane height is determined for client functionality and trunk support. An important factor to consider in back cane height and angle is interference with the client's posterior shoulder and axilla area. If a rigid back support is added to provide the client with postural support, the angle of support must be determined in relation to the seat. This angle may be achieved by mounting the

back to straight back canes, 8-degree bend canes, or angle adjustable back canes. If the rigid back support is mounted on straight, or even 8-degree bend canes, the top of the back support may recline beyond the back cane itself and allow contact of the cane with the client's upper back. In this instance, angle adjustable back canes may be required to open up the seat to back angle. The back support can then be moved forward to the required position. This will also allow the caregiver better access to the push handle. Ultimately, education and providing tips to the caregiver with respect to pushing a wheelchair is of great benefit in preventing caregiver back injuries. For example, it is recommended that using leg power to gain the forces to push the chair will reduce back strain, rather than using a bent back and extended arm pushing posture.

Maximizing the ability to push the chair is also dependent on the rear wheel and front caster size and style. As with standard self-propulsion, the choice of solid tires versus pneumatic tires will be dependent on location of majority of use, and as such, solid tires are used more indoors and pneumatic more outdoors. Often we find that the dependent client mainly uses his or her chair indoors. However, if the client is often left sitting still vs being pushed within the home, the majority of pushing time may be when she is outdoors. In this situation, pneumatic wheels may be required to accommodate outdoor terrains. It is also important to consider the walking speed of the caregiver and the terrain

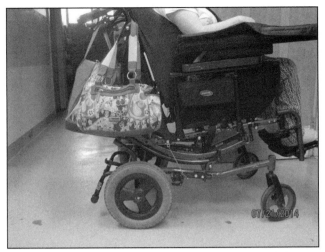

Figure 14-18. Center of gravity set up to accommodate supply bags.

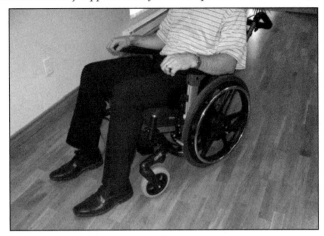

Figure 14-19. Foot-loading on the floor.

the client is being pushed on. Faster speeds over rough ground may create more vibration and shearing issues for the client and pneumatic tires minimize these issues.

When determining rear wheel and caster size, other factors must be considered above and beyond the seat to floor height. With respect to caster size, it is critical to assess the foot space of the client, which may be limited by tight hamstrings or ankle and foot asymmetries. This foot space is determined by the front rigging and footplate position, use of solid foot boxes, caster position and size, and potential interference with caster rotation. Therefore, wheel size should be determined after the seating system is prescribed to ensure proper heights for transfers and foot positioning. Smaller rear wheels (12- or 16-inches) may create a lower overall center of gravity and mass of the chair and client. This can improve stability for clients who demonstrate rocking behavior. Additionally, smaller rear wheels may be used for clients whose hands may get caught in a larger rear wheel due to extraneous movement or maladaptive behaviors. Smaller rear wheels often have foot-braking systems, which may be easier for the caregiver to access.

Balance

Balance is critical for those clients who may demonstrate agitated or destructive behaviors. A longer base will reduce the likelihood of the chair tipping backward or forward. This balance is achieved by placing the rear wheel further back on the axle plate, as well as placing the front caster in a leading position (see Figure 14-16A). Additionally, a wider chair or cambered wheels may reduce the sideways tipping of a chair (e.g., a client who may pull on wall mounted railings). These adjustments will require an adjustable frame. Balance is also affected by placing large and weighted backpacks on the rear of the frame. If this additional weight is always present, this must be taken into account in determining the client's center of mass.

In Figure 14-18, multiple bags of client supplies are carried on the back of this chair frame. The weight of the bags offsets the center of client mass, which is forward in the chair. When the bags are in position, there is no front-loading of the casters, and the chair is balanced. When the bags are removed, and the client is in an upright position, he will be front-loading the casters making the chair harder to push. In this scenario, it is recommended to push the chair in a tilted position to bring the center of mass back toward the rear wheel and reduce caster-loading when the bags are not present.

Foot-Loading

Having foot contact with the ground may provide critical support for the client even though he or she is dependent for mobility. Allowing the feet to reach the floor may provide the client with added stimulation from the rocking movement he or she may gain by pressing his or her feet against the floor. Additionally, this allows the feet to be positioned in more than one set spot, preventing the feet from hanging off the end of a footplate. Foot-loading can improve postural control and prevent sliding out of the seating system. Getting the proper seat to floor height will be dependent on cushion height and seat frame angles, and therefore a vertical adjustable rear axle and front caster fork is required. The use of footrests will still be required when the client is being pushed. Using 60-degree hangars and depth-adjustable footplates will maximize loading of the thighs on the cushion when the feet are placed on the footplates. Before prescribing this setup, it is important to assess the client's hamstring length and knee ROM to allow the foot to sit comfortably on a 60-degree footplate. If the range of the knee is limited, the pelvis will be pulled into posterior pelvic tilt, resulting in the client sliding out of the wheelchair.

The client seen in Figure 14-19 becomes very agitated when placed in regular nontilting wheelchair with footrests. He then begins sliding out of the chair to reach the ground with his feet. By placing him in a tilt chair and lowering the seat to floor height, his feet are placed flat on the floor. By flexing his knees, he is able to rock the chair forward and backward. This stimulation decreases his agitated behavior. The seating system provides postural support and thigh-loading, which also reduce sliding.

Seating System

Back support thickness, or the mounted position of the back support on the back canes, will change where the center of mass of the client is located. A thicker back will push the client forward on the seat frame and therefore move his or her center of mass forward. Seat cushion thickness will also change the vertical height to the floor, affecting foot-loading or finished seat to floor heights for table/activity access. Seating may need to be modified or replaced before the wheelchair frame, requiring growth or replacement. This may be due to growth, postural support changes, or pressure issues. It is therefore critical to determine the client's current seating needs and the potential for change. Once these needs are determined, the frame adjustability components are chosen to maintain a comfortable, functional, supportive, and pressure reduced resting posture. Shearing, pressure management, and postural control are often of more concern with the dependent user because the client may not have the physical, sensory, or cognitive capacity to understand or address the need for a body position change within the seating system. In this situation, the wheelchair frame has become more than four wheels and is now a full pressure management and postural control system in combination with the seating provided. Therefore, all seating components, directions of force, center of mass, center of gravity, and midline positioning are critical to maintain a safe resting posture that will be sustained while being pushed by a caregiver.

Orientation in Space

Changes in orientation in space can impact respiratory and circulatory functioning, as well as functional tasks, such as swallowing and visual regard of the environment. If the client is unable to reposition him- or herself, then the chair and seating system must do this for him or her via a tilt-in-space option to redistribute pressure. The seating system includes several angles that affect orientation in space. These include the seat to back angle, any fixed tilt of the seating system (in relation to the ground), and any tilt-in-space option. These angles may be critical for basic quality of life functioning. The client's respiratory status may be altered with changes in upright positioning, trunk rotation, extension, or flexion. These changes can often be assessed by using pulse oximetry while placing the client in a variety of trunk or orientation-in-space positions. Swallowing capacity may be altered based on trunk and cervical positions. Circulatory concerns may include edema of the lower extremities, impingement behind the knees from a cushion or seat depth that is too long, and overall peak pressure points, which can result in skin breakdown.

SUMMARY

Ultimately, manual mobility applications for the dependent user should address similar concerns as the independent user with respect to postural control in a resting posture. Additionally, the assessment needs to include the potential for independent ADL not related to propulsion. Just because the client is unable to wheel him- or herself does not mean that his or her basic bodily functioning is forgotten. Adjustability, weight, and setup of the seating and wheelchair will make a significant difference in quality of life functioning. Adjustability considerations based on prognosis, weight changes, and change in basic body functioning are critical. The main difference in prescribing manual mobility for the dependent vs independent user is that the actual ergonomics of the caregiver pushing and transporting the system must also be considered. Heights, weights, and chair setup will ensure an easy and smooth moving wheelchair that works for both the client and the caregiver.

BIBLIOGRAPHY

Bach, J. M., & Waugh, K. (2014, March). *Biomechanics and its application to seating.* Presented at the 30th International Seating Symposium Proceedings, Vancouver, Canada.

Buck, S. (2011). *More than 4 wheels: Applying clinical practice to seating, mobility and assistive technology* (2nd ed.). Milton, Canada: self-published.

DiGiovine, C., Berner, T., Roesler, T., & Kilbane, M. (2013, June). *Manual wheelchair selection, configuration and training.* Presented at the International Seating Symposium Proceedings, Nashville, TN.

Engstrom, B. (2002). *Ergonomic seating. A true challenge. Wheelchair Seating and Mobility Principles.* Stallarholmen, Sweden: Posturalis Books.

Helander, M. G., & Zhang, L. (1997). Field studies of comfort and discomfort in sitting. *Ergonomics, 40,* 895-915.

Monette, M., Weiss-Lambrou, R., & Dansereau, J. (1999, June). *In search of a better understanding of wheelchair sitting comfort and discomfort.* Paper presented at the RESNA Annual Conference, Long Beach, CA.

Rehabilitation Engineering & Assistive Technology Society of North America. (2013). *Position on the application of wheelchairs, seating systems, and secondary supports for positioning vs. restraint.* Retrieved from http://www.resna.org/resources/positionpapers/RESNARestraintPositionPaperFinal02032014.pdf

Scherer, M. J. (1994). *Matching person and technology (MPT). A series of assessments for selecting and evaluating technologies used in rehabilitation, education, the workplace & other settings.* Webster, NY: self-published.

Ward, D. (1994). *Prescriptive seating for wheeled mobility: Vol. 1. Theory, application and terminology.* Pasig City, Philippines: Health Wealth International.

Alternate Drive Mechanisms for Manual Wheelchairs
Bridging the Gap Between Manual and Power Mobility

Carmen P. DiGiovine, PhD, ATP/SMS, RET and Theresa F. Berner, MOT, OTR/L, ATP

Alternate drive mechanisms for manual wheelchairs play an important role in the continuum of wheeled mobility for individuals with disability. The continuum ranges from handrim-propelled manual wheelchairs to power wheelchairs. Alternate drive mechanisms fall squarely in the middle, meeting a need for individuals who want better mechanical efficiency than can be attained with a handrim manual wheelchair, but do not want to lose the transportability, versatility, and aesthetics of a manual wheelchair. Alternate drive mechanisms include lever drives, arm-crank drives, geared hubs, reverse pushrim drives, and pushrim-activated power-assist drives. Each drive mechanism has advantages and disadvantages; therefore, one size does not fit all. The stakeholders in the service delivery process must consider the individual's unique characteristics, the activities the individual wants to perform, and the environment in which the activities will be performed (Arledge et al., 2011; Armstrong et al., 2008; Cook & Polgar, 2008). The individual's characteristics, activities, and context inform stakeholders in the selection of the appropriate alternate drive mechanism. Often, alternate drive mechanisms are one of many tools that an individual will use for effective community mobility, whether in a rural or city setting or an industrialized or developing country. The purpose of this chapter is to provide an overview of the alternate drive mechanisms to best meet the mobility needs of individuals with disabilities.

BIOMECHANICS AND PHYSIOLOGY OF MANUAL WHEELCHAIR PROPULSION

The progression of wheeled mobility for individuals with mobility impairments typically starts with canes, crutches, and walkers and ends with scooters and power wheelchairs. In between, an individual may use a manual wheelchair, with or without an alternate drive mechanism. Individuals may enter this progression at any point, but as they age, they tend to move up the chain. This is often due to an increased incidence of upper extremity injury and pain, decreased cardiopulmonary reserves, strength, and endurance, and changes in posture. The biomechanics and physiology of manual wheelchair propulsion (MWP) are critical to understanding the progression and the transition across propulsion mechanisms.

MWP has a significant impact on the upper extremities, especially given that the upper extremities, compared with the lower extremities, are not designed as primary mobility generators. This is evidenced by the fact that numerous studies have identified pain and injury due to overuse of the upper extremities. A review of upper extremity musculoskeletal injuries by Copper et al. (2006) found that the prevalence of shoulder pain ranges from 31% to 73% of individuals who use a manual wheelchair. Furthermore, a review by Boninger et al. (2005) found that between 49% and 73% of individuals who use a manual wheelchair

Lange, M. L., & Minkel, J. L.
Seating and Wheeled Mobility: A Clinical Resource Guide
(pp. 251-260). © 2018 SLACK Incorporated.

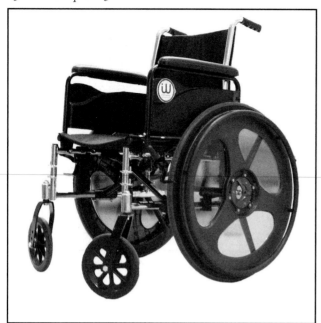

Figure 15-1. Forward propulsion geared wheel.

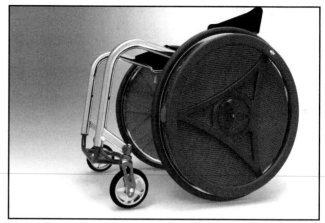

Figure 15-2. Rearward propulsion geared wheel.

experience carpal tunnel syndrome at some point in their life. Although transfers and other upper extremity activities have been identified as potential culprits for the development of pain and injury, pushrim propulsion is the primary activity for most individuals in the development of overuse injuries.

To mitigate the development of injury and pain, numerous recommendations have been developed for manual wheelchair propulsion, independent of the propulsion mechanism. The recommendations center around performing long, smooth motions (or strokes in the case of pushrim propulsion), minimizing the frequency of these motions, and minimizing the force generated during the motion, while maintaining functional speed and maneuverability. Furthermore, to facilitate the attainment of these recommendations, individuals should use the lightest weight, adjustable wheelchair possible. In regard to pushrim propulsion, Boninger et al. (2005) summarized these recommendations in a review of investigations from the Collaboration on Upper Limb Pain in Spinal Cord Injury. These recommendations provide the basis for manual wheelchair propulsion independent of the mechanism of propulsion.

ALTERNATE METHODS FOR MANUAL WHEELCHAIR PROPULSION

Traditionally, individuals have used the wheel, itself, or the handrim to propel the wheelchair. This method is convenient, both for propulsion and for transporting the wheelchair, but presents barriers in terms of overall

efficiency and overuse injuries. Alternate drive mechanisms include lever drives, arm-crank drives (also known as *hand cycles*), geared hubs, reverse pushrim drives and pushrim-activated power-assist drives.

Geared Systems

The geared systems use the standard handrim interface and place a gear system between the handrim and the wheel. Geared systems include both geared hubs and reverse pushrim drives. The geared system provides a mechanical advantage over the 1:1 ratio that is in place for conventional handrims. Most geared systems are set up with a 1:1 ratio for standard wheelchair propulsion and a 1:2 ratio for propulsion on inclines or across terrains with high rolling resistance (e.g., carpet with padding). The geared systems are set up either so that forward propulsion on the handrim elicits forward motion (Figure 15-1) or reverse propulsion on the handrim (pulling back on the handrim) elicits forward motion (Figure 15-2). The geared systems have demonstrated an ability to reduce the muscular effort in the upper extremities on all ramps and abdominal activity on steep ramps (Howarth, Polgar, Dickerson, & Callaghan, 2010; Howarth, Pronovost, Polgar, Dickerson, & Callaghan, 2010). Furthermore, the geared systems have showed the potential to reduce pain when used to overcome challenging environments (Finley & Rodgers, 2007). The opportunity for making it easier to traverse obstacles and ramps is counteracted by the potential for increased stokes, and thereby muscle overuse for multigear systems. The forward propulsion geared systems are appropriate for individuals with reduced upper arm strength who would not be able to traverse obstacles using a conventional handrim. The reverse propulsion geared systems are appropriate for individuals who have appropriate trunk stabilization, either through core muscles or through extrinsic supports (e.g., anterior chest support, abdominal binder), and want to use a motion similar to rowing.

Key to the success of the multigeared systems is the ability to recognize the need to change gears and the ease

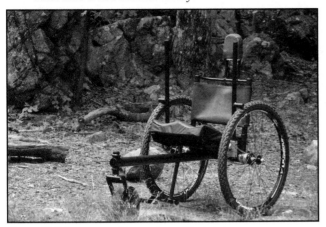

Figure 15-3. Lever propulsion system with chain/gear.

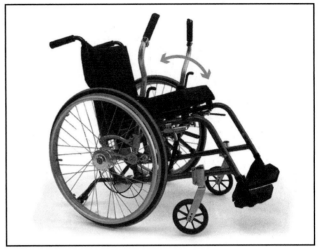

Figure 15-4. Lever propulsion system with multiple gears.

of changing gears. Leaving the geared system in a low gear while traversing flat surfaces could be as detrimental as not having the low gear to travel up inclines. Furthermore, the geared systems add weight; although the majority of the weight is located near the center of the hub, minimizing its effect on propulsion. However, this could have significant impact on transfers in and out of vehicles, even if the wheels are quick-release wheels. Geared systems provide a non-powered option to decrease the force necessary to traverse inclines, minimize the rollback when going up inclines, and reduce the force required to brake when traversing a decline. Pull propulsion (also known as *reverse propulsion*) geared systems provide an alternative method for propelling the wheelchair that takes advantage of larger muscle groups and minimizes impact on the handrim.

Lever Systems

Lever propulsion systems use a lever arm to increase the torque that an individual can generate for forward or reverse propulsion, compared with a conventional handrim. Lever propulsion systems typically include two lever arms, one on each side the wheelchair. The lever arms are placed between the frame and the wheel (Figures 15-3 and 15-4) or outside the wheel (Figure 15-5). The systems have advanced to the point that they add very little width to the overall wheelchair footprint. The increased torque is due to the longer lever arm and, for some systems, due to a gearing system that is built into the lever propulsion system. Furthermore, lever propulsion systems provide a better interface for the individual because it is easier to grasp the handhold on a lever mechanism than it is to grasp the handrim on a conventional handrim. One of the most challenging components of a lever system is the turning mechanism. Some designs use differential motion of the drive wheels, similar to handrim propulsion or power wheelchairs, whereas others incorporate a dedicated steering mechanism, similar to tillers on scooters (McLaurin & Brubaker, 1986; Mukherjee & Samanta, 2001a). Differential motion consists of pulling

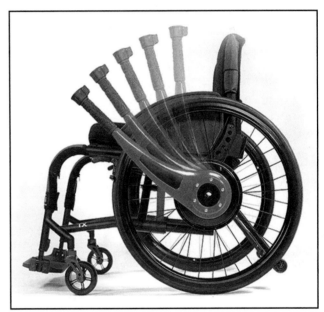

Figure 15-5. Lever propulsion system with lever mounted outside the wheel.

back on the right wheel and pushing forward on the left wheel in order to turn right. Likewise, pushing forward on the right and pulling back on the left will cause an individual to turn left. The push-pull motion of lever propulsion, similar to a rowing motion, that is inherent to the lever system, is easier to generate than the circular motion that is inherent to the handrim propulsion. Furthermore, the individual does not have to focus on properly grabbing and releasing the handrim when using a lever propulsion system as his or her hands are in constant contact with the lever.

Lever propulsion systems provide physiological advantages in comparison to handrim propulsion systems. Lever propulsion systems are more mechanically efficient than conventional handrim propulsion (Lui et al., 2013; Mukherjee & Samanta, 2001a; van der Woude, de Groot, Hollander, van Ingen Schenau, & Rozendal, 1986; van der

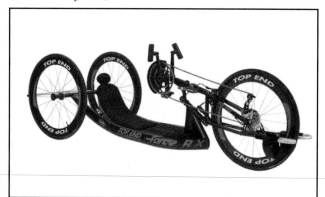

Figure 15-6. Recumbent handcycle.

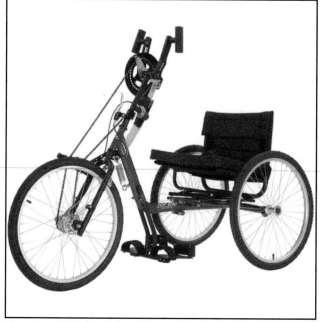

Figure 15-7. Upright handcycle.

Woude, Veeger, de Boer, & Rozendal, 1993). The self-selected speed is higher and heart rate and oxygen consumption are lower for lever drive systems. However, simultaneous turning and propulsion is difficult because of the need for one hand for propulsion and the other for steering in some systems (Mukherjee & Samanta, 2001a). The lever drive is physically less demanding, less strenuous, and more efficient. The lever drive system is especially well-suited for outdoor use, sports, and recreation (van der Woude et al., 1986, 1993). Lever propulsion systems provide an alternative to conventional handrims for generating higher speeds over longer distances, more efficient and less strenuous propulsion, and greater ease of traversing rough terrain.

Arm-Crank Systems

Arm-crank propulsion systems are typically incorporated in handcycles for outdoor recreation and as an alternate mechanism for propulsion in rural areas. The arm-crank systems are modeled after bicycle gearing systems and allow individuals to change gears in order to match his or her capacity and environment. Arm-crank systems, also known as *handcycles*, are described by the position of the individual and the mechanism for generating power (i.e., upper extremities only vs trunk and upper extremities combined). Individuals may use the arm-crank systems in a recumbent position (Figure 15-6), an upright position (Figure 15-7), or any of a number of positions in between (Figure 15-8). The downsides to using the arm-crank system is the size/bulkiness of the system, the limited maneuverability of the handcycle, and the esthetics. Arm-crank systems include both synchronous and asynchronous systems. Initially, the majority of arm-crank systems were asynchronous, that is the left and right crank arms are positioned opposite of each other (i.e., 180 degrees out of phase), similar to the foot pedals on a bicycle. However, the majority of arm-crank systems today are synchronous, with the left and right arm cranks next to each other, because they are more efficient and less strenuous (Dallmeijer, Ottjes, de Waardt, & van der Woude, 2004). Furthermore, synchronous systems produce higher peak-power output and are

easier to steer and brake (Hettinga et al., 2010). The synchronous systems are typically used in outdoor sports and recreation activities because of the ability to travel at higher speeds for longer distances in comparison to conventional handrim propulsion.

Handcycling provides a clear mechanical advantage compared with handrim propulsion. The circular movement of the hands and the continuous force application exhibited in handcycling is mechanically less straining than handrim propulsion (Arnet, van Drongelen, van der Woude, & Veeger, 2012). Handrim propulsion has higher physiological response and lower propulsion speed than handcycles. Handcycles allow the users to go longer distances at higher speeds, most often in outdoor environments. The various handcycles allow numerous options in terms of sitting style and trunk posture, which allows for a lower profile with respect to the upright posture typically used for handrim propulsion. Given the higher speeds, the lower profile is important because the air resistance increases as the square of the velocity. That is, the air resistance increases by 4 times every time the velocity doubles. Therefore, the lower frontal area (see Row 7 of Figure 15-8) that is seen with recumbent, long-seat, and knee-seat handcycles will have a significant reduction on the air resistance. The use of larger wheels makes it easier to travel rough environments that are encountered in both industrialized and developing countries. Finally, the handcycle is easily repairable, especially in developing countries where bicycle parts are readily available (Hettinga et al., 2010; Mukherjee & Samanta, 2001b). Arm-crank systems are more efficient and less straining on the upper extremities; however, they are not as maneuverable as handrim propulsion systems.

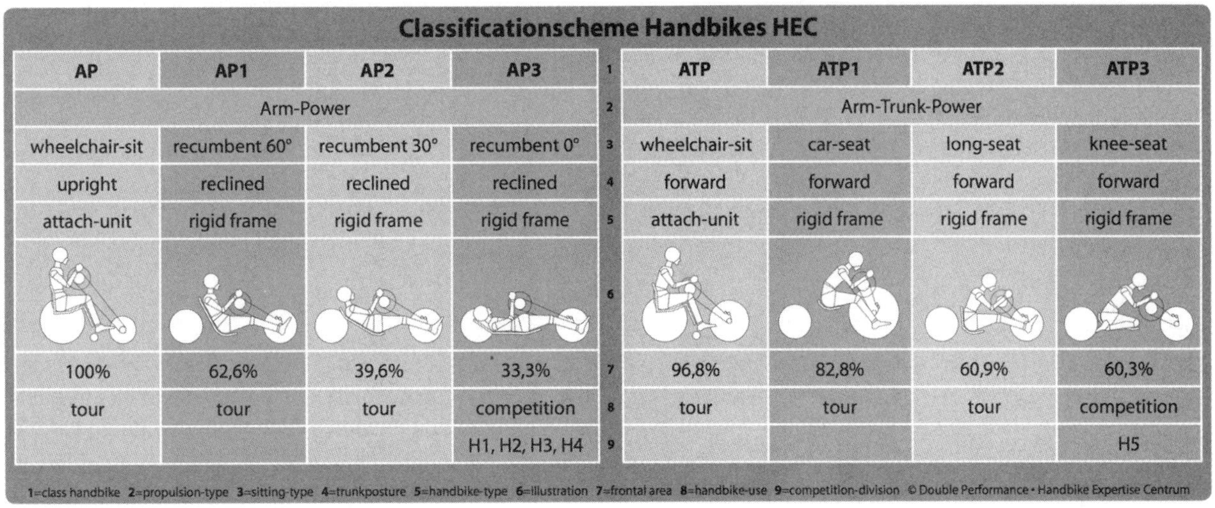

Classificationscheme Handbikes HEC								
AP	**AP1**	**AP2**	**AP3**		**ATP**	**ATP1**	**ATP2**	**ATP3**
Arm-Power					Arm-Trunk-Power			
wheelchair-sit	recumbent 60°	recumbent 30°	recumbent 0°		wheelchair-sit	car-seat	long-seat	knee-seat
upright	reclined	reclined	reclined		forward	forward	forward	forward
attach-unit	rigid frame	rigid frame	rigid frame		attach-unit	rigid frame	rigid frame	rigid frame
100%	62,6%	39,6%	33,3%		96,8%	82,8%	60,9%	60,3%
tour	tour	tour	competition		tour	tour	tour	competition
			H1, H2, H3, H4					H5

1=class handbike 2=propulsion-type 3=sitting-type 4=trunkposture 5=handbike-type 6=Illustration 7=frontal area 8=handbike-use 9=competition-division © Double Performance · Handbike Expertise Centrum

Figure 15-8. Classification of handcycles based on the position of the individual and the type of propulsion (arm power vs arm-trunk power). (Reprinted with permission from Double Performance BV, Gouda, The Netherlands.)

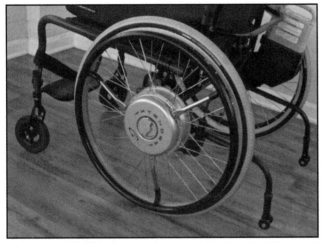

Figure 15-9. PAPAW with the motor mounted in the hub of the wheels and batteries mounted on the back of the wheelchair. (Reprinted with permission from Sunrise Medical, Longmont, CO.)

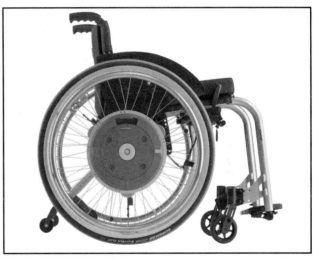

Figure 15-10. PAPAW with the motor and batteries mounted in the hub of the wheel. (Reprinted with permission from Frank Mobility, Oakdale, PA.)

Pushrim-Activated Power Assist

The Pushrim-Activated Power Assist (PAPAW) is a hybrid system that measures the force an individual imparts on the pushrim and then amplifies this force through the application of an electromechanical system. The measurement of the force may be directly through the handrims (Figures 15-9 through 15-11) or indirectly through a fifth wheel that is attached to the back of the wheelchair (Figure 15-12). The PAPAW uses a battery to power motors that are typically included in the hub of the wheels or are external to the frame of the wheelchair (Cooper et al., 2006). The key functional characteristics of the PAPAW is that it uses a manual wheelchair frame; registers the amount of force an individual imparts on the system, either directly or through algorithms based on the system acceleration; and then amplifies the propulsion phase and extends the recovery phase (or *coast-down*) of manual wheelchair propulsion.

PAPAWs are designed to meet the functional mobility needs of individuals who propel a manual wheelchair. Two styles of PAPAWs currently exist, PAPAWs with an intermittent mode only (see Figure 9-11), and PAPAWs with both an intermittent mode and a continuous mode (see Figure 15-12). Both styles amplify the propulsion phase and recovery phase, but the second style also has a continuous mode that allows the individual to turn on the motor via an external switch or a Bluetooth input device (e.g., wristband). This allows the person to travel in a relatively straight line for long distances, while only interacting with the handrims for course corrections. This type of system is ideal for community outings, and college and work

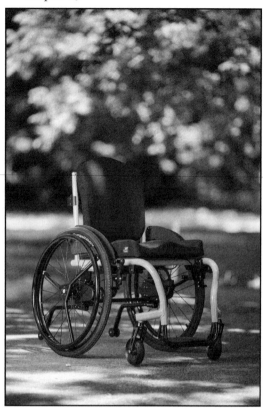

Figure 15-11. PAPAW with motor and batteries mounted under frame of wheelchair. (Reprinted with permission from Clinton River, Auburn Hills, MI.)

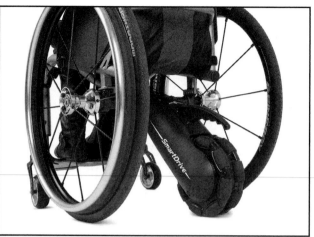

Figure 15-12. PAPAW with motor mounted to a fifth wheel attached to the rear of the wheelchair, and the battery mounted to the underside of the frame. (Reprinted with permission from Maxx Mobility, Nashville, TN.)

campuses. Both systems have their assets and liabilities and may not work for all individuals; therefore, a trial period is critical when evaluating a PAPAW.

Initially, PAPAWs were used by individuals who were unable to effectively propel a manual wheelchair but did not want to transition to a power wheelchair. However, this trend is changing as individuals recognize the importance of upper extremity injury prevention and the need for improved community mobility while maximizing endurance. Research documenting the high prevalence of upper extremity pain and injury for these individuals, has caused many individuals to consider a PAPAW system as a tool to mitigate the likelihood of these injuries. Maintaining the strength and integrity of the shoulder complex is critical to all activities of daily living (ADL; e.g., transfers) for individuals who use a wheelchair as their primary mode of mobility. Limiting the fatigue associated with manual wheelchair mobility is critical to performing ADL other than manual wheelchair mobility.

PAPAWs have been investigated by numerous researchers over the past 2 decades. Compared with individuals' own manual wheelchairs, individuals tend to travel farther when using a PAPAW. Individuals also found it easier to traverse difficult terrains and obstacles (Ding et al., 2008). Furthermore, individuals prefer the PAPAW to their own wheelchair. They indicate that the device is intuitive and the

PAPAW handrim is more comfortable than their own manual wheelchair, although replacing or removing the battery was a difficult task (Algood, Cooper, Fitzgerald, Cooper, & Boninger, 2005). Individuals demonstrated a decreased physical exertion while maintaining, or even improving, propulsion velocity in comparison to a handrim-propelled manual wheelchair. Even as the difficulty of trials increased (speed and resistance), the individual's stroke frequency and ROM stayed the same (Algood, Cooper, Fitzgerald, Cooper, & Boninger, 2004). Furthermore, at higher speeds and higher user power inputs, there is a larger absolute gain from the motors, resulting in greater efficiency (Arva, Fitzgerald, Cooper, & Boninger, 2001). This demonstrates the effectiveness of the PAPAW to bridge the gap between the individual's capacity and the requirements for performing a task. The metabolic energy cost and heart rate for propelling a PAPAW was lower than when propelling an individual's personal wheelchair. The PAPAW showed a reduction in metabolic demand that is greater than geared hubs and lever drive systems, and comparable to arm-crank systems (Cooper et al., 2001). The biomechanical and physiological advantages of the PAPAW allow individuals to travel further at faster speeds, using less energy compared with any other self-prolusion system.

Although overall speed and distance are important, the maneuverability is equally important. A lack of maneuverability has hampered the acceptance of many other alternative drive systems. PAPAWs have been found to be comparable to both power wheelchairs and conventional handrim manual wheelchairs in both activities and performance. The equivalency has been demonstrated both in the lab with a standardized wheelchairs skills test, and in the community (Best, Kirby, Smith, & MacLeod, 2006; Giesbrecht, Ripat, Cooper, & Quanbury, 2011; Giesbrecht, Ripat, Quanbury, & Cooper, 2009). Best et al. (2006) demonstrated that an individual with a disability can complete similar skills in the wheelchair skills test with both a conventional handrim and a PAPAW. Furthermore, the PAPAW was found to be more effective when completing skills that require larger handrim forces, such as pushing up a ramp. The conventional handrim manual wheelchair (without the PAPAW) was more effective on skills that required greater control, such as turning around in a small space (Best et al., 2006). Giesbrecht et al. (2009) conducted a study that examined the effect of replacing an individual's power wheelchair with a PAPAW. The individuals were dual users (i.e., they used both a manual and a power wheelchair). For these individuals, the PAPAW provided an alternative to the power wheelchair because they were able to maintain participation in community-based activities.

Giesbrecht et al. (2011) conducted a focus group of the same dual-users described in the previous study and identified three themes: relative advantages and disadvantages, environmental factors that affect accessibility, and evaluation of mobility device (Giesbrecht et al., 2011). In terms of advantages compared with their manual wheelchair, the PAPAW was easier to propel, especially when encountering environmental challenges (e.g., inclines and soft terrain), and it increased speed and efficiency. Compared with the power wheelchair, the PAPAW was easier to transport. Although it must be noted that PAPAW is more difficult to transport than a conventional handrim manual wheelchair given the added weight of the system, and the additional components (e.g., motor, batteries) that must be removed when placing the wheelchair in a sedan, crossover, or sports utility vehicle. Consistent with Best et al. (2006), concerns about the ability to control the PAPAW while performing high-skill maneuvers, such as popping a wheelie, arose. Furthermore, the individuals were concerned about the ability to propel the PAPAW if the batteries were completely discharged. The participants in this study did not perceive the PAPAW as a replacement for their power wheelchair, even though it allowed them to perform the majority of community activities. They proposed engaging in more activities and environments because of reduced dependence on power wheelchair or manual wheelchair. The PAPAW provides an alternative option to the conventional handrim manual wheelchair or power wheelchair for some individuals.

The PAPAW has numerous biomechanical, physiological, and functional advantages, which are summarized in a systematic review of the literature before May 2012 by Kloosterman, Snoek, van der Woude, Buurke, and Rietman (2013). The review concluded that there are number of advantages and disadvantages to the PAPAW.

Advantages

The advantages of PAPAWs include:

- Reduction of the load on the upper extremities (the upper extremities did not have to work as hard, compared with handrim manual chairs)
- Decrease in cardiopulmonary demand
- Increase in propulsion efficiency
- Maintained benefit of exercise
- Easy access of challenging environments
- Relatively lightweight and easy to transport compared with power wheelchairs

Disadvantages

The disadvantages of PAPAWs include:

- Difficulty performing tasks that require greater control (e.g., wheelie)
- Difficulty with car transfers due to additional weight and width compared with manual wheelchairs
- Difficulty with accessibility to certain environments (e.g., home) due to additional width
- Still performing a repetitive motion, although at decreased forces compared with manual wheelchair propulsion

Given the advantages and disadvantages of a PAPAW, a thorough understanding of the unique characteristics of the individual, activities he or she wants to perform, areas of participation that interest him or her, and context that surrounds the potential use of the PAPAW are critical for a successful outcome. PAPAWs provide a unique solution for individuals who want to reduce the wear and tear on their shoulders and increase access to the physical environment.

SUMMARY

Alternate drive mechanisms for manual wheelchairs play an important role in the continuum of wheeled mobility for individuals with disabilities. The continuum ranges from conventional handrim-propelled manual wheelchairs to power wheelchairs. Alternate drive mechanisms fall squarely in the middle, meeting a need for individuals who want better mechanical efficiency and increased long-distance mobility than can be attained with a conventional handrim manual wheelchair, but do not want to lose the transportability, versatility, and aesthetics of a manual wheelchair. Alternate drive mechanisms include lever drives, arm-crank drives, geared hubs, reverse pushrim drives (a subset of geared hubs), and pushrim activated power-assist drives. Lever drives, arm-crank drives, and geared hubs all use mechanical advantage through levers and gears to improve mobility. PAPAWs utilize advanced algorithms and improved battery and motor technology to improve mobility. The field of alternate drive mechanisms is ripe for further advancement as technologies from the biking and rowing industries trickle down to the manual wheelchair propulsion and as battery and motor technology improve through advancements in consumer electronics and automotive industries. Alternate drives provide a unique opportunity for new and experienced manual wheelchair propellers and also for marginal manual wheelchair propellers to continue using a manual wheelchair in both indoor and outdoor activities.

CASE EXAMPLE

Tony is a 28-year-old male with tetraplegia as a result of a diving injury 5 years ago. Tony has C4 incomplete American Spinal Injury Association C injury. Other diagnoses include neurogenic bladder/bowel, spasticity, and autonomic dysfunction. Tony has been hospitalized with renal stones, suprapubic surgery, and appendectomy.

Tony has an ultralight manual wheelchair with a skin protection and positioning cushion. He has been using this equipment for the past 4 years and reports that he currently has difficulty accessing uneven terrain, carpet, and inclines/declines indoors and any long distances outdoors.

Tony lives with his girlfriend in a one-story home and relies on public transportation. His girlfriend works full time, and he needs to be independent in his wheelchair at all times. He has an aide that helps him with his self-care. He is fully dependent for transfers to his wheelchair, so his aide also assists with this. Once he is in his wheelchair, he remains there for up to 14 hours before he returns to bed. Tony is extremely active and is in the community for a large part of his day. He reports that he and his girlfriend attend many social functions as part of her job, and he needs to be able to access multiple environments.

He is not interested in a power wheelchair because he has enough strength and endurance to push himself for most of his needs. His environment is not set up for power mobility, and he is not ready to transition to power. He needs some form of PAPAW to allow him to maintain his active lifestyle and continue at his level of independence.

During the examination, he presents with moderate spasticity, which is greater in his lower extremities than in his upper extremities. He has poor to fair sitting balance. He has good trunk control in his wheelchair, which is equipped with solid back support. He is able to perform functional weight shifts and uses the push handles for hooking his arm for increased trunk stability. He has good skin integrity with no history of breakdown. His active upper extremity ROM is limited to 90 degrees due to a lack of strength. He has no active grasp but good tenodesis function. He wears palm gloves for assistance with manual wheelchair navigation.

During manual wheelchair propulsion, he exhibited scapular winging and elevation. In his manual wheelchair he was able to perform most all wheelchairs maneuvers on flat surfaces, but he was not able to navigate a ramp greater than 5 degrees without assistance. His endurance is limited for long-distance propelling, and he is unable to get himself around in a timely manner; thus, he needs increased pushing assistance the longer the distance traveled. By the end of the day, he exhibits significant fatigue, has difficulty performing ADL, and experiences significant pain in his shoulders. A propulsion analysis demonstrated that he was only able to propel his current wheelchair at a speed of 0.88 meters/second on tile and 0.7 meters/second on carpet (*Note:* Average walking speed is 1.4 meters/second) (Table 15-1). He scored a 58% on the wheelchair skills test (Table 15-2).

Tony trialed two PAPAWs. The first trial was a fifth wheel system with the additional motorized wheel and battery mounted under the wheelchair frame, similar to the system pictured in Figure 15-12. The second was a system with the motor and batteries mounting in the hub of the wheel (i.e., integrated hub system), similar to the system pictured in Figure 15-10. He indicated that the fifth wheel system was lighter, he could have a friend take it on and off his wheelchair throughout the day, and it would not significantly change the weight or the look of his wheelchair. He indicated that the advantages of the integrated hub system was the ability to independently fine-tune the wheels to his strength and ability.

During the trial of the fifth wheel system, Tony found it difficult to manage the speed and responsiveness of the system due to his limited stability and limited hand function. He really liked the portability of the system and aesthetics of the product. He was frustrated he was not able to control the chair as fluidly as he expected.

During the trial of the integrated hub system Tony felt more in control. The system he used allowed him to adjust the responsiveness of the system to his strength and gave him time to respond. He did not like how the wheels changed the look of his wheelchair, and his girlfriend did not like the weight of the wheels and batteries when she disassembled it for transportation in her sedan.

Tony conducted an extended evaluation of both systems during multiple clinical appointments and was able to use them indoors in open and small spaces and on various terrains (e.g., tile, carpet, sidewalk, uneven surfaces). He took both systems outdoors and navigated around the building and parking lot. He finally arranged for a demonstration at his home and was able to maneuver both pieces of technology in and around his apartment complex. His girlfriend was able to trial disassembling each piece of equipment for transportation in her car.

After evaluating both pieces of technology, he chose the integrated hub system because he felt more in control. The use of this technology minimized the scapular winging that was observed when he propelled his current manual wheelchair. He was able to propel faster (see Table 15-1) and complete more skills (see Table 15-2) compared with his current manual wheelchair. His lack of hand dexterity and limited trunk balance prevented him from having

TABLE 15-1

RESULTS FROM WHEELCHAIR PROPULSION TEST (VERSION 1.0)

	CURRENT WHEELCHAIR		PAPAW—INTEGRATED HUB SYSTEM	
	Tile	*Carpet*	*Tile*	*Carpet*
Distance	10 m (32.8 ft)	10 m (32.8 ft)	10 m (32.8 ft)	10 m (32.8 ft)
Able to successfully complete the 10-m distance?	Yes	Yes	Yes	Yes
Direction of travel	Forward	Forward	Forward	Forward
Extremities contributing to propulsion, steering or braking	Bilateral UE	Bilateral UE	Bilateral UE	Bilateral UE
Total number of propulsive cycles	10	12	7	9
Speed	0.88 m/s (2.0 mph)	0.7 m/s (1.6 mph)	1.1 m/s (2.5 mph)	1.0 m/s (2.2 mph)
Begin the contact between the hands and the handrims behind the top dead center of the rear wheel?	Yes	Yes	Yes	Yes
Push frequency	0.88 cycles/s	0.84 cycles/s	0.77 cycles/s	0.9 cycles/s

UE = upper extremity

TABLE 15-2

RESULTS FROM WHEELCHAIR SKILLS TEST (VERSION 4.2)

	CURRENT WHEELCHAIR	PAPAW—INTEGRATED HUB SYSTEM
Raw Score	29	40
Testing Errors or Not Possible	7	7
Total Capacity Score	58%	80%

consistent reactions to the fifth wheel system. Although he recognized the benefit from both pieces of equipment through multiple trials in the clinic and in his home environment, he felt the integrated hub system provided more options for personalizing the system to match his unique mobility requirements. Specifically, he indicated that the most important feature was the customized responsiveness of the integrated hub system.

Tony returned to clinic 3 months after the equipment was dispensed and reported satisfaction with his choice. He indicated that the PAPAW allowed him to manage his energy better so that he could join his girlfriend at her evening work events. He no longer has the shoulder pain that would prevent him from participating in evening activities and felt more in control of his navigation. He reports he is able to ascend and descend most all environmental ramps and does not need to rely on others for assistance with these surfaces.

REFERENCES

Algood, S. D., Cooper, R. A., Fitzgerald, S. G., Cooper, R., & Boninger, M. L. (2004). Impact of a pushrim-activated power-assisted wheelchair on the metabolic demands, stroke frequency, and range of motion among subjects with tetraplegia. *Archives of Physical Medicine and Rehabilitation, 85,* 1865-1871.

Algood, S. D., Cooper, R. A., Fitzgerald, S. G., Cooper, R., & Boninger, M. L. (2005). Effect of a pushrim-activated power-assist wheelchair on the functional capabilities of persons with tetraplegia. *Archives of Physical Medicine and Rehabilitation, 86,* 380-386.

Arledge, S., Armstrong, W., Babinec, M., Dicianno, B., DiGiovine, C. P., Dyson-Hudson, T. A.,...Stogner, J. (2011). *RESNA wheelchair service provision guide.* Arlington, VA: Rehabilitation Engineering & Assistive Technology Society of North America. Retrieved from http://www.resna.org/dotAsset/22485.pdf

Armstrong, W., Borg, J., Krizack, M., Lindsley, A., Mines, K., Pearlman, J.,...Sheldon, S. (2008). *Guidelines on the provision of manual wheelchairs in less-resourced settings.* Geneva, Switzerland: World Health Organization. Retrieved from http://www.who.int/disabilities/publications/technology/English%20Wheelchair%20Guidelines%20(EN%20for%20the%20web).pdf?ua=1

Arnet, U., van Drongelen, S., van der Woude, L. H., & Veeger, D. H. (2012). Shoulder load during handcycling at different incline and speed conditions. *Clinical Biomechanics, 27,* 1-6. http://doi.org/10.1016/j.clinbiomech.2011.07.002

Arva, J., Fitzgerald, S. G., Cooper, R. A., & Boninger, M. L. (2001). Mechanical efficiency and user power requirement with a pushrim activated power assisted wheelchair. *Medical Engineering and Physics, 23,* 699-705.

Best, K. L., Kirby, R. L., Smith, C., & MacLeod, D. A. (2006). Comparison between performance with a pushrim-activated power-assisted wheelchair and a manual wheelchair on the Wheelchair Skills Test. *Disability and Rehabilitation, 28,* 213-220. http://doi.org/10.1080/09638280500158448

Boninger, M. L., Koontz, A. M., Sisto, S. A., Dyson-Hudson, T. A., Chang, M., Price, R., & Cooper, R. A. (2005). Pushrim biomechanics and injury prevention in spinal cord injury: Recommendations based on CULP-SCI investigations. *Journal of Rehabilitation Research and Development, 42*(Suppl. 1), 9-20.

Cook, A. M., & Polgar, J. M. (2008). Framework for assistive technologies. In *Cook & Hussey's Assistive Technologies: Principles and Practice* (3rd ed., pp. 34-53). St. Louis, MO: Mosby.

Cooper, R. A., Boninger, M. L., Spaeth, D. M., Ding, D., Guo, S., Koontz, A. M.,...Collins, D. M. (2006). Engineering better wheelchairs to enhance community participation. *IEEE Transactions on Neural Systems and Rehabilitation Engineering, 14,* 438-455. http://doi.org/10.1109/TNSRE.2006.888382

Cooper, R. A., Fitzgerald, S. G., Boninger, M. L., Prins, K., Rentschler, A. J., Arva, J., & O'Connor, T. J. (2001). Evaluation of a pushrim-activated, power-assisted wheelchair. *Archives of Physical Medicine and Rehabilitation, 82,* 702-708. http://doi.org/10.1053/apmr.2001.20836

Dallmeijer, A. J., Ottjes, L., de Waardt, E., & van der Woude, L. H. V. (2004). A physiological comparison of synchronous and asynchronous hand cycling. *International Journal of Sports Medicine, 25,* 622-626. http://doi.org/10.1055/s-2004-817879

Ding, D., Souza, A., Cooper, R. A., Fitzgerald, S. G., Cooper, R., Kelleher, A., & Boninger, M. L. (2008). A preliminary study on the impact of pushrim-activated power-assist wheelchairs among individuals with tetraplegia. *American Journal of Physical and Medical Rehabilitation, 87,* 821-89.

Finley, M. A., & Rodgers, M. M. (2007). Effect of 2-speed geared manual wheelchair propulsion on shoulder pain and function. *Archives of Physical Medicine and Rehabilitation, 88,* 1622-1627. http://doi.org/10.1016/j.apmr.2007.07.045

Giesbrecht, E. M., Ripat, J. D., Cooper, J. E., & Quanbury, A. O. (2011). Experiences with using a pushrim-activated power-assisted wheelchair for community-based occupations: A qualitative exploration. *Canadian Journal of Occupational Therapy, 78,* 127-136.

Giesbrecht, E. M., Ripat, J. D., Quanbury, A. O., & Cooper, J. E. (2009). Participation in community-based activities of daily living: Comparison of a pushrim-activated, power-assisted wheelchair and a power wheelchair. *Disability and Rehabilitation: Assistive Technology, 4,* 198-207. http://doi.org/10.1080/17483100802543205

Hettinga, F. J., Valent, L., Groen, W., van Drongelen, S., de Groot, S., & van der Woude, L. H. V. (2010). Hand-cycling: An active form of wheeled mobility, recreation, and sports. *Physical Medicine and Rehabilitation Clinics of North America, 21,* 127-140. http://doi.org/10.1016/j.pmr.2009.07.010

Howarth, S. J., Polgar, J. M., Dickerson, C. R., & Callaghan, J. P. (2010). Trunk muscle activity during wheelchair ramp ascent and the influence of a geared wheel on the demands of postural control. *Archives of Physical Medicine and Rehabilitation, 91,* 436-442. http://doi.org/10.1016/j.apmr.2009.10.016

Howarth, S. J., Pronovost, L. M., Polgar, J. M., Dickerson, C. R., & Callaghan, J. P. (2010). Use of a geared wheelchair wheel to reduce propulsive muscular demand during ramp ascent: Analysis of muscle activation and kinematics. *Clinical Biomechanics, 25,* 21-28. http://doi.org/10.1016/j.clinbiomech.2009.10.004

Kloosterman, M. G., Snoek, G. J., van der Woude, L. H., Buurke, J. H., & Rietman, J. S. (2013). A systematic review on the pros and cons of using a pushrim-activated power-assisted wheelchair. *Clinical Rehabilitation, 27,* 299-313. http://doi.org/10.1177/0269215512456387

Lui, J., MacGillivray, M. K., Sheel, A. W., Jeyasurya, J., Sadeghi, M., & Sawatzky, B. J. (2013). Mechanical efficiency of two commercial lever-propulsion mechanisms for manual wheelchair locomotion. *Journal of Rehabilitation Research and Development, 50,* 1363-1372. http://doi.org/10.1682/JRRD.2013.02.0034

McLaurin, C. A., & Brubaker, C. E. (1986). Lever drive system for wheelchairs. *Journal of Rehabilitation Research and Development, 23,* 52-54.

Mukherjee, G., & Samanta, A. (2001a). Energy cost and locomotor performance of the low-cost arm-lever-propelled three-wheeled chair. *International Journal of Rehabilitation Research, 24,* 245-249.

Mukherjee, G., & Samanta, A. (2001b). Physiological response to the ambulatory performance of hand-rim and arm-crank propulsion systems. *Journal of Rehabilitation Research and Development, 38,* 391-399.

van der Woude, L. H., de Groot, G., Hollander, A. P., van Ingen Schenau, G. J., & Rozendal, R. H. (1986). Wheelchair ergonomics and physiological testing of prototypes. *Ergonomics, 29,* 1561-1573. http://doi.org/10.1080/00140138608967269

van der Woude, L. H., Veeger, H. E., de Boer, Y., & Rozendal, R. H. (1993). Physiological evaluation of a newly designed lever mechanism for wheelchairs. *Journal of Medical Engineering & Technology, 17,* 232-240.

Documentation of the Seating and Mobility Assessment

Julie Piriano, PT, ATP/SMS

Documentation of the clinical evaluation and the technology assessment that identifies the product recommendations, to meet the identified needs of an individual with mobility impairments is an essential and required component of the process for the provision of seating and wheeled mobility products and services, regardless of the payer. Documentation of the clinical evaluation and product recommendations should:

- "Be client specific and refer to the client's identified problems and goals;
- Provide a clear picture of the client's physical, functional, and environmental needs;
- Include limitations of any equipment currently used by the client;
- Include intended goals of the new wheelchair and seating technology;
- [State] the recommendations made based on the assessment; and
- [Document] the rationale for [each of] those recommendations" (Arledge et al., 2011).

For consumers to be afforded the opportunity to make informed decisions about their health care, which includes their financial obligation to pay for the recommended products and services, they must be at the center of the team approach. There must be an accurate written record of each encounter, even when the individual is paying privately.

Third-party payers expect an accurate written record that supports the provision of and payment for the recommended equipment. Some third-party payers remit payment for seating and wheeled mobility products and services upon receipt of a claim. Following payment, these payers may audit files to ensure the accuracy of payment, after the fact (referred to as a *postpayment audit*). They may also recoup funds if they determine the medical need has not been established in accordance with their coverage policies. Other third-party payers require prior authorization of the recommended equipment before a claim may be submitted. However, these payers also have a right to audit the files to ensure accuracy of payments made. Typically third-party payers have a clause in their information that says, "Prior authorization is not a guarantee of payment." If the audit department determines that there is insufficient evidence to validate the medical need for the seating and wheeled mobility products and services provided, they will recover payments that have already been approved and made. In either case, the claim may be appealed through a designated process, but the evidence to establish medical need must be dated before the delivery of the equipment to the consumer.

Lastly, proper documentation is your best defense in the unlikely event of any legal action. In these rare but possible instances, the written record of the physical, functional, and environmental evaluation and treatment plan, along with the rationale for the product recommendations, are part of the legal record and will be used as evidence in a legal case.

Lange, M. L., & Minkel, J. L.
Seating and Wheeled Mobility: A Clinical Resource Guide
(pp. 261-277). © 2018 SLACK Incorporated.

MEDICAL/CLINICAL EVALUATION AND DOCUMENTATION METHODS

The problem-oriented medical record is a comprehensive approach to documenting health care encounters developed by Dr. Lawrence Weed in the late 1950s. It focuses on specific client problems, is completed in a narrative format and is often referred to as *focus charting*.

The SOAP (subjective, objective, assessment, plan) note is one such documentation method used by health care professionals to capture the details of a client encounter in the medical record. If done properly, a SOAP note will support the services provided by the health care professional as well as the decisions made in the provision of the recommended solutions to address the client's identified needs. When performing a seating and wheeled mobility evaluation and/or any follow-up related to the trial/simulation, fitting, delivery, or wheelchair skills training with the equipment the documentation of the encounter should include all four components of a SOAP note, which are as follows.

S = Subjective

All information documented in the subjective section of a SOAP note is communicated to the health care professional by the client and/or caregiver and is in his or her own words.

"At minimum, this should include the client's primary problems/issues related to his/her mobility status, postural support, health, safety, and ability to function within the environment. Assessment should also include the treatment strategies previously used to address the mobility impairments and the outcomes of that intervention" (Arledge et al., 2011).

Health care professionals may document the following:

- The client's story, chief complaint(s), past medical and mobility history
- The reason the client is seeking your assistance, advice, or intervention
- The client's response to specific questions about his or her current health, function, and/or environment

O = Objective

The objective section of a SOAP note contains data that is factual and can be measured or is observed during the client encounter. "The client's functional abilities should be assessed with regard to his or her current and desired level of activity and participation" (Arledge et al., 2011) and may include but is not be limited to the following:

- Primary diagnosis, secondary medical conditions, and onset

- The purpose of the encounter (e.g., wheelchair evaluation, trial/simulation, final fitting, modifications, wheelchair skills training, etc.)
- Observations or evaluations/assessments that can be measured and/or quantified
  - Height and weight
  - Body functions and structures—review of systems responsible for or contributing to the mobility deficit and/or postural deviations
    - Neuromuscular system (e.g., muscle tone, balance, motor control, coordination)
    - Musculoskeletal system (e.g., strength, range of motion [ROM], posture, pain)
    - Integumentary system (e.g., skin integrity, sensation)
    - Cardiovascular system (e.g., heart rate/pulse, blood pressure)
    - Respiratory system (e.g., O_2 liters/minute, respiratory rate, pulse oximetry)
  - Anthropometric measurements
  - Current equipment inspection, condition and use
  - Product demonstration/trial/simulation and outcome
    - Equipment that was tried and failed
    - Equipment that was considered and ruled out
  - Home environment/physical layout/accessibility
  - Mode of transportation
- Activities performed (level of assistance currently needed to perform/participate in activities of daily living [ADL] and instrumental ADL [IADL]—including the movement from point A to point B where the activity is typically performed)
  - Social and community activities participated in and/or attempted
  - Education and/or training provided

A = Assessment

The assessment section of a SOAP note is where the health care professional pulls it all together. It is the assimilation of the subjective report and the objective findings from the physical, functional, and environmental evaluation that forms the rationale for the equipment recommendation. This section "should be used to generate a list of the client's functional requirements, and accordingly, a list of seating and mobility goals. Products that have the desired capabilities/features to address these goals are then discussed and reviewed as options" (Arledge et al., 2011).

Completion of this section may include but is not be limited to the following:

- Your impression/interpretation/what you think
- Equipment recommendations and rationale
  - Including equipment trials/simulation outcomes and the reason(s) why the current and/or less costly, or lower level options were ruled out
  - Features, benefits, advantages, and disadvantages of available options
  - Pros and cons of available options
  - Trade-offs and compromises of available options
- Expected outcome or potential change/improvement with intervention

P = Plan

The plan should include anything that will be done as a result of the assessment. It may include, but is not limited to:

- Next steps
- Follow-up instructions

A SOAP note is just one format for capturing the details of the encounter in a narrative note. Seating and wheeled mobility evaluation forms and templates are also an effective manner in which to document the clinical evaluation, technology assessment, and recommended intervention. In addition, they can serve as a guide to ensure all aspects of the encounter are considered and addressed. Regardless of the format, a comprehensive evaluation for seating and wheeled mobility services is inclusive of the following components:

- Why is the client seeking your service/advice/intervention?
- What objective findings did you evaluate to guide your decision making?
- How did you synthesize the client's story and your evaluation results to determine a treatment plan/recommended product options?
- What next steps are necessary to meet the client's needs through implementation of your plan of care?

Health care records are increasingly being moved from a paper to electronic record. As you are documenting, in any system, be sure each of the four components of the SOAP note are included, even if this means adding comments and free text when using a documentation collection tool, such as a form or template, as part of the process.

WHAT TO WRITE

For the client to come away from the evaluation and recommendation process feeling empowered by the decisions that were made, the communication among the client, caregivers, health care professionals, and the durable medical equipment (DME) provider must be ongoing, open, and honest. This conversation becomes the framework for the information contained in the documentation. When the decision-making process is an open dialogue, with all team members engaged, it is much easier to capture the details of the encounter in a written format at the time it is happening than trying to recall the encounter and documenting the details later. Not only does this assist the client in understanding the relevant aspects of the final recommendation, it also helps paint the picture for team members, such as third-party payers, who were not present.

To establish the medical need for seating and wheeled mobility products and services, it is easiest to approach documentation in a systematic or algorithmic manner. It does not matter whether you document the need for the mobility base first, and then address the options, accessories, seating, and positioning components that will be used with it second, or if you document the individual's need for postural support components first and then address the mobility base it will be used on. The important thing to remember is to document what was considered and ruled out, what was tried and failed or tried and successful, and why—especially if the current, or least costly option is not appropriate.

For the purposes of this chapter, I approach the evaluation, documentation of a client encounter, and recommendation from the perspective of the individual's need for a mobility base first, followed by the need for its related accessories. The reason for this is that most third-party payers require the medical need for a wheelchair to be established as the first step in meeting coverage criteria for any options, accessories, seating or positioning components. Even in cases where there is substantial documentation detailing an individual's significant, non-reducible postural asymmetries and unique shape, if the need for a wheelchair is inferred, assumed, or implied, as opposed to established, it may be grounds for a denial of the entire mobility system.

REASON FOR REFERRAL AND IDENTIFICATION OF NEED

Asking open-ended questions and capturing the client's responses to those questions is likely to elicit the information you need to detail why he or she is seeking your services. This can be done as part of a screening protocol before the appointment, at the start of the encounter, or both. Depending on the situation it may also be the baseline for documenting the outcome measurement of the intervention. Questions may include, but not be limited to the following:

- Do you have a permanent need for a wheelchair?

- What is your primary diagnosis or medical condition for which you are seeking a wheelchair?

- What other conditions or diagnoses do you have or have you been treated for?

- What types of intervention/treatment have you undergone to address your medical condition(s), or are there any treatment plans in place for the future?

As a reminder, diagnosis alone is never sufficient to support the prescription for or the provision of any type of wheeled mobility device, referred to by some payers as mobility assistive equipment (MAE). A comprehensive evaluation detailing the physical and functional presentation of the individual with any diagnosis is the key to establishing the medical need for the recommended intervention, as no two people are alike, and the need for MAE cannot be implied or inferred. Knowing what body system or systems are responsible for, or contributing to, the client's mobility challenges helps to determine the complexity of the individual's needs and treatment plan most effectively.

For example, an individual whose primary diagnosis is a spinal cord injury (SCI) at the T10 level, American Spinal Injury Association (ASIA) A, that was sustained 35 years ago at age 18 years is not likely to change in his neurological presentation. However, this individual is aging with a disability. Therefore, his ability to continue self-propulsion in a manual wheelchair may be significantly limited by changes to the musculoskeletal system, cardiovascular system, and/or pulmonary system at age 53. In planning the physical and functional evaluation, it will be important to keep these body systems in mind when quantifying the mobility limitation.

Specifically in this scenario, the team would want to know about any shoulder pain, shortness of breath or self-identified limitations when the client is pushing the current manual chair. For example, does the client report difficulty pushing up a ramp or across carpet (quantified by limitations in strength or ROM) or for distances longer than 100 feet (perceived level of exertion), due to shoulder pain (rated on a pain scale) or shortness of breath (quantified by respiratory rate or changes in oxygen saturation)?

PAST EQUIPMENT HISTORY AND CURRENT MOBILITY ASSISTIVE EQUIPMENT

Many individuals with chronic medical conditions and complex medical needs change over time as a progression of their primary medical condition, as a result of secondary medical conditions/complications, or due to a new medical condition that was not present at the time the original wheelchair was dispensed. As a result, they may have used, or have experience with, a variety of mobility devices. Never assume that the device the individual is using when he or she arrives at the evaluation is his or her own personal mobility device, or that it is his or her primary/only mode of mobility. To determine a client's past equipment history and current MAE it is important to ask and document his or her response to questions such as the following:

1. **Do you have, or have you ever used, a gait or ambulation aid such as a cane or a walker?**

   a. If yes, what is/was your experience with it?

   b. If no, do you have any concerns with trying/using one?

2. **Do you have, or have you ever used, a manual wheelchair?**

   a. If yes, what is/was your experience with it?

   i. What type of wheelchair did you use?

   ii. Are there any features of the manual wheelchair that you like or that we need to make sure we keep the same?

   iii. Are there any features that you do not like or that are not working properly that need to be addressed?

   b. If no, do you have any concerns with trying/using one?

3. **Do you have, or have you ever tried, a scooter?**

   a. If yes, where did you try it, and what was your experience?

   b. If no, do you have any concerns with trying/using one?

4. **Do you have, or have you ever tried, a power wheelchair?**

   a. If yes, what was your experience with it?

   i. Are there any features of the power wheelchair that you like, or that we need to make sure we keep the same?

   ii. Are there any features that you do not like, or that are not working properly that need to be addressed?

   b. If no, do you have any concerns with trying/using one?

It is also important to note that for many individuals who use MAE, their perception of changes in their own mobility status is often slow. As a result of slow recognition of change, the individual may make accommodations for the mobility challenges by changing his or her activities and participation over time without noticing the impact of those changes.

CASE EXAMPLE

For example, a 76-year-old woman with a diagnosis of chronic obstructive pulmonary disease (COPD) and osteoarthritis in the hips and knees may be able to carry out all of her ADL safely, timely, and independently using a cane for a number of years after these diagnoses. During the course of her medical management, her medications and dosages are changed; she is placed on oxygen, which is increased over time; and she has participated in outpatient physical therapy to decrease her pain and increase her strength, ROM, and endurance.

With the progressive decline of her pulmonary function and the gradual deterioration of her joints, however, she begins to forego nutrition and hydration to limit the number of trips she has to make to the kitchen and bathroom each day. This is not because she can no longer walk but because of the high physiological cost (e.g., pain, fatigue, shortness of breath) to do so. She has fallen three times in the past month due to syncope and is now being seen for a wheelchair evaluation because she has fractured her hip and is nonweightbearing postsurgery. She arrives at the evaluation in a manual wheelchair but may have no experience in using one, and in fact it may be medically contraindicated for her to do so. Hence, it is important to listen to and document the individual's subjective report of her mobility history to plan for your physical and functional evaluation. Likewise, it is equally important for the health care professional to document the objective findings that are relevant to the mobility limitations for a remote reviewer to understand what is specifically limiting the patient's mobility.

For individuals who currently have or use a manual wheelchair, scooter, or power wheelchair, "particular attention should be given to the set-up of the client's current equipment and its components. When a client has been using equipment long term, he or she may adapt to the configuration of the equipment and seemingly small changes in equipment can result in significant functional changes for the client" (Arledge et al., 2011). Digging a little deeper into the current mode of mobility may include questions such as the following:

5. **What is your primary means of mobility inside your home?**

   a. If a current wheelchair user:

   i. How long are you able to sit in your wheelchair during the day?

   ii. Are you able to change your body position/relieve pressure as needed?

   iii. Are you able to set the wheelchair up and transfer to/from it?

   b. Does it allow you to move throughout your home in a timely manner, with or without assistance, or difficulty throughout the day?

   i. Are there any distances you are having trouble negotiating?

   ii. Are there any surfaces or obstacles (i.e., doors, thresholds, turns) you are having trouble navigating?

   iii. Are there any rooms you are having trouble accessing? If yes, why?

   c. Does it allow you to carry out the tasks you need to accomplish throughout the day, each day of the week, every week?

   i. Are you able to get to and move about in the bathroom, bedroom, and kitchen for toileting, bathing, grooming, dressing, and eating? If no, how do you compensate for the difficulty?

   ii. Are you able to reach all surfaces (floor, level, and overhead) and do laundry, prepare meals, clean house, for example? If no, how do you compensate for the difficulty?

   d. Are you having any health issues as a result of your current mode of mobility?

   i. Have you fallen or been injured as a result of your mobility challenges? If yes, what are the circumstances of the fall?

   ii. Do you have any cuts, bruises, sores, or pressure ulcers? If yes, how did they develop?

   iii. Are you experiencing any problems breathing, chewing, or swallowing? If yes, when does this occur and what happens?

   iv. Do you have any pain or fatigue when trying to move about your home? If yes, what brings it on, and what alleviates it?

In the United States, many third-party payers' coverage criteria for MAE are predicated on the need for its use in the home. Therefore, it is important to capture the details of the current mobility situation from the client's perspective to establish that there is a mobility limitation. It does not matter whether the individual is not using MAE, or if he or she is using a cane, walker, manual wheelchair, scooter, or other powered mobility device; you are trying to ascertain whether he or she is safe, timely, and independent with the current mode of mobility in his or her home. If he or she is, then you will want to determine other reasons for the referral. For example, the primary limitation is longer distance mobility within a community setting. If the person is not functional within the home, you will want to determine whether traditional therapy services will mitigate the mobility deficits or if a seating and wheeled mobility evaluation or wheelchair skills training is warranted.

For some payers, if there is no documented need for use of the wheelchair in the home, it is not considered a covered benefit. However, if there is an established need for its use in the home, it is recognized that the individual will also need to use the equipment outside of the home. Therefore, it is also important to determine the other settings of anticipated use.

6. **What is your primary means of mobility outside the home? This may include, but not be limited to, the community, school, and/or work.**

   a. Are you able to get to and participate in all activities you want and need to?

   b. Are there any environmental limitations, such as distances, surfaces (level and unlevel), obstacles (e.g., ramps, curbs) or terrains (e.g., grass, gravel) you are having difficulty negotiating?

   c. Are there any issues or challenges with transportation (e.g., public, private)?

Remember, not all payers restrict coverage criteria to use in the home. In some cases, community mobility must be specifically addressed, but in all cases, it should be considered for the safety of the wheelchair user.

Regardless of the payers coverage criteria, the client should be informed of all the options available to meet his or her mobility needs in the home and community. For some clients, the best answer to this question is the identification of two different devices. For others, the same device will meet the needs both in the home and in the community. If the client has a need that is not met by a covered benefit, then he or she is in a position to make an informed decision about identifying and using other resources to purchase the solutions that meet his or her identified needs.

CONDITION OF THE CURRENT MOBILITY ASSISTIVE EQUIPMENT

The technology assessment may include an evaluation and safety check of the client's current wheelchair to determine whether it will be safe and operable until a new wheelchair is received. If the current wheelchair needs to be repaired, or if modifications to the existing device will meet the individual's mobility needs, then those decisions need to be documented. When assessing the person's current mobility device, the following should be noted:

- Manufacturer, make, and model

- Age and condition of mobility base device

- Specific features and dimensions (i.e., seat height, width, and depth, back height, overall chair width, depth and configuration)

- Safety and reliability of key components (i.e., frame, tires, batteries, mechanical components)

- All options, accessories, seating, and positioning components used with the base

If the device is not in good working order or is placing the client in harm's way, repairs to the current equipment may be necessary to keep it safe and operational during its reasonable useful lifetime, which is typically 5 years. If the chair has been in use for 5 years or more, it may also require repairs while the individual is going through the process to obtain a new wheelchair. This is especially true with complex rehabilitation manual and power wheelchairs that are designed to fit and function for the individual user, as a temporary, replacement device is typically not available to meet their unique needs. However, if the current wheelchair is less than 5 years old and is irreparably damaged or the repairs exceed the replacement cost of a new wheelchair, it will be important to thoroughly document the extent and cost of the repairs as a critical part of the record needed to document the need for a new chair.

If the current wheelchair is in good working order but no longer meets the medical needs of the individual user, consideration may be given to whether the base can be modified to meet the new medical needs of the individual. If it can be modified, then the evaluation should proceed with capturing the details of the physical and functional changes that are observed due to the change in condition. If it cannot be modified to meet the new medical need of the individual, the specific reason(s) preventing modification should be reflected in the details of the technology assessment. This may include, but not be limited to, an incompatibility of new components interfacing with an older model wheelchair structurally or electrically.

PHYSICAL AND FUNCTIONAL EVALUATION

When performing a comprehensive seating and wheeled mobility evaluation, "it is important to consider both body functions and impairments" (Arledge, et al., 2011). According to the *Rehabilitation Engineering and Assistive Technology Society of North America Wheelchair Service Provision Guide*, "the evaluation should include consideration of anatomical alignment, postural control (sitting balance), skin integrity, the neuromuscular system (strength, ROM, tone, coordination, and sensation), vision, cognition, speech and language, as well as the cardiovascular, respiratory, digestive, and urinary systems. The following aspects of body function and structures should be assessed:

- The neuromuscular system including muscle strength, gross and fine motor control and coordination, muscle tone and spasticity, and sitting and standing balance;

- Range of motion and flexibility of the full body including pelvis, hips, knees, ankles and spine, and presence of skeletal alignment/asymmetry, such as a…[reducible or non-reducible] postural scoliosis;

- Current and past skin integrity issues such as persistent redness, pressure ulcers, open areas, or scar tissue; and

- Current mobility skills, including client's ability to functionally ambulate, propel a manual wheelchair and/or operate a power wheelchair. These skills include such factors as independence, safety, timeliness, quality of the client's ability as related to his or her daily activities, and his or her ability to move safely and efficiently through the environment. Visual processing, cognitive awareness of the environment, and motor control should be taken into account." (Arledge et al., 2011)

QUANTITATIVE EVALUATION INFORMATION VERSUS SUBJECTIVE ASSESSMENT INFORMATION

When capturing the detail of this information, it is important to do so in quantitative terms. Not only does this demonstrate that a direct, in-person evaluation took place, it may provide the evidence needed to support why the mobility base was selected over a less costly, or lower level device on the mobility hierarchy. As part of the specialty evaluation for wheelchair options and accessories, quantitative findings may also provide the reasons or evidence for the recommendations being made.

Figure 16-1 is an example of the quantitative information health care professionals may include in the objective section of a seating and wheeled mobility evaluation. This information is then used to relate the equipment recommendations from the technology assessment to the individual's identified needs and goals in his or her home and community.

The quantitative details of the evaluation should provide the objective measure to substantiate the client's subjective assessment of his or her mobility limitation. Quantifiable data also provide the basis for the equipment justification and, when necessary, demonstrate a change in medical need for seating and wheeled mobility products and services due to a change in the individual's presentation, even when the diagnosis does not change.

CASE EXAMPLE

A 35-year-old woman with a diagnosis of multiple sclerosis (MS) who is evaluated for a seating and wheeled mobility device initially presents with 4/5, or good static and dynamic sitting balance, and 3/5, or fair static standing balance, and the ability to transfer to and from a chair independently using a modified sit-pivot technique leading with either her right or her left side. She requires moderate assist to ambulate 15 feet with a walker due to fair minus (3–/5) dynamic balance and 3/5 fair strength in her quadriceps, hamstrings, and gastrocnemius muscles. She walks 0 feet independently. Upper extremity strength is 4/5 or good overall, and grip strength is measured 25 kg bilaterally (within 1 standard deviation of normal for age). Use of a manual wheelchair requires maximum assist. She is not capable of performing the repetitive motion necessary to self-propel because of a perceived exertion level of 5 (heavy) after pushing less than 5 minutes on a level tile floor using her upper extremities. Other surfaces, such as carpet, were not tested as perceived exertion increases to a 7+ (very heavy) in the afternoon and prevents her from preparing a meal because she needs to conserve her energy to use the bathroom and transfer to bed. ROM is within normal limits, and skin and sensation are intact. Client is able to attain anatomical sitting alignment, and no postural deviations were noted. Client transferred to and from a scooter independently and was able to sit in and operate it safely, timely, and independently in all four directions.

Twenty-four months later, after an exacerbation of her MS, she presents with fair (3/5) head control, poor (2/5) sitting balance, and is dependent in standing. She requires maximal assist to transfer and is nonambulatory. Strength is 2/5 (poor) in the lower extremities and 3–/5 (fair–) in the upper extremities. She sits with a posterior pelvic tilt, increased thoracic kyphosis, and forward head position. Her asymmetry is reducible to neutral alignment with postural supports. ROM is within normal limits, sensation and skin are intact; however, she is unable to perform a functional weight shift due to her strength limitations, poor sitting balance and inability to stand/transfer. A manual wheelchair was previously ruled out, and her scooter cannot meet her new medical need due to her inability to sit upright against gravity.

As a reminder:

- The evaluation should be tailored to the individual, not the diagnosis. If the respiratory system is compromising an individual's mobility, then the evaluation would focus more heavily on the impact ambulation and self-propulsion has on O_2 saturation and respiratory rate and may include a respiratory therapist as part of the evaluation team.

Quantitative Evaluation Information	Subjective Assessment Information
1. Balance (Sitting / Standing) (Static / Dynamic) – 0, 1, 2, 3, 4, 5 Dependent, Poor, Fair, Good, Normal	1. Unsteady, falls, history of falls
2. Strength – 0/5, 1/5, 2/5, 3/5, 4/5, 5/5(+ / -) No movement, Trace, Poor, Fair, Good, Normal Within Normal Limits (WNL) or Within Functional Limits (WFL)	2. Generalized weakness, weak decreased or limited strength
Grip strength measurement of_____#	Weak grasp, poor grip
3. Range of motion (PROM / AROM) – Goniometric Measurement (-40 degrees, 20 – 110 degrees) WNL (within normal limits) WFL (within functional limits)	3. Decreased or limited range of motion, poor reach
4. Tone and Reflexes – Hypertonic, Spastic, Hypotonic, Flaccid, Fluctuating tone, Athetoid, Ataxic, Tremors ATNR, STNR, Extensor Thrust, Clonus Modified Ashworth Score of _____ (0 – 5)	4. Stiff, Limp, Uncoordinated, Shaky, Jerky
5. Sensation – Intact, Impaired or Absent to: light touch, sharp/dull, deep pressure with a description of the dermatome or size and location	5. Numbness, tingling
6. Skin integrity – Stage, location and size of pressure injury Location, size and condition of scars, cuts, tears	6. Pressure injury, Compromised skin, open area on (body part)
Braden scale score of _____	At risk for skin breakdown
7. Pain rates 0 – 10 on the pain scale	7. Painful, has pain, experiences pain
8. Respiratory – _____liters O_2/ minute, O_2 saturation levels, Pulse oximetry readings, Vital capacity, Respiration rate pre/post mobility attempts	8. Short of breath, gasping, wheezing
9. Blood pressure___/___, heart rate or pulse	9. Chest pain, light headed
10. Exertion rates 0 – 10 a perceived exertion scale	10. Poor endurance
11. Posture – Pelvic tilt, Pelvic obliquity, Pelvic rotation Kyphosis, Lordosis, Scoliosis Abduction/Adduction, Flexion/Extension, Rotation	11. Leaning, Slouching

Figure 16-1. Evaluation vs assessment information. (PROM = passive range of motion; AROM = active range of motion; ATNR = asymmetrical tonic neck reflex; STNR = symmetrical tonic neck reflex.) *(continued)*

12. Transfers to/from wheelchair by Stand-pivot, sit pivot, sliding board Requires max. (75%), mod. (50%), min. (25%), stand by assistance, contact guard assistance, supervision or dependent (uses a mechanical lift)	12. Needs assistances, used to be able to do.
13. Ambulates_____feet with_____device Dependent/non-ambulatory/(100%) assistance Requires max. (75%), mod. (50%), min. (25%), stand by assistance, contact guard assistance or supervision to ambulate on _____surfaces Timed up and go test at _____ sec.	13. Not an independent ambulator Not a functional ambulator Not a safe ambulator Slow
14. Propels a manual w/c_____feet with Both or bilateral upper extremities (BUE) Both or bilateral lower extremities (BLE) Right upper and lower extremities (RUE/RLE) Left upper and lower extremities (LLE/LLE) Dependent/(100%) assistance Requires max. (75%), mod. (50%), min. (25%), stand by assistance, contact guard assistance or supervision to propel on _____ surfaces Timeliness? Efficiency? Settings of anticipated use?	14. Can use a MWC (if recommending a MWC) Non-functional MWC propulsion (if ruling out a MWC)
15. Transfers to/from a scooter independently and Utilizes the tiller/controls independently or Dependent/(100%) assistance Requires max. (75%), mod. (50%), min. (25%), stand by assistance, contact guard assistance or supervision to transfer, sit in, or operate a scooter on _____surfaces/in _____direction	15. Able to use a scooter/POV (if recommending a scooter/POV) Unable to use a scooter/POV (if ruling out a scooter/POV)
16. Safely operates a power w/c_____ feet Forward, Backward, Right turn, Left turn with a: • Standard joystick • Upgraded proportional joystick • Alternative proportional drive control _____ • Non-proportional drive control _____ Requires max. (75%), mod. (50%), min. (25%), stand by assistance, contact guard assistance or supervision to _____	16. Able to drive a power wheelchair (if recommending a PWC)

Figure 16-1 (continued). Evaluation vs assessment information. (POV = power-operated vehicle.)

- Not all MAE must be tried to prove it will not be appropriate for a particular individual. If a device is ruled out as medically contraindicated, a brief statement as to why there is a contraindication should be included. For example, a gait aid is ruled out for our client with an SCI at the T10 level, ASIA A, because he has no sensory or motor control below the level of injury.

Accurate height, weight, and anthropometric measurements of the individual are also important components of the basic seating and wheeled mobility evaluation. Hip width (O), thigh depth (L), lower leg length (P), and elbow height (K) measurements are recommended on each client. It does not matter who takes the measurements as long as they are done correctly. Often it is the DME provider who is documenting this as part of the technology assessment.

These person-specific measurements are used to identify the size and dimensions of the products being recommended to address the mobility and seating interventions. These measurements can also serve to demonstrate physical changes that warrant a modification to the client's current chair or the provision of a new chair in the event the current chair cannot be modified to meet the person's new size or shape.

For example, one client with an SCI may have experienced atrophy, lost muscle mass, and require a much narrower wheelchair 1 or 2 years postinjury, whereas a second client may show no weight gain on the scale but physically become wider across the hips, necessitating a wider frame. The only way to prove this to a third-party payer is to have the client's measurements at initial issue and subsequent measurements, which illustrate the change in the individual's size.

An outline such as the following may be used to remind the team which measurements to take. The following is a list of the basic set of measurements for hands-free sitters:

- Hip width (External knee width should be measured if wider than hip width.)
- Chest width
- Shoulder width
- Buttock/thigh depth
- Lower leg length
- Elbow height
- Shoulder height (Scapula height or axilla height can be taken as an alternative to shoulder height, depending on the planned style of back support, to help determine desired back support length and height (Waugh & Crane, 2013).
- Maximum sitting height

Figure 16-2 is a chart of full set of measurements for persons with more complex needs.

Quantifying a Mobility Limitation

As of 2005, the Centers for Medicare & Medicaid Service (CMS) National Coverage Determination for MAE uses the following description of a mobility limitation.

"A mobility limitation is one that:

- Prevents the beneficiary from accomplishing the MRADLs [mobility-related ADL] entirely [*Independently*];
- Places the beneficiary at reasonably determined heightened risk of morbidity or mortality secondary to the attempts to participate in MRADLs; [*Safely*]

- Prevents the beneficiary from completing the MRADLs within a reasonable time frame [*Timely*]." (CMS, 2005)

Therefore, if an individual requires any level of assistance (i.e., maximum assist, moderate assist, minimal assist, stand-by assist, contact guard, or supervision) to move from point A to point B, he or she is not independent. If you are documenting that the person can ambulate (or propel) 1000 feet with moderate assistance, it is helpful to further clarify that he or she ambulates (or propels) 0 feet independently. Although this may seem unnecessary, based on the definition of the levels of assistance, remember that there is no guarantee the reviewer for the third-party payer has an intimate working knowledge of the levels of assistance. It is better to paint the picture by stating what you have observed and document it.

Safety is not just about a fall risk. An individual who is at risk for falls would be deemed not independent, which was addressed earlier. Safety also refers to the physiological response to moving from point A to point B. For example, our 76-year-old female with COPD and osteoarthritis may be able to ambulate without assistance once her hip fracture is healed, according to the orthopedic surgeon. However, on further examination you find that her pulse oximetry reading drops to 78% O_2, while on 3L of continuous oxygen, when she stands up from a seated position. This puts her at significant risk for complications secondary to her attempts to ambulate. In this case, it would be important to state that ambulation and manual wheelchair propulsion are medically contraindicated as a result of this finding. There is no need to place her in harm's way to confirm these findings.

Lastly, if timeliness in moving from point A to point B is compromised, documenting this in a quantitative manner by performing the Timed Up and Go (TUG) test may be appropriate. To calculate walking, or self-propulsion speed, simply plug in the distance the client walks (or pushes his or her wheelchair) and the amount of time (in seconds) it took him or her to cover the distance into the formula in Figure 16-3.

Although there is no validated TUG test for manual wheelchair propulsion, it may be necessary to demonstrate the difference in self-propulsion between a standard high-strength, lightweight manual wheelchair and an ultralightweight manual wheelchair in a quantitative manner. To do this, mark a fixed distance on the floor with tape. When you say "go," have the individual push the standard lightweight/high-strength lightweight wheelchair from one tape line to the next. Count the number of strokes and time it takes to cover the distance. Repeat the test with the ultralightweight wheelchair that is optimally configured for the individual. (For more on this, refer to Chapter 9.) Again, count the number of strokes and the time it takes to reach the second tape line. If it takes less time and fewer strokes to cover the distance it may quantitatively substantiate a more generalized statement that

MEASUREMENTS	LEFT	RIGHT		LEFT	RIGHT
A Max. sitting height		_____	**J** Forearm depth	_____	_____
B Occiput height		_____	**K** Elbow height	_____	_____
C Head width		_____	**L** Thigh depth	_____	_____
D Shoulder width		_____	**M** PSIS height	_____	_____
E Chest width		_____	**N** Ischial depth	_____	_____
F Trunk depth		_____	**O** Hip width*		_____
G Shoulder height	_____	_____	External knee width		_____
H Axilla height**	_____	_____	**P** Lower leg length	_____	_____
I Scapular height**	_____	_____	**Q** Foot depth	_____	_____
_____	_____		_____	_____	_____

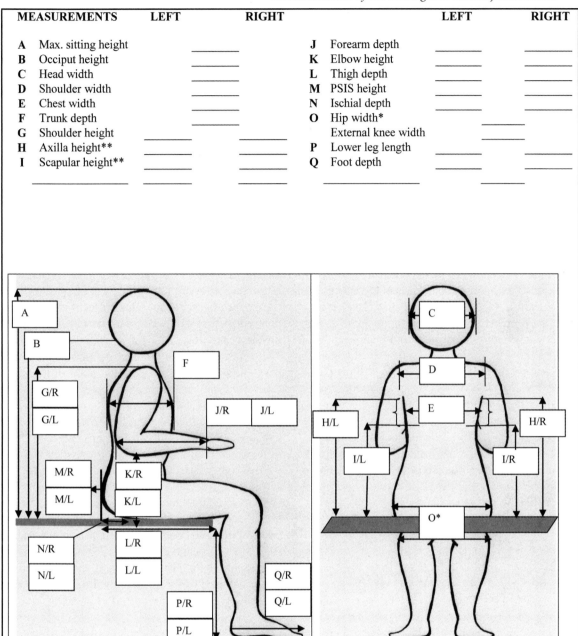

Figure 16-2. Seating anthropometric measurement guide. (PSIS = posterior superior iliac spine.)

$$\frac{X\ ft.}{Y\ sec.} \times \frac{3600\ sec.}{5280\ ft.} = Z\ miles\,/\,hour$$

As a result:

- 4 miles / hour = 5.86 ft. / sec.
- 3 miles / hour = 4.40 ft. / sec.
- 2 miles / hour = 2.93 ft. / sec.
- 1 mile / hour = 1.46 ft. / sec.
- .5 miles / hour = 0.73 ft. / sec.
-

(Note: Average walking speed for an adult is approximately 2.5 – 3.0 miles / hour)

Figure 16-3. Walking speed calculation formula.

says, "Client needs an ultralightweight wheelchair for increased efficiency in propulsion." It may also support the point that an ultralightweight wheelchair is necessary to reduce the risk of repetitive strain injury in the upper extremities as outlined in the publication "Preservation of Upper Limb Function Following Spinal Cord Injury: A Clinical Practice Guideline for Health-Care Professionals" (Paralyzed Veterans of America Consortium for Spinal Cord Medicine, 2005).

A timed test for manual wheelchair propulsion may be an effective way to demonstrate to a payer, and our 53-year-old gentleman who is 35 years postSCI, ASIA A, at the T10 level, that it is time to transition to a power wheelchair or power assist wheels. Although he is likely still able to push and make the chair advance in all directions the following questions arise, "At what speed?" "At what cost?" and "In which environments?" In conducting the propulsion test, it may be important to document the client's pain rating on a scale of 1 to 10, his O_2 saturation level, respiratory rate, blood pressure, heart rate, and/or pulse in light of his secondary medical conditions and complications. If there is an adverse physiological response or the inability to push a manual chair at least as fast as a walking person beside the wheelchair user, that is mitigated by a trial use of a power wheelchair, or power assist wheels, this may help quantify the difference.

In a situation where the individual is able to independently self-propel but has significant weight added to the chair from medically necessary postural support components, a timed manual wheelchair test may also demonstrate the ineffectiveness of such a system.

Detailing the Postural Evaluation

By most payers' standards, if the individual qualifies for a wheelchair, he or she qualifies for a basic seat cushion and back support to use on the mobility base. However, to configure the wheelchair so that it fits and functions for your client, a comprehensive postural evaluation should be conducted to ensure his or her seating needs are met.

In sitting, there are numerous bony prominences that may come in contact with the wheelchair support surfaces, including seating and positioning components. When postural asymmetries are noted, the position and significance of these bony prominences can change and skin breakdown can occur in less likely places, such as the spinous processes. Therefore, a thorough inspection of the client's skin and sensation is warranted, even if there are no reported decubitus ulcers documented, as it gives the team a baseline measure. Often the right wheelchair may afford the individual independent mobility, such that he or she spends a significantly greater portion of his day in the seated

position. If the skin is intact, it should be documented to ensure that skin integrity was addressed. Any scars, cuts, tears, redness, discoloration, or open wounds should be notated with regard to the location, size, condition, and stage, as appropriate. In addition, numbness, tingling, and absence or impairment of sensation in the dermatomes may also be noted.

If a postural asymmetry is identified, quantify the degree of the deviation to the best of your ability. Often taking a picture of the client (with permission) sitting in his or her typical, unsupported posture and then again in a supported posture, helps the reviewer (and at times the client) see the degree of asymmetry present. If the asymmetry is reducible or partially reducible, it is important to convey reducibility as a clinical finding. However, if the asymmetry is not reducible, you do not want to indicate to a third-party payer that the asymmetry is fixed. In fact, a non-reducible asymmetry may progress and worsen due to the effects of gravity and other influences. Using the term non-reducible as opposed to fixed may avoid an unintended misunderstanding.

It is also important to detail the impact the asymmetry has on the client's ability to maintain his or her health and ability to function in the environment. For example, our now 37-year-old woman with MS, whose postural tendency is to sit with a posterior pelvic tilt, increased thoracic kyphosis, and forward head position, may have significant difficulty in taking a deep inspiration, effectuating a productive cough, managing her saliva, chewing her food, or swallowing safely as a result of her posture. Her postural evaluation may include other nontraditional members of the health care team, such as nurses, speech and language pathologists, and respiratory therapists as the team evaluates and documents the best positions for her to sit in, and the support components necessary to achieve them. This is best accomplished by performing an equipment trial and simulation.

Documenting Equipment Trials and Simulation

Information derived from the subjective and objective components of the process are used to develop the treatment plan. This may include, but not be limited to, a list of equipment parameters and requirements that are necessary to meet the identified seating and mobility goals of the client.

"After reviewing the possible product options, a product trial should be arranged for the client to determine whether the product meets the client's needs and to assist him or her in selecting the final product. If a product is readily available, a trial may occur during the assessment session itself" (Arledge et al., 2011).

If the most appropriate trial equipment is not readily available, separate sessions in the clinic or in other environments may be needed. The treatment plan, including number of visits and location of service, will be dependent on the complexity of the client's needs, the range of readily available trial equipment, and consideration of specific environments of use.

The device "trial and selection process should be an educational experience for the client/caregiver(s) to assist them in making informed decisions. This process should include a discussion of options, including the range of products available to meet the client/caregivers' specific needs and goal(s)" (Arledge et al., 2011). In documenting the success or failure of equipment that is tried or simulated, it is important to capture the positive or negative impact the trial has on the individual. From the client's perspective, discussing what the mobility base, option, accessory, seating, or positioning component does or using generic statements about its intended use are ineffective. Nonspecific discussions about product features can leave the client feeling like he or she received a product "because it's what 'they' told me I needed" and leave the client feeling like an outsider from the therapist and supplier team.

For example, power tilt, power recline, and power leg elevation with articulation is often recommended for individuals who cannot perform a functional weight shift, and hence are more susceptible to the development of a decubitus ulcer. Unfortunately, the evaluation finding details in support of such a statement may be omitted from the conversation and documentation, leaving the client confused and a reviewer with the opportunity to deny the power wheelchair with multiple power options. If the client is unable to perform an independent transfer to and from his or her chair, it is highly likely he or she is also unable to shift his or her weight an adequate number of times for a sufficient duration to allow reperfusion of blood to the weightbearing area to occur. Therefore, it is important to follow a statement such as, "He is unable to perform a functional weight shift" with *because*, and list all the reasons identified during the physical and functional evaluation. These reasons may include, but are not limited to, upper extremity strength issues, compromised balance, and the inability to unweight the pelvis, similar to the action of performing a transfer. To further demonstrate the efficacy of the recommended power seat functions document the individual's response to the trial of his or her use in relation to all issues identified during the physical and functional evaluation.

Although power seating functions may be the most effective way for the individual with complex medical needs to independently manage her position in space and redistribute pressure at the bony prominences, he or she is still at risk for the development of decubitus ulcers due to the length of time spent in the wheelchair. Appropriate, properly placed postural support components, and a cushion that promotes envelopment, reduces interface temperature, and wicks away moisture may all provide additional aid in mitigating the development of a pressure ulcer of the skin on weightbearing areas while seated. During the trial and simulation process, an inspection of the client's skin and its reaction to the proposed intervention is important. Bony prominences, scars, cuts, tears, redness, discoloration, or open wounds that were noted during the physical examination should be monitored for changes as various seating and wheeled mobility devices are mocked up and tried.

Lastly, if any tools (e.g., pressure mapping, pulse oximetry) are used to quantify the individual's issues with his or her current seating and wheeled mobility device or in response to proposed interventions that are tried, it is important to document and interpret the results of these tests in the client's file.

"Ultimately these measures can be used to determine the success of the outcome of the chosen technology intervention. These objective measures should identify and quantify problem areas at baseline and at reevaluation and may include digital photography, skills performance (transfers and/or propulsion), propulsion analyses, and pressure analyses. Assessments may also be used to compare and contrast wheelchairs, seat cushions, back supports, and positioning components, or to compare control systems for powered wheelchairs regarding comfort, safety and client acceptance of use" (Arledge et al., 2011).

CONSIDERING THE ENVIRONMENT AND TRANSPORTATION

The Durable Medical Equipment, Prosthetics, Orthotics and Supplies (DMEPOS) Quality Standards, issued by CMS in 2008, states that the DME provider "shall, as applicable, ensure that the beneficiary and/or caregiver(s) can use all equipment and item(s) provided safely and effectively in the settings of anticipated use" (DMEPOS Quality Standards, 2008).

"In addition to collecting information regarding the client's home, school, work and other community environments, the client's transportation requirements, characteristics of indoor/outdoor terrain, and typical weather conditions should also be addressed. An environmental assessment should include [the client's]:

- Ability to enter/exit settings of routine use
- Ability to maneuver within the current/anticipated environments
- Ability to reach and/or access all items, furnishings, and surfaces necessary to carry out daily activities
- Ability to transfer to/from the wheelchair
- Ability to use personal or public transportation" (Arledge et al., 2011)

ASSESSMENT AND PLAN

A letter of medical necessity (LMN) is often used to summarize the client's identified problems and provide the rationale for the recommended equipment. When this information is presented in a standalone document, it may not be considered part of the medical record. This is especially true if the LMN contains statements or justification for the wheelchair or its related accessories that is not substantiated in the written report of the evaluation encounter. However, regardless of whether the SOAP note format is followed or an evaluation and justification documentation collection tool is used, the equipment justification is documented as the assessment component of the encounter.

The assessment should be client-specific and detail how the intervention addresses the identified problems. For example, stating that our 37-year-old female with MS requires power recline to manage her spasticity may be accurate, but there is no evidence that she has spasticity or that it is an identified problem. Therefore, although spasticity management may be one indication for use of this power seat function, per a payers' coverage criterion, its use is not supported in the client's current medical record. However, if spasticity is an identified issue and it was evaluated and documented in a quantitative manner, such as a modified Ashworth score, then the rationale may state, "Power recline will be used to provide a controlled stretch to the identified muscle(s) to manage spasticity brought on by changes in temperature, humidity, and prolonged sitting."

WHAT IS THE LEGAL HEALTH RECORD AND DESIGNATED RECORD SET?

"The legal health record is the documentation of health care services provided to an individual during any aspect of health care delivery in any type of health care organization. The legal health record serves:

- To support the decisions made in a patient's care;

- To support the revenue sought from third-party payers;

- To document the services provided as legal testimony regarding the patient's illness or injury, response to treatment, and caregiver decisions; and

- As the organization's business and legal record.

Historically, reports, or findings, on which clinical decision-making is based, are parts of the legal health record. The determining factor in whether information is to be considered part of the legal health record is not where it resides or the format it takes but rather how it is used and whether it may be reasonably expected to be routinely released when a request for a complete medical record is received" (American Health Information Management Association [AHIMA], 2011).

Clinicians, physicians, and other health care professionals actively engaged in the evaluation and recommendation process for seating and wheeled mobility equipment rarely question their legal obligation to provide a written record of their encounter(s) with the client. However, the documentation to substantiate the medical need for the device(s) may be viewed as lacking sufficient detail to warrant the provision of the recommended item(s) by third-party payers.

DME suppliers, including complex rehabilitation technology suppliers, often state that their technology assessment, which is a key component in matching the identified needs of the individual with the recommended technology solutions to address their needs, is not considered part of the medical record. As a result the supplier's file may be viewed as lacking sufficient detail to support prior authorization or payment for a wheelchair base and related accessories by third-party payers. However, the fact that DME providers submit claims to third-party payers for seating and wheeled mobility products and services, as recommended by health care professionals and prescribed by a physician, places them in the continuum of medical care as a covered entity. Hence, their records are, at a minimum, considered part of the designated record.

"The HIPAA (Health Insurance Portability and Accountability Act of 1996) privacy rule defines the designated record set as a group of records maintained by or for a covered entity that may include:

- Patient medical and billing records;

- The enrollment, payment, claims, adjudication, and case management or medical management record systems maintained by or for a health plan; or

- Information used in whole or in part to make care-related decisions.

If external records and reports are used to make decisions about an individual, they become part of the designated record set. If those decisions are care decisions, in most cases those same records and reports will also be included in the provider's legal health record" (AHIMA, 2011). Therefore, health care professionals and providers should be mindful of the concept that *if you did not document it, it was not done* as they approach the documentation details of their seating and wheeled mobility evaluations.

FUNDAMENTALS OF MEDICAL RECORD DOCUMENTATION

From the U.S. Code of Federal Regulations, often referred to as the *Federal Register*, 42 CFR Section 482.24(c)(1), states that "all patient medical record entries must be legible, complete, dated, timed, and authenticated in written or electronic form by the person responsible for providing or evaluating the service provided, consistent with hospital policies and procedures" (CMS, 2012). Medical records that are not legible may be misread or misinterpreted and could lead to inappropriate recommendations, inaccurate decisions, or contribute to an adverse medical outcome, and medical records that are incomplete may delay access to care or cause medically necessary equipment to be denied by third-party payers for failure to meet stated coverage criteria.

CMS interpretive guidelines of 42 CFR Section 482.24(c)(1) explains that "a medical record is considered complete if it contains:

- Sufficient information to identify the patient;
- Support the diagnosis/condition;
- Justify the care, treatment, and services;
- Document the course and results of care, treatment, and services; and
- Promote continuity of care among providers." (CMS, 2009)

"For medical review purposes, Medicare requires that services provided/ordered be authenticated by the author. The method used shall be a handwritten or electronic signature. Stamped signatures are not acceptable" (CMS, 2013a, p. 35). The signature must be legible or accompanied by a signature log to authenticate the author and should be dated to validate when the services were performed or ordered. "Providers using electronic systems need to recognize that there is a potential for misuse or abuse with alternate signature methods. For example, providers need a system and software products that are protected against modification, etc., and should apply adequate administrative procedures that correspond to recognized standards and laws" (CMS, 2013a).

With these criteria in mind, a health care professional's entry in the medical record, together with the provider's entry in the client's file that captures the details of the wheelchair evaluation, trial/simulation, and recommendation process, should contain sufficient evidence to establish the consumer's medical need for the mobility base and all related accessories. It should also confirm the recommended technology will address those needs and explain why less expensive options were either tried and failed or considered and ruled out.

LEGAL IMPLICATIONS

The client's legal health record is admissible in court. As such, it is important for health care professionals and providers to understand that there is a significant difference between *documents* and *documentation*. Documents, according to the *Oxford Dictionary* (n.d.), are simply the "written, printed, or electronic matter that provides information or evidence or that serves as an official record" (Oxford, n.d.). For example, a detailed product description (DPD) provides a line-by-line description of a configured wheelchair. The DPD is a document within a beneficiary's record. Whether or not the prescribed chair was ordered, delivered, and fitted to the client will need to be *documented* by the service provider who provides the service.

Accurate documents and documentation can provide crucial legal protection for the author and the company/facility he or she works for when they are complete, accurate, clear, concise, logical, written in a timely manner, signed, and dated.

In the event that the documents that comprise a beneficiary's designated record set, including the legal health record, are used as evidence in any legal proceeding, whether that is the appeal of a denied claim or in conjunction with a lawsuit, the documents must be complete and accurate. The absence of detailed documentation can result in a reviewer or judge ruling in favor of the petitioner (third-party payer) in the denial of an appealed claim or for a judge and jury to rule in favor of the defendant in an action due to insufficient evidence in the file.

Changing a medical record is a serious offense and may be construed as fraud if it is not handled correctly. If a health care professional or provider is presented with his or her record of the events that occurred during a client encounter and finds that the documentation does not completely or accurately describe the encounter to the fullest extent possible, he or she may be inclined to make changes to describe the event more completely. The proper method of documentation in this type of a situation is to record an *addendum* or an *amendment* to the file that more fully details the situation or encounter at a later date. Although falsification of medical records is a criminal offense punishable by fines and incarceration, in many states, addendums, amendments, corrections, and delayed entries may be acceptable to set the record straight.

Addendums, Amendments, Corrections, and Delayed Entries

State laws vary on how medical records can be amended. Legally and ethically, health care professionals and providers are expected to report all necessary information completely, honestly and truthfully. If there is an error in, or omission of, information there are appropriate ways to manage these limited occurrences. However, the best way to avoid the situation is to do it right the first time.

For clarification Business Dictionary defines an *addendum* as a "document or information attached or added to clarify, modify, or support the information in the original document or written work" (Business Dictionary, n.d.a).

An *amendment* is a "change in a legal document made by adding, altering, or omitting a certain part or term. Amended documents, when properly executed (signed by all parties concerned), retain the legal validity of the original document" (Business Dictionary, n.d.b).

"[Although] providers are encouraged to enter all relevant documents and entries into the medical record at the time they are rendering the service [CMS and other third-party payers recognize that] occasionally, upon review, a provider may discover that certain entries, related to actions that were actually performed at the time of service but not properly documented, need to be amended, corrected, or entered after rendering the service [and]…shall consider all submitted entries that comply with the widely accepted Recordkeeping Principles" (CMS, 2013b).

"Regardless of whether a documentation submission originates from a paper record or an electronic health record (EHR), documents containing amendments, corrections or addenda must:

- Clearly and permanently identify any amendment, correction, or delayed entry as such

- Clearly indicate the date and author of any amendment, correction, or delayed entry

- Not delete but instead clearly identify all original content

Paper Medical Records: When correcting a paper medical record, these principles are generally accomplished by using a single-line strike through so that the original content is still readable. Further, the author of the alteration must sign and date the revision. Similarly, amendments or delayed entries to paper records must be clearly signed and dated upon entry into the record.

Electronic Health Records: Medical record keeping within an EHR deserves special considerations; however, the preceding principles remain fundamental and necessary for document submission. Records sourced from electronic systems containing amendments, corrections, or delayed entries must:

a. Distinctly identify any amendment, correction or delayed entry

b. Provide a reliable means to clearly identify the original content, the modified content, and the date and authorship of each modification of the record. (CMS, 2013b)."

Recommended Documentation Dos and Don'ts

Do

- Make certain you are writing in the correct chart or file.

- Put the date and reason for the encounter on the first page of a paper record.

- Put the client's first and last name and the date on each page of a paper record.

- Use a black ink pen for all paper records.

- Write legibly and professionally.

- Log on to an EHR system with your user name/password only.

- Use people-first language (e.g., "Evaluated 6 y/o CP for a new chair" should be written "Evaluated a 6 y/o boy with a diagnosis of CP for a new chair").

- Be clear, concise, and accurate in all statements.

- Use widely accepted terminology and abbreviations that cannot be misconstrued.

- Identify the specific measurement scales used and write in quantitative terms for all test and measures (e.g., ROM expressed in degrees of movement).

- Write N/A, for *not applicable*, when information to be gathered on a form or template used for recording the encounter does not pertain to your client; leaving a section blank appears as if it was not addressed or was overlooked.

- Draw a single line through an error, notate the error, and sign and date the change on a paper record.

- Sign (legibly) and date all paper entries and ensure all electronic entries are recorded as signed and date stamped when closing out the record.

- Mark "late entry" if you recall and document information after you have signed and dated the original entry. Sign and date the late entry for the date and time it was written or recorded.

Don't

- Date an entry so that it appears to have been written at an earlier time.

- Misspell words, use poor grammar, or write illegibly.

- Use shorthand, abbreviations, or terminology that are not typically used in medical dictionaries and/or medical references.

- Use vague (e.g., nonfunctional, unsteady) or subjective (e.g., weak, slow) language to describe anything that can be measured quantitatively.

- Use words with a negative connotation or that may convey a negative attitude.

- Offer or document your opinion outside of your professional assessment.

- Document tests or measures that were not performed or responses to trials or simulations that were not conducted.

- Cover up anything by scribbling through the information, drawing across it with marker or use a white correction fluid designed to look like there is nothing written on the paper beneath it.

- Delete any information in a manner that is not clearly visible and annotated properly or recoverable in an EHR system.

- Add information at a later date without annotating it properly, as an addendum, amendment, or late entry.

SUMMARY

The record of any encounter between a clinician, rehabilitation technology supplier, and a consumer for the purpose of evaluating and recommending MAE, as well as the options, accessories, and seating and positioning components to be used with it is a legal document. The saying "if it isn't documented, it didn't happen" is the well-known reply of every third-party payer looking to deny a prior authorization request or claim and prosecuting attorney looking to find fault on behalf of her client in the event of an adverse occurrence or dispute. Hence, keeping good, accurate records is an essential professional and legal requirement for all parties involved in the provision of seating and wheeled mobility products and services, regardless of the payer or service delivery model.

REFERENCES

American Health Information Management Association. (2011). Fundamentals of the legal health record and designated record set. *Journal of AHIMA, 82*. Retrieved from http://library.ahima.org/xpedio/groups/public/documents/ahima/bok1_048604.hcsp?dDocName=bok1_048604

Arledge, S., Armstrong, W., Babinec, M., Dicianno, B., DiGiovine, C., Dyson-Hudson, T.,...Stogner, J. (2011). *RESNA Wheelchair service provision guide*. Retrieved from http://www.resna.org/sites/default/files/legacy/resources/position-papers/RESNAWheelchairServiceProvisionGuide.pdf

Business Dictionary. (n.d.a). *Addendum*. Retrieved from http://www.businessdictionary.com/definition/addendum.html

Business Dictionary. (n.d.b). *Amendment*. Retrieved from http://www.businessdictionary.com/definition/amendment.html

Centers for Medicare & Medicaid Services. (2005). Medicare national coverage determinations (NCD) manual (CMS Pub 100-03). National Coverage Determination (NCD) for Mobility Assistive Equipment (MAE) (280.3). Retrieved from http://www.cms.gov/medicare-coverage-database/details/ncd-details.aspx?NCDId=219&ncdver=2

Centers for Medicare & Medicaid Services. (2009). CMS manual system. State operations provider certification (CMS Pub 100-07; Rev. 47, June 5, 2009). Retrieved from http://www.cms.gov/Regulations-and-Guidance/Guidance/Transmittals/downloads/R47SOMA.pdf

Centers for Medicare & Medicaid Services. (2012). 42 CFR Section 482.24(c)(1). Retrieved from http://www.gpo.gov/fdsys/pkg/CFR-2011-title42-vol5/pdf/CFR-2011-title42-vol5-sec482-24.pdf

Centers for Medicare & Medicaid Services. (2013a). CMS manual system. Program integrity manual, chapter 3, section 3.3.2.4 (CMS Pub 100-08; Rev.465, 06/18/13). Retrieved from http://www.cms.gov/Regulations-and-Guidance/Guidance/Manuals/downloads/pim83c03.pdf

Centers for Medicare & Medicaid Services. (2013b) CMS manual system, CMS Pub 100-08, Program Integrity Manual, Chapter 3, Section 3.3.2.5 (Rev. 442, 01/08/13). Retrieved from http://www.cms.gov/Regulations-and-Guidance/Guidance/Manuals/downloads/pim83c03.pdf

Durable Medical Equipment, Prosthetics, Orthotics and Supplies Quality Standards, (2008). Retrieved from http://www.cms.gov/Medicare/Provider-Enrollment-and-Certification/MedicareProviderSupEnroll/downloads/dmeposaccreditationstandards.pdf

Oxford Dictionary. (n.d.). *Document*. Retrieved from http://www.oxforddictionaries.com/definition/english/document

Paralyzed Veterans of America Consortium for Spinal Cord Medicine. (2005). Preservation of upper limb function following spinal cord injury: A clinical practice guideline for health-care professionals. *Journal of Spinal Cord Medicine, 28*, 434-470. Retrieved from https://www.ncbi.nlm.nih.gov/pmc/articles/PMC1808273/

Waugh, K., & Crane, B. (2013). *A clinical application guide to standardized wheelchair seating measures of the body and seating support surfaces* (rev. ed.). Denver, CO: University of Colorado Denver. Retrieved from http://www.assistivetechnologypartners.org

V

Putting It Together
Specialty Applications

17

Considerations When Working With the Pediatric Population

Jan Furumasu, PT, ATP

The most important concepts that distinguish pediatric from adult seating and mobility are growth and play. This refers to not only physical growth; children with disabilities are changing developmentally, as well as growing cognitively, emotionally, and socially. Physical growth in children with weakness or asymmetry in strength or tone can potentially cause orthopedic asymmetries of the extremities, spine, and pelvis. Pediatric seating systems and wheelchairs have growth adjustability and support systems to maintain trunk and pelvis alignment while the growing body is gaining control or to prevent asymmetries in alignment if control is inadequate. The pediatric wheelchair must not only support growing, changing bodies but also facilitate improvement of motor control, allow for cognitive growth by ensuring age-appropriate interaction with the environment, and allow peer interaction and participation to promote social and emotional growth and development.

Play is important for young children to be able to develop cognitively, emotionally, and psychosocially. For children with disabilities, wheelchair seating is crucial in supporting the child's body in an upright posture so that he or she can concentrate on play, vocalize, interact, and explore using his or her eyes, head, and upper extremities. By providing a wheeled or powered mobility device, children are able to initiate mobility, spontaneously explore the environment, satisfy their curiosity, and interact in play. The positive effects include improved self-confidence, self-esteem (Guerrette, Furumasu, & Tefft, 2013) and personal social skills (Jones, McEwen, & Neas, 2012). Children with disabilities were compared with able-bodied children

on the playground. The children with disabilities were observed to be less involved in cooperative play, played a lower status or passive role, or were more of an observer, rather than involved in interactive play. Restricted mobility in play leads to frustration, apathy, decreased social development, self-esteem, and identity formation (Missiuna & Pollock, 1991; Tamm & Skar, 2000).

Finally, children are growing socially and emotionally. Social and emotional growth occurs through peer interaction and communication (Butler, 1991; Tamm & Skar, 2000). Children need to interact with their friends and peers. The chair should also allow the child to interact with peers in different settings, including going over grass or playgrounds, going down to the floor for participation in circle time, elevating the seat, or even standing, if appropriate. Provision of early powered mobility has demonstrated increases in social interaction and facilitates developmental growth and self-confidence (Guerette, Furumasu, & Tefft, 2013; Jones et al., 2012; Livingstone & Field, 2014). Mothers reported that the powered wheelchair impacted their children's social skills by allowing them to be more independent and to better engage in age-appropriate, meaningful activities with their peers (Wiart, Darrah, Hollis, Cook, & May, 2004). Assistive technology is the key to unlocking children's potential and compensating for disability. Pediatric seating and wheelchair mobility can empower children with disabilities to be recognized as individuals of value and to build the self-confidence necessary to interact positively with the world at large.

Lange, M. L., & Minkel, J. L.
Seating and Wheeled Mobility: A Clinical Resource Guide
(pp. 281-296). © 2018 SLACK Incorporated.

Shift From Traditional Model of Skill Acquisition to Using Parallel Forms of Mobility

The neuromaturational theory, the dominant traditional practice model of motor development, encouraged intervention strategies that aspired to normalize movement patterns by changing the child through repetitive training, whereas newer contemporary approaches to intervention encourage children with physical disabilities to use their most efficient movement strategies to explore their environment and participate in meaningful activities. The dynamic systems theory considers the effect of interactions between person, task, and environment on motor development. Learning to use a variety of flexible patterns to accomplish a task leads to rich, complex brain organization adapting to environmental demands. This approach suggests using different mobility options in different environments, and also encourages therapists to consider various mobility options with the family that match the child's ability. Focusing on task accomplishment allows for an array of mobility solutions depending on the environment and the context. For example, in a survey, 45% of children with cerebral palsy (CP) used floor mobility as a functional independent mode of home mobility (rolling, scooting, or crawling). At school, 34% of the children may use a walker to walk in their classroom. Out on the playground, 21% use their power wheelchair to be able to play with their peers on the playground or grassy field. The focus is on function, task accomplishment, and the ability to participate in society as opposed to what society views as normal development (Tiemen et al., 2014).

Traditionally, power mobility has been perceived as a last resort or failure of walking. The client was expected to walk as much as possible even though ambulation was not the most functional method of mobility. More current practice encourages children to explore their environments in all settings and participate in meaningful activities, which positively contributes to their confidence and self-esteem (Wiart & Darrah, 2002).

Early Intervention for Seating and Mobility

Early provision of appropriate seating for children with physical disabilities provides a means to increase head, trunk, and extremity control; prevent skeletal asymmetries; and improve socialization by providing access to the child's environments. Postural stability affects feeding, sensory input, hand use for play, and access to computers, switch toys, and communication. There is a critical window of learning that children may miss if they do not experience the ability to sit in an upright stable posture, interact with their surroundings, and experience some form of independent mobility. These cognitive, social, and psychological skills may be difficult to acquire later in life. Research has demonstrated the importance of providing early seating interventions and the influence of proper seating on function (Harris & Roxborough, 2005; Roxborough, 1995; Stavness, 2006). Effectiveness of adaptive seating in children with cerebral palsy has demonstrated short-term improvement in pulmonary function, active trunk extension, and improved performance on the Bayley Mental Scale, improving sitting posture, vocalization, and some oral-motor skills (Roxborough, 1995).

Ryan and colleagues (2009) evaluated the short-term impact of two adaptive seating devices on the activity performance and satisfaction in children with CP, as observed by their parents in their home setting. Thirty parents of children with CP, mean age of 4 years and 6 months, with Gross Motor Function Classification System Levels III and IV participated. Two special purpose seating devices, one for sitting support on the floor or on a chair and the other for postural control on a toilet, were provided to the families for a 6-week intervention. Changes in activity performance and satisfaction were measured through parent ratings on the Canadian Occupational Performance Measure. Parents reported that their children were more able to engage in self-care and play activities when using specific adaptive seating devices in their homes and that their child's activity performance decreased after the seating devices were removed from their homes (Ryan et al., 2009) (Table 17-1).

Preventing Orthopedic Asymmetries in Growing Children

Scoliosis is a curvature of the spine and is common in all children with a physical disability who are nonambulatory. Muscle weakness, asymmetry in tone or strength, and a growing spine contribute to spinal asymmetries. It is estimated that 80% to 98% of children who sustain a spinal cord injury (SCI) before skeletal maturity develop a scoliosis. Research has found that 93% of children with SCI injured before 11 years of age and 9% of children older than 11 years had at least one subluxed or dislocated hip (McCarthy, Chafetz, Betz, & Gaughan 2004). Early bracing of the spine, using an orthosis such as a thoracic lumbar sacral orthosis (TLSO), may delay the onset of spinal curvature and the age that surgical intervention is required. In curves less than 20 degrees, an orthosis may reduce the possibility of a surgical fusion. One in five children with CP will have scoliosis (Lubicky & Betz, 2011). Rotational

	TABLE 17-1	
PEDIATRIC MOBILITY EQUIPMENT: ROLE OF ASSISTIVE TECHNOLOGY IN THE CHILD'S DEVELOPMENT		
DEVELOPMENTAL TASKS	**APPROXIMATE AGE RANGE**	**MOBILITY EQUIPMENT**
Rolling supine to prone	5 to 6 months	Large wedges
Prone activities: • Crawling on abdomen • Assumption on all fours • Reciprocal creeping	 • 6 to 7 months • 8 months • 9 to 10 months	Wedges: promote head extension, shoulder stability, upper extremity weightbearing Prone scooters or crawlers: prone mobility
Sitting activities: • No head lag • Flexion of head/trunk pull to sit • Propped sitting • Hands-free sitting	 • 4 months • 5 months • 6 to 7 months • 8 months	Corner seats: static support for upper extremity activities Bolsters, balls, or peanuts: trunk control Caster casts: floor mobility
Standing: • Standing with support • Walking with support	 • 8 months • 10 to 12 months	Prone or supine stander (tilt table) Mobile stander
Walking	≥ 12 months	Walkers: ring, front-wheeled, rear-wheeled Forearm crutches, canes Orthotics: parapodiums, reciprocating gait orthosis, hip knee ankle foot orthosis, knee ankle foot orthois, ankle foot orthosis
Wheeled mobility	≥ 12 months	Adapted tricycles Manual wheelchair: front-wheeled, rear-wheeled Powered toys Powered wheelchairs

asymmetries of the spine, in the transverse plane, are the most difficult to control in children with strong asymmetrical tonic neck reflex posturing. Maintaining a midline pelvis and head are key in preventing rotation of the pelvis and spine and inhibiting asymmetrical tonic neck reflex posturing. A windswept posture of the thighs caused by a rotated pelvis can be prevented by stabilizing the pelvis with abduction of the adducted thigh. Abducting the thigh will block rotation of the still flexible pelvis and therefore the spine. Maintaining a midline and symmetrical posture of the upper extremities and keeping the head midline will also assist in preventing rotation of the upper spine. Conservative treatment of a mild scoliosis in the frontal plane includes three points of control: lateral hip support on the concave side, lateral trunk support at the apex of the convex curve, and a higher trunk support on the opposite concave side as counter pressure (Figure 17-1).

A flexible scoliosis can be corrected with the supports, but a fixed scoliosis must be accommodated with offset trunk and thigh supports or a custom-molded system. As with all seating, functional movement must be prioritized and may be the reason scoliosis prevention is not successful. Seating supports may be too restrictive of movement and may interfere with the client's ability to function, specifically to lean, pick up objects, dress after self-catheterization, or transfer. In active children, if the supports are custom molded to the body or are not able to swing away, these will interfere with functional activities and therefore not be used.

In nonambulatory children with CP, it is often difficult to prevent hip contractures. Typically, asymmetrical pull

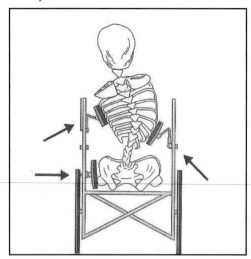

Figure 17-1. Opposing forces of a three-point control system (Reprinted with permission from Furumasu, J. (2008). Seating and positioning for disabled children and adults. In J. Hsu & J. Fisk (Eds.), *Atlas of orthotics and assistive devices* (4th ed.). Shannon, Ireland: Elsevier Science Ireland).

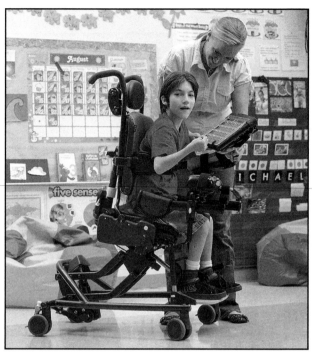

Figure 17-2. Active seated posture in a Rifton Activity chair. Photo © 2014 by Rifton Equipment. Used with permission.

on the hip joints is caused by an asymmetrical tonic neck reflex type posturing, which can lead to rotation of the pelvis and adduction of one hip and abduction of the other hip (windswept posture). This asymmetrical muscle pull or strength imbalance around the hip joint causes acetabular dysplasia and the head of the femur may become subluxed or dislocated (the head of the femur sliding out of the socket). These are problems historically managed by a surgeon with tendon lengthening or a joint realignment surgery. Postoperatively, the child will need seating accommodations to maintain joint range of motion into abduction and to accommodate for any residual asymmetries, such as a shorter thigh or seat depth length.

In a prospective study, Pountney, Mandy, Green, and Gard (2009) compared early seating to a historical control group and demonstrated that early provision of postural management equipment played a role in reducing the number of hip problems, and therefore the need for treatment of hip subluxation/dislocation in children with CP at 5 years of age. The study followed 39 children who began using postural management equipment when younger than 18 months of age. Levels of ability, type and amount of equipment use, and treatments were recorded every 3 months. At 30 and 60 months, the hips were x-rayed, and the hip migration percentage was measured. The results were compared with the historical control group and demonstrated that surgical intervention, use of a hip and spinal orthosis, and/or botulinum toxin injections in the intervention group were significantly less compared with the historical control group (Pountney et al., 2009). Early postural management in children with disabilities is important in preventing asymmetries and promoting stable midline alignment. This

is addressed further in Chapter 7 of this volume, "Posture Management 24/7."

DYNAMIC SEATING

Dynamic seating can have different conceptualizations when used in seating and wheelchair mobility. One concept of dynamic seating is active seating. Active seating allows the flexibility for a client to move forward within a seating system. The seated posture is not static or rigid, but allows a child's base of support, the pelvis, to move into a position of readiness or an active learning posture. A position for active learning is an anteriorly tilted pelvis, either allowing the pelvis freedom to tilt forward by placing the seat belt below the pelvis, adjusting the back angle forward 5 degrees or anteriorly tilting the seat itself. The ability to tilt wheelchairs or adaptive chairs in a slightly forward 5-degree tilt shifts the pelvis into an anterior posture, activating weight-bearing in the lower extremities and increasing extensor tone in the trunk (Figure 17-2). This muscle activation is the result of the body's reaction to gravity through the vestibular system and proprioceptors. This is frequently referred to as *active holding* or *coactivation*. It increases alertness and provides a readiness for interactive activity of the head and upper extremities (Kangas, 2002). This active positioning has been shown to improve upper extremity function and task performance in a classroom setting. Ten studies that investigated the effect of seat inclinations were reviewed.

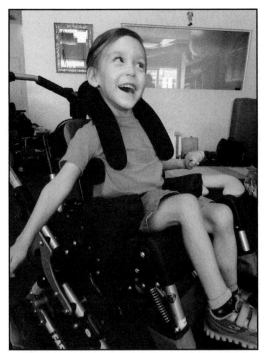

Figure 17-3. A 4-year-old boy with CP and dystonia-type movement, using the dynamic seating system of a Kids UP wheelchair. The wheelchair allows extension of his hips and knees and returns to a stable seated posture to allow access to a communication device using a switch at his head.

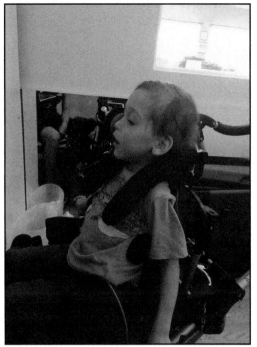

Figure 17-4. The dynamic movement option can be locked out, giving the client or caregiver the option of choosing when to use these features.

Improved postural control and a reduction in pathological movements were achieved in anterior tilt and arm and hand function were improved in the functional sitting position, as opposed to a posterior seat incline (McNamara & Casey, 2007).

A second concept of dynamic seating is the ability of the positioning equipment to move dynamically when the child initiates movement. When the child relaxes, the positioning system returns to a stable, neutral pelvic position. The frame of the wheelchair or the seating system has springs, hydraulics, or pistons to allow movement into hip, knee or trunk extension. Dynamic seating can be viewed as a therapeutic tool, allowing a child to initiate movement for sensory or vestibular input. A goal of dynamic seating is to use the energy in the hydraulics or springs of a seating system to channel the fluctuating muscle tone, spasticity or hypotonia of a child into purposeful movement or to diffuse force, increase sitting tolerance and prevent hardware breakage (Figures 17-3 and 17-4). Generally, children who struggle in their static seating systems may benefit from dynamic movement, which is typically extension, and returning to a neutral position of rest. A seat or backrest that moves dynamically can accommodate involuntary extensor thrusts, absorb the extensor tone, and, through the movement of the seating system, dampen the overall impact of hypertonia on the body. Evidence suggests that using a dynamic backrest reduces sacral sitting caused by the trunk sliding down with repeated extensor thrusting (McNamara & Casey, 2007).

Research shows that dynamic seating improved range of motion (ROM) of the trunk, limited loss of position of the trunk, and decreased dystonia and dyskinesia in children with dystonic tetraparesis. Control of upper extremity movement was actually improved as well (Cimolin et al., 2009).

The stability of the seating may be necessary for certain functions (e.g., accessing a communication device, feeding), but when the child needs to move, the system can be unlocked, allowing him or her to extend. It is becoming increasingly recognized in the rehabilitation field that active sitting is also relevant for wheelchair users and adaptive seating (Sturgeon, 2010).

Thirdly, dynamic seating or movement describes movement in space. Dynamic powered seating, such as tilting back in space, reclining, seat elevation, seat to floor or sit-to-stand, are options on some power wheelchair bases. These features may allow the seat to go to the ground for floor access for play and interaction with peers and then back and up to a standing position. This dynamic movement allows the child the independent experience of interacting with his or her environment and peers on all levels as any child would be able to do.

Prime Engineering's KidWalk Dynamic Gait Mobility System is a dynamic walking system (Figure 17-5). The child initiates the movement and the dynamic component of the seat assists the weight shift so one leg is unweighted

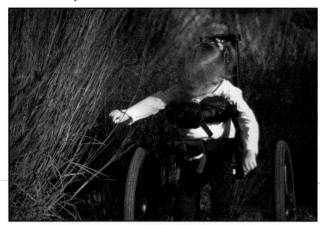

Figure 17-5. KidWalk dynamic mobility system.

and able to take a step. The child's trunk and pelvis are supported while the seat facilitates reciprocation of the lower extremities by moving side to side and up and down.

All dynamic movement in rehabilitation equipment encourages self-initiated change in position to promote upper extremity function, alertness, pressure relief, peer interaction, facilitation of balance, strengthening, and weightbearing.

PHYSIOLOGICAL DEMANDS OF MOBILITY

Physiological Demands of Ambulation

In the traditional model, the expectation was to encourage the child to walk as much as possible, even though ambulation was not the most functional method of mobility. Studies have demonstrated that pathological gait patterns increase muscular demands and energy expenditure. The ability to ambulate declines as a child grows older and heavier (Johnston, Moore, Quinn, & Smith, 2004; Rose, Gamble, Medeiros, Burgos, & Haskell, 1989; Waters, Hislop, & Campbell, 1983). The typical crouched gait of a child that has CP or spina bifida increases energy demands, stance time, and decreases velocity and efficiency. In children with spastic diplegia, walking uses three times higher than normal energy expenditure, even at a slower than normal walking speed (Campbell & Ball, 1978; Rose et al., 1989). The effects of ambulation on children with spina bifida were studied on three measures of school performance. The results suggest that the high energy cost of walking may have a negative effect on certain aspects of school performance (Franks, Palisano, & Darbee, 1991). Ambulation energy costs for children with spina bifida have been shown to be 218% higher than their nondisabled peers and walking is twice as strenuous as propelling a wheelchair (Williams et al., 1983).

Physiological Demands of Manual Wheelchair Propulsion

Manual wheelchair propulsion requires upper extremity strength and coordination, handgrip, head and trunk control, endurance, and higher oxygen consumption than ambulation in the typical child (Luna-Reyes et al., 1988). Manual wheelchair mobility may be inefficient for kids with compromised respiratory capacity, impaired coordination, or muscle weakness. Pediatric aluminum folding frames weigh greater than 50% of a 4- to 6-year-old child's body weight. Rigid titanium frame wheelchairs weigh as little as 12 pounds, or less than 30% of the mean weight for a 4- to 6-year-old child. The size and weight of the wheelchair, the child's shorter upper extremities, and other issues, such as trunk and upper extremity weakness, compromised respiratory system, and motor control impairments, all affect manual wheelchair propulsion efficiency. When prescribing a manual wheelchair system, the wheelchair and seating system weight to child weight ratio should be considered. The average pediatric ultralight wheelchair weight ranges from 12 to 30 pounds, depending on size, without seating and accessories. The average adult weighs 150 pounds, giving us a 5:1 ratio. The average child under 6 years of age weighs 30 to 40 pounds, bringing the ratio closer to 1:1 or 1:2. Manual wheelchair propulsion should be energy efficient and not considered exercise for the upper extremities. Instead, wheeled mobility needs to provide mobility similar to the child's ambulatory peers in a school-based setting.

Young children from 8 months to about 4 years old, depending on their disabilities, may have shorter arms, which limit the range of a propulsive stroke. The child may also have limited strength with which to propel a wheelchair in a standard rear wheel configuration. Front-wheel drive manual wheelchairs (sometimes referred to as *reverse configuration*) have the drive wheel positioned in front to allow better efficiency in wheel propulsion for the very small or young child (Figures 17-6 through 17-8).

PEDIATRIC EQUIPMENT SPECIFICS

Dependent Stroller-Type Push Wheelchairs

Push wheelchairs or dependent stroller-style bases come with customizable seating, and some bases also include tilt-in-space and recline functions for changing positions (Figures 17-9 and 17-10). Tilt allows a position change with a fixed seat-to-back angle, whereas a back recline function opens the thigh to trunk angle (e.g., allowing for a diaper change in the stroller or respiratory management). Adapted seating in strollers allows adjustment of the postural components on a lighter weight, more convenient, compact,

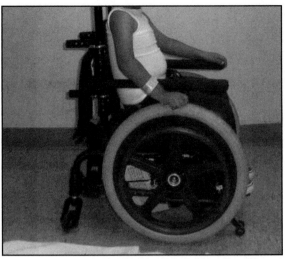

Figure 17-6. Front-wheel drive manual wheelchair for child with C7 tetraplegia.

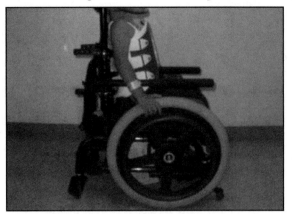

Figure 17-7. Same child with C7 tetraplegia sitting with thoracic lumbar sacral orthosis to prevent kyphoscoliosis.

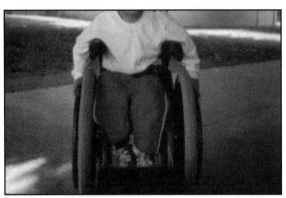

Figure 17-8. A 3-year-old child with osteogenesis imperfecta with short arm length secondary to multiple fractures propelling front-wheel drive manual wheelchair.

foldable frame. Dependent push wheelchair bases have become more streamlined and lighter weight, provide seating supports, and are easy to load into a vehicle. Overall, these bases may be perceived as more parent- and child-friendly and more convenient than standard wheelchairs.

Standing Frames

For individuals who are seated in wheelchairs most of the day, periodic episodes of standing can prevent joint contractures, such as hip and knee flexion contractures and equinus of the ankles. Various standing devices exist on the market. Prone, supine, and multiposition standers provide complete support and adjustability of upright or vertical positioning. Prone standers provide support on the chest and anterior body, stretching the hip flexors, and challenge the child to extend his or her head against gravity to improve head and trunk control. The prone position is also gravity dependent, making functional tasks with the upper extremities more difficult. Supine standers support the individual on the back until he or she reaches an upright position where he or she can balance his or her head and use the upper extremities (Figure 17-11). Tables or trays can be placed in front of these standers to engage the child in activities. Sit-to-stand standers provide a seat or strap beneath the pelvis that lifts the client from a seated position (from the wheelchair) to an upright standing position. These devices work well with larger, heavier youth who have good head and trunk control.

Dynamic or mobile standers provide all of the benefits of standing while also allowing the individual to be independently mobile, propelling the wheels with her upper extremities (Figure 17-12). The Rehabilitation Engineering and Assistive Technology Society of North America (RESNA) supports the incorporation of standing devices into school settings, with proper medical professional supervision (Dicianno, Morgan, Lieberman, & Rosen, 2013). Standing adds significant vertical access and functional reach. As the seat surface moves to vertical, the vertical access is equal to the user's seat depth. This allows a greater functional reach to access the environment, such as sinks, countertops, and blackboards in the classroom. The standing position places a mechanical stretch on the hip, knee, and plantar flexors, increasing passive ROM to these joints and reducing the risk of contractures from long-term sitting. Full upright standing fully relieves pressure from the ischial tuberosities, decreasing the risk for pressure ulcers. Bone density loss may be decelerated in certain populations. Weightbearing promotes improved bone density (Glickman, Geigle, & Paleg, 2010). Subjectively, many individuals report improvements with bowel and bladder function, as well as with circulation and respiration after beginning a standing program. Eye-to-eye contact with peers increases socialization, emotional development, confidence, and self-esteem. When standers are incorporated into school programs of younger children, care should be taken to ensure a slightly abducted position to promote normal development of the femoral-acetabular joint and decrease the risk for hip dislocation.

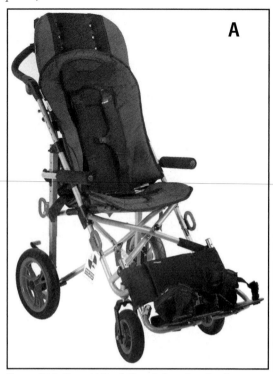

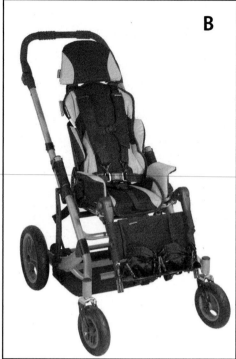

Figure 17-9. Convaid fixed tilt and tilt-and-recline bases.

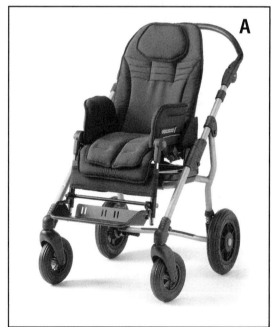

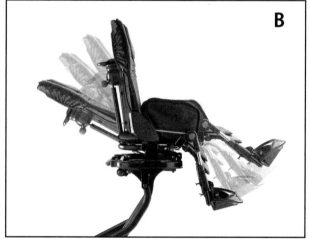

Figure 17-10. Ormesa Bug tilt-in-space and recline base.

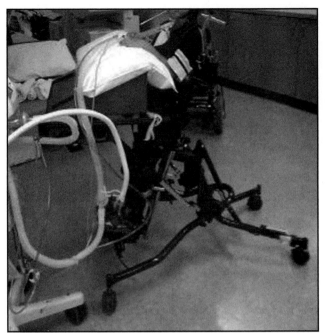

Figure 17-11. A 5-year-old child with incomplete tetraplegia secondary to transverse myelitis, using a ventilator, standing in Prime Engineering Superstand.

Adapted Tricycles

Adapted tricycles frequently offer trunk support and pedals with straps that secure the rider's feet (Figure 17-13). Some tricycles are hand pedaled to assist or replace leg-based propulsion. Adapted tricycles allow children with disabilities to participate in age-appropriate mobility with family, siblings and friends out on the playground or in parks. Children, teens, and adults with CP and similar disorders can use adapted tricycles to increase strength and coordination. Research using stationary bikes for children with CP examined the effects of a stationary cycling intervention on muscle strength, locomotor endurance, preferred walking speed, and gross motor function in children with spastic diplegia. Sixty-two ambulatory children aged 7 to 18 years with spastic diplegic CP and Gross Motor Function Classification System levels I to III participated in this study over 12 weeks. Significant improvements in locomotor endurance, gross motor function, and some measures of strength were found for the cycling group but not the control group, providing preliminary support for use of cycling for lifelong cardiorespiratory fitness for this population (Fowler et al., 2010).

PEDIATRIC CONSIDERATIONS IN POWERED WHEELCHAIR MOBILITY

For children with severe physical disabilities, the lack of self-initiated mobility increases the risk for developmental,

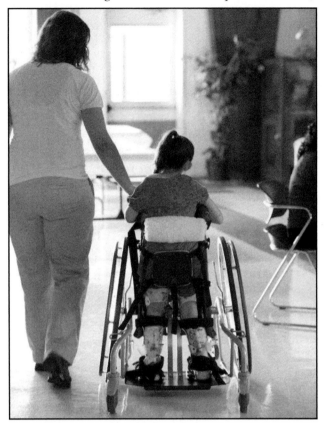

Figure 17-12. Mobile stander. Photo © 2014 by Rifton Equipment. Used by permission.

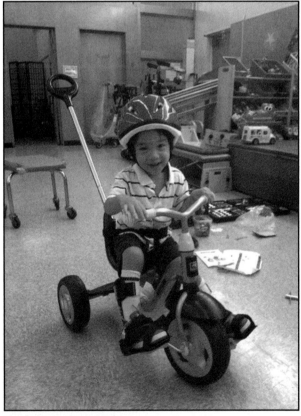

Figure 17-13. Adapted tricycle.

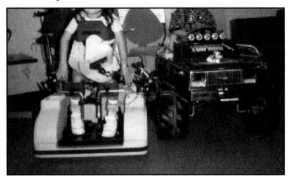

Figure 17-14. Transitional powered mobility aid and an adapted powered toy.

cognitive, and psychosocial delays. Early provision of powered mobility is believed to facilitate and enhance learning, socialization and self-esteem by enabling independent movement, interactive play and allowing children to spontaneously move to satisfy their curiosity. Increasing evidence supports the benefits of early powered mobility. Benefits that have been documented include improvements in psychosocial and cognitive developmental skills, increase in alertness in severely cognitively involved children, as well as increases in interaction levels with objects in the environment and with people (Butler, 1986; Bottos, Bolcati, Sciuto, Ruggeri, & Feliciangeli, 2001; Guerrette et al., 2013; Nilsson & Nyberg, 2003; Nisbet, 2002; Wiart et al., 2004).

Philosophical and Historical Attitudes Toward Power Mobility and Parental Acceptance

In a review article on powered mobility, Field (1999) emphasized the need for the assistive technology provider to take into account many factors in the evaluation process for a successful powered wheelchair experience. These factors include issues relating to the client e.g., cognitive, sensory, and motor abilities), specific features of the wheelchair (e.g., different types of input devices and wheelchair processors), and the social and physical environments in which the wheelchair might be used.

These and other factors, such as a child's developmental readiness and behavior, level of parental support, background and level of expertise of the provider, and availability of a wheelchair for an extended trial period, may influence the assessment process and the ultimate provision of a powered wheelchair for a young child. In a national survey of suppliers and therapists, reasons that a child who was ready for powered mobility was not given a powered wheelchair were funding issues, lack of family support, and transportation issues. Educating the family was just as important as educating the third-party payers (Guerette, Tefft, & Furumasu, 2005). Allowing the family to grieve

over the diagnosis and prognosis of their child's disability is also a step in the provision of early powered mobility. It is important to educate the family on the importance of using a mobility device not only for mobility, but also as a therapeutic intervention.

Traditionally, doctors, therapists, and parents were hesitant in advocating powered mobility because it might make the child "lazy" or unmotivated to work on ambulation skills. Bottos et al. (2001) demonstrated that providing powered mobility did not impede the development of ambulatory skills. They found that ambulation potentials can often be predicted by age 3 years and were interested in powered mobility for those children who were not able to ambulate efficiently.

Early Exploratory Movement

Powered, off-the-shelf mobility toys suit children who have sufficient trunk control to sit unsupported and coordinate use of both hands. Some power toys can be adapted with seat inserts for those children who need more pelvic and trunk support. Depending on a child's motor control, most off-the-shelf power toys are inadequate for children with severe disabilities in terms of seating and access. Power toys can be adapted with switch access, but usually for the hand. Typically, power toys are meant for outdoor use. The Go Bot was an innovative transitional powered mobility device designed in 1996 by Christine Wright-Ott (1997) as a tool for providing children exploratory or transitional mobility experiences, which may lead to functional mobility (either walking or in a powered wheelchair) (Figure 17-14). Galloway, Ryu, and Agrawal (2007) have introduced self-initiated movement through robotic devices to a 7-month-old normally developing infant and a 14-month-old child with Down syndrome. Hsiang-Han and Galloway (2012) have also modified toy mobile vehicles for switch access.

Powered Mobility

Independent mobility is important in the development of a number of cognitive and psychosocial skills, including spatial relations, verbal skills, and social interactions with peers. For a young child with mobility impairments, the opportunity for early powered mobility enhances the development of skills that may otherwise develop more slowly or not at all (Guerette et al., 2013; Jones, McEwen, & Hansen, 2003; Jones et al., 2012; Livingstone & Field, 2014; Lynch, Ryu, Agrawal, & Galloway, 2009).

Self-initiated mobility powerfully affects a child's development, self-confidence, social acceptance, and ability to participate with peers. A child's inability to move leads to a self-perception of incompetence and a sense of learned helplessness. Learned helplessness, instilled by 4 years of age, results when the child has no control or ability to

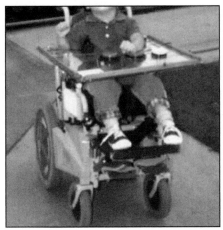

Figure 17-15. A 3-year-old boy started using switches for powered mobility until age 6, when his hand control improved well enough to use a proportional joystick controller.

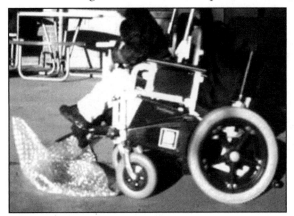

Figure 17-16. Motivational play allows children to experience and practice movement in a power wheelchair.

interact with his or her environment, causing a sense of passivity and decreased motivation and curiosity. Early independent mobility allows the child to form a sense of identity and confidence. It reduces apathy and depression and improves self-esteem and confidence (Guerette et al., 2013).

Children with physical disabilities, as young as 18 to 24 months, can learn to drive power wheelchairs in very short periods of time (Butler, Okamoto, & McKay, 1983, 1984; Furumasu, Guerette, & Tefft, 1996). However, children with complex developmental delays and cognitive limitations have also successfully developed independent power mobility skills, but with longer training times (Bottos et al., 2001; Deitz, Swinth, & White, 2002; Huhn, Guarrera-Bowlby, & Deutsch, 2007), or use of additional technologies, such as smart wheelchairs or robotic mobility devices (Galloway et al., 2007).

How early is a child ready for powered mobility? Chronological age and IQ are not good determinants of a child's ability to operate a powered wheelchair. Children as young as 7 months have experienced self-initiated mobility in a mobile robotic type device (Galloway et al., 2007). Children as young as 18 to 20 months have learned to drive a powered wheelchair within a period of 2 to 4 weeks (Butler, 1986; Butler et al., 1983, 1984; Jones et al., 2003; Tefft, Guerette, & Furumasu, 1999).

The Pediatric Powered Wheelchair Screening Test (PPWST) (Teft et al., 1999) can determine a cognitive developmental age. A child must demonstrate the ability to use an access method (joystick or switch), as well as exhibit cognitive, sensorimotor, and coping skills (Figure 17-15). Cognitive abilities include cause and effect, directional concepts, problem solving, and spatial relationships. Sensorimotor abilities include perception, processing, motor planning, and reaction time. Coping abilities include

attention span, motivation, and persistence. Children understanding spatial relations at 25 months in combination with understanding problem solving at 20 months demonstrated the ability to learn basic powered wheelchair skills of intentional directional control, starting and stopping to play games, and speed control of a proportional joystick. Learning specific skills to negotiate doorways, hallways, ramps, sidewalks, and curb cuts required a slightly higher understanding of problem solving seen at 30 months in combination with their spatial awareness seen at 25 months (Tefft et al., 1999). See the Resources at the end of the chapter for availability of the PPWST screening test and the Powered Mobility Program.

The training approach for powered wheelchair mobility in infants and young children is to incorporate the child's own motivation and curiosity (Figure 17-16). Curiosity sparks spontaneous exploration of the newly found ability to move. Experimenting with going forward and learning directional control of the joystick was reinforced with one child who was trying to follow pigeons walking along a patio. Gradual introduction of more functional skills through games and play, like follow the leader, will reward the child with successful intentional exploration. The amount and type of training will vary with the individual based on his or her needs, cognitive and physical impairments, motivation, and learning style (Bottos et al., 2001; Deitz et al., 2002; Huhn et al., 2007; Livingstone & Field, 2014). Generally, a child who demonstrates emerging skills and motivation to drive from one location to another, with limited hands on assistance, is ready for powered mobility.

Other pediatric considerations when recommending powered mobility include power seat functions including tilt, recline, seat elevation, and powered standing. RESNA does recommend early utilization of powered mobility for appropriate candidates as medically necessary to promote psychosocial development, reduce learned helplessness, and facilitate social and educational integration and independence (Rosen et al., 2009).

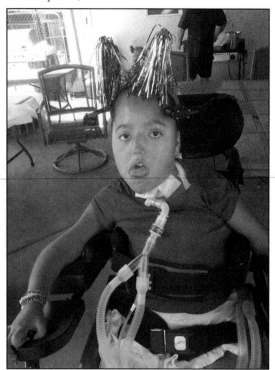

Figure 17-17. A 10-year old girl with nemaline rod myopathy using a proportional micropilot controller to drive her power wheelchair, control a computer, and use her communication device.

Ruth Everard of Dragonmobility, who had been a pediatric power wheelchair user herself and now manufactures powered mobility devices, summarizes her thoughts on considerations for pediatric seating and wheeled mobility:

> A wheelchair should not be thought of or designed as a vehicle in the mainstream sense. It is mobility, not transportation, so it should tap into natural instincts and understanding of the physical world rather than involve a conscious learning process. This opens up its use to people with cognitive limitations. The mobility system should be usable by a child of 9 months of age (i.e., when crawling/walking might normally be expected). It should allow access to the environment…it should provide feedback to all the senses about the environment (floor surface, up/downhill, etc.)—which incidentally enables use by the visually impaired. Its electronics should be able to interpret tremor or other unintentional movement of the user. It should be as compact as possible. It should provide access to the floor and to a height at which the user can look people in the eye (this is not only a need for reaching things, but for social and developmental purposes). It should move in three dimensions at once and not limit performance according to configuration. It should enable the user to stand if at all possible. Its battery life should exceed the stamina of its user and should re-charge in the time the user sleeps. It should be possible for a skilled bicycle mechanic to service it and do basic repairs (and the manufacturer's service operation should allow for this). The mobility system should be agile enough to "dance" and powerful enough for hiking. Its design should draw the eye to the face of the user and not draw attention to the seat or machine. It should be custom-built because nobody who uses a wheelchair has standard needs.

CASE EXAMPLE

Loli is a 10-year-old girl with a diagnosis of congenital nemaline rod myopathy (Figure 17-17). She has a tracheostomy tube and is dependent on a ventilator full time; however, she is able to breath off her ventilator for 30 minutes during bathing. Loli is dependent for all transfers, mobility, and activities of daily living. She is able to hold a pen and draw if the paper is held vertically to allow her wrist and fingers to drop down with gravity. Her mother is able to understand her speech; however, at school it is difficult for others to understand her, so she uses a Dynavox speech-generating device (SGD). She accesses this with eye gaze, and her mother reports that it is not always successful. She is able to self-feed if her plate is high enough. She is hypotonic and has significant weakness more proximally than distally, typical for a patient with a muscle disease. She has fair head control, poor facial muscle strength, and is unable to keep her lips closed. She has absent trunk control. She has weak movement of her thumb and fingers in all directions, and her right hand is stronger than her left. Loli developed scoliosis at a young age, requiring spinal fusion surgery at age 7 years. She no longer wears a body jacket (TLSO); however, she has a residual right thoracolumbar curve, and her pelvis is in posterior tilt with a left pelvic obliquity. Her left ischial tuberosity is painful, and she intentionally laterally leans to her right to unweight her left hip. Loli was referred for a power wheelchair evaluation and to address her seating to decrease pressure under her coccyx and ischial tuberosities.

Loli was positioned on an adult demo Quantum Q6 Edge, using a ROHO Quatro seat cushion and back pad to modify the seat depth. Positioning of a demo Micropilot mini proportional joystick needed be accurate to provide consistent access using just her right thumb over the top of the joystick. Foam support was mocked up to support her forearm and wrist. She was seen for five sessions to evaluate optimal setup and to practice. Final recommendation was for the Quantum Q6 Edge powered wheelchair and the SWITCH-IT Micropilot mini proportional joystick for driving. The Quantum Q-Logic electronics can function as a Bluetooth mouse emulator for access to the SGD

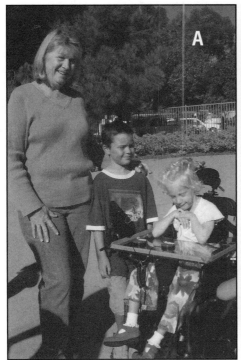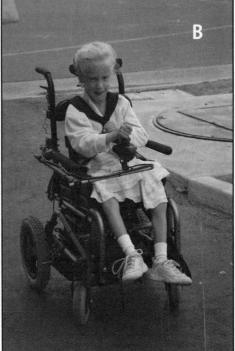

Figure 17-18. At age 4, this little girl initially had dynamic cognitive processing issues that were teased out from cognitive developmental readiness skills tested by the PPWST. Dynamically, it was easier for her to (A) understand switches first and quickly progressed to a (B) proportional joystick controller.

and a computer through the drive control. The wheelchair electronics can also send infrared signals to control devices such as the TV, lights, and a fan. She was most comfortable on a ROHO Contour Select cushion, which relieved her sitting pressures under her ischial tuberosities.

CASE EXAMPLE

Alexa has CP and had been part of pediatric powered wheelchair mobility project at age 4 (Furumasu, Guerette, & Tefft, 2004) (Figure 17-18). The PPWST assesses problem-solving and spatial relations skills found to be valid for learning powered wheelchair skills for children with disabilities (including CP) using a powered wheelchair with a joystick controller. At 3 years old, she did not yet have the understanding of spatial relations at the 25-month level, although her understanding of problem-solving skills was at the 20-month level. She worked on her spatial relations skills, eventually passing the cutoff points in both areas, demonstrating readiness to learn powered wheelchair skills. Alexa began practice in a pediatric powered wheelchair, and although she demonstrated cognitive developmental understanding of problem solving and spatial relations, dynamically she had cognitive processing problems when she was trying to learn to functionally control the wheelchair. She was physically able to manipulate a proportional

joystick well (she already used a mouse on a computer), but it seemed confusing to her. Dynamically and cognitively she understood single switches better than the proportionality of the joystick.

After 6 months of practice, her powered wheelchair was ordered with a proportional joystick through her father's insistence. When the power wheelchair was received, she did not do well learning to drive the proportional joystick controller. She attempted the joystick, but eventually shut down and was frustrated and unmotivated. The joystick was exchanged temporarily for switches. She was gradually introduced to a single switch to move forward. Within 2 weeks, right and left directional switches were added. After 2 months of practicing with switches, she demonstrated directional understanding, and the proportional joystick was tried again, this time successfully. Her mother provided the assistance and supervision she needed until she was ready to use the powered wheelchair at school (which took another year of practice at home). She has been using a powered wheelchair for all mobility at home, school, and in the community for the past 6 years. For Alexa, motor access and developmental readiness were not her issues in being successful in maneuvering a power wheelchair. The dynamic processing, perceiving her environment, motor planning, and physically coordinating the movement were the components she needed to work on. So for her, dynamic practice was important to develop those skills.

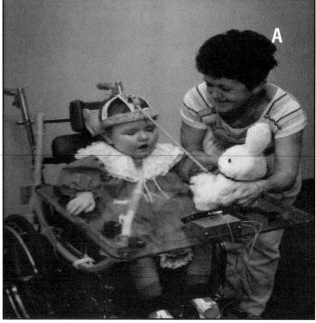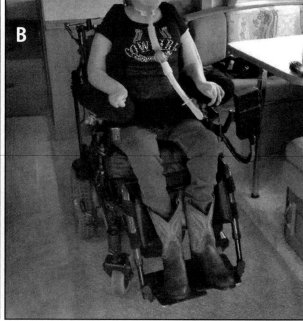

Figures 17-19. (A) Ashley as a 3-year-old with C1,2 tetraplegia from a birth injury. (B) Ashley as a 27-year-old county-western fan who travels to Nashville with her family in her RV.

CASE EXAMPLE

A 3-year-old at the time of this evaluation, Ashley had a C1,2 spinal cord birth injury that resulted in her being dependent on a ventilator (Figure 17-19). She was cognitively age-appropriate and has a supportive and loving grandmother who was her primary caregiver. She was very curious about her surroundings and very verbal. Ashley had very good head control and used a head pointer to play with dolls and to pick up miniature toys to put in her dollhouse. She was using a TLSO to give her the circumferential support she needed to sit upright. Without the body jacket, she would be more reclined and that would be a more difficult position from which to reach and use her head pointer in play. Once she was positioned in a trial power wheelchair, she immediately knew how to use the joystick and maneuver the wheelchair. She was ready to learn by exploring her environment independently. She used a chin proportional joystick controller and had a switch by her cheek to tap when she wanted to tilt back to change her position in space independently. She is now 27 years old. She has preferred the chin joystick controller when other methods were tried over the years and has a power tilt and recline for pressure relief and bladder management. She was recently seen in clinic to problem solve sitting pressure problems exacerbated by pelvic obliquity and weight loss. She loves country music and she, her grandmother, and mother make annual road trips to Nashville in their RV.

REFERENCES

Bottos, M. C., Bolcati, Sciuto, L., Ruggeri, C., & Feliciangeli, A. (2001). Powered wheelchairs and independence in young children with tetraplegia. *Developmental Medicine and Child Neurology, 43,* 769-777.

Butler, C. (1986). Effects of powered mobility on self-initiated behaviors of very young children with locomotor disability. *Developmental Medicine and Child Neurology, 28,* 325-332.

Butler, C. (1991). Augmentative mobility. Why do it? *Physical Medicine and Rehabilitation Clinics of North America, 2,* 801-815.

Butler, C., Okamoto, G. A., & McKay, T. M. (1983). Powered mobility for very young disabled children. *Developmental Medicine and Child Neurology, 25,* 472-474.

Butler, C., Okamoto, G. A., & McKay, T. M. (1984) Motorized wheelchair driving by disabled children. *Archives of Physical Medicine and Rehabilitation, 65,* 95-97.

Campbell, J., & Ball. J. (1978). Energetics of walking in cerebral palsy. *Orthopedic Clinics of North America, 9,* 347.

Cimolin, V., Piccinini, L., Avellis, M., Cazzaniga, A., Turconi, A. C., Crivellini, M., & Galli M. (2009). 3D-Quantitative evaluation of a rigid seating system and dynamic seating system using 3D movement analysis in individuals with dystonic tetraparesis. *Disability and Rehabilitation Assistive Technology, 4,* 422-428.

Deitz, J., Swinth, Y., & White, O. (2002). Powered mobility and preschoolers with complex development delays. *American Journal of Occupational Therapy, 56,* 86-96.

Dicianno, B., Morgan, A., Lieberman, J., & Rosen, L. (2013). *RESNA position on the application of wheelchair standing devices: 2013 Current state of the literature.* Arlington, VA: Rehabilitation Engineering and Assistive Technology Society of North America. Retrieved from https://www.resna.org/sites/default/files/legacy/resources/position-papers/RESNAStandingPositionPaper_Dec2013.pdf

Field, D. (1999). Powered mobility: A literature review illustrating the importance of a multifaceted approach. *Assistive Technology, 11,* 20-33.

Fowler, E. G., Knutson, L. M., Demuth, S. K., Siebert, K. L., Simms, V. D., Sugi, M. H.,…Azen, S. P. (2010). Pediatric endurance and limb strengthening (PEDALS) for children with cerebral palsy using stationary cycling: A randomized controlled trial. *Physical Therapy, 90*, 367-381.

Franks, C., Palisano, R., & Darbee, J. (1991). The effect of walking with an assistive device and using a wheelchair on school performance in students with myelomeningocele. *Physical Therapy, 71*, 570-535.

Furumasu, J., Guerette, P., & Tefft, D. (1996). The development of a powered wheelchair mobility program for young children. *Technology and Disability, 5*, 41-48.

Furumasu, J, Guerette, P., & Tefft, D. (2004). Relevance of the pediatric powered wheelchair screening test for children with cerebral palsy. *Developmental Medicine and Child Neurology, 46*, 468-474.

Galloway, J. C., Ryu, J. C., Agrawal, S. K. (2007). Babies driving robots: Self-generated mobility in very young infants. *Intelligent Service Robotics, 1*, 123-134.

Glickman, L. B., Geigle, P. R., & Paleg, G. S. (2010). A systematic review of supported standing programs. *Journal of Pediatric Rehabilitation Medicine, 3*, 197-213

Guerette, P., Furumasu, J., & Tefft, D. (2013). The positive effects of early powered mobility on children's psychosocial and play skills. *Assistive Technology, 25*, 39-48.

Guerette, P., Tefft, D., & Furumasu, J. (2005) Pediatric powered mobility: Results of a national survey of providers. *Assistive Technology, 17*, 144-158.

Harris, S., & Roxborough, L. (2005). Efficacy and effectiveness of physical therapy in enhancing postural control in children with cerebral palsy. *Neural Plasticity, 12*, 143-229.

Hsiang-Han, H., & Galloway, J. C. (2012). Modified ride-on toy cars for early power mobility: A technical report. *Pediatric Physical Therapy, 24*, 149-154.

Huhn, K., Guarrera-Bowlby, P., & Deutsch, J. (2007). The clinical decision-making process of prescribing power mobility for a child with cerebral palsy. *Pediatric Physical Therapy, 19*, 254-260.

Jones, M. A., McEwen, I. R., & Hansen, L. (2003). Use of power mobility for a young child with spinal muscular atrophy. *Physical Therapy, 83*, 253-262.

Jones, M. A., McEwen, I., & Neas, B. (2012). Effects of power wheelchairs on the development and function of young children with severe motor impairments. *Pediatric Physical Therapy, 24*, 131-140.

Johnston, T. E., Moore, S. E., Quinn, L. T., & Smith, B. T. (2004). Energy cost of walking in children with cerebral palsy: Relation to the gross motor function classification system. *Developmental Medicine and Child Neurology, 46*, 34-38.

Kangas, K. (2002). Seating for task performance. *Rehab Management.*

Livingstone, R., & Field, D. (2014). Systematic review of power mobility outcomes for infants, children and adolescents with mobility limitations. *Clinical Rehabilitation, 28*, 954-964.

Lubicky, J. P., & Betz, R. R. (2011). Spinal deformity in children and adolescents after spinal cord injury. In R. R. Betz & M. J. Mulcahey (Eds.), *The child with a spinal cord injury* (pp. 363-370). Rosemount, IL: American Academy of Orthopedic Surgeons.

Luna-Reyes, O. B., Reyes, T. M., Sol, M. L., Florian, Y., Matti, B. M. S., & Lardizabal, A. A. (1988). Energy cost of ambulation in healthy and disabled Filipino children. *Archives of Physical Medicine and Rehabilitation, 69*, 946-949.

Lynch, A., Ryu, J. C., Agrawal, S., & Galloway, J. C. (2009) Power mobility training for a 7 month old infant with spina bifida. *Pediatric Physical Therapy, 21*, 362-368.

McCarthy, J. J., Chafetz, R. S., Betz, R. R., & Gaughan, J. (2004). Incidence and degree of hip subluxation/ dislocation in children with spinal cord injury. *Journal of Spinal Cord Medicine, 27*(Suppl. 1):S80-S83.

McNamara, L., & Casey, J. (2007). Seat inclinations affect the function of children with cerebral palsy: a review of the effect of different seat inclines. *Disability and Rehabilitation Assistive Technology, 2*, 309-318.

Missiuna, C., & Pollock, N. (1991). Play deprivation in children with physical disabilities: The role of occupational therapist in preventing secondary disability. *American Journal of Occupational Therapy, 45*, 882-888.

Nilsson, L. M., & Nyberg, P. J. (2003). Driving to learn: A new concept for training children with profound cognitive disabilities in a powered wheelchair. *American Journal of Occupational Therapy, 57*, 229-233.

Nisbet, P. D. (2002) Assessment and training of children for powered mobility in the UK. *Technology and Disability, 14*, 173-182

Pountney, T. E., Mandy, A., Green, E., & Gard, P. R. (2009). Hip subluxation and dislocation in cerebral palsy—a prospective study on the effectiveness of postural management programmes. *Physiotherapy Research International, 14*, 116-127.

Rose, J., Gamble, J. G., Mederios J., Burgos, A., & Haskell, W. L. (1989). Energy cost of walking in normal children and with those with cerebral palsy. *Journal of Pediatric Orthopaedics, 9*, 276-279.

Rosen, L., Arva, J., Furumasu, J., Harris, M., Lange, M. L., McCarthy, E.,…Wonsettler, T. (2009). RESNA position on the application of power wheelchairs for pediatric users. *Assistive Technology, 21*, 218-225.

Roxborough, L. (1995). Review of the efficacy and effectiveness of adaptive seating for children with cerebral palsy. *Assistive Technology, 7*, 17-25.

Ryan, S. E., Campbell, K. A., Rigby, P. J., Fishbein-Germon, B., Hubley, D., & Chan, B. (2009) The impact of adaptive seating devices on young children with cerebral palsy and their families. *Archives of Physical Medicine and Rehabilitation, 90*, 27-33.

Stavness, C. (2006) The effect of positioning for children with cerebral palsy on upper-extremity function: A review of the evidence. *Physical and Occupational Therapy in Pediatrics, 26*, 39-53.

Sturgeon, J. (2010). Dynamic seating poised to move mobility market forward. *Mobility Management*. Retrieved from https://mobilitymgmt.com/articles/2010/05/05/dynamic-seating-tech.aspx?admgarea=pediatrics

Tamm, M., & Skar, L. (2000). How I play: Roles and relations in the play situations of children with restricted mobility. *Scandinavian Journal of Occupational Therapy, 7*, 174-182.

Tefft, D., Guerette, P., & Furumasu, J. (1999). Cognitive predictors of young children's readiness for powered mobility. *Developmental Medicine and Child Neurology, 41*, 665-670.

Tiemen, B. L., Palisano, R. J., Gracely, E. J., Roesenbaum, P. L., Chiarello, L. A., & O'Neill, M. E. (2004). Changes in mobility of children with cerebral palsy over time and across environmental settings. *Physical and Occupational Therapy in Pediatrics, 24*, 109-128.

Waters, R. L., Hislop, H. J., & Campbell, J. (1983). Energy cost of walking in normal children and teenagers. *Developmental Medicine and Child Neurology, 25*, 184-188.

Wiart, L., & Darrah, J., (2002). Changing philosophical perspectives on the management of children with physical disabilities—their effect on the use of powered mobility. *Disability & Rehabilitation, 24*, 492-498.

Wiart, L., Darrah, J., Hollis, V., Cook, A., & May, L. (2004). Mothers' perceptions of their children's use of powered mobility. *Physical & Occupational Therapy in Pediatrics, 24*, 3-21.

Williams, L. O., Anderson, A. D., Campbell, J., Thomas, L., Feiwell, E., & Walker, J. M. (1983). Energy cost of walking and of wheelchair propulsion by children with myelodysplasia: Comparison with normal children. *Developmental Medicine and Child Neurology, 25*, 617-624.

Wright-Ott, C. (1997) The transitional powered mobility aid: A new concept and tool for early mobility. In J. Furumasu (Ed.), *Pediatric powered mobility: Developmental perspectives, technical issues, clinical approaches* (pp. 58-69). Arlington, VA: Rehabilitation Engineering and Assistive Technology Society of North America.

SUGGESTED RESOURCES

The Pediatric Powered Wheelchair Screening Test: https://itunes.apple.com/us/book/ready-set-go-powered-mobility/id991600558?mt=13

Considerations When Working With the Geriatric Population

Deborah A. Jones, PT, DPT, GSC, CEEAA, ATP and Joanne Rader, RN, MN

Individualized seating means identifying the person's body contours, range of motion, and orientation in space and implementing a seating system that best positions and supports the person for comfort and function.

AGE-ASSOCIATED CHANGES

Physical changes commonly found in older people can affect their posture and functioning; therefore, seating and mobility needs differ from those of younger persons. There is a great deal of debate about what changes are part of the normal aging process and what changes occur as a result of disuse or disease. Common age-associated changes related to seating and mobility needs include the following:

- Decreased body fat and fluids, so there is less padding over bony prominences

- Thinner, more fragile skin that is prone to injury

- Visual changes resulting in problems with glare and need for more light

- Changes in bladder and kidney function resulting in urinary urgency and frequency

- Cardiovascular changes resulting in a drop in blood pressure upon standing and a longer recovery period after exercise

- Respiratory changes resulting in increased energy expenditure for breathing, diminished cough reflex, fatigue and shortness of breath with exertion, and increased susceptibility to pneumonia and other respiratory infections

- Diminished muscle mass, increased osteoporosis, and limited range of motion (ROM)

In addition to these age-associated changes, older people may have one or several health problems, such as osteoporosis or diseases affecting the respiratory system, the heart, or the nervous system, such as cerebral vascular accident, falls, orthopedic fractures or trauma, chronic obstructive pulmonary disease, and systemic diseases, such as Parkinson's disease, rheumatoid arthritis, diabetes, and Alzheimer's disease. Other comorbidities, such as osteoarthritis, osteoporosis, obesity, and dementia, have an effect on the body's ability to maintain its bony structure and skin integrity. These chronic conditions and changes in the musculoskeletal and neuroendocrine systems with nutritional and immunological deficits can lead to frailty. Accompanying these may be mental changes, such as dementia and depression. Osteoporosis, which is particularly common in elderly women, makes the bones more fragile and at risk for breaking (Fried, et al, 2001; Guralnik, Ferrucci, Simonsick, Salive, & Wallace, 1995; Xue, 2011).

Osteoporosis can also alter posture, creating a kyphosis or curved spine. Heart disease can affect exercise tolerance and general energy levels. Dementia affects the person's memory, insight, and judgment, increasing the risk of injury. Multiple diseases create the problem of disease interactions, which create further disability. While assessing for wheelchair seating and mobility, considerations of the primary diagnosis, as well as the comorbidities, will affect the long-term outcome, function, and skin integrity. Seating

Lange, M. L., & Minkel, J. L.
Seating and Wheeled Mobility: A Clinical Resource Guide
(pp. 297-316). © 2018 SLACK Incorporated.

and mobility choices should be made with the future prognosis in mind (Kemp, Brummel-Smith, & Ramsdell, 1990).

The majority of people admitted to nursing homes have lower extremity weakness and inability to walk safely. A wheelchair is often required for transportation and is a standard issue upon admission to a nursing home because of frailty and increased fall risk. Often these chairs have been issued or purchased without a clear understanding of the user's wants, needs, and desires. When wheelchairs do not fit the person using them, it causes pain, discomfort, inhibited mobility, poor posture, and unnecessary restraint use. For many years frail elders were issued a wheelchair as if one size fits all when it comes to seating. The typical wheelchair had sling-style upholstery with little to no adjustment for the person's size or mobility needs. Often, the wheelchair did not have a seat cushion or back support. The standard sling seat, slingback, collapsible wheelchair was designed to transport people short distances, for short amounts of time, to assist the person pushing the chair, and to make storage easy. The chair works for the caregiver but very poorly for the person in it, particularly if it is used for long periods of time and as the primary seating system for the individual. This predictable negative outcome is particularly true when the chair is used for long periods of time and as the primary seating system for the individual. This type of wheelchair creates poor postural stability resulting in increased posterior pelvic tilt, trunk kyphosis, and forward head position. After a short period of time in a wheelchair without supportive seating, the individual may begin leaning forward, sometimes to the point of falling out, leaning to one side with one arm hanging over the armrest, or sliding forward toward the floor. Some caregivers resort to restraining, wedging, or restricting movement, because they think that these interventions will help. Yet actually, the only result of these actions is that the person continues to be uncomfortable and unable to move. The poor positional position with lack of stability increases energy consumption while attending to simple activities of daily living (ADL) and wheeled mobility. These types of wheelchairs were originally designed for brief transportation but are uncomfortable when used for long-term sitting and self-mobilization.

What is needed is individualized seating and wheeled mobility for the older adult. This begins with a comprehensive seating assessment involving an interdisciplinary team and the person using the wheelchair. Individualized seating and wheeled mobility means identifying the client's body contours, ROM, and orientation in space, and implementing a seating system that best positions and supports the person for comfort and function and improved mobility. From the evaluation and measurements, seating and wheeled mobility equipment can be selected to meet the person's individual needs for postural control and mobility with the goal of increasing independence in activities and mobility. How people sit is fundamental to their health.

There are seating and wheeled mobility manufacturers who have designed specific seating and wheeled mobility products to meet the needs of the elderly. For instance, these specialized products are more adjustable, lighter weight, and designed to accommodate for common aging changes and needs. When frail elders are properly seated in chairs designed to meet their particular needs, improvements can occur in the following areas:

- Posture
- Comfort, leading to increased sitting tolerance and less time in bed
- Skin condition
- Ability to care for self
- Efficient use of limited energy and endurance
- Socialization
- Quality of life
- Caregiver burden

Improved Posture

Improving posture can enhance a number of functions in the elderly; however, as a result of illness or orthopedic changes, many elders have postures that cannot be corrected and can only be supported. The first step in achieving proper seating is a seating assessment. A seating assessment by a physical or occupational therapist is required to determine whether the person needs accommodation of fixed posture and/or support of flexible posture. The assessment should include a physical evaluation, in which the person is transferred out of the wheelchair and onto a treatment mat or firm surface. The out-of-chair assessment allows the therapist to evaluate the person both lying down and in a seated position for fixed joints, spasticity, pain, and skin problems. With better positioning and/or support through proper seating, physiologic functions such as breathing, swallowing, digestion, and elimination are improved. Respiratory function improves in several ways. The chest cavity more easily expands if the person is not slumped forward. Many frail elders have a delayed swallow that places them at risk for choking or aspirating (taking food or fluid into the lungs). It is essential that the person sit upright for meals so that food and particularly liquids can be better controlled and to aid the normal gravitational flow into stomach. Needless to say, if a person is constantly choking, food may often be refused. The ability to move the bolus of food in the mouth may be improved if the person with a normal swallow and kyphotic or curved back (resulting in a forward head and neck position) is properly supported and positioned so that gravity can assist in getting the food to the back of the mouth. Also, elongating the abdominal region through proper positioning allows food to move more easily through the digestive tract and better utilize gravity to facilitate digestion and elimination.

Good positioning can also improve eye gaze, that is, the visual field created by the position of one's head. If older persons have stooped posture while sitting, the eyes naturally fall lower, sometimes to the floor, requiring a considerable effort to raise the eyes or head to see what is in front of them. Even if the posture is fixed, as with a kyphosis or curved spine, improvements can occur. For example, positioning the wheelchair at even a 15-degree recline may bring the eye gaze level, making it easier for the person to attend to what is going on around him or her and socialize.

Improved Comfort and Wheelchair-Sitting Tolerance

Comfort is an important concern of frail elders. Comfort is achieved or improved through proper support and positioning. Wheelchair-sitting tolerance, or the amount of time the person feels able to be up in the chair, can be used as a practical indicator of comfort. That is, comfort is directly related to wheelchair tolerance. If the person is uncomfortable in the wheelchair, he or she will often ask to go to bed sooner and refuse to become more involved in activities. Older adults experience more pain than younger people for many reasons. They often suffer from arthritis or other chronic illnesses that have pain associated with them. Often pain is unidentified or undertreated in the frail elderly. Many frail elders have diagnosed or undiagnosed spinal fractures that can be a source of pain. Often with proper positioning and support, this type of pain can be dramatically reduced.

Persons with dementia may not have the verbal or cognitive ability to express their pain in words or even respond appropriately when asked if they are in pain. However, their behavior, particularly increased agitation, is often a good indicator of pain.

Prevention of Skin Breakdown

Proper cushions and support prevent skin and tissue breakdown by more evenly distributing pressure, thus allowing the individual to be up for longer periods without causing damage. Some fabric cushion covers wick away moisture and fluid from the skin. Heat buildup may also contribute to skin breakdown, and some cushion materials (e.g., air, fluid) are cooler than foam. The optimal microenvironment is close to normal body temperature to allow good blood flow and tissue health.

Improved Ability to Care for Self

A properly fitted wheelchair can improve the person's ability to care for him- or herself in many ways. For example, correct armrest length and height allow the chair to get under the table so that at meals the person can be close enough to reach the food and feed him- or herself. It gives the person a level eye gaze so he or she can see in the mirror for grooming. Further, with the proper chair, many people can wheel themselves from place to place.

Better Use of Limited Energy and Endurance

Frail elders often have limited stamina, endurance, and energy. When one is not positioned properly, energy is required simply to remain upright. When properly equipped, the ability to self-propel is enhanced and requires less expenditure of energy. Choosing a wheelchair where the rear wheel can be adjusted forward or back can distribute the person's weight and improve wheeled efficiency. Also, the standard wheelchair weighs between 40 and 50 pounds, a lightweight chair weighs 24 to 28 pounds, and an ultralight chair can weigh even less (18 to 21 pounds). Choosing a lighter weight chair can save energy for use with other activities. Having the seat low enough so that the person who ambulates is able to foot propel efficiently because his or her feet can get a good heel strike (connection of the foot to the floor) also improves efficiency. Providing a chair with the proper width so that the person can easily access the handrims on the wheels is another way to better conserve limited energy. Being comfortably seated and positioned for eating may mean that the person will eat more because he or she is not too fatigued to finish the meal. With proper support, the person can relax and focus on other activities, such as eating or conversing.

Improved Socialization

Improved socialization can result from a combination of the factors already mentioned, such as level eye gaze, the ability to move oneself in and out of social situations, and increased comfort. Improved socialization may also be related to eliminating restraints. Individuals often find restraints uncomfortable, humiliating, and degrading, causing them to shrink from social situations.

Improved Quality of Life

What might be considered obvious, but should not be underestimated is that if a person is more comfortable, more independent, and has better physiologic function, that person will have improved quality of life and self-esteem.

Easing of Caregiver Burden

When properly seated, frail elders may be easier to transfer, or able to transfer themselves and to feed or toilet themselves; they may require less repositioning (creating less back and shoulder stress for the caregiver), tolerate being up for longer periods, and have fewer behavioral problems. All of these positive outcomes ease the caregiver's burden.

The following case example illustrates many of the benefits of proper seating.

CASE EXAMPLE

Ninety-seven-year-old M.P. was in the typical wheelchair with a sling back and a sling seat with an inexpensive foam cushion. Her thighs were rolled inward, and her pelvis was in a posterior pelvic tilt, which made her trunk collapse and her movements limited, affecting her breathing and circulation. Consequently, M.P. suffered from considerable back pain, making her irritable, as manifested by crying, angry outbursts, and refusing all activities. A physical therapist conducted an evaluation, including a physical assessment on the mat to assess her needs. She discovered that M.P. had the following:

- A fixed posterior pelvic tilt or forward thrust of pelvis
- Hip ROM (thigh to trunk angle) limited to 90 degrees
- Shortened hamstring muscles
- A fixed thoracic, kyphotic spine, causing her head to be positioned forward

The therapist recommended a smaller, lightweight chair and a solid, contoured back and seat system. Putting M.P. in a wheelchair with smaller diameter (20-inch) wheels provided her access to the wheels because she did not have to flex her shoulder or elbow as much as when trying to access the standard 24-inch wheels; thus M.P. has enough ROM to bring her elbows back far enough to have full excursion on the wheel so she could more easily propel her wheelchair. The stability and contoured support that M.P. received from the new seating system also protected her skin with better distribution of pressure. Finally, the system stabilized her pelvis, allowing elongation of her trunk and resulting in better upright sitting, energy conservation, and comfort.

The overall results were dramatic. Before, because of her pain, M.P. had been very withdrawn, not talking to people or attending activities. Following the improvements in her seating, she became clearer cognitively and moved easily through the facility talking to others. She was more comfortable, aware, and pleasant. Her son was amazed and pleased with the differences. M.P. lived another 4 years, continuing to use her individualized wheelchair and maintaining her improved comfort and mobility (Pitts, 1995).

Restraint and Secondary Support Use

Restraint use in long-term care facilities has declined due to changes in policy and practices. In the past, restraints were used as standard practice to prevent falls, sliding out of chairs, interference with treatments, and disruptive behaviors such as wandering and aggression. It was found that in many cases, restraining a person was unnecessary, ineffective, and in some cases dangerous; it was also frequently done for the convenience of staff members and not the safety of the resident. This realization prompted the National Citizens Coalition for Nursing Home Reform to seek change in practice by passing the Omnibus Budget Reconciliation Act (OBRA) of 1987 requiring all nursing homes to rethink the practice of restraint use and mandated the reduction of physical restraints. When the OBRA went into effect in 1990, more than 40% of long-term care residents were physically restrained with devices such as geri chairs, bedrails, lap devices, and/or vests that tied them to beds and chairs.

The definition most commonly used for restraints comes out of the Nursing Home Reform Act:

> "Physical restraints" are defined as any manual method or physical or mechanical device, material, or equipment attached or adjacent to the resident's body that the individual cannot remove easily which restricts freedom of movement or normal access to one's body. "Physical restraints" include, but are not limited to, leg restraints, arm restraints, hand mitts, soft ties or vests, lap cushions and lap trays the resident cannot remove. Also included as restraints are facility practices that meet the definition of a restraint, such as:

- Using bed rails to keep a resident from voluntarily getting out of bed as opposed to enhancing mobility while in bed;
- Tucking in a sheet so tightly that a bed bound resident cannot move;
- Using wheelchair safety bars to prevent a resident from rising out of a chair;
- Placing a person in a chair that prevents rising; and
- Placing a person who uses a wheelchair so close to a wall that the wall prevents the person from rising (Health Care Financing Administration, 1995).

Key points to remember in the definition of restraints are these: the individual cannot easily remove the device, and the device restricts freedom of movement or normal access to one's body. Numerous negative consequences related to restraint use have been documented in the literature (Blakeslee, 1989; Evans & Strumpf, 1989, 1990; Jones & Rader, 2015; Miles & Meyers, 1994; Parker & Miles, 1997) . No studies have shown that restraints increase safety (Table 18-1).

Common Asymmetries

Even though age-associated changes plus the lack of activity make an elderly person more prone to asymmetries, one should not assume that all asymmetries are fixed. In

TABLE 18-1

CONSEQUENCES OF RESTRAINT USE DOCUMENTED IN THE LITERATURE

NEGATIVE CONSEQUENCES

- Withdrawal, humiliation, depression, regressive behavior, resistance, anger, agitation
- Complications of restricted mobility, including circulatory obstruction, edema or swelling, pressure ulcers, muscle wasting, joint contracture, osteoporosis, respiratory problems, infection, increased incontinence, and a drop in blood pressure when standing
- Increased confusion
- Decreased appetite, dehydration
- Changes in body chemistry due to response to stress
- Injuries and deaths related to restraint use

POSITIVE CONSEQUENCES

- None

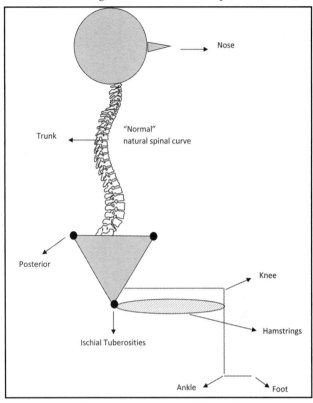

Figure 18-1. Parts of the body affecting sitting posture.

fixed skeletal asymmetries, permanent changes have taken place in the bones, muscles, and ligaments that restrict normal ROM (Cook & Polgar, 2008). Often, increased tone and muscle tightness cause a person to assume certain postures and he or she may appear to have an asymmetry. If the asymmetry can be returned to a more normal position with support, than it would be considered a flexible asymmetry (Figure 18-1). The approach toward fitting the person with a flexible joint will be different than for a fixed asymmetry. Fixed joints need to be accommodated whereas flexible joints need to be corrected within the person's tolerance. *To accommodate* means that a therapist determines through a physical assessment that fixed (unmovable) joint positions exist and a seating system is selected that matches the person's fixed position, rather than trying to move his or her joints and support him or her in a normal position he or she can no longer achieve.

Frequently seen fixed asymmetries that can affect seating include:

- Abnormal spinal curvatures (e.g., kyphosis or scoliosis)
- Limited hip ROM (thigh to trunk angles >95 degrees)
- Limited knee ROM (thigh to lower leg angles <85 degrees)
- Posterior pelvic tilt

Abnormal Spinal Curvatures: Kyphosis or Scoliosis

A kyphosis occurs when the spine is overly curved into a C-shape from a side (sagittal) view and is often the result of osteoporosis. With kyphosis and the resulting muscular imbalance and effects of gravity, the neck and head respond with increased flexion, so the person routinely looks down into his or her lap (Figure 18-2A). If there is flexibility, the person may lift his or her head into extension or slide down into the chair to maintain the ability to see forward (Figure 18-2B).

The seating goal for a person with a fixed spinal asymmetry is to accommodate the curve with a standard back system that has a similar curve (Figure 18-3) or with a custom-molded back system for more severe asymmetries. A corrective back system uses gravity to assist in positioning, allowing the trunk to recline to create a more level eye gaze. A similar intervention would be used with a spinal

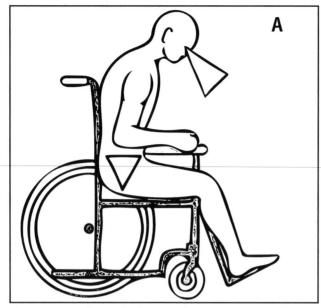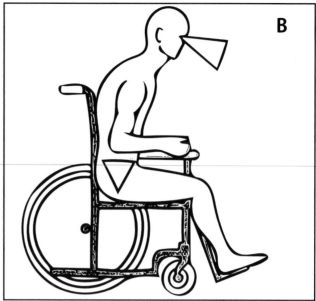

Figure 18-2. (A) Thoracic kyphosis. (B) Thoracic kyphosis with flexible neck.

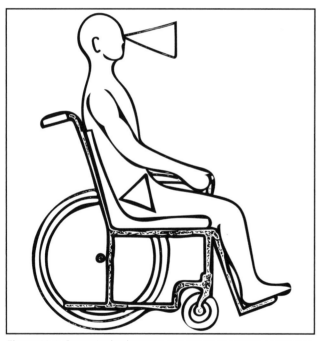

Figure 18-3. Corrective back system uses gravity to assist in positioning.

asymmetry know as *scoliosis* (where the spine makes an S-shaped curve to the side) (Figure 18-4). Providing lateral trunk support assists in holding the person in a more upright position (see Figure 18-4). Adjusting the wheelchair seat and back angles to use gravity also assists a weak trunk to stay in a more upright position.

Limited Hip Range of Motion (Open Trunk to Thigh Angle)

Limited hip ROM is common in frail elders, especially those who walk infrequently or not at all. It is important not to overflex (bend) a tight hip joint because this pulls the pelvis forward and creates a sacral sitting position with the pelvis thrust forward in the chair seat, causing the person to slide out. Positioning the person with limited hip ROM, in a seated position that requires a tighter angle between the trunk and the thigh may result in more severe tilting of the pelvis into a sacral sitting position to accommodate for the lack of hip range (Figure 18-5). The increased pelvic tilt in turn will cause increased pressure on the lumbar spine, resulting in discomfort and decreased wheelchair tolerance. To accommodate limited hip ROM, the chair seat and back should be adjusted with an open seat to back support angle, to the individual's specific needs.

Limited Knee Range of Motion Because of Tight Hamstring Muscles

The hamstring muscles are located behind the knee, and they extend up the back of the leg to the pelvis. The hamstrings tend to become tighter in frail elders who walk infrequently, resulting in decreased knee ROM. As a result, they are unable to straighten their legs or sit in the standard wheelchair with footplates and legrests (Figure 18-6).

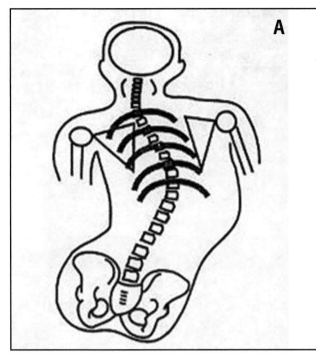

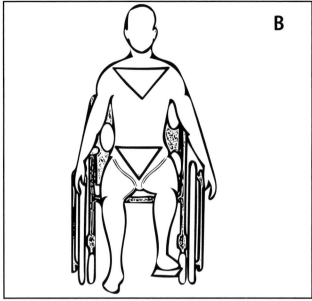

Figure 18-4. (A) Problem: scoliosis of the spine. (B) Solution: use lateral support for trunk.

When the person's legs are forced out to the footplates with heel loops, boards, or tie-downs, the person may respond by sliding out of the chair to decrease the stretch of his or her hamstrings, or the feet may fall off the footplates (Figure 18-7). Such individuals will need a custom footplate or angle-adjustable footplates, or their feet should be placed on the floor to reduce the pull or pressure on the hamstrings (Figure 18-8).

Fixed Posterior Pelvic Tilt

A fixed posterior pelvic tilt is common among frail elders and is caused by bony changes in the spine. The pelvis of an elderly client tends to respond to the spinal changes by moving into a posterior tilt position so that the head and neck come increasingly forward. This position helps to balance the person during walking. As the person begins to sit more than walk, the tendency for the pelvis to progress into further poor pelvic position increases. The seating goal for posterior pelvic tilt is to stabilize the pelvis with a seating system that includes a large well space for the buttocks, adequate femoral support, and posterior stabilization of the pelvis. In addition, a properly placed seat belt placed over the upper thighs may be necessary to assist in femoral pressure to stabilize the pelvis (Figure 18-9).

FUNCTIONAL GOALS FOR SEATING

Functional goals for seating include the following:
- Independent mobility
- Maximizing head and upper extremity function

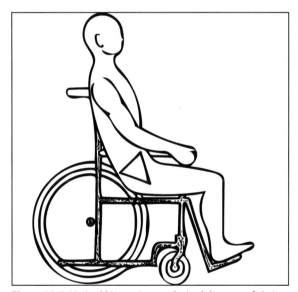

Figure 18-5. Limited hip motion results in sliding out of chair.

- Minimizing trunk asymmetry and maximizing function
- Minimizing abnormal foot position
- Maximizing head control to facilitate interaction
- Preventing skin breakdown
- Achieving reasonable wheelchair tolerance (Brienza, Karg, Geyer, Kelsey, & Trefler, 2001; Jones, 1995a, 1995b)

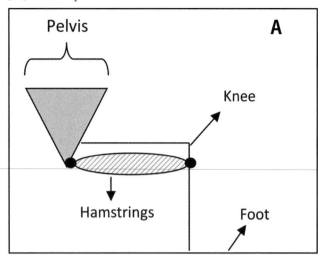

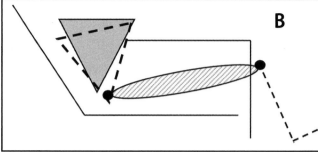

Figure 18-6. (A) Problem: shortened hamstring muscles can influence lower leg and pelvis position (feet falling off footplates). (B) When hamstrings are maximally lengthened, both the pelvis and lower leg can be influenced.

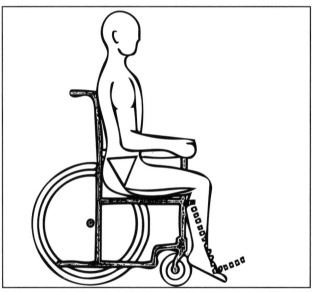

Figure 18-7. Problem: Tight hamstrings may result in feet falling off of footplates.

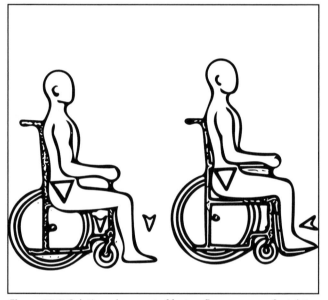

Figure 18-8. Solution: placement of feet on floor or proper footplates.

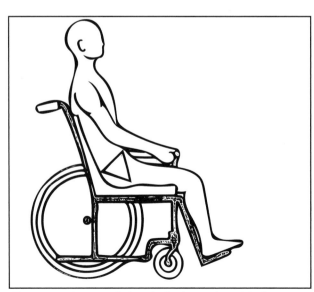

Figure 18-9. Accommodation of a fixed posterior pelvic tilt.

GOAL 1: INDEPENDENT MOBILITY

When individuals are placed in a good position with the correct wheelchair and seating system, they have the potential for improved wheeled mobility. It is important to enable frail elders to move in the most efficient way. Some will use both legs for mobility, others will use both arms, and still others a combination of arms and legs. Providing proper lightweight and adjustable wheelchairs that have been optimized for the individual needs to be the standard of practice when working with elders of wheelchair mobility.

Optimal Method of Mobility

Arms-Only Propulsion

When an individual is using both arms for propulsion it is important to make sure the wheelchair is the correct width for the person. This is determined by measuring the width of the person's hips and then selecting a wheelchair

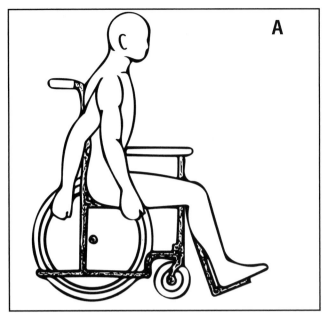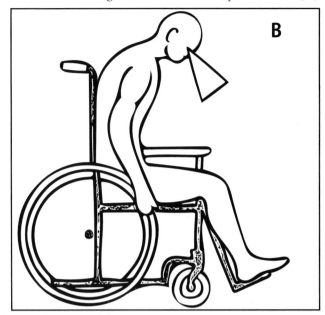

Figure 18-10. (A) Problem: inefficient propulsion. (B) Solution: modifications to enhance propulsion.

width that fits. The rule of thumb is to allow just enough space between the hips and the side of the wheelchair for the person to easily slip his or her hands between the sides of the wheelchair (maybe the inside of the armrest) and the hips. Wheelchair width is important because the handrims should be located in a plumb line under the person's shoulders. The person will then be able to achieve the most effective push. A wheelchair that is too wide is difficult to propel.

Once the proper wheelchair width is selected and the feet are fully supported on the footrest, without undue pressure under the thighs, the wheel axle placement should be looked at to determine how efficiently the chair can be propelled. If the rear axle is placed too far behind the person's back, the chair will be more stable, but self-propelling will be hindered because the person will be unable to reach the wheel for a full push (Figure 18-10A). The optimal placement of the rear axle is directly in line with the spine line or slightly behind it (Figure 18-10B). This position of the rear wheel is not always possible on a nonadjustable, standard wheelchair. If the standard wheelchair rear position cannot be adjusted far enough forward for optimal position, consider trialing a wheelchair with an adjustable rear axle to test the improvement in self-propulsion. Following optimal rear wheel adjustment, if the wheelchair appears too likely to tip backward, adding anti-tippers to the back of the chair is advised.

Other things to take into consideration include the following:

- A small, 20-inch rear wheel may be easier to rotate than a large, 24-inch wheel. When the arms are used for mobility, the arms should move not only forward but also down and backward and then up. This

motion will stimulate trunk extension and breathing (see Figure 18-10B).

- The handrims may be easier to grip if they are covered with a grip-ease material; gloves with leather in the palms also help to increase friction for propulsion, and they keep hands clean and protect hands from callousing.

- A lightweight wheelchair is easier to propel, especially for the elderly, who often have upper extremity weakness.

CASE EXAMPLE

An 87-year-old woman with fixed thoracic kyphosis living in a long-term care home was sitting in an 18-inch-wide standard wheelchair with standard 24-inch rear wheels. She had to abduct her shoulders to reach the wheels, and then, due to her fixed forward trunk kyphosis and head, her arms were lower and more forward when trying to access the rear wheel for propulsion. She was unable to flex her elbows and extend her shoulders to reach the top of the handrims. To propel the wheelchair, she placed her hands forward on the handrims and gave a light push resulting in little forward movement of the wheelchair. She would push the wheelchair a few feet and then waited to be pushed or asked for help. To individualize her seating, a 16-inch-wide wheelchair was selected with 20-inch rear wheels. She was issued a supportive back and seat cushion to accommodate her fixed trunk posture. This configuration allowed increased ability to use her upper extremities with improved position and efficiency for self-propulsion. She then was able to

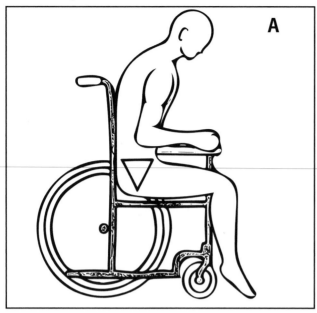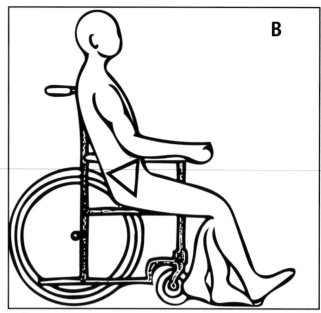

Figure 18-11. (A) Problem: feet do not reach floor. (B) Problem: sliding to reach the floor.

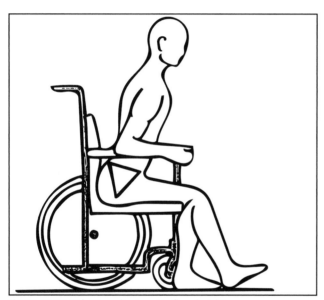

Figure 18-12. Solution: adjust seat to floor height.

propel her wheelchair independently using both arms from her room to the dining area (approximately 55 feet) with ease, stopping for rest but not asking for help or waiting for a push.

Legs-Only Propulsion

Arthritic changes in upper extremities, pain, weakness and/or cardiac conditions can be indicators for legs only propulsion or as an adjunct to upper extremities propulsion. If a person is using the legs for propulsion, then both feet must reach the ground easily while the pelvis stays back in the chair. Figure 18-11 illustrates problems that occur when feet do not reach the ground easily.

To achieve the proper seat to floor height, the length from the back of the knee to the floor should be measured, making sure to add in the cushion thickness, before wheelchair selection or adjustment. Several adjustments can be made to the chair. For example, a wheelchair can be ordered as a hemi-height chair, which allows the frame of the chair's seat to floor height to be 2 inches closer to the floor. Also, the wheel size can be altered on certain wheelchairs; instead of the standard 24-inch wheel, a 22- or 20-inch wheel can be used, which will also lower the seat to floor height of the frame, allowing the person's feet to reach the floor with full support. If the rear wheel size is reduced, the front casters will need to be smaller to prevent a downward slant of the seat. The person's hips should be positioned to the back of the chair with the trunk leaning forward. This will allow for the downward pressure toward the floor that is necessary for forward movement (Figure 18-12).

If the person is wedged backward into the seat for stability, this will hinder self-mobilization, because it is difficult to foot propel when the hip to back angle is decreased. The person will move more easily if he or she is able to lean slightly forward. It is more efficient to have a flat seat or to angle the seat slightly forward to promote forward movement and to encourage the trunk to align in a more upright position.

A major advantage to having the feet on the floor is that the person then has the option to rock him- or herself back and forth in the chair. This repetitive motion is not only good for exercising the legs but also produces a calming effect. In addition, when elderly persons have their feet on the ground, they can change not only their foot position but also their pelvic position. We all change our positions often to alleviate pain and discomfort. We need to allow the elderly this opportunity as well (Kong, Evans, & Guevara 2008).

Tip: When front foot supports are removed from the wheelchair to allow for foot propulsion, the wheelchair can easily tip forward. This is especially true for someone who leans forward. For safety, the foot supports can remain on the wheelchair with the individual footplates removed to provide a forward stability. Another method is to add front anti-tip riggings to decrease potential of forward tipping of the wheelchair.

Combination of Upper Extremity and Lower Extremity Propulsion

Combination of One Arm and One Leg

For people who use one arm and one leg to move the wheelchair, the approach is the same as those already described, except that the cushion may need to be altered so that one leg is supported on a foot support while the other leg is on the floor. To make this adjustment, a cushion should be considered that can be shortened or scooped out for the thigh of the leg that will be contacting the floor for mobility. Using one arm and one leg is necessary for users who have weakness or flaccid extremities from a cerebral vascular accident or head trauma.

Transfer To and From the Wheelchair

If the person has difficulty getting in and out of the wheelchair, there are several possible solutions:

- Remove or flip up foot supports to allow enough space for the resident to place his or her feet slightly under the wheelchair.
- Remove the armrest that interferes with the resident when he or she is transferring from the side of the wheelchair to another surface, with or without the use of a sliding board.
- Consult a physical therapist for an evaluation to identify the best transfer solutions.

GOAL 2: MAXIMIZING HEAD AND UPPER EXTREMITY FUNCTION

Correct Hip or Pelvis Positioning

The pelvis and the angle of the hips with the upper leg (trunk to thigh angle) form the base for the upper body and the head. It is therefore extremely important that the pelvis and the hips are aligned and supported. As mentioned earlier, the most common observation is that the person's hips are sliding out of the wheelchair. This position can cause a great deal of discomfort—low back pain, increased pressure on the sacral area, and poor trunk alignment leading to poor head position and decreased ability to use the upper extremities. Sometimes when a person has slid forward in the chair, it is because he or she is trying to reach the floor to use his or her feet for mobility or to change his or her position in order to relieve discomfort. But quite often frail elders are too weak to reposition themselves and they are then at risk for skin breakdown, slipping out of the chair, and injuring themselves by falling.

When an individual has thoracic kyphosis and the hips are positioned to the back of the chair, the trunk is pushed forward and he or she ends up looking at his lap (see Figure 18-12). The client then needs to scoot his or her hips forward to have a more level eye gaze or to reach the floor for propulsion.

There are several solutions to this problem. First, a comprehensive assessment is necessary to determine the pelvic mobility and hip ROM as it pertains to seating:

- Accommodate contractures and support flexible postures
- If the person has fixed posterior pelvic tilt, support the posterior aspect of the pelvis in the best position toward neutral.
- With a posterior pelvic tilt, the additional length of the pelvis and legs will need to be accommodated with a longer supportive seat cushion to take advantage of full femoral support.
- If the person continues to migrate or slide toward the front of the wheelchair after the preceding interventions, sometimes a positioning seat belt (either push-button or latch type) is needed to keep the hips in the proper position. A seat belt is not a restraint if the person can take it off at will. However, if the person cannot remove the seat belt independently, it is considered a physical restraint, and less restrictive interventions should be considered.
- If the person's hips can be relocated to the back of the chair, see that his or her feet are supported—either flat on the floor or on foot supports with adequate support under the thighs. If the feet are not supported, a simple footrest adjustment may support the feet better. A different wheelchair with a lower seat to floor height may be indicated for the person who is a foot mobilizer and needs feet flat on the floor.
- To accommodate a kyphotic spine, the back of the wheelchair needs to be reclined enough to allow for the asymmetry without compromising pelvic positioning (Figure 18-13).

Correct Equipment (Seating)

A common reason for improper pelvic positioning is sling seating. This type of seating does not provide a

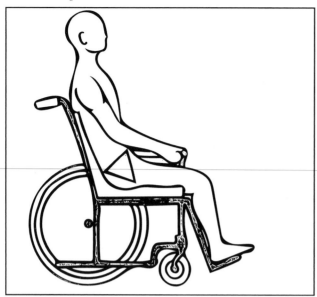

Figure 18-13. Accommodated fixed posture results in level eye gaze and improved comfort.

level base on which to align the pelvis and thighs. Instead it tends to roll the person's legs inward and support the buttocks and thighs unevenly. Many older wheelchairs have sling upholstery that is stretched out, increasing the hammocking effect and causing discomfort, pain, and sitting intolerance. As mentioned earlier, sling seating was intended for transportation purposes and to allow folding of the wheelchair, not for the long-term sitting in the way that many elderly clients use them. There are two ways to address this problem:

1. Sling seating can be replaced with sturdier fabric or solid seating. Some solid seats are adjustable and can be lowered to reduce the seat to floor height; some also can be adjusted to angle the seat backward or forward to achieve an upright pelvis and position the pelvis back in the seat.

2. A solid seat insert can be added across or between the seat rails of a wheelchair that has sling seating. Most solid seat inserts can be placed under the cushion or inside the cushion cover; this consolidates the pieces and may prevent improper placement. A cushion over the solid seat insert is necessary for comfort and positioning.

When the pelvis and hips are positioned in the back of the wheelchair and the lower trunk is supported to achieve upper trunk and head control, then the armrest height should be adjusted to support the forearms comfortably. Unfortunately, many wheelchairs have fixed armrests that cannot be adjusted; although, if the fixed-length armrests are removable, adjustable height armrests can be purchased. The length of the armrests also needs to be considered. Full-length armrests provide greater support for transfers.

A desk-length armrest, however, allows the resident to pull up closer to a table or sink, which facilitates ADL.

GOAL 3: MINIMIZING TRUNK ASYMMETRY, MAXIMIZING FUNCTION

Need for Trunk Support

Once the hips are in the proper position, it is time to observe the trunk. If a person has poor trunk control, the trunk tends to collapse, the shoulder girdle becomes rounded, and the arms are more difficult to raise—all of which make it more difficult to use the upper extremities. Improper trunk position can also affect head position, breathing, swallowing, eye gaze, and socialization.

After the hips and pelvis are supported in the optimal position to the back of the chair, observe the trunk position. Is the person leaning to one side, or is he or she falling forward? Usually leaning is caused by weakness, upright spatial orientation problems, or improper pelvis positioning (Figure 18-14).

- The pelvis should be positioned as level and upright as possible on a solid contoured seating surface and against a solid contoured supportive back support.

- A slight recline (a seat to back support angle > 90 degrees) in the back of the wheelchair will decrease the gravitational forward pull and support the trunk better. This can be accomplished by replacing the back upholstery of the wheelchair with a contoured back that can recline but maintain posterior pelvic stabilization.

- Lateral trunk supports may be necessary to assist a weak trunk. Lateral trunk supports can be attached to the sides of the wheelchair or ordered as an option with the back support component of a seating system.

- Sometimes trunk weakness is severe enough to require a combination of opening the seat to back support angle and add the lateral trunk support for proper positioning and improved functioning.

Remember: The pelvis is the starting point. Make sure the pelvis is properly positioned before attempting to support the trunk. Installing a lap tray to help achieve an upright position is not appropriate. The enormous pressure this places on the arms and shoulder joints can cause pain, skin breakdown, and shoulder joint limitation over a period of time. Also, fatigue occurs from trying to hold up one's trunk weight with one's arms.

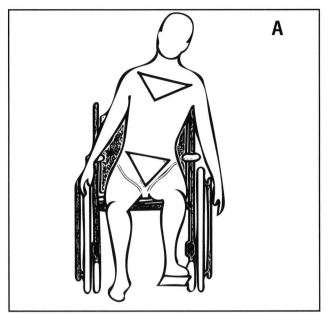 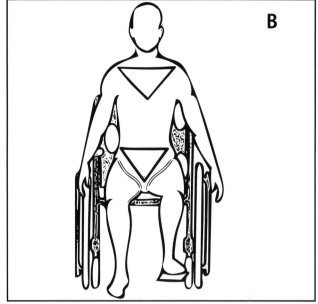

Figure 18-14. (A) Leaning of the trunk. (B) Trunk supported.

GOAL 4: MINIMIZING ABNORMAL FOOT POSITION

Assess Foot Position

Feet need to be properly supported to maintain the position of the pelvis (with the hips to the back of the chair) and have effective mobility. Wheelchair foot supports are used to support the feet, but they may not be high enough or low enough to enhance positioning and function. A change in the position of the feet or the pressure on the feet can negatively affect trunk and pelvis position. For instance, if the footrests are too high, the thighs are inadequately supported and more pressure is placed on the bony prominences of the pelvis (ischial tuberosities), which may lead to discomfort and skin breakdown. If the foot supports are too low, there is too much pressure on the thighs and circulatory problems can occur, as well as skin breakdown. If the foot supports are placed too far out or if elevated legrests are used, the resident may scoot out toward the edge of the wheelchair to decrease the stretch on tight hamstrings. If the person is a foot mobilizer and the seat is too high, he may scoot out to the edge of the chair to get the full foot support needed to achieve efficient mobility.

First, make sure the pelvis is all the way back in the wheelchair, because this affects the position of the feet. Then try one of the following solutions to the problem:

- Depending on the wheelchair, the foot supports can be adjusted up or down. If the footrests cannot be adjusted to the proper height, a different wheelchair may be needed.

- If the angle of the footrest hangers needs to be altered because of hamstring limitations, another set of hangers can be ordered (if available), or a solid footplate can be attached with brackets to the foot supports. The solid footplate can be positioned to support the feet at the position of knee flexion needed to allow the tight hamstrings some slack. Now the hamstrings no longer pull the pelvis forward from their origin, the ischial tuberosities.

- If the person cannot reach the floor without full foot contact for mobilization, the seat can be replaced with a solid drop seat to reduce the seat to floor height and allow better floor contact. A hemi-height wheelchair can also be considered for persons who use their feet for mobility. The hemi-height chair can be used in combination with a dropped seat (allowing for the seat cushion thickness, which can add 2 to 4 inches to the seat to floor height). If the wheelchair is still not low enough, it may be necessary to use a smaller wheel size, such as a 22- or 20-inch wheel, and a smaller caster wheel, to lower the chair closer to the floor. Very short people who need to reach the floor may need to use a combination of a hemi-height wheelchair and a dropped seat and smaller wheels to achieve the proper seat to floor height (Figure 18-15). This type of arrangement is referred to as a *superhemi wheelchair*.

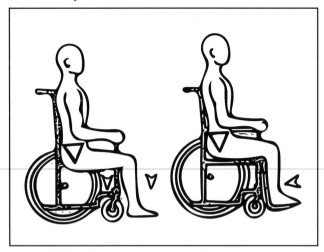

Figure 18-15. Solution: proper footplates or feet placed on floor.

GOAL 5: MAXIMIZING HEAD CONTROL TO FACILITATE INTERACTION

Need for Head Support

Once the hips and trunk are positioned properly, the head should be positioned properly. If the head is weak, proper head support is necessary for level eye gaze, orientation, and socialization. If the individual appears to have poor head control, a headrest and seat to back support angle opened to greater than 90 degrees could be considered.

GOAL 6: PREVENTING SKIN BREAKDOWN

Pressure injuries can be caused by improper seating and prolonged sitting, especially among individuals who have poor sensation and are unable to reposition themselves. It is important to check the buttocks and back of the person's trunk for persistent redness (lasting longer than 20 minutes) and any open skin areas. Individuals who have existing open sores need special attention if they sit in a wheelchair. Here are three approaches to preventing pressure injuries:

1. Always check the skin thoroughly after transferring the resident from the wheelchair. Pay close attention to the ischial tuberosities, sacrum, coccyx, and spinous processes.

2. When a person is just beginning to use a wheelchair, start slowly until the person has built up a tolerance for wheelchair sitting. This is especially necessary for cognitively impaired person who cannot tell you what is wrong and cannot reposition him- or herself.

3. Pressure distributing cushions are available for wheelchairs. These types of cushions allow the person to sit with minor open skin areas or sensitive skin that is susceptible to skin breakdown. Again, constant skin monitoring is necessary to ensure that healing is promoted. A good pressure-distributing cushion needs to be used in combination with regular pressure relief, such as shifting weight off of the buttocks.

GOAL 7: ACHIEVING REASONABLE WHEELCHAIR TOLERANCE

It is important to note the individual's wheelchair tolerance. How long does he or she sit in the chair, and what are his or her reasons for wanting to get out of the chair? If the person is agitated, irritable, crying, or asking to go back to bed, the person is probably uncomfortable and cannot tolerate sitting any longer. Long periods of sitting, especially when one is unable to move, may cause increased pressure on bony prominences, which in turn may lead to discomfort, pain, and skin breakdown, because of decreased circulation to skin areas.

Another reason for poor sitting tolerance could be undiagnosed fractures and especially compression fractures in the spine. Supporting the pelvis posteriorly will support the lumbar and thoracic spine and reduce pressure that causes pain from compression fractures.

Many times the seating arrangement is the problem. To solve this problem, a comprehensive seating and mobility evaluation will need to be completed. This would include a physical assessment of the skin integrity, joint ROM, and seated posture. The current seating and mobility device will need to be inspected for correct product, placement, and configuration for the individual.

POWER MOBILITY DEVICE

Power wheelchair mobility is an area of growth with the aging population. For those who cannot walk or maneuver a manual wheelchair, power mobility is an option to maintain desired independence. Power mobility enables the user to conserve energy, reduce pain, and improve ability to reach household and community goals. The special concerns when introducing power mobility to an older person is his or her past experience of driving a motor vehicle and the willingness to try something new. Some people do not like the power or speed of a power mobility device (PMD).

The basic criteria are as follows:

- Ability to release hand from power controls for stopping
- Adequate vision
- Ability to rotate neck and head for safety
- Ability to maneuver small spaces
- Ability to maintain batteries
- Ability to address general maintenance of PMD

Some people may need additional training, reprogramming of power controls and/or caregiver assistance to achieve these goals. The control settings that should be considered for initial trial is slow onset of forward movement, slow forward, and reverse speed to adjust for environmental changes, increased speed for turning and adjustment to enable a quick stop. If the person is going to use the PMD outside, safety and rules of operating a PMD on the road will need to be tested and addressed before issue. The Wheelchair Skills Test for Power Mobility is available to determine ability and training goals for the power wheelchair user (www.wheelchairskillsprogram.ca).

To enhance posture and improve function, it is important to assess each wheelchair user for his or her individual needs, wants, and desires. A mat assessment is an important part of that process. A through orthopedic and neurological examination followed by a supine and seated assessment to determine fixed vs flexible joint ROM. If the client has fixed joints, the seating needs to accommodate the shape and distribute pressure to maintain skin integrity and comfort. If the client has flexible joint ROM, the seating can support and assist with the correct posture while protecting the skin.

COMMON SEATING PROBLEMS

Sliding Out of the Wheelchair

Often wheelchair users are seen sliding out of their wheelchairs. The user and/or caregivers complain of constant repositioning, discomfort, and fear of skin issues and falls. Sliding can be prevented and corrected with individual seating assessment followed by correct equipment to support or accommodate the user without using restraints.

The mat assessment should reveal the biomechanical features causing the sliding. It is usually poor pelvic support and position due to posterior pelvic tilt fixed or flexible, followed by tight hamstring muscles pulling the pelvis further into posterior tilt, along with incorrect foot placement causing further stress on the shortened hamstring muscles. Having these structural problems in combination with poorly selected wheelchair and gravity can cause sliding.

To prevent or reduce the sliding potential a combination of a seat cushion and back support with the proper angles can support the user and reduce sliding. The back support needs to have posterior pelvic control to assist with best upright position for the pelvis. The seat cushion needs to have contours to allow the pelvis to reach the rear of the wheelchair with a well space and pelvic shelf to block the forward movement of the pelvis. The seat cushion also needs to be long enough from buttocks to behind the knees to fully support the femurs.

Once the contours of the body have been supported with an appropriate cushion and back support, gravity may still influence forward sliding and posterior pelvic tilt. If this is the case, a seat belt can be used to stabilize the pelvis, prevent pelvic migration, and reeducate the muscles and joint tissue. Correct placement of the seat belt is crucial to successful stabilization of the pelvis. The belt should not be placed across the abdomen, but high across the thighs with a downward and slightly backward pull. This will provide optimal control of the pelvic migration without causing pain and pressure across the abdomen. Elderly clients cannot tolerate a seat belt across their abdomen because of fixed postures, compromised abdominal space, and lack of trunk elongation, but their thighs can tolerate increased pressure from the belt because of the abundance of muscle tissue and lack of bony prominences. The seat belt can be removed once the muscles are re-educated and the body becomes accustom to the new position. The time required for muscle re-education depends on the individual, and this should be reassessed at regular intervals.

Inadequate Hip Flexion

The equipment parts that correspond with the hip range (thigh to trunk angle) are the seat to back angle of the wheelchair frame and seating system. The hip joint needs to be able to reach 90 degrees without influencing the pelvic position. If the hip(s) cannot reach 90 degrees, then the cushion will need to be adjusted or the seat to back angle opened to accommodate for the lack of hip range. To accommodate inadequate hip flexion (unable to achieve a 90-degree thigh to trunk angle), foam cushions can be modified by carving out the section where the femur lies, and air cushions can be modified by adjusting the air level to drop the leg down. This modification can be used for open thigh to trunk angles up to 105 degrees (Figure 18-16).

For more severe asymmetries (>105-degree thigh to trunk angle), a combination of cushion modification and

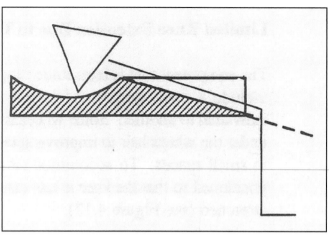

Figure 18-16. Cushion can be altered for increased hip to thigh angle.

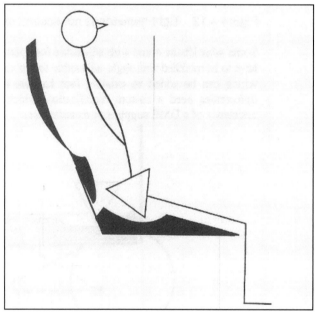

Figure 18-17. If more hip to thigh angle is required, the seat and back angle can be increased.

an open seat to back support angle will be necessary. The pelvis must still be supported posteriorly while accommodating for hip flexion to maintain proper pelvic control and lumbar positioning. A tilt-in-space system shifts the seat and back simultaneously, maintaining the hip angle and pelvic support while reducing the effects of gravity (Figure 18-17).

Limited Knee Extension Due to Tight Hamstrings

The equipment that effects knee ROM is the lower leg support and foot support system, often referred to as *front riggings*, to include a hanger (the tubing connecting the seat to the foot support). Foot placement differs from one individual to another. Some wheelchair users choose to have their feet placed under the wheelchair to improve accessibility and maneuverability, especially in small spaces. To accommodate tight hamstrings, the foot must be positioned so the knee is less extended and the hamstring muscles are not stretched. Elevating legrests are rarely, if ever, appropriate for older adults due to lack of knee range and hamstring length influencing pelvic position into posterior tilt resulting in sliding, skin shearing, discomfort, and poor wheelchair sitting tolerance (Figure 18-18).

Some wheelchairs come with adjustable foot supports and hangers, but most standard chairs have to be modified with angle-adjustable footplates of modified footplates, which can be added to existing foot hangers (Figure 18-19). Some asymmetries need custom modifications, which can

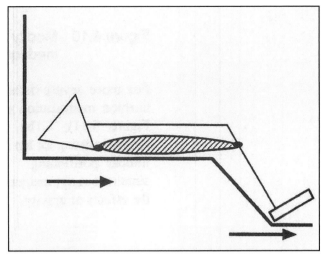

Figure 18-18. Problem: shortened hamstring muscles can pull pelvis forward, especially when feet are placed on footplates.

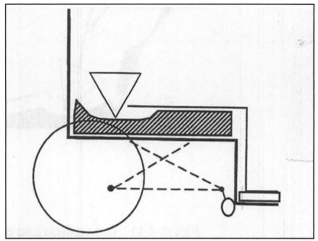

Figure 18-19. Solution: change the footplate placement to accommodate shortened hamstrings.

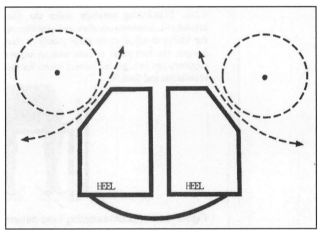

Figure 18-20. Solution: footplate accommodates for caster swivel.

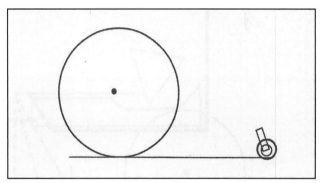

Figure 18-21. Solution: smaller casters to allow caster swivel.

be created with the assistance of a durable medical supplier or manufacturer.

The problem with placing the feet directly under the front edge of the seat is that the foot supports can interfere with the front casters ability to rotate (see Figure 18-19). Either the foot supports must be modified to allow caster movement (Figure 18-20), smaller casters should be used, or both modifications can be made. If small casters are used, the rear wheel will also have to be adjusted to realign the seat surface (Figure 18-21).

Ankle Contractures

A normal ankle position is in neutral. When a contracture is present, the foot still needs full support. Some foot supports can be adjusted to accommodate supinated, pronated, dorsiflexed, or plantar flexed contractures (Figure 18-22). Distributing pressure under the foot decreases potential skin breakdown, improves comfort, and provides

stability. Wheelchairs without the ability to adjust at the ankle can be modified by using wedges to fully support the foot, replacing either the hanger, the footplate, or both with an angle adjustable foot support. Durable medical equipment suppliers can help get the correct match for the existing chair and help with installation and final fit.

If the person is a foot propeller, the feet should be positioned on the floor with the posterior aspect of the thighs supported with adequate space behind the lower leg to allow for full excursion (Figure 18-23).

Flaccid or Nonfunctioning Lower Extremity

A flaccid or nonfunctioning lower extremity should be supported with a cushion that provides adequate posterior thigh support. The foot support must be adjusted up or down to ensure contact of the thigh with the cushion (Figure 18-24). A full footplate that extends from heel to toe is recommended to keep the foot and toes in a neutral position.

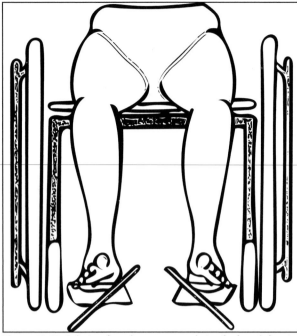

Figure 18-22. Solution: footplate accommodation for foot deformity.

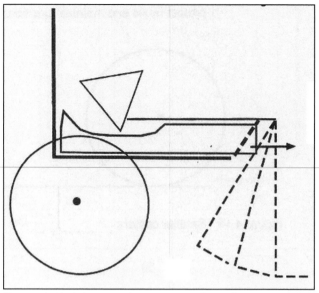

Figure 18-23. Solution: cushion accommodation for improved foot excursion.

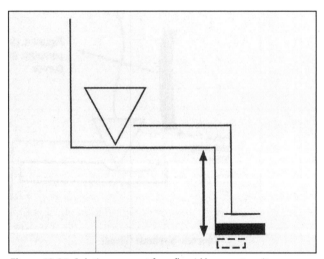

Figure 18-24. Solution: support for a flaccid lower extremity.

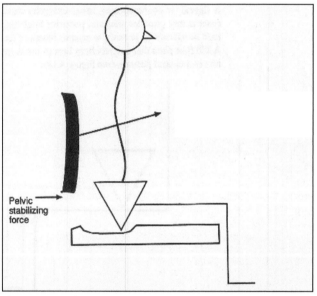

Figure 18-25. Solution: supporting trunk using a cushion with posterior pelvic stabilization.

Trunk and Head

Once the pelvis, hips, and knees have been supported or accommodated, the trunk can be positioned. The trunk and head should be viewed together because changes in the trunk position will cause changes in the head position.

If the trunk is flexible, support it and bring into the best upright posture that the person can tolerate without losing pelvic stabilization (Figure 18-25). This can be done using a contoured back support that is comfortable for the user. In addition to using a seat cushion, it may be necessary to open up the seat to back support angle of the wheelchair to gain gravity assistance with trunk control—again being careful not to lose pelvic stabilization.

Thoracic Kyphosis (Fixed)

A fixed thoracic kyphosis is common among older adults, and accommodation is needed for this. There are back supports designed to accommodate kyphosis (Figure 18-26). Many of these back supports can be modified if necessary by carving the foam insert, by adjusting the air in the air inserts, or by placing supplementary pads of foam. If the kyphosis is severe, a custom-molded system may be an option. A slight opening of the seat-to-back angle allows gravity to assist with and enhance trunk control and provides enough stability for upright sitting and upper extremity functioning. If a greater opening of the seat to backrest

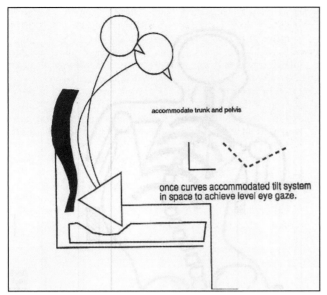

Figure 18-26. Solution: accommodation of a kyphotic curve.

angle is needed to accommodate the kyphosis, a headrest may be necessary to maintain head control.

Asymmetrical Trunk: Scoliosis

With severe trunk control problems, where leaning or asymmetry is observed, a deeper than usual back system with lateral control is necessary to maintain trunk stability. If enough control is not provided with a deeper back, a combination of a lateral trunk support and gravitational control, using a fixed or angle-adjustable tilt-in-space system is recommended. If tilting the person limits access to table activities or propulsion, then a compromised solution could include using more aggressive lateral trunk supports such as a three-point system (Figure 18-27). A three-point system consists of three lateral supports. The first one is placed in the thoracic region at the largest point of the scoliotic curve. Find the largest point of the curve, follow those ribs down to the lateral trunk region, and place the first lateral support. The other trunk supports are placed on the opposite side, one just under the axilla (careful to not place pressure on the axilla area) and the second low at the pelvis. This system supports the trunk and prevents, corrects, or delays further migration of the scoliotic curve. The supports are attached to the back of the chair or to the back support system. They should be large, padded supports to distribute pressure and contoured to fit the persons shape.

Head

Usually problems with the head position can be fixed by stabilizing the pelvis and trunk; head supports are rarely needed. They are needed, however, when a person is reclined or tilted in the seating system.

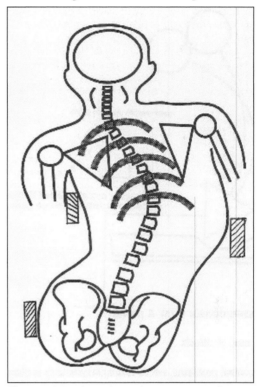

Figure 18-27. Lateral trunk supports, such as a three-point system.

SUMMARY

When providing or assessing seating and wheeled mobility for the geriatric person, a mat assessment is necessary to find joint and muscle strength limitations. Once body shape and contour are identified, a seating and wheeled mobility device can be created to support a person while sitting. When supported properly, a seating and wheeled mobility device can provide comfort, increased tolerance, and function with less need to add extra devices, such as tie-on restraints to hold a person into his or her chair. Remember that proper seating does not replace the need for a person to move, exercise, and stand, if possible.

REFERENCES

Blakeslee, J. (1989, December 4). *Untie the elderly: quality care without restraints.* Symposium before the Senate Committee on Aging, Washington, D.C. Retrieved from www.aging.senate.gov/imo/media/doc/reports/rpt589.pdf

Brienza, D. M., Karg, P. E., Geyer, M. J., Kelsey, S., & Trefler E. (2001). The relationship between pressure ulcer incident and buttock-seat interface pressure in at-risk elderly wheelchair users. *Archives of Physical Rehabilitation Medicine, 82,* 529-533. http://dx.doi.org/10.1053/apmr.2001.21854

Cook, A., & Polgar, J. (2008). *Cook and Hussey's assistive technologies: Principles and practice.* St. Louis, MO: Mosby-Elsevier.

Evans, L., & Strumpf, N. (1989). Tying down the elderly: A review of the literature on physical restraints. *Journal of the American Geriatrics Society, 37,* 65-74.

Evans, L., & Strumpf, N. (1990). Myths about elder restraint. *Image: Journal of Nursing Scholarship, 22,* 124-128.

Fried LP, Tangen, C., Walston J., Newman, A., Hirsch, C., Gottdiener, J.,...McBurnie, M.; Cardiovascular Health Study Collaborative Research Group. (2001). Frailty in older adults: Evidence for a phenotype. *Journal of Gerontology: Series A. Biological Sciences and Medical Sciences, 56,* M146-M156.

Guralnik, J., Ferrucci, L., Simonsick, E. M., Salive, M., & Wallace, R. (1995). Lower extremity function in persons over the age of 70 years as a predictor of subsequent disability. *New England Journal of Medicine, 332,* 556-561

Health Care Financing Administration. (1995). State operations manual: Guidance to surveyors. F tag 221-222, 483.13(a).

Jones, D. (1995a). Real solutions. *Team Rehab Report.* Retrieved from http://www.wheelchairnet.org/WCN_ProdServ/Docs/TeamRehab/ RR_95/9509art1.PDF

Jones, D. (1995b). Regaining independence. *Team Rehab Report.* Retrieved from http://www.wheelchairnet.org/WCN_ProdServ/ Docs/TeamRehab/RR_95/9508art4.PDF.

Jones, D., & Rader, J. (2015). Seating and wheeled mobility for older adults living in nursing homes: What has changed clinically in the past 20 years? *Topics of Geriatric Rehabilitation, 31,* 10-18.

Kemp, B., Brummell-Smith, K., & Ramsdell, J. (1990). *Geriatric rehabilitation.* Boston, MA: College Hill Press.

Kong, E., Evans, L., & Guevara (2008). Nonpharmacological intervention for agitation in dementia: A systematic review and meta-analysis. *Aging & Mental Health, 13,* 4.

Miles, S., & Meyers, R. (1994). Untying the elderly—1993 update. *Clinics in Geriatric Medicine 10,* 513-524.

Pitts, M. (1995). Gray matters. *Team Rehab Report 6*(2), 14-19.

Xue, Q. (2011). The frailty syndrome: Definition and natural history. *Clinics in Geriatric Medicine, 27,* 1-15. Retrieved from http://www. geriatric.theclinics.com/article/S0749-0690%2810%2900083-2/full-text

19

Considerations When Working With the Bariatric Population

Stephanie Tanguay, OT/L, ATP

Clinicians can expect to find bariatric clients within almost any diagnoses or patient population. Persons of significantly larger size sustain spinal cord injuries, traumatic brain injuries, experience cerebral vascular accidents, have amputations, and are diagnosed with multiple sclerosis and other neurological and orthopedic conditions. The term *bariatric pediatric* has even become prevalent as the incidence of childhood obesity has increased. According to the World Health Organization's 2014 report citing the global health observation data for that year, 41 million children under the age of 5 were overweight or obese. For adults age 18 and above, 1.9 billion were overweight and more than 600 million were obese.

Body mass index (BMI) is just one measure of obesity. Originally developed by Belgian statistician Adolphe Quetelet in 1832 (and then known as the *Quetelet Index*), it became known as the *body mass index* in 1972 when Ancel Keys first referred to it by that name (Eknoyan, 2008).

The BMI Formula: weight (kg) / [height (m)]^2

With the metric system, the formula for BMI is weight in kilograms divided by height in meters squared. Because height is commonly measured in centimeters, divide height in centimeters by 100 to obtain height in meters.

Example: Weight = 70.3 kg, Height = 173 cm (1.73 m)

Calculation: $70.3 \div (1.73)^2 = 23.5$

The BMI Formula: weight (lb)/[height (in)]^2 x 703

An alternative to the metric system enables calculation of BMI by dividing weight in pounds (lbs) by height in inches squared and multiplying by a conversion factor of 703.

Example: Weight = 155 lbs, Height = 5 feet 8 inches (68 inches)

Calculation: $[155 \div (68)^2] \times 703 = 23.56$

Several websites include BMI calculators including the Centers for Disease Control and Prevention (www.cdc.gov) and the National Heart Lung and Blood Institute (www.nhlbi.nih.gov) in the United States and in other countries. On an Internet search engine, enter "BMI calculator."

The Centers for Disease Control and Prevention recommendations delineate the BMI in this manner:

- BMI < 18.5 = Underweight
- BMI 18.5 to 24.9 = Ideal
- BMI 25 to 29.9 = Overweight
- BMI ≥ 30.0 = Obese
- BMI ≥ 40.0 = Morbidly Obese

BMI is still used as a simple calculation guideline for weight. There are other tests that can be used to determine percentage of body fat. BMI certainly has questionable validity for very muscular body types and during pregnancy. Percentage of body fat is generally higher for women than men with the same BMI. Age and race are also variables in body fat percentage. For the purposes of this text, BMI is referenced as a long accepted and easy computation. BMI is not a deciding variable in mobility or seating device warranties, nor is it used in diagnosis qualifications for equipment coverage. However, statistics of increased average BMI worldwide reflect the need for seating and mobility devices for clients with higher weight ranges.

Many bariatric clients are fragile ambulators, perhaps only independently mobile within their home environments and occasionally for very short distances in the community. For these clients, a minor incident, such as a fall or

Lange, M. L., & Minkel, J. L.
Seating and Wheeled Mobility: A Clinical Resource Guide
(pp. 317-332). © 2018 SLACK Incorporated.

several days of bed confinement from the flu, can lead to a rapid decrease in strength and mobility. This deconditioning may prompt short inpatient hospitalization or perhaps referrals for home-based occupational and physical therapy services. Obesity has become very common as a secondary diagnosis or preexisting condition. Finding appropriate equipment to meet the requirements of bariatric clients can be challenging. Although more commercially manufactured bariatric cushions, back supports, and manual and powered mobility devices are available today than ever before, properly measuring the client and configuring the equipment are necessary to achieve successful results.

Working with bariatric clients poses some unique challenges (especially persons who weigh 500 pounds or more), and it is critical to maintain a professional demeanor. As with all interactions, the clinicians and team members should be respectful of the client's privacy. Measurements, weighing of the client, and other aspects of the assessment process should be performed with as much privacy as possible. Being sensitive to the client's situation will build trust and a better rapport. Significantly larger clients are often disrespected and embarrassed by the comments and actions of strangers, including health care personnel. Many facilities are ill-prepared to meet the needs of persons with bariatric presentation. Calling "all hands on deck" for transfers because an appropriate assistive lifting device is not available creates a degrading experience for the client and potentially dangerous situation for all persons involved.

BARIATRIC BODY TYPES

Several different bariatric body types are described by Michael Dionne (2006) in his book *Among Giants; Courageous Stories of Those Who Are Obese and Those Who Serve Them*. Each of these body shapes presents with a different weight distribution—so much so that, if not considered, the equipment selection could be completely nonfunctional for the client.

Pear-Shaped Bodies

Gluteal/femoral obesity is described as the *pear shape*. This client carries most of his or her adipose tissue below the waist and above the knees. It is important to note whether the distribution of redundant tissue is more medially or laterally distributed.

Excessive medial femoral tissue distribution will prevent the femurs from achieving a neutral alignment in sitting. Masses of redundant tissue in the inner thighs can force the lower extremities into abduction. Lower extremity support may be a challenge.

Excessive lateral femoral tissue distribution can require larger seat widths for accommodation. In this circumstance,

the knees and feet are able to rest in a more neutral alignment closer to midline.

Apple-Shaped Bodies

Abdominal obesity (described commonly as the *apple shape*) is characterized by primary excessive weight distribution in the belly area. As weight distribution is more anterior, this can lead to more anterior instability of the wheelchair. This forward instability can be problematic for many manual wheelchair bases as well as some mid-wheel and front-wheel drive power bases.

SECONDARY DIAGNOSES AND CONDITIONS

Secondary and commonly occurring conditions associated with long-term obesity include cardiovascular disease, hypertension, diabetes mellitus, and sleep apnea. Each of these conditions affect the client and decisions related to wheeled mobility. Some bariatric clients may not be physically able to attempt manual wheelchair mobilization because of their cardiac status. Clients with circulation and sensory complications from diabetes mellitus have an increased risk of serious injury to their lower extremities if using foot propulsion. Other bariatric clients may require supplemental oxygen when in their wheelchair. Several other secondary diagnoses are discussed in the following sections.

Lymphedema

One of the secondary risks of long-term morbid obesity is the potential for severe lower body lymphedema to develop. As the bariatric client's mobility becomes more restricted and the client spends greater amounts of time in a seated position, the lymphatic system may be occluded in the groin region. This type of lymphedema is characterized initially by asymmetrical or unilateral lower extremity swelling. Sometimes lower extremity lymphedema can become so severe that ambulation is greatly limited and wheeled mobility is required.

Due to the asymmetrical nature of lymphedema, measurement for mobility devices can be challenging. For example, a severely involved lower extremity can be double the circumference and weight of an uninvolved extremity. The size of one lower extremity may take up two thirds of the seat width. The size or shape of the lower extremity may cause asymmetrical seated postures including rotation, more lateral orientation of the less involved lower extremity, and even obliquity of the pelvis.

Lower extremity lymphedema can affect the functional seat depth and anterior cushion shape and length as the shape and size of one or both lower extremities changes and increases. Additional complications, such as cellulitis or lipoma, pose further challenges.

Unfortunately, some people who experience lymphedema as a complication of obesity are not diagnosed in a timely fashion. As a result, the condition can progress for an extended period of time, resulting in extreme size and shape of the involved extremities. Not all doctors or clinicians are experienced in addressing the needs of clients with lymphedema. The mobility and positioning challenges are only one aspect of the needs of this population. Persons with this condition should be seen by an occupational or physical therapist who is certified in lymphedema management.

Cellulitis

A bacterial infection of the skin and subcutaneous tissue is a frequent secondary complication and can become chronic and recurrent. Morbidly obese clients are at greater risk of developing cellulitis and obesity increases the chance of cellulitis reoccurring. Deep cutaneous folds create moist warm areas that are difficult to clean and where bacteria can thrive. History of cellulitis is a common risk factor for the reoccurrence of cellulitis.

Lipoma

Lipoma are benign tumors composed of fatty tissue that can occur with adiposis dolorosa. Adiposis tissue is fat tissue that is commonly found beneath the skin (although it can also form around the internal organs). Adiposis dolorosa may also be referred to as *Dercum's disease.* Clients may experience severe pain with this condition, which can make sitting and contact with any support or surface very uncomfortable.

Panniculus

A pannus is a hanging flap of tissue. When the abdomen is involved, it is called a *panniculus* (Figure 19-1). This mass consists of skin, fat, and sometimes contents of the abdominal cavity as part of a hernia. A panniculus can become very large, even hanging down to or below the knees when the client is in a standing position.

The following is grading of abdominal panniculi (Igwe et al., 2000.).

Grade 1: Panniculus barely covers the hairline of the mons pubis but not the genitalia

Grade 2: Extends to cover the genitalia

Grade 3: Extends to cover the upper thigh

Grade 4: Extends to cover the midthigh

Grade 5: Extends to cover the knees or beyond

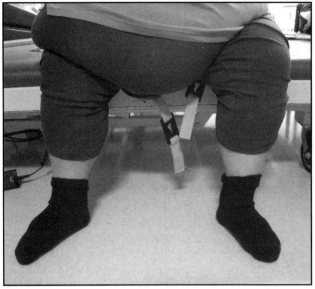

Figure 19-1. When sitting, a panniculus can limit functional seat depth.

When the client is seated, the mass may hang below the seat. If the panniculus is large enough, the posterior aspect of the tissue mass contacts the front seat edge and will significantly limit the amount of functional seat depth. The weight of the pannus tissue is anterior and below the waist, often forcing the client into some degree of anterior pelvic rotation and/or spinal lordosis. This not only influences the client's seated posture but her ability to transfer and ambulate as well.

It is imperative to pad all edges and sharp points of contact. If a tilting system is prescribed, anticipate where gravity may displace tissue during the shift (e.g., front seat edge).

The extra tissue of a hanging panniculus can make personal hygiene difficult; fungal infections are common in the deep folds of the skin and cellulitis can also occur. Because of these risks, covers should be removable for washing or at least covered with a material that can be disinfected and wiped down.

The increased tissue mass that can develop with lower body lymphedema or a panniculus can make mobility base and seating system prescription difficult. With the client in a seated position, the lymphatic lower extremities or excessive abdominal tissue mass create a forward weight distribution and can result in anterior instability. This is a risk with prescription of manual or power wheeled mobility systems for clients with significant anterior weight and tissue distribution in the seated position.

Lymphorrhea

Lymphorrhea is the seeping of lymph fluid through the skin from ruptured lymphatic vessels. This condition can occur with lymphedema and impedes the use of compression garments and multilayer bandaging. With regard to the seating and mobility system, porous fabric covers should be removable or easily cleaned. Risk of fungal infection and cellulites is increased with lymphedema and great care should be taken to utilize fabrics with moisture barriers to prevent draining fluids from permeating foam materials.

PEDIATRIC BARIATRIC

The incidence of childhood obesity has increased globally in the past 25 years. In a study published in 2010 in the *American Journal of Clinical Nutrition,* De Onis, Blössner, and Borghi estimated that 43 million preschool-age children worldwide were overweight and obese. As with the bariatric adult population, these children can sustain injuries and experience the same variety of disease processes as their nonobese peers. Meeting the wheeled mobility needs of a bariatric pediatric client can be challenging because of the unique dimensions and weight capacities required in the equipment. Children under 10 years who exceed 100 pounds may require a wheelchair that is 14 or 16 inches wide. While body weight and width exceeds average range, the bariatric pediatric client's height is typically within average range. As a result, the wheelchair requires a shorter seat depth, greater width, and higher weight capacity.

Additional components such as contoured upper extremity supports present similar issues. Pediatric bariatric clients may present with age-appropriate forearm lengths, but due to excessive weight, forearm width and circumference requirements may exceed pediatric size arm troughs. Seat cushions that are wider yet shorter in depth may be considered custom by manufacturers and can require special fabrication, increasing costs and additional provision time. Any components that are custom in size, configuration, or weight capacity may cost more.

ASSESSMENT

Weight

The first step to providing appropriate equipment is to complete a thorough evaluation. This should start with an accurate history, including a weight history. The assessment team should determine recent weight loss or gain, and if that can be attributed to illness, medications, or surgical intervention. Also, an accurate current weight is crucial. This can be difficult for some morbidly obese clients who may not have access to a scale that can measure their weight. Some clinicians have used two scales, one under each foot, and combined the total weights. For clients who are unable to stand unsupported, platform scales are available onto which a wheelchair can be rolled. The same chair is then weighed without the client and the chair weight is deducted from the combined total. Unfortunately, many platform scales are only large enough to hold an 18- or 20-inch-wide manual wheelchair. Some transfer and lift systems have scale options—a smart option for hospitals and rehabilitation facilities to consider. A less convenient solution is finding a facility that has a loading dock where material is weighed. These scales are usually easily accessible (embedded in the floor) and most can accommodate the weight of a person in a power chair. Somewhat less accurate and infinitely more embarrassing for the bariatric client would be use of a commercial laundry scale or a meat processing scale, either of which is often floor based and accessible to a device on wheels. In extreme instances, a weigh station used for trucks has been used. The last three methods listed should only be used as a final resort when other problem-solving options have been exhausted and absolutely no other choice is available.

Seated Postures and Tissue Distribution

Tissue distribution will often dictate seated postures. A seated lateral view will reveal the clients' weight distribution and how the bariatric client's posture is affected by that tissue distribution. A large dense mass of belly tissue (associated with the apple body type) can prevent a client from sitting with 90 degrees of hip flexion. This bariatric client may sit with his or her pelvis forward on the seat surface, essentially maintaining a position of less hip flexion. Attempts to position the client with a more neutral hip angle often results in the belly tissue being forced against the thighs, causing abduction of the lower extremities.

The bariatric body type of pear shape can present with excessive tissue on the lateral aspects of the pelvis and femurs (adducted type) or with significantly more tissue distribution on the medial aspects of the thighs (abducted type). Both of these presentations require wider seat surfaces and narrower back supports. Support and positioning of the lower extremities can be the greatest challenge for this bariatric client. Many clients have posterior pelvic tissue distribution. Extreme amounts of this redundant soft tissue can create a gluteal shelf (Figures 19-2 and 19-3).

Lateral views of clients in the seated position (Figure 19-4) reveal tissue distribution in relation to anterior and posterior orientation and can be helpful in the mobility base selection and overall configuration of the wheelchair system.

Measurements

Measurement of the client is the next vital component to the prescription process. Depending on the client's diagnosis and endurance, this may require two or three people to safely and accurately complete. It is important to measure the client in a sitting position on a firm planar surface. This will ensure the most accurate dimensions. Avoid measuring anyone in bed, on a sofa, or in an easy chair, because

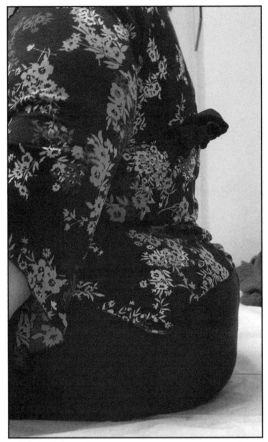

Figure 19-2. Posterior pelvic tissue will contact an enclosed back support before the client's posterior torso reaches stability. Accommodate the pelvic tissue by mounting the back support above the posterior distribution.

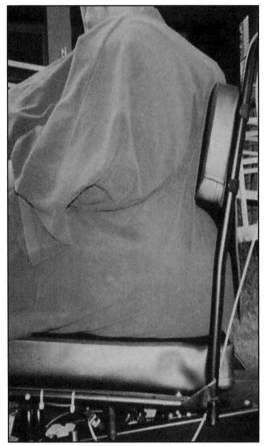

Figure 19-3. Posterior pelvic tissue will contact an enclosed back support before the client's posterior torso reaches stability. Accommodate the pelvic tissue by mounting the back support above the posterior distribution.

the soft surfaces accommodate tissue, making it difficult to account for as wheelchair specifications are selected. Ideal for this activity is a height adjustable therapy mat; the height adjustment allows femur support on the table surface while the feet can be in contact with the floor. An adjustable height table also makes sit-to-stand transfer assessment safer (see Transfers later in this chapter).

Measurements should be taken with a rigid measurement device: a metal tape measure, sturdy yardstick, carpenter's ruler, or pair of sliding calipers. Callipers can make measurements easier and reduce errors. These need to be large enough to accommodate the client's width.

Supplemental Measurements

Clinicians who are experienced in evaluation and prescription for seating and mobility are certainly familiar with typical body measurements. Some additional measurements of the bariatric client can enhance the prescription

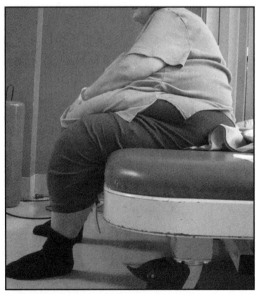

Figure 19-4. Imagine the center of mass in the lateral view. Observe the lateral view of the client in his or her wheelchair for a concept of weight distribution within the mobility device.

ADDITIONAL MEASUREMENTS FOR BARIATRIC CLIENTS

Current weight:_____   Weight history:_____

_____

_____

_____

_____

_____

_____

1. Back of knee/calf to back of buttocks (seat pan depth) _____

2. Back of knee/calf to thoracic-lumber trunk (for seat depth) _____

3. Seat pan to under forearm (armrest height) _____

4. Seat pan to top of gluteal tissue (lower aspect of back support height) _____

5. Width at toes (lateral aspect) _____

6. Width from lateral calf to lateral calf (at widest aspect) _____

7. Overall hip width _____

8. Lateral elbow to lateral elbow _____

9. Back of head scapula _____

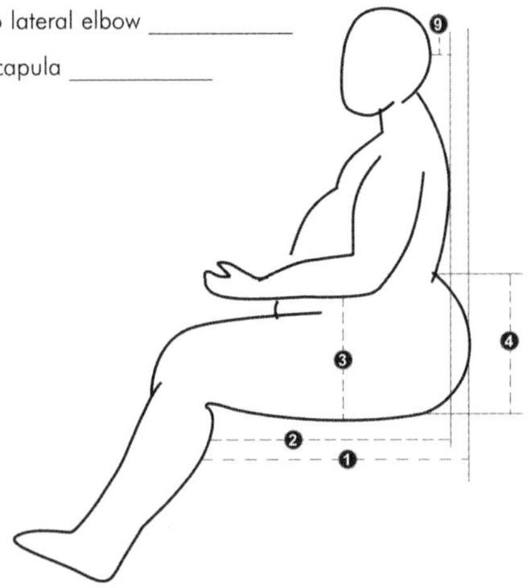

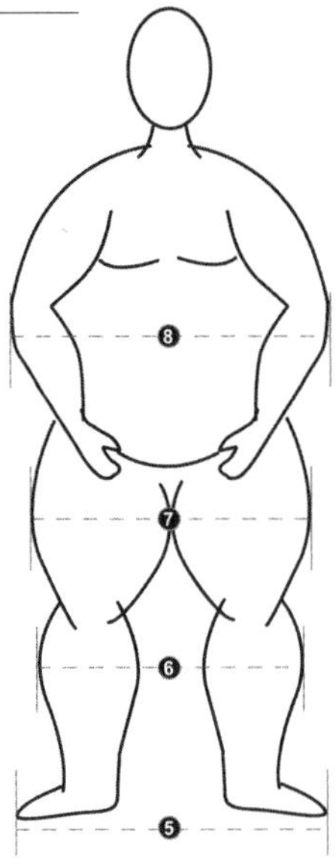

Figure 19-5. Additional Measurements for Bariatric Clients worksheet. Originally created by Jane Fontein, OT and Stephanie Tanguay, OT; graphics by Sofiya Kagan.

process and make equipment configuration more effective. Please refer to the Additional Measurements for Bariatric Clients worksheet (Figure 19-5). These additional measurements are critical for bariatric clients because of the shape and distribution of tissue, which can make it difficult to configure a mobility device for seat depth and width, back support, and lower leg position.

Excessive posterior pelvic tissue distribution requires at least three specific measurements (see Figure 19-5) with the client seated: posterior aspect of the tissue at the calf to the posterior aspect of gluteal tissue on the pelvis (Measurement 1), posterior aspect of the tissue at the calf to the posterior aspect of client's trunk (Measurement 2), and from the seat surface (mat table) to the top of the gluteal tissue on the posterior aspect of the pelvis (Measurement 4).

Bariatric clients may have large amounts of adipose tissue on the posterior trunk or flanks. This tissue distribution increases the distance from the back support surface to the occiput. If a bariatric client with this presentation requires a head support, longer horizontal mounting hardware may be required (refer to Measurement 9 on Figure 19-5).

Variance of trunk width and pelvic width is certainly not exclusive to the bariatric population. Most prevalent is the need for wider seat surfaces and narrower trunk supports to address the tissue distribution of the pear body shape. A wheelchair with a narrower back than seat is commonly referred to as an *endomorph back* (Figure 19-6). It may be possible to have a back 2, 4, or 6 inches narrower than the seat width, or perhaps even more. This allows a more neutral midline orientation for the client's trunk without the interference of a wider back behind the upper extremities. The armrests may be able to mount in closer to the torso for a more neutral position of the upper extremities.

When a client has a significantly wider trunk than pelvis (more common with the apple-shaped body type), a wheelchair with a narrower seat width and wider back support

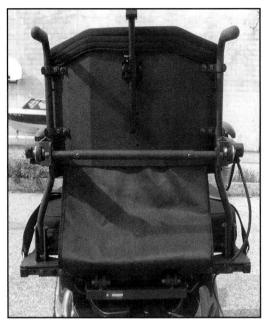

Figure 19-6. Endomorph back canes accommodate a narrower trunk compared with hip width.

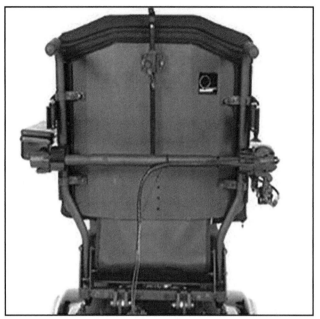

Figure 19-7. Mesomorph back canes accommodate a wider trunk compared to hip width.

is indicated. Commonly referred to as a *mesomorph back* (Figure 19-7), these configurations are more frequently available on power wheelchairs than manual wheelchairs. With this configuration, the narrower pelvis is in a midline orientation while the wider upper body is accommodated. The alternative would be a chair width based on the upper body width resulting in amounts of space on each side of the pelvis for lateral deviation.

Transfers

Many bariatric clients are physically able to perform standing or modified standing transfers. However, physically repositioning themselves in relation to their seat surface can be difficult or impossible. It is not uncommon for bariatric clients to transfer onto a surface and find themselves on the anterior two thirds of the target. From the seated position, they may be physically unable to scoot themselves more posteriorly. This can result in very uncomfortable seated postures as well as front-loaded casters in a wheelchair.

An elevating mat table is ideal for sit-to-stand assessment and to determine seat to floor height parameters. If the client is physically able to perform a standing or modified standing transfer, it is important to determine the lowest and highest seat to floor height from which he or she can safely complete that transfer. If the client is currently using a wheeled mobility device and is able to transfer onto the assessment surface, it is wise to start with the mat table at the same height as the client's existing wheelchair. By lowering the table in small increments and asking the client to stand from those lower surface heights, it is possible to

determine the seat to floor height from which it is too low to safely rise. In similar fashion and from the original start position, raise the mat table in small increments and ask the client to stand from each until he or she cannot move from sit to and from stand independently. In this manner, the range of possible finished seat to floor height will be established. Power or mechanical height adjustment evaluation surfaces should be size- and weight-appropriate. Note where the bariatric client places his or her hands and where he or she pushes or pulls from, in addition to any postural compensation, such as extreme upper body flexion and/or rotation. Placement of the lower extremities is also important: Are the feet closer to midline or abducted and lateral?

Bariatric clients who are physically unable to transfer or assist with transfers may use some type of mechanical transfer system. Once again, it is important to determine the exact style of transfer device not only to confirm that it is weight-appropriate but to ensure that a floor-based transfer device will be accessible around the dimensions of the new wheelchair. This will ensure that the lower extremity supports of the new chair will not obstruct the use of an existing floor-based transfer device.

Gluteal Depth and Height

Excessive adipose tissue in the gluteal region can prevent bariatric clients from sitting with adequate spinal support, which can contribute to incidence of back pain for this population (see Figures 19-2 and 19-3). Measurement from the evaluation support surface to the top of the gluteal tissue can help determine the height at which a back support surface is mounted, perhaps allowing some of the redundant

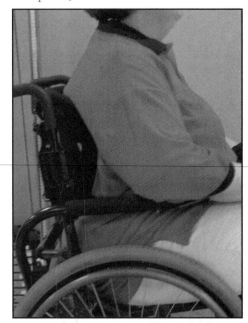

Figure 19-8. Example of a back support mounted above the gluteal tissue although posterior pelvic rotation is evident with the back support providing minimal support.

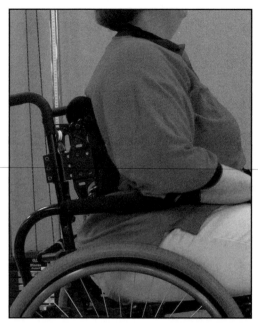

Figure 19-9. Note the back mounted above the gluteal tissue and anterior, providing more lumbosacral support and reducing posterior pelvic rotation.

tissue to stay below the back support and posterior of the back canes. Obviously, seat cushion thickness must also be taken into account with this approach. The depth of excessive gluteal tissue, measured in the lateral view as the difference from the popliteal to the posterior aspect of the gluteal tissue and from the popliteal to the posterior aspect of the trunk above the gluteal shelf, should be considered in the specification of the seat pan and cushion depth. This is one of the most frequent errors in configuration of mobility equipment for clients with significant posterior pelvic tissue distribution. In Figure 19-8, the client is sitting in a chair configured with a seat length that is too deep for her. As a result, her popliteal is in contact with the front of the upholstery and she must posteriorly rotate her pelvis to achieve contact with the back support. Figure 19-9 shows a more anterior mounting of the back support to provide more appropriate support with a neutral pelvis. Adjustable depth orientation of the back support with adjustable depth of the back canes or back support mounting hardware can improve postural seated position for the bariatric wheelchair user.

LOWER EXTREMITY ISSUES

Some clients' hip flexion may be limited, or their abdominal tissue may exert pressure on the femurs, forcing the upper legs into an abducted or even externally rotated position. This in turn can make the use of footrests on a wheelchair very difficult, because the lateral aspect of the knees or lower legs may be in constant pressure against the footrest hangers. The bariatric client with the apple-type tissue distribution or a panniculus, will typically sit with his feet in a more widely spaced orientation (laterally in relation to midline). Traditional footrests that attach on the lateral aspects of the wheelchair seat frame are often more appropriate than a center-oriented foot platform for this client.

Excessive medial thigh tissue distribution (commonly seen with the pear body type with abduction) presents some of the greatest challenges for lower extremity positioning (Figure 19-10). This bariatric client's widest point of tissue distribution is typically the most lateral aspects of the knees, often exceeding the width measurement of the hips. This client can benefit from a wider seat than back support. Flared or offset lower extremity supports may be necessary to prevent direct contact of the lower extremities with the wheelchair legrests. Several manufacturers offer this option, which is more commonly available on power wheelchairs (Figure 19-11).

On most manual wheelchairs and many power wheelchairs, the lower extremity supports are usually attached at the front of the side frames on each side, which means the foot plates are spaced out to the width of the chair. Clinicians should note orientation of the feet when evaluating for mobility devices. Some manual wheelchairs include options that can bring the foot supports closer to the

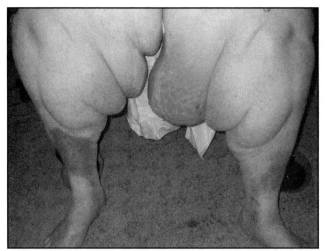

Figure 19-10. Excessive tissue distribution in the medial thigh region dictates an abducted lower extremity orientation with the lateral knee width often presenting as the widest point.

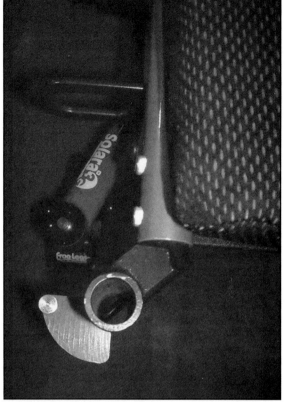

Figure 19-11. Example of an offset receiver for a right legrest. Offset receivers move the legrest out, providing some additional space for the lower extremity.

midline of the seat width. Many mid-wheel and front-wheel drive power chairs have options for center-mount foot supports or platforms. In some instances, a support can be fabricated to bridge the span between the plates.

Excessive lateral thigh tissue distribution (commonly seen with the pear body type with adduction) requires a more midline orientation for foot support (Figure 19-12). This client is able to maintain his or her femur alignment and may be able to easily use a center-mounted foot platform or foot supports that mount along the horizontal anterior aspect of the wheelchair (Figure 19-13).

Bariatric clients may present with excessive tissue distribution on their lower extremities. Several secondary diagnoses within the bariatric population can increase the potential for greater amounts of tissue to be distributed in the lower body. The circumferential size and overall weight of the lower extremities can limit the range of motion and prevent the possibility of full lower extremity elevation (Figure 19-14) due to pinch points where tissue can become entrapped and compressed. Many of the manual and power elevating mechanisms are not weight- or size-appropriate and simply will not support a significantly larger lower extremity (Figure 19-15).

Distribution of tissue that shortens the possible seat depth is a frequent challenge. Adipose and lymphatic material can form large masses on the posterior of the client's thigh (Figures 19-16 and 19-17), creating issues with seat depth. The seat pan may need to be shortened to accommodate this tissue (Figure 19-18). Keep in mind that a mass of this nature should be properly wrapped and supported, perhaps with a padded shelf or a hammock (Figure 19-19).

If these masses are exceptionally large, some mid-wheel and front-wheel drive power wheelchairs may not have enough open space for accommodation of this tissue. A larger panniculus (Grade 4 or 5) can also have the same issue. In those situations, a rear-wheel drive power chair or a custom manual chair may be the only options available.

PANNICULUS AND SEAT DEPTH

The excessive amount of tissue that forms a panniculus often limits the seat depth available to the client in much the same manner as the hanging folds of adipose tissue on the posterior thighs. These tissue masses stop the client from moving farther back onto the seat surface as the panniculus contacts the front of the seat (Figure 19-20). Some custom solutions have been explored (Figures 19-21 and 19-22), but careful measurement of the client with this condition is imperative if a custom mobility device is prescribed. (Refer to the panniculus measurement form, Figure 19-23.)

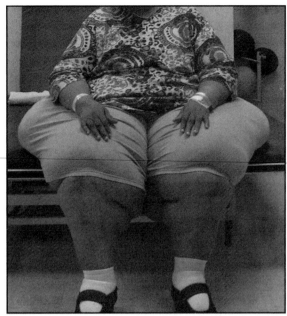

Figure 19-12. Femurs aligned and good knee to foot alignment with excessive tissue distribution in the lateral thigh region.

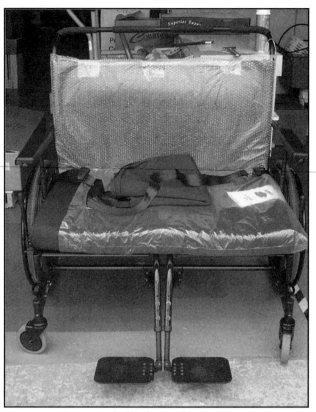

Figure 19-13. An example of a midline lower extremity support on a manual wheelchair.

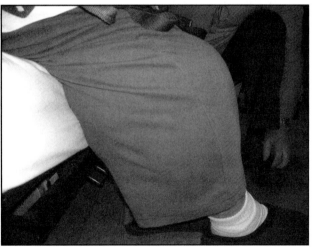

Figure 19-14. Lateral view illustrates the size of the lymphatic tissue mass, which limits right knee flexion and affects this clients' seat depth.

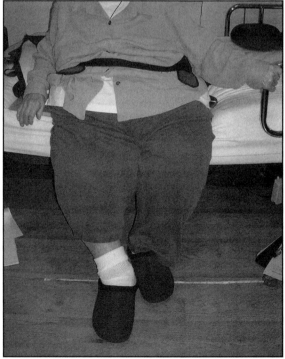

Figure 19-15. In this example, lymphedema in the right lower extremity limits the client's knee flexion, resulting in asymmetrical position of the feet and must be addressed with a more anterior support for the right foot.

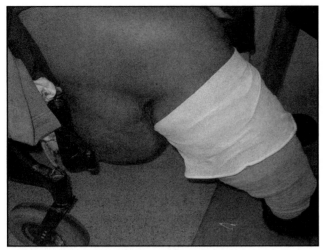

Figure 19-16. A lymphatic mass on the posterior thigh in a seated position. Note the effect of gravity on the tissue.

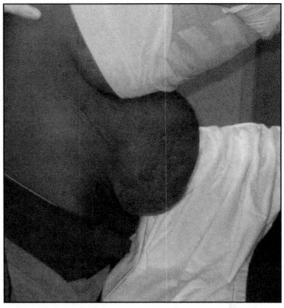

Figure 19-17. A lymphatic mass on the posterior thigh in a position of posterior tilt with knee orientation above the pelvis. Note the effect of gravity on the tissue in this orientation.

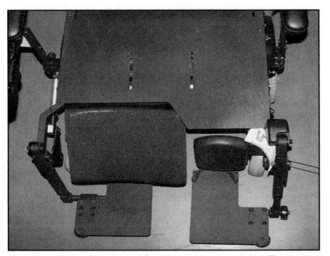

Figure 19-18. Leg-length modification to the seat pan, an offset legrest receiver, and a padded support for the tissue mass.

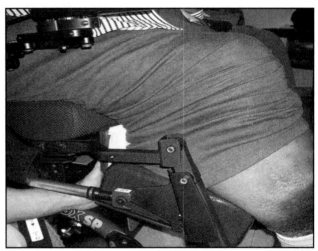

Figure 19-19. An additional pad was mounted beneath the seat pan to prevent the tissue from touching the edge of the pan or seat frame.

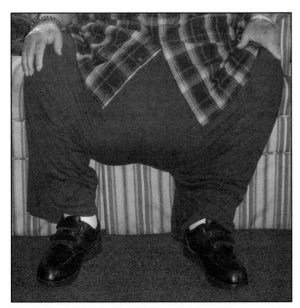

Figure 19-20. An example of a Stage 4 panniculus.

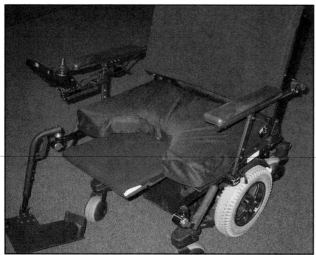

Figure 19-21. An example of a powered support for a Stage 4 panniculus.

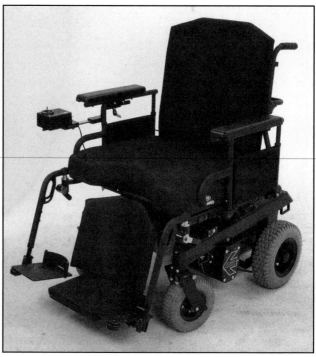

Figure 19-22. An example of a static support for a Stage 5 panniculus.

Specifically, with the client sitting at the edge of the assessment mat as much as possible, measure the depth from the front of the mat edge to the posterior aspect of the pelvis to determine the maximum depth of pelvic support posterior to the mass of hanging tissue. Then measure both the right and the left lower extremities from the popliteal to the posterior aspect of the pelvis to determine the depth of seat support under each femur. The higher grade panniculus will require modifications to the seat cushion surface as well as the seat pan (and possibly the frame) for less length in the center. Supporting under the femurs will improve weight distribution and increase anterior sitting balance. The panniculus mass can range from soft with loose skin to very dense and firm to the touch. Be attentive to padding edges and surfaces and be mindful of pinch points, especially if using a powered seating system or other type of moving components. For the larger size panniculus, padded shelves can be used. Some clinicians have had success with custom abdominal supports for moderate size panniculi.

Equipment Selection

Prescribing appropriate mobility bases for bariatric clients is not simply a matter of getting the width right. Many options are available for bariatric clients: both manual and power wheelchairs, as well as seat support surfaces and back supports. Taking the time to carefully evaluate and measure the client and problem solve some of the challenging aspects can ensure more successful outcomes and greater client satisfaction.

Stability and Weight Distribution

Bariatric clients who require or use wheeled mobility devices benefit from optimal performance from their equipment, just like any other person who uses a wheelchair. The key to maximizing the function and performance of any wheelchair is the distribution of weight in relation to the chair's drive (propulsion) wheels. The client's weight distribution will affect the center of gravity and ultimately the wheelchair's overall performance.

Although posterior instability or "tippy-ness" is a challenge for clients using ultralightweight manual wheelchairs, anterior instability is frequently a greater risk for the bariatric client. Belly and lower extremity weight distribution move the seated center of mass anteriorly. Lower extremity edema or lymphedema may require some degree of extended or elevated lower extremity support, which accentuates the anterior distribution of weight. Reaching forward, especially while seated in a manual wheelchair, can shift the center of mass anteriorly enough to result in tipping the wheelchair forward.

Excessive gluteal tissue can prevent the client from sitting in contact with the back support surface as described earlier. It can also keep the client's center of mass more forward in relation to the mobility base, promoting anterior instability and limiting effective manual chair propulsion. Bariatric clients with a forward center of mass place more weight on the front casters of the manual wheelchair, which limits the forward mobilization and turning of the chair.

In a power wheelchair, excessive anterior weight can overload front casters or pivot the chair forward onto front antitip wheels, especially when driving down sloped surfaces. Strategies to address center of gravity vary from manual wheelchairs, power wheelchairs, and the seating system itself. Adjustability is necessary for successful outcomes.

PANNICULUS MEASUREMENTS

Current weight:_____   Weight history:_____

_____

_____

_____

_____

Pannus weight:_____

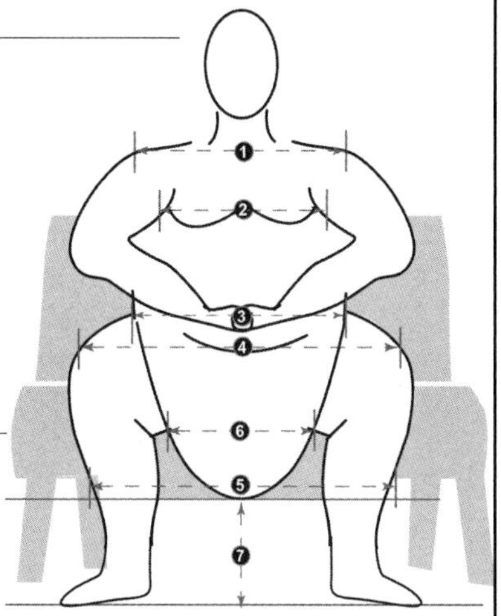

1. Overall shoulder width (at widest aspect) _____

2. Overall chest width _____

3. Overall hip width _____

4. Width at lateral thigh distal (at widest aspect) _____

5. Width at lower leg (at widest aspect) _____

6. Pannus width (at widest aspect) _____

7. Pannus to floor _____

8. Pannus depth (arterior to posterior) _____

9. Posterior pelvis to popliteal:
   Left Side: _____   Right Side: _____

10. Posterior pelvis to posterior pannus:
    Left Side: _____   Right Side: _____

11. Supported (lifted) height to floor _____

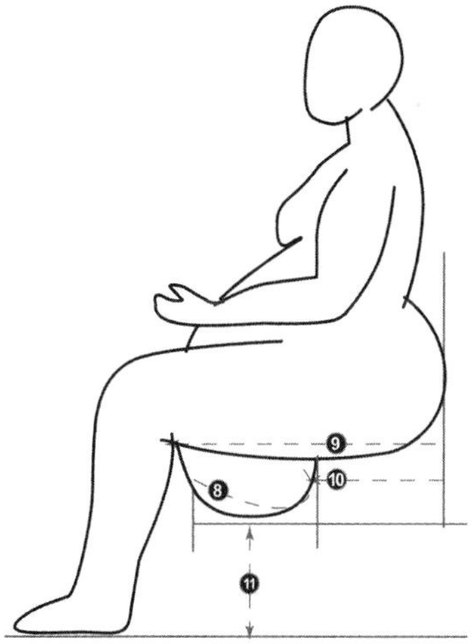

Figure 19-23. Panniculus Measurement worksheet. Originally created by Stephanie Tanguay, OT/L, ATP; graphics by Sofiya Kagan.

Manual Wheelchairs

Many manual chairs have a nonadjustable rear axle integrated with the rear frame and back post component of the chair. Bariatric clients who have excessive adipose tissue in the posterior gluteal area or the posterior trunk struggle with propulsion of a manual wheelchair with this configuration because their body position is anterior in relation to the rear wheels. This wheel position also places less weight over the propulsion wheel and more weight over the front castors, contributing to poor mobility of the chair. Many bariatric clients encounter more issues with anterior tipping of manual wheelchairs than posterior tipping. Some manual wheelchairs are designed with the ergonomics of bariatric weight distribution in mind. More anterior adjustment of the rear wheels can help, as can having the casters further forward to accommodate for the anterior center of mass of the bariatric client, thus providing greater stability and better mobility of the wheelchair.

Seat to Floor Height

Very often, clients with obesity use manual wheelchairs and attempt to propel using combinations of upper extremity and lower extremity motility. To improve lower extremity contact with the floor, the client may abandon footrests and seat cushions. This can result in extremely high areas of pressure, particularly at the front edge of the seat surface. Lower seat to floor height configurations are often necessary to optimize manual wheeled mobility.

It is important to note signs of high pressure because circulation can be compromised in this population. For mobility devices with fabric or sling seat materials, watch for stretching and tearing over time. Some wheelchairs have reinforced seat materials as standard or perhaps as additional charge options. If a client is using his or her lower extremities for manual wheelchair propulsion, ideally the seat to floor height, including a cushion, must reflect this. Optimal configuration of a size-appropriate manual wheelchair should be accessed but may not be adequate. Overall width eventually precludes the ability to access the propulsion wheels. The weight of the mobility device combined with the consumer's weight might exceed the client's ability to self-propel.

The client's ability to perform propulsion and sustain mobility is frequently limited by poor endurance related to obesity and comorbidities. Compromised respiratory function is a common secondary complication for this population. Watch for labored breathing with mild exertion. These clients are often independent with standing transfers and may be able to ambulate somewhat within their household. However, power mobility may be required for longer distances and functional mobility.

Power Wheelchairs

The vast majority of power wheelchairs available today include a power base with seating system and/or power repositioning seat systems mounted on top of the base. The base includes the drive wheels, motors, casters, and possibly stabilizing wheels. The batteries that provide power to the wheelchair are mounted within the base as well. The seat and back support frame is above this and, for some bariatric applications, may extend beyond the width of the power base. Due to the base style of power wheelchairs, it is common for a power wheelchair to be narrower overall than a manual wheelchair with the same seat width. The bariatric client's access may be greatly improved within some environments with use of a power wheelchair.

As with manual wheelchairs, center of mass is also an issue with power wheelchairs. It is important to consider the client's weight distribution in relation to the drive wheels, as well as the length of the wheelbase, for anterior stability. Short wheelbases with suspension stabilizers in the front (common in mid-wheel drive power bases) can compress with excessive anterior weight loads, pitching the system forward. This is most likely to be an issue with weight load on the anterior aspect of the seat during transferring and with navigation down inclines.

Seat Surfaces

Finding seat support surfaces and back supports that are size and weight appropriate can be difficult. If the bariatric client requires increased postural support, it may be impossible to find off-the-shelf seating solutions. Although many more heavy-duty options are available today, the greater the width of the equipment needed and the higher the weight capacity required, the fewer options that are available.

Bariatric seat surfaces must support higher weight capacities. Some heavy-duty cushions are significantly thicker in an attempt to compensate for the compression of the product materials. These thicker cushion designs result in higher seat to floor heights and can be detrimental for bariatric clients who use their lower extremities for manual wheelchair mobility. Higher seat to floor heights may also interfere with standing transfers. Seat cushions often show compression and collapse along the anterior (front) aspect, especially when the client is foot propelling or when the client discards use of the lower extremity support—a common attempt at improving maneuverability within a household.

Seat cushions are required for pressure distribution as well as pelvic support and stability. Bariatric clients may have need of these features for various conditions and diagnoses, just like their average-size counterparts. When looking at the design of cushions with wider proportions, it is worth noting that the pelvic structure of an adult who weighs 140 pounds is the same as a person who weighs 400 or even 650 pounds. This means the width between the ischial tuberosities does not change with weight gain. The pelvic contouring and lateral pelvic support of wider cushions should reflect attention to this anatomical fact as well as accommodate the additional soft tissue surrounding the pelvic structures.

Alignment of the femurs while seated can vary with body shape and tissue distribution. Clients with the apple body type or the pear abduction body type may have difficulties sitting with parallel alignment of the femurs. Many cushions have adduction contours that cannot influence or support the abducted and externally rotated femurs of these bariatric clients. For these clients, especially the bariatric person with significant amounts of medial thigh tissue, the cushion may require modification to allow the femurs to rest in a more lateral, abducted orientation.

Inappropriately long seat depths can cause contact and pressure in the popliteal region. This occurs frequently for bariatric clients as their lower extremity tissue distribution can change with fluid retention and weight gain. Great attention must be placed on proper seat depth during the prescription and fitting of wheeled mobility devices. Although seat depths that are too long can cause problems, seat depths that are significantly short can pose an even more serious issue for the bariatric population. When the client's higher weight is distributed on an inadequate seat depth, the pressure at the front edge of the seat surface can limit or disrupt the return of fluids from the lower extremities. With the bariatric client already at greater risk for lymphedema, this additional pressure on the posterior aspect of the thighs can cause fluid to pool in the legs at the point of seat edge contact. Large masses can develop on the posterior lower extremities as a result.

Back Supports

Excessive posterior pelvic tissue distribution (or *gluteal shelf*) can be difficult to measure and address. When the excessive posterior gluteal tissue contacts the back upholstery or back support surface, the posterior trunk is typically several inches forward and unsupported. This lack of posterior pelvic and trunk support can cause back pain as the client sits in a somewhat lordotic posture as he or she attempts to lean against the back support. Some clients place small pillows above the posterior gluteal tissue in an attempt to achieve some amount of back support by filling in this space. Accommodation of the unique posterior shape created by this redundant tissue is required. A back support can be mounted above the gluteal tissue to contact the client's posterior thoracic region. When this approach is used, the back support is frequently much shorter then typically prescribed. As the posterior pelvic tissue is visible below the back support, a cover or privacy flap should be provided. This material should extend below the back support to the seat pan and will assist in maintaining the client's dignity and privacy.

If a power reclining seating system is prescribed for a bariatric client with excessive posterior pelvic tissue distribution, accommodation of the tissue with a back support mounted above the gluteal shelf can be used. However, it is imperative that the recline feature is not a sliding shear compensating mechanism. In that configuration, the back support could compress posterior pelvic tissue and injure the client as the system reclines. A recline without this sliding mechanism is much safer because it eliminates this pinch point below the lower aspect of the back support. It is highly unlikely that any bariatric client would not experience a degree of shear in any reclining mechanism because the additional soft tissue alters the body's proximity to the pivot point of the reclining back.

For clients with abdominal obesity the mass of adipose tissue can prevent the client from sitting completely upright. Evaluation of the client's tolerance for seat to back angle is very important for the apple-type weight distribution for comfort, respiration, and function. A chair or back support that allows adjustment to open the back angle greater than a 90-degree orientation from the seat may be required.

HOUSEHOLD EGRESS

The Americans with Disabilities Act mandates commercial doorway widths to be a minimum of 36 inches for access. Newer residential construction must feature at least one external access doorway of 36 inches as well. Unfortunately, most manual wheelchairs with a seat width greater than 24 inches will not fit through that space. Making a home accessible for a bariatric wheelchair user requires extreme and costly structural modifications. Often the client may be limited to access of a single room. For the client's safety, at least one point of egress is recommended, and even that modification may be quite costly. Replacement of a sliding glass door with a set of French doors that would accommodate much wider wheelchairs is an example of a modification to create an accessible entrance.

The weight of a power wheelchair, including the batteries and the seating system, combined with the weight of a bariatric client, can exceed the weight capacity of aluminum ramps often used for household access. Weight-appropriate devices and accessories are required to ensure safety for bariatric clients and their families and caregivers. Some ramp products have weight capacities greater than 800 pounds. Width of the ramping must also be considered because many modular ramps are not wide enough to accommodate bariatric wheelchairs.

TRANSPORTATION

The physical transportation of a bariatric client in a wheelchair is frequently impossible. The weight of a power wheelchair, including the batteries and the seating system combined with the weight of a bariatric client, can exceed the weight capacity and width dimensions of most commercially available lift gates used to access vans and forms of public transportation. If the client is able to safely transfer into a motor vehicle, his or her wheelchair may be transported separately. Small trailers with flip-down doors can be modified with tie-downs for transportation of bariatric power wheelchairs. Manual wheelchairs are often perceived as easier to transport. Again, due to the overall weight and width of the bariatric client in his or her wheelchair, it may be necessary and safer for the client to transfer into the seat of a motor vehicle. Cross-braced folding frame manual wheelchairs wider than 24 inches are rather large even when they are folded and may not fit in the trunk of some cars. Due to the height of these wider chairs when folded, hoist devices (which mount in the trunk or cargo space of a vehicle and are used to load and unload the mobility device) may not be compatible with bariatric wheelchairs. Bariatric rigid frame manual wheelchairs are sometimes easier to disassemble and transport.

Summary

Seated and wheeled mobility for bariatric clients requires multiple considerations based on the person's medical condition, weight, body type, seated posture, and tissue distribution. It is critical for the clinician to take additional measurements to ensure the person is seated properly and safely in a chair that takes into account his or her specific needs. Lower extremity tissue distribution should be a factor in the selection of a mobility base, and the clinician may need to consider custom options to support or accommodate all tissue. Many bariatric clients present with a number of secondary conditions that can further complicate the prescription of assistive mobility systems. Taking some additional measurements and problem solving through some unique secondary considerations are necessary steps to providing a successful mobility device and avoiding complications for bariatric clients.

References

De Onis, M., Blössner, M., & Borghi, E. (2010). Global prevalence and trends of overweight and obesity among preschool children. *American Journal of Clinical Nutrition, 92*, 1257-1264.

Dionne, M. (2006). *Among giants. Courageous stories of those who are obese and those who care for them* [self-published].

Eknoyan, G. (2008). Adolphe quetelet (1796-1874)—The average man and indices of obesity. *Nephrology Dialysis Transplantation, 23*, 47-51.

Gurunluoglu, R., Williams, S. A., Johnson, J. L. A classification system in the massive weight loss patient based on skin lesions and activity of daily living. *Eplasty,* 12: e12.

Igwe, D., Stanczyk, M., Tambi, J., Fobi, M., Lee, H., & Felahy, B. (2000). Panniculectomy adjuvant to obesity surgery. *Obesity Surgery, 10*(6), 530-539. doi: 10.1381/096089200321593742

Ogden, C. L., Carroll, M. D., Kit, B. K., & Flegal, K. M. (2014). Prevalence of childhood and adult obesity in the United States, 2011–2012. *Journal of the American Medical Association, 311*(8), 806–814.

World Health Organization. (2014). World Health statistics report 2014 and WHO Media Centre statements on obesity and overweight children & adults. Retrieved from http://www.who.int/gho/publications/world_health_statistics/en/

Suggested Reading

Modolin, M. L., Cintra, W., Jr., Paggiaro, A. O., Faintuch, J., Gemperli, R., & Ferreira, M. C. (2006). Massive localized lymphedema (MLL) in bariatric candidates. *Obesity Surgery, 16*, 1126-1130.

20

Considerations When Working With Degenerative Neurological Conditions

John "Jay" Doherty, OTR, ATP/SMS

No matter whether an individual is newly diagnosed with a degenerative neurological condition or has lived with one for some time, many aspects need to be considered in everyday life and care. With so many different conditions that teams may come across, there is not just one way to treat a client's seating needs. The team also has to consider that seating and mobility is only one aspect of this client's life when working with a person who has a degenerative neurological condition; a variety of aspects—including medical, physical, psychological, and emotional—must also be addressed. Decisions regarding a person's seating system and mobility device often get put off for long periods of time, especially when the client can still ambulate.

Some of the degenerative neurological conditions clinicians and suppliers may see include amyotrophic lateral sclerosis (ALS), multiple sclerosis (MS), and spinal muscular atrophy (SMA). ALS is a degenerative neurological condition with no known cause. It affects the upper and lower motor neurons and is often associated with spasticity, increased weakness, and muscle atrophy. Getting clients who have ALS into power mobility early on can significantly lengthen their independence and safety with mobility (ALS Association, 2015).

MS is a chronic immune-mediated process where the body attacks the myelin sheath around the nerve cells in the brain and spinal cord, causing permanent damage and resulting in an interruption of nerve conduction (National Multiple Sclerosis Society, 2015). A multitude of symptoms can occur from sensory to motoric issues. The progression of MS is unique for each person. Some people live with few effects from the disease for years, and others may experience very rapid progression of the disease. For this reason, seating and mobility needs of these individuals will vary greatly.

SMA is a group of hereditary genetic disorders that attack the nerve cells in the spinal cord. This disease causes weakness and wasting away of voluntary muscles. Because there are four types of SMA, how the individual presents varies significantly from person to person (Muscular Dystrophy Association, 2015). These degenerative neurological conditions are just a few of the more common conditions that an assistive technology professional and therapist may see; there are a variety of less common conditions you may come across that all manifest in different ways.

One of the major challenges when working with individuals who have a degenerative neurological condition is the rapidity with which you may see decreased functional movements, increased postural support needs, and the changing ability to control a power chair using the original driving method. This chapter covers some of the common progressions seen in this population, including the supports needed within the seating system, the changes in access to the power wheelchair's drive control device and power seat functions, the changes in the client's overall independence, and how all these factors can affect the health and well-being of the individual you are working with.

SEATING ISSUES

Seating is hardest to maintain with anyone who has a degenerative neurological condition. A person's positioning

Lange, M.L., & Minkel, J. L.
Seating and Wheeled Mobility: A Clinical Resource Guide
(pp. 333-344). © 2018 SLACK Incorporated.

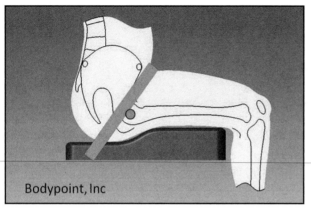

Figure 20-1. This picture demonstrates the typical 45-degree angle found on seating systems. (Reprinted with permission of Bodypoint Inc.)

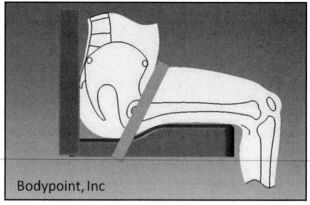

Figure 20-2. Pelvic belt shown at 60 to 70 degrees to the body. (Reprinted with permission of Bodypoint Inc.)

can often change due to the degeneration of his or her condition. This begs the question of how often the client needs to be reevaluated or have follow-up. Unfortunately, there is no perfect answer to this question. The therapist and supplier need to remember that every client is different, and because of those differences, the changes they see will be different as well. When working with people who have degenerative neurological conditions, the best practice is to follow up with the client every 1 to 3 months with a phone call to determine whether intervention is needed. Keep in mind that because progression is often slow, the client or care providers may not recognize the need for seating changes.

THE PELVIS

The pelvis is one of the single most important parts of the overall seating picture. We all get the greatest stability from a properly positioned pelvis; however, stable does not mean "no movement." A client can have functional pelvic movement and still have a stable pelvic position during a variety of activities.

When looking at the pelvis, the team has to keep in mind that the client may be moving around in his or her seating system, at least initially. This means the seating system should not restrict all movement but be as supportive as the individual needs. We still need to provide a good base of support to provide the stability the individual needs to maximize function. The surface from which the client works (the seat cushion) needs to provide stability and pressure distribution (envelopment). Stability will be most important initially for function to occur, but as atrophy occurs, pressure distribution needs to be closely monitored. Many degenerative neurological conditions spare sensation, which means that envelopment will not only affect skin integrity but also sitting tolerance from a comfort perspective. For this reason, pressure distribution and the ability

to shift position become paramount to the client's ability to remain in the wheelchair.

There are a variety ways to provide pelvic stability. As stated previously, the seat cushion is key to providing stability. Another important piece of equipment is the pelvic belt. The most common angle a pelvic belt is mounted at is 45 degrees to the frame of the chair (Figure 20-1). Although the juncture between the seat and back frame is a convenient point of attachment, it does not allow for the appropriate angle of pull relative to the person. The pelvic belt should always be angled to the individual's body while seated in the chair. With the belt mounted to the seat rail, a 45-degree angle across the pelvic notch may provide sufficient support to allow for mobility and stability of the client. However, this position should not be an automatic go-to or default placement location. When choosing the pelvic belt angle, team members need to think about what they are trying to achieve. If pelvic mobility is important, then a 60- to 70-degree or 80- to 90-degree angle to the individual should be considered. The 60- to 70-degree angle provides a downward and slightly back pull to minimize the pelvis from tilting posteriorly, while still allowing the individual to lean forward for a reaching activity. A steeper angle (80 to 90 degrees) allows the pelvis to tilt anteriorly for forward leaning activities (Figure 20-2). If an 80- to 90-degree angle is desired, then a four-point pelvic belt must be used. With a four-point belt, the larger strap should be angled at 90 degrees to the individual and the smaller pelvic belt strap should pull back at about 45 degree to the individual (Figure 20-3). This allows the greatest anterior tilt angle for forward leaning activities to be achieved, yet still prevents the pelvis from tilting posteriorly and the ischial tuberosities from migrating forward on the seat cushion. For this reason, a 60- to 70-degree angle or an 80- to 90-degree angle is most ideal to allow the client with a degenerative neurological condition to remain as mobile and functional as possible for as long as possible. As the person's neurological condition progresses, the team should consider greater stability at the pelvis to prevent undesired movement. At

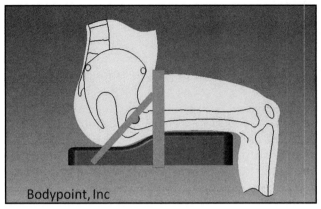

Figure 20-3. Pelvic belt shown at 80 to 90 degrees to the body with a four-point attachment. (Reprinted with permission of Bodypoint Inc.)

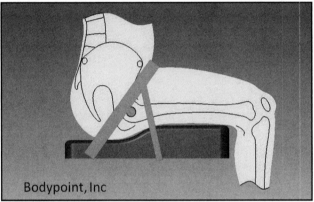

Figure 20-4. Four-point pelvic belt setup for 45-degree angle to the body to prevent anterior tilt of the pelvis and provide maximal stability. (Reprinted with permission of Bodypoint Inc.)

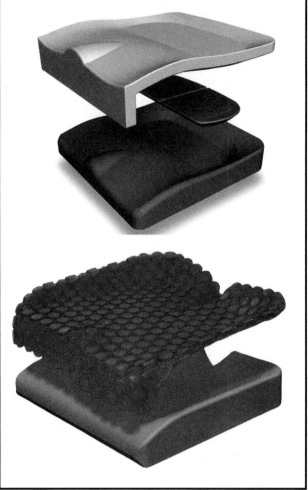

Figure 20-5. Examples of seat cushions that use combination of materials.

this point, a 45- to 60-degree pelvic belt angle may be considered to provide greater stability. A four-point pelvic belt should be setup with the larger strap at approximately 45 to 60 degrees to the individual's body, and the smaller narrower strap should be attached to the seat rails and set as close to 90 degrees to the thighs as possible. This position minimizes anterior pelvic tilt, which in turn should create greater trunk stability (Figure 20-4).

The pelvic belt provides only one aspect of pelvic stability for clients with degenerative neurological conditions. We must consider all directions of support needed for stability at the pelvis. The seat cushion must provide a base of support for function. The cushion must also provide sufficient envelopment for pressure distribution, which can be counter to the need for stability to allow the individual to remain highly functional, particularly early on in his or her diagnosis. Materials that provide sufficient envelopment also tend to shift under the client, causing instability. For this reason, a combination of materials may be best suited to meet the client's needs (Figure 20-5). Foam or other types of materials will provide a stable surface to optimize function. A second material, such as an air bladder or gel, will often provide the envelopment needed for pressure

distribution and increased sitting tolerance under the ischial tuberosities. The material needs to meet the needs of the client who has the degenerative neurological condition now and in the future as changes occur. As atrophy occurs, the seat cushion must assist with distributing pressure to protect the skin and prevent pressure injuries from occurring, since the person will likely continue to lose body mass. Other important considerations with clients who have a degenerative neurological condition include heat management and incontinence. Some of these conditions affect bladder control. Even if the condition will not affect bladder control, the decline in functional movement will eventually affect the timeliness or capability of performing transfers, which will affect the client's ability to get to the bathroom in time to void. For this reason, the team should consider protection of the internal material of a seat cushion.

Early on, keeping the pelvis centered on the seat can be a challenge as the client is moving around on the cushion during functional activities. Lateral thigh and pelvic supports will provide a way to keep the pelvis centered on the seat cushion, even as the individual performs transfers in and out of the seating system. As the individual loses function over time, the lateral thigh/pelvic supports maintain the position of the pelvis while driving a power wheelchair over rougher terrain. The lateral thigh/pelvic supports will also guide care providers in centering and properly positioning the individual's pelvis during transfers into the seating system.

The last component of pelvic support is the back support. The back support must provide posterior support to the pelvis. Otherwise, the pelvis will shift into a posterior pelvic tilt, which is detrimental to function and can cause long-term orthopedic problems to arise and have a negative impact on the individual's ability to breathe, chew, swallow, and digest food properly. Teams must ensure that the back support comes down low enough to provide posterior support to the pelvis and work with the pelvic belt to provide stability.

THE LOWER EXTREMITIES

When dealing with positioning of the lower extremities, the team needs to consider present and future circumstances and changes that will likely take place. When thinking about the present, the team needs to look at the following:

- What are the current functional needs of the individual?

- Is the person doing stand-pivot transfers or a modified transfer?

- How do his or her lower extremities need to be positioned currently, and what might his or her needs for lower extremity positioning be in the future?

These are all important considerations. Often the team will look at the prevalence of edema in an individual's lower extremities. Elevation may be recommended to manage any swelling using center mount or swing-away power elevating legrests. If the client is still performing stand-pivot transfers and will be for some time, then the team should strongly consider the swing-away style to allow the individual to move the legrests out of the way to place his or her feet securely on the floor to perform transfer. A second option would be to provide a center mount; although, this type of elevating foot support can at times create a problem, because flipping up the footplates for transfers is difficult and may not remain in position. An available option allows the footplates to lower (telescope) all the way down to the floor so that the individual can stand on the footplates safely during a transfer. Power center-mount foot platforms can also be modified by the manufacturer with an extra actuator added to flip up the footplates by pressing a button.

As some degenerative neurological conditions can cause an increase in spasticity, the team may need to consider securing the lower extremities to the footplates to prevent the feet from falling from this surface and being injured.

This is usually only done for safety purposes because strapping will prevent the client from being able to independently transfer out of the chair. In addition to foot support, the upper portion of the lower extremities may require additional support. If spasticity is causing hip abduction to occur, lateral thigh supports may be required to keep the hips aligned. If there is an increase in spasticity in the hip adductors, then a medial thigh support may need to be considered. This type of support can assist in aligning the lower extremities and preventing long-term orthopedic issues from occurring, which can cause further complications as the neurological condition continues to progress. Keep in mind that when dealing with spasticity, you need to carefully consider the options and don't be afraid to modify the position of seating components further to meet the client's individual needs. If using a power feature to elevate the lower extremities of an individual who has spasticity, then assess whether increased knee extension leads to an increase in spasticity and whether the client has adequate range of motion in the hamstrings.

THE TRUNK

Early in the disease process, even if the client is highly functional, gravity affects the body and can lead to asymmetry of the trunk. These changes may not be noticed until the orthopedic changes are significant and perhaps irreversible. For this reason, early education and intervention is extremely important. Early trunk support should not limit functional movement. These clients will still need to move within the seating system for functional activities until their neurological condition limits this.

The trunk of an individual with a degenerative neurological condition will over time slowly lose muscle control. This can result in an imbalance in muscle control on one side more than the other, which can often lead to a curvature in the spine over time. Gravity will continue to pull on the trunk and worsens the situation, resulting in the curvature progressing over time. The client and his or her family members often do not notice the progression of the curve because it happens slowly over time and they see the person daily. The client also compensates for this curvature as it progresses without realizing it, leading to postures that compensate for the muscle imbalance and the orthopedic changes. These destructive postures often lead to other complications during functional activities (e.g., relying on the armrests and arms to support the trunk position, which prevents freedom of movement of the upper extremities) or medical complications, such as breathing difficulties or pressure injuries. For these reasons, the team needs to address the individual's trunk instability as early as possible.

The first strategy is to allow gravity to assist with sitting upright. This is often accomplished by having the

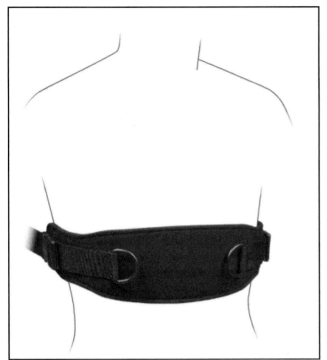

Figure 20-6. Anterior trunk support. An example of a chest strap. (Reprinted with permission of Bodypoint Inc.)

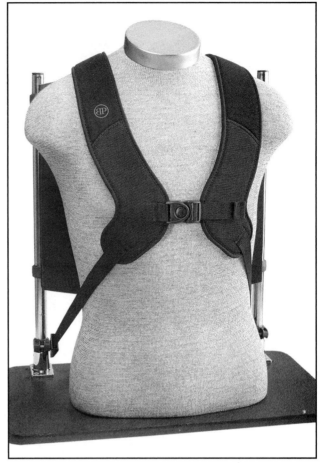

Figure 20-7. Anterior trunk support. An example of an H-style harness. (Reprinted with permission of Bodypoint Inc.)

individual tilt about 5 to 10 degrees in the posterior direction. This can also be accomplished by opening the seat to back angle 5 to 10 degrees, although this can negatively affect function (Dicianno et al., 2009). For this reason, tilt and recline are important seating interventions. The team must educate the individual on how to use tilt and recline to his or her advantage for positioning and for function. The client may need to use tilt or recline when driving down an incline as well as maintain postural control of the trunk. Gravity is something people fight their entire lives when sitting in a wheelchair, but the team can show clients how to use tilt or recline to their advantage.

When tilt and recline are not enough, trunk positioning components are used. These include lateral trunk supports, anterior trunk support, and, of course, posterior trunk support via a back support.

Lateral Trunk Supports

These components provide lateral stability to the individual's trunk when weakness is present. These can be mounted at the same height for balance purposes or offset heights (one higher than the other, the lower lateral trunk support just below the apex of the curvature in the trunk providing support in the plane needed) to reduce or accommodate a curvature in the trunk. A third point of support at the pelvis will be needed when using offset lateral trunk supports (on the same side as the higher lateral trunk support).

Anterior Trunk Support

Chest Strap

This is generally used for balance only. The individual's upper trunk may collapse onto the strap when using this type of anterior support (Figure 20-6).

H-Style Anterior Trunk Supports

These components provide a rearward and upward direction of pull at the anterior trunk and at the shoulders, which will help keep the person from falling or collapsing forward but can also limit the client's ability to reach forward. The upper part of the device should pull up and back (Figure 20-7).

Shoulder Retractors

Retractors are solid anterior trunk supports that come down over the top of the shoulder. These types of trunk supports prevent the individual from falling forward, but can limit forward reaching.

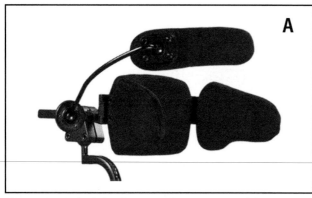
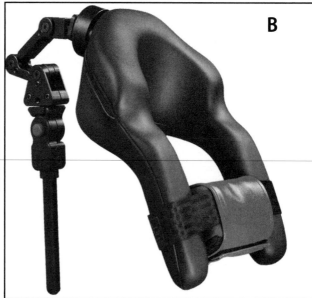

Figure 20-8. Multiple head supports that may assist with head position as neck muscles weaken.

Posterior Back Support

In addition to the preceding supports, the posterior back support is critical. As many of these individuals will lose function over time (some quicker than others), seating teams often provide a higher level of back support. The higher back support is also needed when the client is in a fully tilted or reclined position. Another important factor is the pressure distribution the back support must provide. Although the back support does not seem to support as much force as the seat cushion, a person can develop a pressure injury over the bony prominences of the back. Clients who are experiencing atrophy are predisposed to developing pressure injuries over time. For this reason, the team needs to look closely at the materials to be used in the back support as well as the amount of surface the client is making contact with (the greater the surface area, the more pressure is distributed). Trunk support is just as important to the individual's function as pelvic and lower extremity support. The function and general health of an individual who has a degenerative neurological condition will be significantly affected by the position of the trunk itself. Every part of the body above the trunk (head/neck and upper extremities) is directly impacted by the position of, and stability in, the trunk. As the neurological condition progresses, the needs of the individual will also change, so follow up is extremely important.

HEAD AND NECK

Just like every other part of the body, the need for support of the head and neck will change over time. The position of the head and neck are extremely important to speech production, swallowing, and breathing, all of which are body functions that are often affected by degenerative neurological conditions.

Functional movement is extremely important early on for people who have degenerative neurological conditions. A basic headrest can provide posterior head support when the client is fatigued or tilted/reclined in the seating system. Some degenerative neurological conditions can affect the head and neck very early in the disease process, increasing the need for support.

Tilt and recline can facilitate head and neck positioning as much as it can assist with trunk positioning. Too much tilt or recline can negatively affect a person's head and neck position, causing the individual to pull his or her head forward (due to a righting reaction), limiting the client's ability to safely swallow, manage saliva, and produce speech.

Whenever a client presents with head or neck difficulties, the team must start at the pelvis first, because head and neck position may be stemming from poor positioning in another part of the body. Once the pelvis, lower extremities and trunk have been addressed, if no improvements have been achieved at the head and neck, a more complex type of head support may be needed. Suboccipital support may limit neck hyperextension. The headrest may need to include lateral or even anterior head support. Anterior head supports include collars and anterior forehead supports or a strap. There is nothing perfect on the market when it comes to head and neck support, and because every person that comes into the clinic is going to present with different needs, the head and neck supports will be as individual as the person the team is evaluating (Figure 20-8).

UPPER EXTREMITY SUPPORT

Positioning of the upper extremities will influence the comfort, functioning, and positioning of the client with a degenerative neurological condition. Early on, the position of the upper extremity will affect function and endurance. Height adjustable armrests are essential to meet the changing needs of individuals with degenerative neurological conditions. The seating team needs to teach clients to use the support provided to maximize function and decrease the effects of fatigue throughout the day. Wider armrest pads can provide forearm support and help prevent the client from holding his or her extremities up against gravity during various activities. If the upper extremities are unsupported, the position of the trunk is negatively affected over time, especially as weakness progresses. For this reason, people with a degenerative neurological condition will also rely on their upper extremity supports to assist with controlling their trunk position.

Laptrays provide a flat surface to both support the arms and provide a work surface, but will often prevent independent transfers. The team has to assess whether desk- or full-length armrests will best meet the client's needs. Desk-length armrests will allow a person to pull up closer to a surface, such as a desk or table, and may be beneficial early on. However, desk-length armrests do not provide a long enough hand hold for the client who is performing stand-pivot transfers, commonly done during the early stages of these conditions.

Long term, the team needs to consider weakness that may develop from the degenerative neurological condition, and where the weakness is occurring. If the shoulders are weakening, full-length armrests at the proper height are important to prevent shoulder subluxations from occurring and to maintain the integrity of the shoulder joint, which can decrease pain in the long term as well. Full upper extremity support may allow the individual with shoulder weakness to stabilize against the support, allowing him or her to remain functionally independent for a longer period of time. Solid gel is a good material to consider in full-length armrest pads. Gel pads can provide comfort, help distribute pressure, and minimize the risk of developing a pressure injury, especially over the elbows. As the degenerative neurological condition progresses, arm troughs may be needed to maintain the upper extremities in a functional or comfortable position, especially during tilt or recline. Swivel, adjustable-style mounting hardware may be necessary to position the arm in a midline orientation for function or comfort, especially in later stages of disease progression. In some cases, forearm straps may also be required to keep the arms within the arm troughs.

Keep in mind that some individuals may have great difficulty using upper extremity supports and may choose to rest their upper extremities on their lap (this may be a position of comfort for some individuals). Unfortunately, this position is not the ideal, possibly compromising joint integrity and circulation. Therefore, education of the long-term effects of poor upper extremity support is an important part of the evaluation process.

CONSIDERATIONS BEYOND SEATING

Access to the Power Wheelchair

If a client is using a power wheelchair, which is often the case with degenerative neurological conditions, then access to the electronics can allow the client the greatest level of independence throughout the day. The difficulty for a seating team is determining the best access method, as the individual's condition will progress, but the extent and rapidity of change is unknown. It will depend on the disease process and the team may have to look at the individual's history to best predict what will be needed based on typical disease process.

With electronics, consideration must be given to future needs while the individual is using the power wheelchair. Expandable electronics, no matter which manufacturer is used, will allow a client to start with a proportional joystick control as appropriate and progress to specialty input devices such as switches, a head array, or a sip-and-puff system.

This is a suggested progression of driving methods:

1. Proportional joysticks

2. Other proportional devices (e.g., mini proportional joysticks, chin joysticks, proportional head control, proportional foot control)

3. Switches

4. Head arrays

5. Head array/sip-and-puff combination

6. Sip-and-puff

7. Single-switch scanning

This list is not all inclusive, but a great place to start with progression of input devices. The top of the list offers the quickest, most direct input methods with the greatest amount of control, and the bottom of the list offers input devices with less directional and speed control, and which can be a little more time consuming to use to control the power wheelchair. Please refer to Chapter 11, "Power Mobility: Alternative Access Methods," for further information.

One of the difficult situations teams may encounter is determining when to move from a traditional joystick to an alternative access method. The team should consider introducing a new input method early on, allowing the client to become proficient at using the input device, reducing potential frustration. Many manufacturers have the capability to decrease the throw of a proportional joystick through programming. Decreasing the throw allows the individual to reach maximum speed with less deflection of the joystick, therefore requiring less movement. Throw typically can be reduced to as little as 30% of the standard throw. When an individual requires more than 50% throw reduction, other input methods should be considered, because the client is probably fatiguing quickly with use of a standard joystick and another input method is inevitable. At this point, either a mini proportional joystick or a switch input device is needed. Whether using four switches or only one via scanning, fiberoptic switches may be easiest to access for the longest period of time. Fiberoptic switches often work well when someone only has finger or thumb movement, because only slight movement and zero force is required for activation. Keep in mind that support of the extremity is important for access to remain consistent. As decline in function occurs, single-switch scanning may be a good option for an individual with a degenerative neurological condition. Single-switch scanning, although more time-consuming to use, allows the client to remain independent with control over his or her power wheelchair and power positioning system. Having control over one part of life can be very important to a client who is losing independence in other areas.

As strength declines, the client will likely need tilt and recline more, and access to his or her input device while tilted or reclined may be very challenging. The client needs to be able to access the input device throughout the entire weight shift cycle. This will ensure that the client uses tilt and recline to full capacity to maintain a healthy body. The client may use a toggle switch to control power seating, a separate switch (which can be placed wherever the client has control), or control power seating through the specialty input device. The team must also look at the client's independent access to his or her environment. Infrared signals can be sent through the power wheelchair to devices such as televisions, stereos, and more, allowing the client to control these devices through the driving method. Most manufacturers offer these capabilities standard or as an option. Some degenerative neurological conditions, such as ALS, can affect speech production. When appropriate, access to a speech-generating device (SGD) is possible through the driving method using interfacing. In addition to SGDs, access to a computer and the Internet can allow communication with others when the client may not be able to easily get out into the community. Bluetooth access to control a computer through mouse emulation using the driving method can really enhance someone's daily life and communication with people in other locations. These power wheelchair features are discussed in further detail in Chapter 13, "Power Mobility: Advanced Applications."

Clients with a progressive neurological condition are changing daily, weekly, and monthly. As a result, the appropriate option, accessory, postural support component, position in space, method of operating the power wheelchair, and access to the environment will change just as quickly. Planning for change is key to working with individuals with progressive neurological conditions so that the technology solution can continue to meet changing needs.

Power-Adjustable Seat Height

Powered mobility provides 360 degrees of movement in a two-dimensional plane. Power-adjustable seat height allows for access in the vertical plane and can have a significant impact on the population with a degenerative neurological condition. Many of these clients will perform a stand-pivot transfer; therefore, having the option to elevate the seat of the power wheelchair can allow this type of transfer to continue over a longer period of time. By elevating the seat, the client has less height to overcome in order to stand for the transfer. Less distance to cover means the client is using less effort and energy, which in turn means energy saved for another functional activity during the day. It also allows the chair to be setup so gravity can assist with sit-pivot or sliding board transfers as the disease progresses.

Many wheelchair users spend most of their day looking up at their peers who can stand and ambulate. This places strain on the neck, which can cause pain to develop over a period of time. However, as head control becomes compromised, clients may lose the ability to lift their head and engage in conversation. Raising the height of the seat also provides greater visibility for safe navigation of the power wheelchair in areas where line of sight may be compromised. In addition, elevating the seat also extends functional reach to turn lights on and off and reach for clothing, food, medication, or other necessary items. This decreases the need for assistance throughout the day, promotes independence and a feeling of greater self-worth.

For these reasons, people with progressive neurological conditions benefit significantly from the use of a power adjustable height seat, so if there is a resource to pay for this enabling technology, it should be pursued.

Manual Mobility

Although the majority of people with degenerative neurological conditions will use power mobility to maintain their independence, some may choose or only require a manual wheelchair for a period of time. A good example of this would be a client with MS. Lightweight (ultralightweight), highly adjustable manual wheelchairs can be adjusted and adapted to the client's needs as he or she goes through functional changes. A manual tilt or recline wheelchair may be required to provide adequate postural support and weight shifts. Considering the historical progression of the disease for an individual client will help meet his or her needs now and in the future.

CONSIDERATIONS DURING THE LATER STAGES OF DEGENERATIVE NEUROLOGICAL CONDITIONS

Positioning Needs of the Client

As the client with a degenerative neurological condition has a decline in function, there may come a time when he or she can no longer adequately or safely drive a power wheelchair. However, the client may still have the capability to control power seat functions or his or her environment independently. If the client can no longer drive the power wheelchair safely, then it can be set up with an attendant control for a care provider to drive the chair and a switch for the client to access the power seating, infrared, and Bluetooth functions on the chair during the daytime. This will allow the client to independently maintain his or her skin integrity, comfort, sitting tolerance, and independence throughout the day.

Respiratory Needs of the Client

Some degenerative neurological conditions (e.g., ALS) and some forms of SMA will eventually affect the ability to breathe. In these cases, the team members must ensure that they anticipate the need for a ventilator to sustain the client's life. It is a personal choice to use a ventilator, and some people may change their mind as their condition progresses. The evaluating team should ensure any power base and seating system provided to a client has the capability to support a ventilator and power source.

To complicate things further, a variety of size ventilators are on the market. Over the years, ventilators have decreased in size significantly. The correct ventilator tray must be specified for the wheelchair.

Ventilators can be powered by an internal battery, draw power from the power wheelchair batteries, or use a separate battery, which may be mounted inside the power wheelchair base or attached to the ventilator tray itself. These many factors must be considered when specifying equipment. Education of the client is important so that he or she is able to make an informed decision.

SUMMARY

It cannot be overstated when working with clients who have a degenerative neurological condition that being proactive is very important. It is not a matter of if but when the client will lose function, muscle control, and independence.

To be proactive, the team must educate the client and family as to what options are available, as well as the advantages and disadvantages of each choice. Well-educated clients will choose the best outcome for themselves.

CASE EXAMPLE

A.L. was diagnosed with MS in 1993. Initially, she was diagnosed with lapsing-remitting MS. A few years later, A.L. was rediagnosed with primary progressive MS. A.L. resides in a single-family residence with her husband, who provides care to her in the evenings. She has paid care assistants who assist with her care during the daytime hours.

After her diagnosis, A.L. used a cane for ambulation from 1995 until 1998. In 1998, she moved to a rolling walker, which provided a safer means of ambulation. After many years of using a rolling walker for mobility, she moved to a manual wheelchair for distances in 2002. Then, in 2004, as the MS continued to progress, she started to use a power wheelchair with a van-style seat. She paid for the power wheelchair out of pocket and primarily used it to walk her dog.

Over time A.L. found that she needed to use the power wheelchair for longer periods of time. In 2007, she started to develop greater upper extremity weakness. This additional upper extremity weakness prevented her from weight shifting adequately. It was at this time that she developed a pressure injury on her buttocks. The therapist confirmed that the pressure injury was indeed from sitting on her seat cushion for long periods of time without any relief. The team identified her upper extremity weakness as part of the issue.

After further evaluations, the team decided that the best course of action was to provide a power wheelchair with power seating to allow A.L. to use the power seat functions for a variety of activities, some of which included pressure relief, changing position as fatigue set in, and changing position for transfers in and out of the wheelchair. In 2008, A.L. received her power wheelchair with power tilt, recline, and a power-articulating foot platform, along with a gel seat cushion to assist in managing her positioning, medical, and functional needs.

Not long after receiving her power wheelchair and using the power-positioning seating system, A.L.'s pressure injuries healed. A.L. reports that she uses her power tilt and recline for pressure relief, and her skin has been healthy since she received these power-positioning components. She also reports that over time, she started to develop edema in her lower extremities, and the power-articulating foot platform, along with tilt and recline, has assisted in managing this and preventing swelling from remaining problematic. In 2011, A.L. found that using her arms to assist in holding her trunk upright was becoming a problem, and her arms would become sore over time. She was reassessed and the team found that she could really benefit

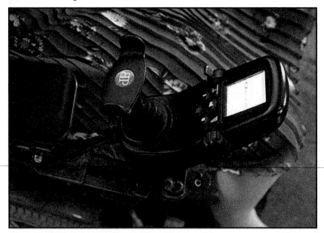

Figure 20-9. Goalpost joystick handle that A.L. now uses to drive and control her power wheelchair.

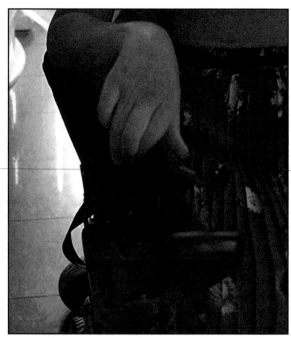

Figure 20-10. Example of how A.L. uses goalpost joystick handle to control tilt and recline while the power positioning system is upright or back.

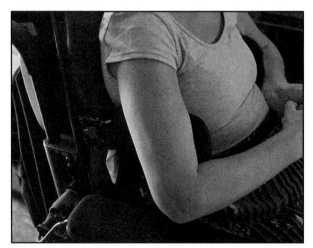

Figure 20-11. The lateral trunk supports that now assist with A.L.'s trunk balance.

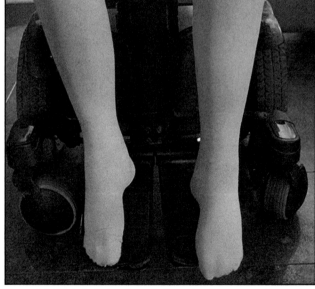

Figure 20-12. Articulating foot platform that A.L. uses to elevate feet throughout the day in order to manage her edema.

from lateral trunk supports, but A.L. was against using lateral trunk supports because she thought they would affect her function and movement while seated in the wheelchair. The team provided her with gel armrest pads to prevent her from developing discomfort in her upper extremities. The team also found that at this time, her upper extremity function and strength was continuing to decline. A.L. reported that she was only able to use her proportional joystick part of the day due to fatigue. The team evaluated A.L. and found that the best match for her was a Magitek input device. The reason this worked best was A.L.'s head control and head position would differ from day to day, and with the Magitek system, head position did not matter. This allowed A.L. to use her proportional joystick until the late afternoon, when she would switch to the Magitek system to control her power wheelchair.

The system worked well for A.L. until 2013, when she decided she needed to try lateral trunk support, so the team added these to her seating system. The lateral trunk supports have allowed A.L. to feel well-supported and no

longer rely on her upper extremities for balance. At this time, A.L. also changed from a custom modified joystick handle to a goalpost style joystick handle. The lateral posts on it allow A.L. ease of use when driving the power wheelchair, and she uses the vertical posts of the joystick handle to bring herself upright out of a tilted or reclined position. Figures 20-9 through 20-13 provide comparison.

Today, A.L. is pursuing a new wheelchair with tilt, recline, and articulating foot platform and wants to explore

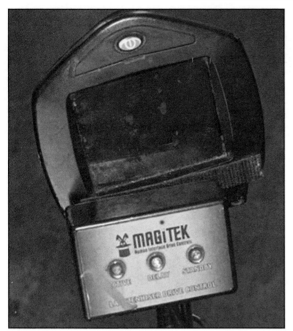

Figure 20-13. The combination of the enhanced display and the Magitek system that A.L. uses when she is too fatigued to use the joystick.

a proportional chin control to independently control the power wheelchair. She reports that her upper extremity function is not as severely affected as it was a few years ago and that without her power seating and wheelchair, her independence would not be what it is today.

CASE EXAMPLE

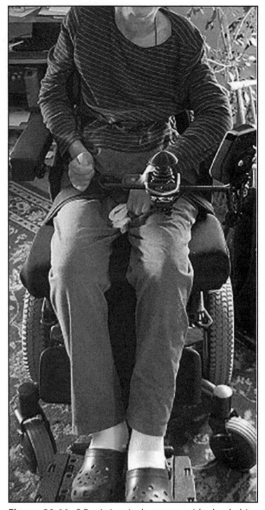

Figure 20-14. S.B. sitting in her new mid-wheel drive power wheelchair.

S.B. is a 59-year-old woman who had an onset of MS symptoms in 1977, but was not diagnosed until 1988 when this was confirmed by magnetic resonance imaging. Originally, her MS was diagnosed as relapsing-remitting, but in 1999, this diagnosis was changed to secondary progressive MS. Her MS over the years has resulted in her current quadriparesis. S.B. also has a current stage II pressure injury on her right ischial tuberosity, a history of a stage II pressure injury at her coccyx, suprapubic catheter, and Baclofen pump to help manage lower extremity extensor spasticity, bilateral foot/ankle edema, impaired sensation in the lower extremities, scoliosis, postural kyphosis in sitting, a right pelvic obliquity, and carpal tunnel syndrome.

At the time of the evaluation, S.B. reported a number of seating and mobility issues. A major problem was that S.B. was leaning heavily on the right armrest pad because the lateral trunk supports were removed from the wheelchair as their bulkiness got in the way of functional activities. She had difficulty with her hand position on the joystick that affected her ability to drive in all directions. When tilted or reclined, S.B. could no longer access the power

seating control switches, which could strand her in a tilted or reclined position (she was unattended for 6 hours a day, so this was a significant issue). S.B. could not turn the chair on and off independently. Various repairs were needed to a chair that was quite old and many of the seating components had worn out (backrest and seat cushion).

S.B. was provided with a mid-wheel drive power wheelchair, which allows her to remain independently functional in all aspects of her mobility (Figure 20-14). The power wheelchair meets her needs indoors and outdoors. The power tilt-and-recline system provides S.B. with the ability to shift weight from her buttocks to protect her skin. She cannot otherwise perform a weight shift due to severe weakness and so uses tilt and recline effectively to maintain her skin integrity throughout the day. S.B. uses the seat elevator to assist with stand-pivot transfers throughout the day. She cannot perform a stand-pivot transfer without use of this feature. The seat elevation feature provides her with the ability to reach items on higher surfaces throughout the day to access food and beverages that have been prepared for her earlier in the day. S.B. uses the center mount foot

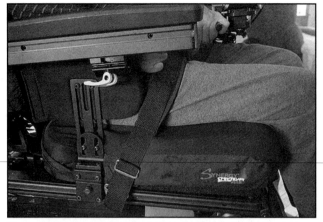

Figure 20-15. Pelvic belt angled at approximately 70 degrees to keep pelvis back on seat cushion but not make contact with suprapubic catheter.

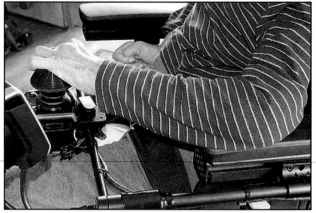

Figure 20-16. S.B. with support needed to access midline-mounted stand-alone joystick.

platform to manage her edema throughout the daytime. S.B also has a padded pelvic belt, which has been placed on her at approximately 70 degrees to her body to prevent it from hitting her suprapubic catheter, yet still maintain her pelvis back in the seating system (Figure 20-15). She also opted to use lateral trunk supports this time to assist with her trunk posture and prevent the discomfort she develops in her elbows from holding up her trunk by pressing against the arm pads. A standalone joystick is used with a midline mount to allow her the greatest access and control over the power wheelchair, yet still be able to swing it out of the way for transfers to occur (Figure 20-16).

In addition, the infrared features of the power wheelchair are programmed to allow S.B. to have independent access to her television, an air conditioner in the summer, and an electric heater in the colder months.

S.B. reports that she is very pleased with the power wheelchair and finds the infrared features beneficial at times when she is alone.

REFERENCES

ALS Association. (2015). *What is ALS?* Retrieved from http://www.alsa.org/about-als/what-is-als.html

Dicianno, B. E., Margaria, E., Arva, J., Lieberman, J. M., Schmeler, M. R., Souza, A.....Kendra L. (2009). *RESNA position on the application of tilt, recline, and elevating legrests for wheelchairs, assistive technology* (pp. 13-22). Retrieved from http://www.resna.org/sites/default/files/legacy/resources/position-papers/RESNA%20PP%20on%20Tilt%20Recline_2017.pdf

Mendoza, M., & Rafter, E. (2002). *Living with ALS manual 4: Functioning when your mobility is affected.* Retrieved from www.alsa.org/assets/pdfs/brochures/als-book4-2016.pdf

Muscular Dystrophy Association. (2015). *Spinal muscular atrophy.* Retrieved from http://www.mda.org/disease/spinal-muscular-atrophy/overview

National Multiple Sclerosis Society. (2015). *What is MS?* Retrieved from http://www.nationalmssociety.org/What-is-MS

BIBLIOGRAPHY

Arva, J., Schmeler, M., Lange, M., Lipka, D., & Rosen, L. (2009). *RESNA position on the application of seat-elevating devices for wheelchair users. Assistive technology* (pp. 69-72) Retrieved from https://www.resna.org/sites/default/files/legacy/resources/position-papers/RESNAPositionontheApplicationofWheelchairStanding.pdf

DiGiovine, C., Rosen, L., Berner, T., Betz, K., Roelser, T., & Schmeler, M. *RESNA position on the application of ultralight manual wheelchairs.* Retrieved from https://www.resna.org/sites/default/files/legacy/resources/position-papers/UltraLightweightManualWheelchairs.pdf

SUGGESTED RESOURCES

BodyPoint, Inc.: www.Bodypoint.com

Quantum Rehab: www.Quantumrehab.com

Stealth Products, Inc.: www.StealthProducts.com

Symmetric Designs Inc.: www.Symmetric-designs.com

21

Considerations When Working With Complex Neurological and Orthopedic Presentations

Elizabeth McCarty, OTR/L and Melissa Tally, PT, MPT, ATP

CHARACTERISTICS OF INDIVIDUALS WITH NEUROLOGIC AND ORTHOPEDIC IMPAIRMENTS

The seating and positioning considerations of individuals with complex physical and medical needs can be complicated, ongoing, and variable. The long-term effects of abnormal tone common with these diagnoses, including cerebral palsy (CP), traumatic brain injury, and movement disorders, can be severe and affect the musculoskeletal system dramatically. Each person is unique, and there is no clear rule book when matching product with physical presentation. The age and developmental level of the child are important factors when trying to maximize participation and socialization. After years of working with complex physical needs, the authors are certain of one thing: Starting early is critical. For a child to participate and have any type of typical experience, he or she needs to be able to interact with the environment. He or she needs to experience visual information, communicate, activate, initiate, and participate. Progressive musculoskeletal and medical consequences will occur if appropriate support from a seating system is not prescribed and monitored. Early intervention and the ability to adjust and make changes to a postural system or mobility base are crucial to the long-term success of any intervention. Starting early better educates the family about the benefits of ongoing compliance with postural equipment. More important, early intervention

allows the child to have the maximum opportunity to develop through age-appropriate experiences.

One of the crucial areas used at our center to evaluate in individuals with neurologic or orthopedic presentations includes the type of muscle tone or tonal patterns of movement present. Understanding the impact of abnormal tone on the musculoskeletal system, as well as having a grasp of available medical considerations and interventions for tone management, are important first steps. Orthopedic management, including pre- and postsurgical considerations, is critical to determining the type of postural or mobility system required and supporting the surgical intervention. Is the individual going to require a thoracic brace, or will the seating system support a spinal curvature or dislocated hip? Factors such as transfers and placement of complex medical equipment need to be considered for the caregiver. The overall goal of any evaluation is to gather enough information to successfully match product with the goals and needs of each client. The end result will be good medical management and a high level of client interaction and participation.

TONE MANAGEMENT

Individuals with CP (and other complex neurological disorders) often present with movement patterns that can be categorized into four types: spastic, dyskinetic, ataxic, and flaccid/mixed. Each of these patterns results in significant abnormal postures, musculoskeletal imbalance, and secondary orthopedic asymmetry (Goodman & Glanzman, 2003; Wollack & Nicher, 2003). Complex seating systems

Lange, M. L., & Minkel, J. L.
Seating and Wheeled Mobility: A Clinical Resource Guide
(pp. 345-362). © 2018 SLACK Incorporated.

and postural supports are required to promote midline orientation, inhibit abnormal patterns, and/or facilitate functional movement and control.

Dyskinesia (further categorized into dystonia and athetosis) is defined as fluctuations between high and low tone, often resulting in spasms (Skogseid, 2014). Dyskinesia can affect the whole body (as in CP) or one region of the body (as in adult onset dystonia) (Evatt, Freeman & Factor, 2011). Although the symptoms are similar, adult-onset dystonia is degenerative, whereas athetoid CP is not. Athetosis may present as uncontrolled, slow, writhing movement of the limbs, or dystonia may affect the trunk, which results in twisted, fixed postures (Skogseid, 2014). Dyskinetic movements can be further described as chorea, chorea-athetoid, or dystonia based on the specific movement dysfunction (Wollack & Nicher, 2003). These fluctuating patterns affect postural control and require dynamic positioning systems to inhibit abnormal patterns while supporting midline stability of the head, trunk, pelvis, and hips (Skogseid, 2014). Occupational and physical therapists are widely taught that proximal stability results in improved distal mobility and control. In our experience with seating and positioning for individuals with dyskinesia, proximal stability of the trunk and pelvis can result in inhibited tonal patterns of movement, improved weightbearing through the pelvis and trunk, and thus improved access and function, as well as alignment.

Spastic (hypertonic) patterns of movement present as increased muscle tone in flexion or extension postures, often resulting in very stiff limbs (Bower, 2009). Damage to the neural-motor pathways in the central nervous system results in increased tightness of the muscle and reduced capacity of the muscle to stretch (Bar-On et al., 2015). Hypertonia is associated with spastic CP, traumatic brain injury, and other associated disorders. Untreated hypertonia can lead to loss of function, loss of range of motion` (ROM), and orthopedic changes (Bar-On et al., 2015). Clients presenting with hypertonia require external supports to facilitate neutral postures and orthopedic alignment to inhibit contractures and asymmetry.

Flaccid muscle tone (hypotonia) is a condition characterized by the weakening or loss of muscle tone as a result of disease or trauma affecting the muscular system, nervous system and the nerves associated with the involved muscles (Bower, 2009). In our practice, we have found our clients with hypotonia are unable to maintain upright functional postures without external supports and seat functions to provide antigravity postures.

Bower describes how primitive reflexes are often associated with abnormal tonal patterns of movement and are persistent as the result of abnormalities within the central nervous system. Most primitive reflexes are integrated by 4 to 8 months of age, but the child with CP or other neurological condition may present these reflexes through adulthood (Bower, 2009). The most common abnormal reflexes that affect postural control of clients with complex neurological conditions are tonic labyrinthine reflex (TLR), asymmetrical tonic neck reflex (ATNR), symmetrical tonic neck reflex (STNR), and clonus. The TLR reflex presents when the head is tilted back while lying supine or with contact to the occipital area and results in the back stiffening and even arching backward; the legs straightening, stiffening, and pushing together; the toes pointing; the arms bending at the elbows and wrists; and the hands fisting or the fingers curling. Severe TLR presentations are referred to as an *opisthotonic reaction*. The ATNR presents when the head is turned to the side, resulting in the arm and leg on the face side extending while the opposing side flexes. This may also be referred to as a *bow-and-arrow presentation*. The STNR presents when the head is extended back and results in the arms extending while the legs flex or, when the head is flexed forward, resulting in the arms pulling into flexion and the legs extending. Clonus is movement marked by rapid contractions and relaxations of a muscle following extension or flexion of a body part, often seen in the foot or hand.

Effects on Seating and Positioning

Understanding how these tone patterns affect the musculoskeletal system is necessary when selecting the appropriate postural supports. The constant movement of a joint and rotation of the spine of a dyskinetic client; the static positioning of the joint and shortening of the muscle fiber for the spastic client; and the lack of support and stability of the hypotonic client all place great strain on the body and can lead to additional medical concerns and functional limitations (Table 21-1).

Ball (2014) discussed how areas of increased pressure and weightbearing lead to increased risk for skin breakdown; poor alignment of the esophagus and trachea result in risk of aspiration; limited ROM results in contracture and scoliosis; decreased gastrointestinal motility results in reflux, poor breakdown of nutrition, and constipation; and limited room for organs in the body cavity (due to rib cage distortion and/or trunk posture) results in poor respiration and overall organ function. It is important to consider these factors when completing the mat assessment of the client and making seating recommendations. Clinical findings of this detailed manual assessment will indicate how tonal patterns are affecting postural stability and overall systems function (Ball, 2014). In addition, we have found that the external supports recommended should correlate to the manual support required during the mat assessment to facilitate more neutral alignment, inhibit abnormal patterns, decrease pressure on bony prominences, improve comfort, and allow for functional access and participation. Refer to Chapter 1 for details on mat assessment.

Although seating can support, assist, and facilitate more neutral postures, it is important to consult with the

Table 21-1
EFFECTS OF ABNORMAL TONE

• Increased risk of skin breakdown	• Impaired mobility
• Increased risk for aspiration	• Impaired respiration
• Decreased ROM	• Increased risk of pneumonia
• Joint contractures and scoliosis	• Constipation
• Impaired body system function	• Poor nutrition
• Pain and discomfort	• Decreased participation

rehabilitation specialist, neurologist, or both in regard to pharmacological tone management. The coordination of pharmacological agents with complex seating can result in more positive outcomes for the client. Some common agents used include injections of phenol and botulism toxin (Botox), and oral medications include baclofen, Dantrium (dantrolene), Sinement (carbidopa/levodopa), and tizanidine (Chung, Chen, & Wong, 2011). Surgical intervention may be suggested as well, including placement of a baclofen pump (intrathecal, intraventricular), soft tissue or tendon releases, and selective dorsal rhizotomy (Bower, 2009). Making referrals for these consults and remaining active as part of the medical team is encouraged and intervention is recommended. Referrals as young as 18 to 24 months of age are appropriate, with surgical consults after 3 years of age. Clients and families living with complex disorders and associated tonal patterns can greatly benefit from early referrals and medical management for these chronic conditions. The medical team can assist with tone management, maintaining or improving ROM, and increased comfort. Medical management can also allow the caregiver increased ease in daily care, more opportunities to connect to his or her loved one, and promote active functional participation across the life span. The medical plan must be reviewed before making any seating changes or recommending new equipment.

ORTHOPEDIC MANAGEMENT

Postural support and alignment are critical for the needs of the client with orthopedic concerns. The goal of positioning is to align joint structures to allow weightbearing and to counter rotational forces and torque that could lead to orthopedic asymmetries. Early positioning is focused on promoting neutral postures and maintaining good ROM for development of joints and structures. As the client moves into adolescence, the focus changes to supporting growth spurts and continuing to promote neutral alignment, which often requires more frequent seating adjustments and modifications. The adult client needs to be supported

to promote participation, accommodate orthopedic asymmetries, and prevent additional complications. Common orthopedic issues include subluxed or dislocated hip, spinal curvatures and rotation, pelvic obliquity and contractures of the elbow, wrist, knee, and ankle (Bower, 2009).

Often the complex client will be a candidate for surgical intervention. The most common orthopedic surgeries (Table 21-2) include soft tissue and tendon lengthening, hip osteotomies, spinal fusion, and rhizotomy (McCarthy, 2011). At our facility, we have found that pre- and postsurgery postural positioning can greatly improve the outcome of a surgery. This leads to the importance of working with the surgical team to create an optimal positioning plan of care postsurgery. Otherwise, the client may have no functional options to adapt his or her posture after the surgery and will be placed in a seating system that does not support or complement the surgical intervention. In our experience, it is typical for a client undergoing spinal rod surgery to grow 4 to 6 inches in back height, and a hip osteotomy client may require a 2- to 4-inch change in seat width to keep the femur seated in the acetabulum.

Tables 21-3 and Table 21-4 show the suggested Orthopedic Seating Protocols for surgical and non-surgical clients with complex neuromotor conditions, developed by The Perlman Center at Cincinnati Children's Hospital Medical Center.

Depending on the funding source, prior authorization of funding for wheelchair modifications or a new chair can be a lengthy process, and each state may have different guidelines. This needs to be worked into the surgical plan. Our protocol recommends for a clinician to see a surgical client 3 to 4 months prior to the surgery date or as soon as surgery is recommended. This allows time for the family, clinician, surgeon, and supplier to become familiar with the upcoming procedure and the expected outcome. If a category of seating can be recommended, such as a molded seating system or new seat and back, the medical team and supplier can initiate the funding process. Typically the client is often not medically able to tolerate an evaluation for up to 4 to 6 weeks after surgery depending on the intervention. The clinician and supplier should arrange to see the client

TABLE 21-2
COMMON SURGICAL INTERVENTIONS
Orthopedic surgery (McCarthy, 2001) • Muscle and tendon lengthening, shortening or transfer: tendon Achilles lengthening, adductor release, split tendon transfer, rectus femoris transfer, splint anterior tendon transfer • Bony osteotomy: periacetabular osteotomy, femoral derotation osteotomy, varus derotation osteotomy, pelvic osteotomy • Single-event multiple-level surgery: combination of soft tissue and bony surgical procedures performed at the same time; this procedure has become increasingly common for clients with CP
Spinal Correction: Neurogenic Scoliosis • Spinal fusion: rod placement • Vertical expandable prosthetic titanium rib; metal rod curved to fit the back of the chest and spine placed in an up-and-down position, can be expanded as child grows (Campbell, 2013)

Neurosurgery
 	
• Baclofen pump: A pump is implanted in the child's abdomen to deliver continuous baclofen into the fluid surrounding the spine to reduce spasticity (Albright & Ferson, 2006)
  ○ Intrathecal baclofen
  ○ Intraventricular baclofen
 	
• Selective dorsal rhizotomy: A procedure in which the nerves are cut to decrease spasticity (Grunt, Fieggen, Vermeulen, Becher, & Langerak, 2014)

acutely after surgery to allow for immediate adjustments to the current equipment, or provide loaner equipment and set a schedule for delivery of new positioning equipment. It is important for the seating recommendations and authorization process to be part of the surgical intervention protocol. This allows the funding sources to understand the significant contributions that seating and positioning have on postsurgical outcome. Our experience has suggested that insurance companies and other funding sources will approve a new seating system as it relates to the change that will likely affect the musculoskeletal system as a result of the surgical intervention.

We additionally recommend that the nonsurgical candidates be referred for complex seating evaluations to explore alternative options to promote neutral positioning, reduce pressure over bony prominences, improve comfort, and inhibit progression of orthopedic distortions. Orthopedic conditions that are not addressed properly in a timely manner can lead to detrimental effects for the client, increasing the level of disability and decreasing life expectancy. Inadequately supported joints experience continued stress, torque, and pull. This can shift the client's center of gravity and promotes pressure points over bony prominences. These joints may become painful, ROM is often lessened, and the surrounding area can be at risk of skin breakdown. This may lessen a client's functional ability; decrease his or her tolerance to remain in upright postures, subsequently reducing ability to participate; and decrease overall health. Often, with aging, muscle mass decreases, and bony prominences become more prominent, particularly in the pelvic area. This can place pressure on the sciatic nerve, resulting in increased pain and discomfort to maintain upright sitting. Using pressure mapping during the evaluation process for any seating system, particularly for clients with orthopedic complications, can decrease future pain and tissue breakdown and assist with product recommendation (Hanson, Thompson, Langemo, Hunter, & Anderson, 2012).

FUNCTIONAL CONSIDERATIONS

The client with severe complex orthopedic considerations will often present with spinal rotation, pelvic obliquity, and lower extremities windswept to one side, which affects the client's ability to interact with technology or participate in his or her environment. What is the priority and why? It is important to remember the reasons behind our recommendations. There are several additional questions that need to be considered. What is the functional task or goal to be achieved? Does he or she need to be supported in a comfortable, manageable position? Does he or she need to have pressure relief over bony prominences? Does he or

TABLE 21-3
RECOMMENDED PROTOCOL FOR OPTIMAL SEATING FOR THE SURGICAL CLIENT
• Medical team has recommended client for surgery: Seating modifications will be needed to allow optimal positioning status postsurgery to accommodate physical and functional changes.
• Preoperative visit: Medical team refers client for seating and positioning consult (optimally 3 months before surgery date) to allow for assessment of recommendations, justification of medical need by therapist, and prior authorization of funding to be initiated.
• Inpatient: Therapist and supplier work with inpatient medical team to assist client with loaner wheelchair for transport or modify current wheelchair to accommodate postsurgical restrictions and positioning.
• 6- to 12-week follow-up (out of casts/bracing and tolerating ROM and upright positioning): Therapist and supplier remeasure client to assess any changes needed to recommendation prior to ordering.
• Schedule delivery of new equipment.
Originally created for the CCHMC Perlman Center Therapists.

TABLE 21-4
RECOMMENDED PROTOCOL FOR OPTIMAL SEATING FOR THE NONSURGICAL CLIENT
• The medical team has determined the client is not a candidate for surgical procedure.
• The medical team refers the client for seating and equipment assessment to determine appropriate 24-hour positioning products to promote functional positioning and access, support asymmetries and contractures, and prevent further impairments.
• Therapist and supplier perform assessment of recommendations; complete all necessary documentation for therapeutic justification and funding.
• Schedule delivery of equipment.
Originally created for the CCHMC Perlman Center Therapists.

she need to access a speech-generating device (SGD) and be able to keep his or her eyes forward to drive a power wheelchair using a head array? If a goal is functional participation in any form, the seating may focus on how the trunk is positioned to allow interaction and participation. This may result in the legs remaining in a windswept position to the side so the client can look at an individual, see where he or she is going, or perhaps access his or her communication device.

VISUAL IMPAIRMENTS

Visual impairments are common in individuals with CP and other neurological impairments. Christine Roman-Lantzy, who has devoted many years developing assessments and interventions for cortical visual impairment (CVI) that has affected children with CP. According to Roman-Lantzy, CVI is now the most common cause of visual impairment in children in the United States and CVI is frequently seen in children who have neurological

disorders or have acquired brain injury. With the exception of power mobility, a visual evaluation is not common when performing a seating and positioning evaluation. Knowing how common visual impairments are with this population, it is an area that needs to be considered (Roman-Lantzy, 2010). Common visual dysfunction of individuals with neurologic conditions includes nystagmus, ocular motor apraxia, and CVI. Nystagmus is involuntary eye movement alternating in a slow and a fast component in two directions. Ocular motor apraxia is impairment of voluntary horizontal saccades, a small rapid jerky movement of the eye, and compensatory jerky head movement to enable fixation. The more significant deficit affecting posture is CVI, and this should be considered when making recommendations for a seating system.

Visual deficits, especially CVI, can affect postural patterns and head position. A client that positions his or her head in a flexed and lateral position with upward ocular gaze may be doing this to gather visual information. He or she may lift his or her head in and out of this position with frequency to gather visual information. It is natural to want

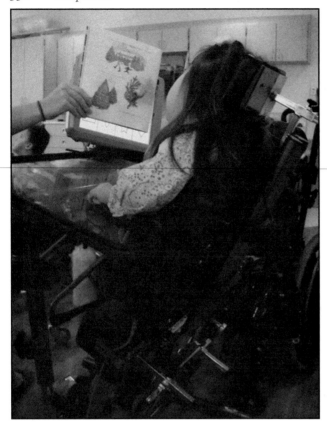

Figure 21-1. Slight head tilt to obtain visual field.

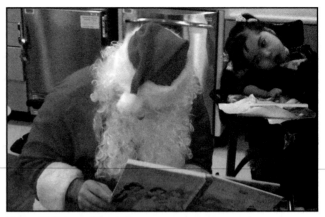

Figure 21-2. Lateral head tilt.

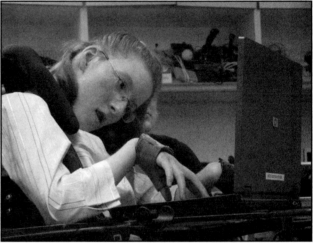

Figure 21-3. Head drop and lateral tilt.

to correct the head to be in a midline and upright position. As a clinician, it is critical to recognize and not limit this movement. Occupational therapist Katherine Engle has worked with a number of children with CVI at the Perlman Center. Some of the interactions with children with CP at the Perlman Center include looking at tonal patterns in relation to their seating and positioning. Clinical observations look at how blocking an ATNR pattern of the arm of a client with CP can prevent him or her from accessing a switch for function. Similarly, altering or limiting the head position of a client with CVI may be altering his or her optimal visual field and how he or she gathers visual information. Roman-Lantzy stated that CVI is often referred to as *cerebral visual impairment* or *cortical visual impairment* and implies damage to the visual cortex of the brain. The visual cortex is rarely damaged on its own, so the broader term, cerebral visual impairment, is gaining wider acceptance as a more accurate term. Chris Roman-Lantzy describes CVI as "a condition in which the eye works but the part of the brain which interprets the signals provided by the eye does not. This will cause the child to have difficulty using visual input he/she is receiving" (Roman-Lantzy, 2010, p. 5). CVI is not an indication of the child's cognitive ability. It differs from ocular forms of visual impairment in that the interference in visual function exists not in the structures of the eye or optic nerve, but in the visual processing centers and visual pathways of the brain.

How does CVI affect postural positions and what considerations should be made when determining final product recommendations? Just like tonal patterns are different for each individual, how visual information is received also varies. On the basis of our observations, a typical head posture seen is a head drop with the client using sideways glances of objects in the environment or the client holding his or her head in a forward flexed posture while activating a switch or operating a power wheelchair (Figures 21-1 through 21-4). This is commonly observed in our clinics, and when children are working on their communication devices or other functional tasks. The individual will lose contact with the head support and frequently have his or her head flexed forward. This is an all too familiar scenario for many professionals determining an appropriate head support. Head positioning is always a frustration and with no easy answers. For an individual who has CVI, it is important to provide both a static and a dynamic system. It is suggested that headrest recommendations should be finalized after the pelvic and spinal supports have been determined.

Dynamic seating components allow for movement and may optimize head control for a client with CVI, allowing for frequent head positioning changes. It has been our experience that providing good shoulder support through anterior trunk support will help maintain the upper trunk and pelvic position while a lap tray will also provide forearm support. A headrest that provides support to the suboccipital area may be helpful and decreases other responses, such as opisthotonic reaction. A forehead pad with a swing-away component can provide the client a period of rest. Anterior head support can be used to limit the active range of neck movement in clients with limited head control. The swing away pad should be contoured and measured according to the height of the forehead and amount of movement the client needs. When the individual needs to be interactive, allowing the headrest supports to be moved out of the way prevents blocking vision. These have been common recommendations used in our clinic with good functional success for the child. These are significant considerations when clients are using augmentative communication, computers, and power mobility. Tilting a client does not always promote the head to rest on the head support. Often the opposite occurs and the client will resist and flex forward. Using anterior tilt may keep the client in an active position and promote neck extension. A client may not be able to maintain this position for long periods of time, however, and needs close supervision.

It is important to allow for a period of exploration when allowing dynamic head movement. Having the individual explore without lateral or anterior static supports on the headrest will provide the experiences in movement the individual may never have had with previous, more restrictive systems. Headrest components should be considered separately to match the functional need and task performance requirement. Separating each component is a good approach. Trial is important to a successful intervention. Vision requirements, tone patterns, and sensory reaction to pressure placed anywhere in the head and neck area are essential considerations to selecting the appropriate headrest. Trial of the various components is an important part of the evaluation process (Clark & Pope, 2015).

EARLY INTERVENTION

Why start early? The simple reason is that research has shown this is a critical period of development. A child's brain is growing rapidly and reaches two thirds of its size by 3 years of age, with most neural connections made during this time (Kolb & Wishaw, 2008). The young child learns best through active exploration and mastery of the environment. By addressing and providing postural control early, we can help prevent learning deficits that may develop due to the inability to interact with the environment and others, as well as combat the severity of physical limitations that present across the life span. Evidence shows that

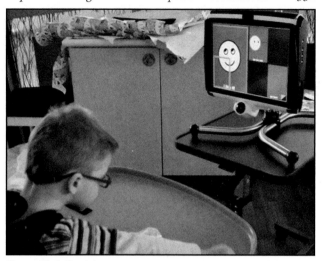

Figure 21-4. Head drop.

deprivation and limited experiences may cause long-term cognitive deficits (Ramey, Campbell, & Blair, 1998).

Development is complex, and it may be difficult to have this conversation with a parent in the early stages of diagnosis. When addressed properly, this discussion can lead to successful intervention and positive outcomes. Sometimes predicting the level of disability is challenging and unknown, but understanding the medical effects of abnormal tone on the musculoskeletal system can be a predictor of long-term postural presentations and need for intervention. The Gross Motor Functional Classification Scale can also be a predictor for long-term needs of the complex client (Rosebaum et al., 2002).

Although we know that development follows a linear progression of skills, there is much variability in the performance and achievement of these milestones. The goal of providing intervention early is to develop consistent skills, nurture learning, and promote participation in play and achievement of milestones. It doesn't matter how the child performs the task but more that he or she has the opportunity to try. A child with complex needs may have no way to explore his or her environment other than on his or her back if he or she is not provided postural support.

However, there is another component equally as important in providing postural support early: the parent or other caregiver (Rigby, Ryan, & Campbell, 2009). Parents and caregivers need to develop confidence and comfort in caring for and nurturing their child. Specifically, caregivers need to gain confidence in parenting, understand their child, bond with their child, see the abilities of the child, and learn the importance of the technology needed to allow him or her to grow and learn. The more confidence and competence caregivers have, the more receptive they will be to the long-term use of postural supports. This can only lead to improved outcomes for clients and hope for a decrease in surgical interventions and medical complications across the life span.

TABLE 21-5
PERLMAN CENTER: 24-HOUR POSITIONING
Developmental Positioning • Postural control, strengthening • ROM, weightbearing • Home exercise programs
Upright Positioning • Activities of daily living: play, feeding, bathing, sleeping • Computer access/augmentative and alternative communication-integrated technology • Vision, sensory processing, participation
Total Mobility: Early Mobility • Gait trainer, stander, wheelchair • Manual vs power • Recreational
Transfers and Transportation • Body mechanics, Hoyer lifts, overhead systems

We educate caregivers that by providing these supports, we are reaching outcomes that matter. The child will be able to actively explore and participate in play, move through the environment, assist with self-help routines, interact with family and friends, participate in community activities (e.g., shopping, restaurants, church, visiting friends and relatives), gain an effective means of communication, and make choices about wants, desires, and needs (Morgan, Novak, & Badawi, 2013). In addition, caregivers learn that positioning and postural control is needed to provide stability for task performance and function, manage spasticity and tone, maintain joint alignment, strengthen antigravity postures, provide weightbearing, and relieve pressure.

For the complex client, our therapists provide support through multiple pieces of equipment for 24-hour positioning (Table 21-5), pharmacological management, therapeutic handling, external bracing, and modalities. Chapter 7 addresses 24-hour positioning in further detail. At this young period of development, the equipment needs to be functional for the child but also address the needs of the family. The team needs to teach parents to lift and carry their child correctly. The team must provide developmental positioning and seating systems for functional daily tasks including bathing, feeding, and sleeping. It is also important to get the child up and moving via standers and gait trainers and provide safe transportation (i.e., car seats). Clinically, key areas of focus are strengthening and weightbearing, gaining and maintaining ROM, improving body awareness, increasing functional endurance, and inhibiting tonal patterns. Therapists need to show the

parent or caregiver how to incorporate these key areas into meaningful tasks (Darrah al., 2011). Meaningful tasks for the very young child include the daily routines of being cared for and nurtured and playing with caregivers. The use of adaptive supports and equipment throughout the typical day allow these natural parenting skills, parent-child bonding, and developmental experiences to occur. It allows the parent to be a parent, the child to bond and experience learning, and fosters lifelong acceptance of equipment for participation.

CONSIDERATIONS FOR EQUIPMENT

Clients often require different positions throughout the day to perform varied tasks. Looking at a typical school- or workday, demands range from passive sitting when being transported to actively participating in a classroom or work setting. The expectation of a seating system is to support the individual throughout the day and offer accommodations in postures and movement. The seating system also needs to provide stability. "Seating for anyone, cannot be a singular posture, and any singular posture without any inherent mobility within that system, cannot assist an individual in becoming independent in any task" (Kangas, 2002). Matching equipment to fit varied functional and physical needs requires careful consideration. As discussed earlier, clients with CP or orthopedic concerns may present with primitive reflexes, abnormal tone, spinal curvature, extensor thrust, hip dislocation, pelvic obliquities, sensation deficits, and general upper and lower asymmetry. Areas where bones are close to the surface (called *bony prominences*) and areas that are under the most pressure are at greatest risk for developing pressure injuries (Model Systems Knowledge Translation Center, n.d.). The weight of the client will affect decisions, because people who are underweight or have decreased body mass will more likely have pronounced bony prominences. Clients who are overweight or have increased body mass may have excessive tissue with reduced bony prominences. This does not mean, however, that people who are overweight are less susceptible to pressure issues. This is addressed further in Chapter 19. Additionally, when considering a seating system, the frame or base is key and should be considered in combination, as these each influence the other. The proper combination of chair and seating will enable a client to sit in a neutral and stable posture and to participate.

Properties of the seating and positioning equipment can be associated with specific functional outcomes. Understanding the characteristics of various cushions and cushion materials is critical in matching client positional needs. Matching the type of cushion to the client's needs will depend on a variety of factors, including how much time he or she spends in his or her chair, how much he or she moves around in the chair, and how stable his or her posture is. Cushions require varying levels of maintenance, inflation, care, installation, and replacement (Schmeler & Buning, 1999). For the client with complex needs, standard or off-the-shelf products have limited ability to assist with tone management, pressure, and postural control, because they are too basic and not supportive to the client's needs. Customized seating or molded systems provide the customization required for medical and functional management.

Seating Systems: Back and Seat Cushions

Off-the-Shelf Products

Off-the-shelf products are rarely appropriate for the complex client due to abnormal tone, curvatures, contractures, respiratory issues, and pressure risk. Off-the-shelf products will not accommodate or support the complex client's muscular skeletal system. Custom products that allow for individual configuration and adjustability or molded systems are typically recommended.

Material and Properties

Viscous Gel

Viscous gel material is often held together in small pockets or sacs within a cushion Sometimes gel is in a concentrated area under the ischial tuberosities or as a thin overlay on top of a foam cushion. Gels and fluid-filled cushions are moderate conductors of heat and have a high heat capacity.

Caution should be taken because gel can also have heat buildup that is not easily released. However, for the complex client, the gel may not provide enough stability or surface contact. Gel tends to allow for motion. If a client requires a controlled and stable pelvis, gel may not be the best option.

Air

Air flotation cushions support the body entirely on air. A typical example is the ROHO cushion, designed with a group of small, interconnected rubber balloons arranged in rows. Pressure is balanced by air shifting out to surrounding sacs or cells, spreading pressure evenly against the buttocks and posterior thighs. The whole system is closed, so air flotation cushions cannot bottom out the way gel cushions can (Karp, 1998). The individual with high tone may have difficulty with air cushions because they may not provide enough stability due to air shifting between cells. These cushions provide excellent air exchange for heat and pressure relief. A combination of air cells and contoured foam can be useful to provide postural support and stability but also provide improved pressure distribution and relief under the ischial tuberosities.

Foam

Many densities of foam are available for seating. Foams range in density and the ability to envelope the body shape of the client (i.e., memory foams). Foams are poor conductors of heat and have a low heat capacity. The biggest concern with foam is the high shear potential. Foam can be easily altered and customized.

Custom contoured cushions typically include three layers of foam in addition to a solid or rigid base. The top layer allows for air circulation and reduces sitting pressure (Figure 21-5). This layer may also provide comfort for clients that have full sensation and provide emersion, allowing the client to sink into the support for added stability. A soft open-cell or reticulated foam, 0.5 to 1.0 inch thick, is recommended. The middle layer controls shearing, reduces pressure, and controls heat (Figure 21-6). Medium- or high-density foams and gel components are typically 1.0 to 2.0 inches thick. The middle layer determines how much emersion and support are provided for the client. The bottom layer supports the properties of the middle layer (Figures 21-7 and 21-8). The base is typically Ethafoam placed on a wood, metal, or a hard plastic board to allow hardware to attach to the mobility base (Ferguson, 1998).

Custom or Modular Seating Systems

Custom or modular seating systems use a variety of primary and secondary supports. These systems are made by many independent sources as well as through manufacturers that allow the clinician and the supplier to specify shape and materials. A custom seating system typically has a separate seat and back that can be independently attached to a mobility base (Figures 21-9 and 21-10). The materials

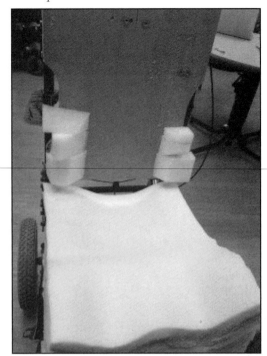

Figure 21-5. Soft top layer.

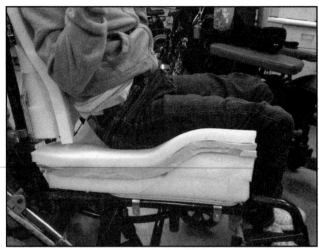

Figure 21-6. Blue middle layer.

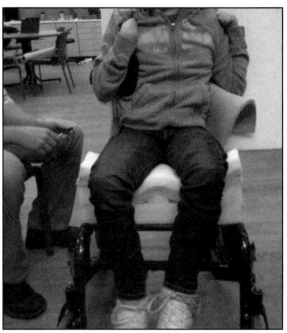

Figure 21-8. Front view of seating material layers.

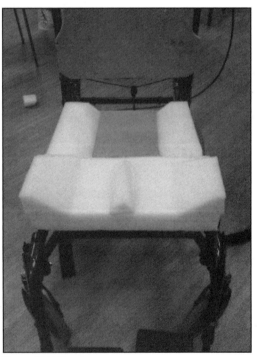

Figure 21-7. Base layer.

can be any combination of foam, air, and gel. Primary support surfaces include the seat and back. Secondary supports include lateral trunk and thigh supports, anterior trunk supports, and head supports. The seating hardware is adjustable and growth options are incorporated. A single seating system may include secondary supports from several manufacturers. Custom backs can accommodate spine distortions if a more aggressive mold is contraindicated. Using a grid back, which has individual blocks of foam that can be carved or reduced in thickness, can accommodate the apex of a curvature. Foam can be cut and a gel or air pad embedded to accommodate a high pressure area. Foam can also be cut to allow for a leg-length discrepancy or a pelvic obliquity. Lateral trunk supports can be adjusted in asymmetric patterns to capture a curvature and provide varied forces on the trunk. The downside of these systems is the complexity and decreased overall surface contact compared with a molded system. This system does allow for growth and frequent adjustments.

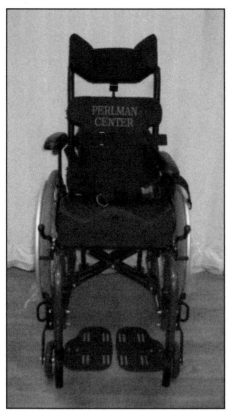

Figure 21-9. Custom seating system.

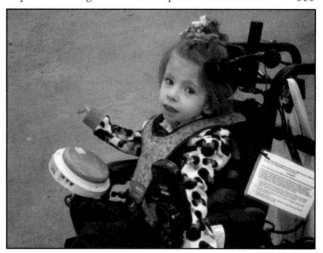

Figure 21-10. Child in custom seating system.

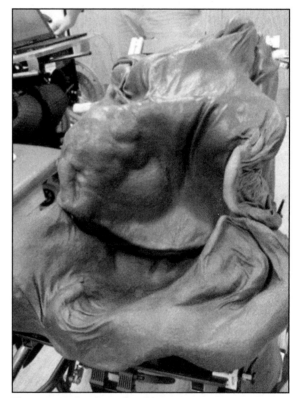

Figure 21-12. Simulator after shape capture.

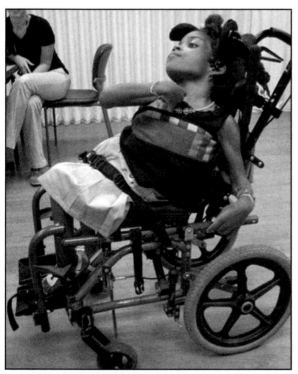

Figure 21-11. Client before molded seating.

Molded Systems

Molded systems are typically formed with varied densities of foam and are an excellent choice for significant spinal curvatures and other orthopedic distortions (Figures 21-11 through 21-13). Molded seating is discussed in further detail in Chapter 5. The molded seating system conforms to the shape of the client and also allows hands-on experience to identify areas of force and counterforce needed to

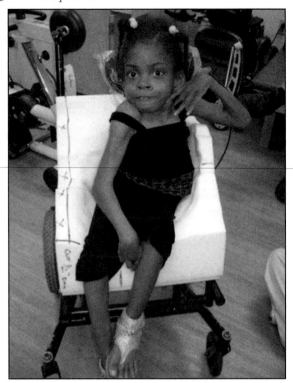

Figure 21-13. Client in unfinished product, prior to final fabrication.

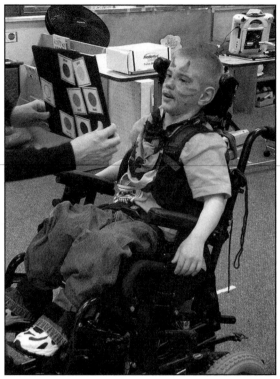

Figure 21-14. Manual tilt-in-space.

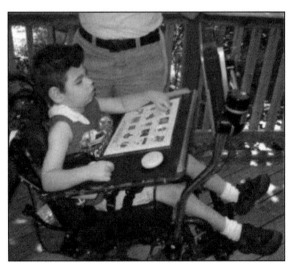

Figure 21-15. Manual tilt-in-space with mounting system.

support a complex presentation. Typically, a custom mold does not allow for much proximal movement of the client. A client using molded seating typically cannot reposition him- or herself or lean to the side to reach items. These clients typically have a current spinal curvature, pelvic obliquity, and other medical issues such as respiratory and swallowing disorders. Custom molds can also provide a very stable base of support to aid in the control of abnormal tone. For the dystonic client, using a molded seat to provide pelvic support and a stable base can be used in

conjunction with a custom back cushion that still allows for upper extremity and trunk movements. We have found some clients with movement disorders, such as dystonia or athetosis, do well in a fully molded system because this significant stability decreases extraneous movement.

Seat Functions: Tilt, Recline, and Elevating Legrests

Using seat features, such as tilt and recline, has many medical benefits, which are discussed in detail in Chapter 10. For the complex client, these features can be critical. Changes in body position are necessary to address issues related to postural alignment, function, physiology, transfers and biomechanical issues, contractures or orthopedic distortions, edema, spasticity, pressure management, comfort, or dynamic movement (Dicianno et al., 2009).

Tilt-in-space is a common recommendation for individuals with multiple medical and physical needs (Figures 21-14 and 21-15). If recline is to be used in combination with tilt, it is important to consider how recline will affect the placement of postural supports. Recline can be useful for managing medical issues, such as catheterization, but can have a negative impact on the posture of the client on return to upright. Due to shear, the position of secondary supports in relation to the client change during recline. Tilting allows frequent positioning changes, provides changes in visual field, and provides a position of rest.

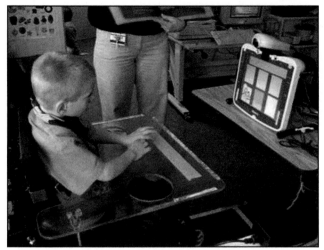

Figure 21-16. Use of tray.

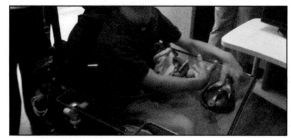

Figure 21-17. Handgrip on tray.

Elevating legrests should be used with caution for clients with significant physical involvement. Complex clients rarely have sufficient ROM in the hamstrings to extend the knee, so using elevating legrests can lead to posterior pelvic tilt and displace the pelvis from the cushion contours.

Two other items that can promote function include a tray (Figure 21-16) and a grip placed on the tray (Figure 21-17). Trays can be used for upper extremity support and stability and can affect trunk posture as the client stabilizes against this surface. The tray can be covered with a black cloth to decrease visual distraction. The tray can provide a work surface and support items such as switches. A grip device can be mounted to the tray and used by clients with dystonic arm movement. The client can learn to grasp the bar or handle to provide stability.

The evaluation and team contributions are critical for the complex client. When possible these clients should be seen in an established wheelchair and seating clinic with skilled clinicians and a multidisciplinary team. The complex client will most likely have other technology that will need to be considered. The following are some questions the team can ask during an evaluation to better understand participation:

- Is the client currently using any type of technology such a computer or communication device?

- What are the primary activities that the client participates in or enjoys?

- How does the client communicate his or her needs to others?

- How does the client access his or her school or work environment?

- Does the client need frequent positioning changes to tolerate a full day of participation?

USING MODALITIES TO ENHANCE SEATING

Occupational therapist Katherine Engle and physical therapist Erin Pope at the Perlman Center have been pairing Kinesio Tape applications with seating systems. Modalities, such as Kinesio Tape and bracing, in conjunction with seating, may provide support that is often difficult to produce with seating products alone. A good example of this is at the rib cage and shoulder blades. Minimal correction of muscle tissue in these areas can often provide support and contact that is difficult to achieve with the seating system. The rib cage often collapses even with significant support provided by a molded seating system. Kinesio taping is a method of functional taping that has a wide variety of applications, including assisting the body to hold a joint or position, increasing proprioception and body awareness, and positioning a part of the body in better alignment.

Kinesio Tape is not permanent and needs to be reapplied. General guidelines used with the clinicians at our center include wearing the tape at least 3 to 5 days/application. The tape is designed to move with the wearer, allows normal ROM, and is elastic. The stretches are on a longitudinal axis and have up to 60% stretch. The tape itself is 100% cotton, latex free, and has similar thickness and weight to skin. When worn, the tape lifts the top layer of the skin, taking pressure off of deeper layers and structures. This, in turn, can lead to increased blood flow, increased lymphatic drainage, decreased edema and pain, and increased kinesthetic awareness (Kase, Wallis, & Kase, 2003).

Kinesio taping techniques can be applied with a wide variety of clients, including those with low- or high-muscle tone. Taping can be used to address many issues including, but not limited to, muscle imbalance, postural insufficiency, circulatory and lymphatic conditions, and pathological movement patterns, making it a unique contributor for seating and positioning (Clark & Pope, 2014).

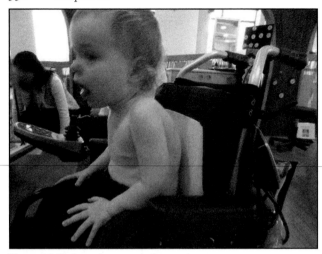

Figure 21-18. Seated posture before taping.

Low-Tone Presentation

This client presents with low trunk tone and has a tendency to flex forward in the chair. Taping can address the low tone and promote spinal extension (Figures 21-18 and 21-19).

High-Tone Presentation

Clients with high tone that is not easily controlled through the seating system can benefit from taping in specific locations to decrease further curvature (Figures 21-20 and 21-21).

CASE EXAMPLE

This case study is adapted from (Clark & Pope, 2014). T presents with significant spastic tone as well as spinal and pelvic curvatures.

Equipment: Zippie TS manual wheelchair by Sunrise Medical with custom-molded seat and back, open back angle.

Presenting problems: Decreased seating tolerance, changes in tone decrease consistent contact with molded seating, constipation, risk for skin breakdown, shallow respiration, and decreased tolerance of upright positioning for access of SGD and age-appropriate activities.

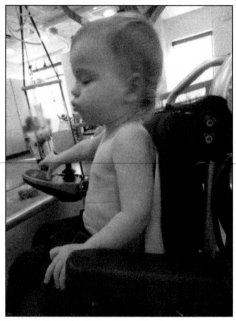

Figure 21-19. Seated posture after taping.

Assessment: Severe scoliosis, right side torticollis, pelvic rotation, pelvic obliquity, decreased rib cage mobility, flexed and adducted lower extremities, and lower extremities windswept to right.

Goals of taping: Increased comfort, increased tolerance of upright positioning in wheelchair, maintain fit in custom-molded seating, maintain posture to prevent further contractures, and increased attention to task for access and participation in age appropriate activities.

The taping provided better postural control of the trunk and rib cage and the client's ability to tolerate being in the molded system (Figures 21-22 through 21-24). The taping reduced the muscle tension, allowing for increased surface contact with the seating system. Additional benefits of the taping included increased rib cage mobility, increased deep breathing, decreased respiration rate, increased regularity of bowel movements, increased comfort, decreased complaint in seating, increased endurance and length of tolerance in seating, maintained fit in custom mold, and increased tolerance of upright positioning for access and peer interaction. The downside to this, according to Clark and Pope (2014) in their experience and also reported by the caregivers, was the need to repeat the placement of the tape every 4 to 5 days. The many benefits, the most important to the caregivers being comfort, provided the incentive to add taping to weekly care.

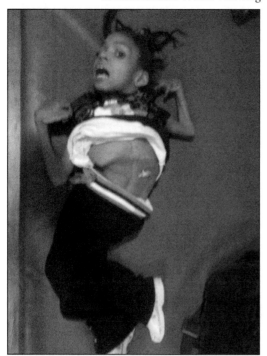

Figure 21-20. Supine posture before taping. *To see this image in color, please visit the companion website at www. healio.com/books/mobility.*

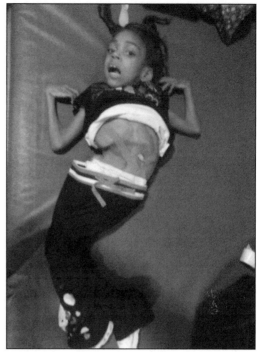

Figure 21-21. Supine posture after taping. *To see this image in color, please visit the companion website at www. healio.com/books/mobility.*

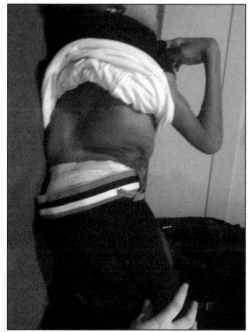

Figure 21-22. Client's posture before taping. *To see this image in color, please visit the companion website at www.healio.com/books/mobility.*

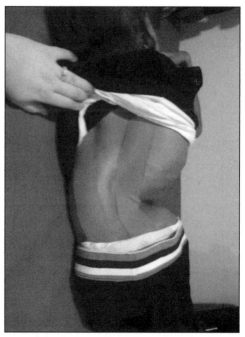

Figure 21-23. Taping locations along the spine to reduce curvature. *To see this image in color, please visit the companion website at www.healio.com/books/ mobility.*

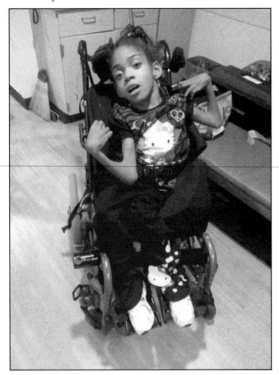

Figure 21-24. Client in her seating post-taping.

TABLE 21-6
FUNCTIONAL CONSIDERATIONS
If a child cannot sit up due to abnormal tone:
• A child cannot visually observe his or her environment.
• A child cannot explore his or her environment.
• A child cannot interact with others.
• A child cannot have opportunities to learn.
• A child cannot be a child.

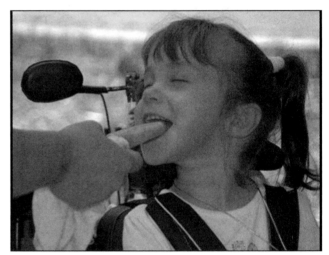

Figure 21-25. Positioning and eating.

FUNCTIONAL POSITIONING: INTEGRATING TECHNOLOGY WITH POSITIONING

Functional positioning is positioning that promotes active movement, participation, and an opportunity to positively affect cognitive function. Piaget viewed action and active engagement as instrumental processes in the cognitive and intellectual development of children (Ginsberg & Opper, 1987). Children with neurologic and developmental disabilities are often unable to explore or manipulate their natural environments independently. This may promote learned helplessness, and the child becomes a passive observer. Seating and positioning equipment should not only provide support for the musculoskeletal system but also promote function and participation across the life span (Table 21-6 and Figure 21-25). A client may be well supported to prevent spinal curvature, but is he or she able to use an SGD or a computer for his or her education? Equipment supports participation by allowing a client to be upright and visually explore the environment. Mobility creates opportunities to make connections with peers and physically explore the environment. All of these experiences will help a child achieve developmental milestones. Postural support is the first step to participation.

Clients with complex positioning needs frequently require other assistive technology. The seating system should optimize the access method used to control this assistive technology (Figures 21-26 and 21-27). Technology such as speech generating devices, computer access and electronic aids to daily living need to be considered when recommending a seating and positioning system. Access can be defined as "how an individual is able to manage an activity of interest with intention, independently" (Kangas, 2002). Postural supports are the precursor to developing functional access. If a client is not supported properly, he or she will struggle to interact with his or her environment. Technology considerations that influence seating and positioning recommendations include SGDs, computers, single-output switches, and mounting equipment.

TRANSFERS

Seating systems can affect how a caregiver transfers the client. The complexity of the individual and the customization of the seating system can increase transfer difficulty. When possible, active assistance from the client should be encouraged and maintained for all transfers. This helps maintain ROM and strength as well as ease caregiver effort. We recommend that a good time to educate families on

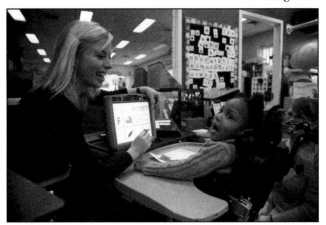

Figure 21-26. Access for communication.

transfer options is when the client is between 8 and 10 years old, because this is the start of a growth spurt and entry into adolescence. Families may also explore home modifications during this time. Other important considerations for transfers include how aggressive the seating system is, such as a molded seating system. The intimate fit may make transfers more difficult. A contoured seating system with removable parts, such as lateral trunk supports, may provide fewer restrictions. The team needs to assist the family in understanding the impact of a new seating system on transfers. If the caregivers cannot perform a transfer from a specific type of seating system, the team may need to consider other options. External lift systems may also be required.

LONG-TERM CONSIDERATIONS

Medical interventions have provided a high quality of life and increased life span for many individuals with complex physical needs. This means clinicians need to develop long-term goals for seating and positioning. Establishing a plan of care for equipment will help to determine the need for ongoing intervention. A seating system should be evaluated at least yearly, depending on the complexity of the individual's needs and key transitional periods across the life span.

SUMMARY

Proper positioning early on and throughout the life span can lead to increased function and participation, as well as the following:

- Movement and exploration
- Strengthening
- Proprioceptive input

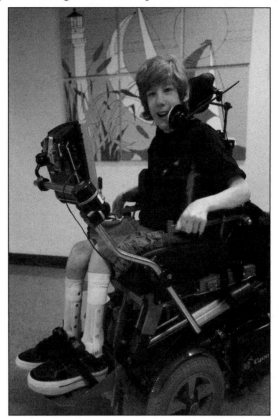

Figure 21-27. Access for communication and mobility.

- Sensory integration
- Visual development
- Learning and development

Providing proper body alignment and both static and dynamic opportunities at all ages can enhance overall development and quality of life for clients with complex needs, facilitating greater activity, participation, and independence. Seating and positioning for functional outcomes enables our clients to be in an age appropriate position, up with their peers, further enhancing cognitive and social development. It is essential that persons with CP and related conditions are able to access such devices as part of their care, treatment, and habilitation across the life span.

REFERENCES

Albright, A. L., & Ferson, S. S. (2006). Intrathecal baclofen therapy in children. *Neurosurgical Focus, 21*(2), 1-6. Retrieved from http://thejns.org/action/showCoverGallery?journalCode=foc

Ball, M. (2014, May). *Ins and outs of seating* [PowerPoint slides]. Symposium conducted by Freedom Designs Inc. and Pindot Custom Seating at the Perlman Center, Cincinnati Children's Hospital and Medical Center.

Bar-On, L., Molenaers, G., Aertbeliën, E., Van Campenhout, A., Feys, H., Nuttin, B., & Desloovere, K. (2015). Spasticity and its contribution to hypertonia in CP. *BioMed Research International*. Retrieved from https://www.hindawi.com/journals/bmri/2015/317047/

Bower, E. (2009). Understanding movement, both typical and in the child with CP. In E. Bower (Ed.), *Finnie's handling of the young child with CP at home* (4th ed., pp. 101-118). London, United Kingdom: Butterworth Heinemann Elsevier.

Campbell, R. M., Jr. (2013). VEPTR: Past experience and the future of VEPTR principles. *European Spine Journal, 22*(Suppl. 2), 106-117. doi:10.1007/s00586-013-2671-2

Chung, C. Y., Chen, C. L., & Wong, A. M. (2011). Pharmacotherapy of spasticity in children with CP. *Journal of the Formosan Medical Association, 110*, 215-222. doi:10.1016/S0929-6646(11)60033-8

Clark, K., & Pope, E. (2014). Use of Kinesio Taping as an adjunct to positioning. *Directions, 5*, 40-43. Retrieved from http://www.nrrts.org/directions/2014%20vol%205/DIRECTIONS_2014.5-Clinical%20Corner.pdf

Clark, K., & Pope, E. (2015) *"Seeing" positioning from a different angle: Functional vision considerations in seating and positioning.* National Registry of Rehabilitation Technology Suppliers webinar. Retrieved from http://www.nrrts.org/teleseminars-1/Webinars/on-demand-webinars-1

Darrah, J., Law, M., Pollock, N., Wilson, B., Russell, D. J., Walter, S. D.,...& Galuppi, B. (2011). Context therapy: A new intervention approach for children with CP. *Developmental Medicine & Child Neurology, 53*, 615-620. doi: 10.1111/j.1469-8749.2011.03959.x

Dicianno, B. E., Arva, J., Lieberman, J. M., Schmeler, M. R., Souza, A., Phillips, K., ...& Betz, K. L. (2009). RESNA position on the application of tilt, recline, and elevating legrests for wheelchairs. *Assistive Technology, 21*, 13-22.

Evatt, M. L., Freeman, A., & Factor, S. (2011). Adult-onset dystonia. *Handbook of Clinical Neurology, 100*, 481-511. doi: 10.1016/B978-0-444-52014-2.00037-9

Ferguson-Pell, M. W. (1998). Technical considerations. Seat cushion selection. *JRRD Clinical Supplement No. 2: Choosing a Wheelchair System.* Retrieved from http://www.rehab.research.va.gov/mono/wheelchair/ferguson-pell.pdf

Ginsberg, H., & Opper, S. (1987). *Piaget's theory of intellectual development* (3rd ed.). London, United Kingdom: Pearson Education Inc.

Goodman, C., & Glanzman, A. (2003). CP. In C. Goodman, K. Fuller, & W. Boissonnault (Eds.), *Pathophysiology for the physical therapist* (2nd ed., pp. 1098-1105). Philadelphia, PA: Elsevier

Grunt, S., Fieggen, A. G., Vermeulen, R. J., Becher, J. G., & Langerak, N. G. (2014). Selection criteria for selective dorsal rhizotomy in children with spastic CP: A systematic review of the literature. *Developmental Medicine & Child Neurology, 56*, 302-312. doi: 10.1111/dmcn.12277

Hanson, D., Thompson, P., Langemo, D., Hunter, S., & Anderson, J. (2012). Pressure mapping. A new path to pressure ulcer prevention. *Wound Care Advisor, 1*, 16-19. Retrieved from http://woundcareadvisor.com/

Kangas, K. M. (2002). Seating for task performance: Creating seating systems that allow weight bearing, pelvic stability and mobility. *Rehab Management, 15*(5), 54-56, 74.

Karp, G. (1998). *Choosing a wheelchair: A guide for optimal independence.* Cambridge, MA: O'Reilly.

Kase, K., Wallis, J., & Kase, T. (2003). *Clinical therapeutic applications of the Kinesio taping method.* Tokyo, Japan: Ken Ikai Co. Ltd.

Kolb, B., & Wishaw, I. (2008). *Fundamentals of human neuropsychology.* New York, NY: Worth.

McCarthy J. (2011, August). *The orthopedic evaluation and treatment of children with CP* [PowerPoint slides]. Presentation at the Fourth Annual CP Conference, Cincinnati Children's Hospital and Medical Center.

Model Systems Knowledge Translation Center. (n.d.). *Skin care & pressure sores: Areas at high risk of developing pressure sores.* Retrieved from http://www.msktc.org/sci/factsheets/skincare/Areas-of-the-Body-at-High-Risk-for-Pressure-Sores

Morgan, C., Novak, I., & Badawi, B. (2013). Enriched environments and motor outcomes in CP: Systematic review and meta-analysis. *Pediatrics, 132*(3), e735-e746.

Ramey, C., Campbell, F., & Blair, C. (1998). Enhancing the life-course for high-risk children: Results from the Abecedarian Project. In J. Crane (Ed.). *Social programs that really work* (pp. 163-183). New York, NY: Sage.

Rigby, P. J., Ryan, S. E., & Campbell, K. A. (2009). Effect of adaptive seating devices on the activity performance of children with CP. *Archives of Physical Medicine and Rehabilitation, 90*, 1389-1395. doi:10.1016/j.apmr.2009.02.013

Roman-Lantzy, C. (2010). *Cortical visual impairment: An approach to assessment and intervention.* New York, NY: AFB Press.

Rosenbaum, P. L., Walter, S. D., Hanna, S. E., Palisano, R. J., Russell, D. J., Raina, P.,...& Galuppi, B. E. (2002). Prognosis for gross motor function in CP: Creation of motor development curves. *JAMA, 288*, 1357-1363. doi:10.1001/jama.288.11.1357

Schmeler, M. R., & Buning, M. E. (1999,). *Strategies for documenting the need for assistive technology.* Retrieved from www.wheelchairnet.org/wcn_wcu/SlideLectures/MS/8Documentation.pdf

Skogseid, I. M. (2014). Dystonia—New advances in classification, genetics, pathophysiology and treatment. *Acta Neurologica Scandinavica, 129*(Suppl. 198), 13-19. doi: 10.1111/ane.12231

Wollack, J., & Nicher, C. (2003). Static encephalopathies. In C. Rudolph, A. Rudolph, M. Hostetter, G. Lister, & N. Siegel (Eds.), *Rudolph's pediatrics* (21st ed., pp. 2197-2202). New York, NY: McGraw Hill Medical.

VI

Additional Considerations

22

Considerations When Working With a Person Who Is Aging With a Disability

Susan Johnson Taylor, OTR/L, RESNA Fellow

HISTORY OF REHABILITATION AND DISABILITY

Seating professionals who work in the field of complex rehabilitation must be aware of the early effects aging can have on people with physical disabilities. It is also important to understand that the client has attitudes that were partially shaped by how and when he or she went through rehabilitation.

Life expectancy increased about 60% between 1900 and 2000—from about 47 to 77 years of age. As recently as 1945, the life expectancy of an able-bodied person was 55 years, whereas life expectancy was only 2 years for someone who had sustained a spinal cord injury (SCI). Nowadays, the life expectancy of most individuals with acquired disabilities is 85% of those without physical disability. It is estimated that about 12 million people in the United States are disabled (Kemp & Mosqueda, 2004).

Until about 1945 (World War II), no organized rehabilitation existed. During the 1940s, rehabilitation was born as a profession to reintegrate those who sustained injuries in the war back into society. During that era, the prevalent attitude was that one could overcome anything if he or she tried hard enough. Society was not set up for those with disabilities, so people were encouraged to fit in and be productive in society (Kemp & Mosqueda, 2004).

The 1960s and early 1970s saw the rise of the disability rights movement, which paralleled other rights movements of the same era. It became imperative that access to society literally become accessible. The passage of the Americans With Disabilities Act in 1991 was a first step in this process. At the same time, more people were surviving serious accidents and incidents. As time moved into the 1970s and early 1980s, large numbers of people with disabilities were living into middle and older ages, and it became clear that signs of early aging were evident and could not be ignored. Keep in mind that this was not anticipated, and many clients were, and continue to be, caught off guard by the changes that they experienced. These clients were taught that hard work would overcome all and that one must rely on oneself. Their lives had revolved around exerting huge efforts on a daily basis, as if one had to run a marathon every day. The attitude was "Use or Lose It."

This attitude did not show appreciable change until the 1980s, when clients and professionals alike realized that there were consequences to this philosophy. Studies of the physical, psychological, and sociological aspects of aging revealed some troubling trends. From the late 1990s through the present, enough information is available to incorporate into everyday clinical practice.

Lange, M .L., & Minkel, J. L.
Seating and Wheeled Mobility: A Clinical Resource Guide
(pp. 365-372). © 2018 SLACK Incorporated.

THE AGING PROCESS

Recent theory in the field of aging delineates several types of aging.

Successful

These are people who have what we would call "good genes." Little change in function is noted until the age of early- to mid-70s, with no chronic disease to limit function.

Usual

This type is defined as positive or neutral genes that unfold in a neutral or slightly negative environment. Although there may be some disease, this does not impair the individual's ability to function.

Pathologic

These people are at serious risk of major functional limitations with severely limited independence, although it is not well understood how each person's genetics and the presence of a disability intersect (Rowe & Kahn, 1998).

These concepts apply to all individuals, with and without physical disabilities. Obviously, the addition of a disability has a large effect on the person's aging process. Also, where it was once thought that after rehabilitation the client would go out into the work with few changes, it is now known that functioning over time is quite a dynamic process.

SPECIFIC AGING PROBLEMS

Going back to the beginning, it is imperative that wheelchair seating and mobility professionals understand an individual client's diagnoses and conditions and the effects that aging can have on function. More and more studies are diagnosis-specific and can be generalized as well. Many of these studies are directly related to factors that can be screened during a seating evaluation, and other studies indicate when the clinician should refer the client for other services.

Clients often return to seating professionals for four areas of concern:

1. Pain

2. Fatigue

3. New weakness

4. New or recurring pressure ulcers

Often, these symptoms have reached a point where the client can no longer ignore them. It has been noted over and over by clients and seating professionals that pain, fatigue, and weakness can be insidious, changing function here and there over time until the client has cut his life down to the necessities.

Pain

Musculoskeletal changes are the most obvious external signs of aging and are particularly affected by aging with a disability. In SCI, this includes the presence and increase in upper extremity pain, decreased strength due to atrophy, and increased risk for fractures (Hitzig et al., 2011; Moore et al., 2015). The most frequently reported pain occurs at the shoulder and wrist. The longer someone has been injured, the more common this becomes, as increased physical demands and overuse of certain muscle groups intersect. Incidence of upper extremity pain in people with SCI is between 30% and 70% (Klingbeil, Baer, & Wilson, 2004; Pentland & Twomey, 1994; Sie, Waters, R. L., Adkins, R. H., & Gellman, 1992; Waters & Sie, 2001).

In 1992, Sie et al. looked at 239 people with SCI who were an average of 12 years postinjury. Fifty-five percent of those with tetraplegia had upper extremity pain and 65% had shoulder pain; 64% of those with paraplegia had upper extremity pain, mostly shoulder and carpal tunnel pain (Sie et al., 1992). The Pentland and Twomey study in 1994 demonstrated similar results. They found that 58% to 60% of males with paraplegia had shoulder pain that was related to time since injury, rather than age (Pentland & Twomey, 1994). It should be noted that the same types of overuse syndromes of the upper extremities have been identified in clients with spina bifida (Klingbeil et al., 2004).

As one can appreciate, the incidence of pain in those aging with cerebral palsy (CP) may be significant after years of functioning with joints that are malaligned or not well-formed, and in postures and using movements that lead to these orthopedic issues. Soft tissue limitations leading to joint distortion over time can also increase pain and discomfort. Andersson and Mattson (2001) found that 79% of individuals with varied types of CP had pain that was primarily in the hips, back, and shoulders. Voglte (2009) noted that 67% of clients with CP had one or more pain sites and identified back, hip, and lower extremities as the biggest pain sources. Haak, Lensik, Cooley Hidecker, Li, and Paneth (2009) stated that although there is not a huge amount of objective information on adults aging with CP, anecdotal reports do indicate that many clients feel the effects of aging in their 20s, with decreasing function, increased spasticity, and, if walking, decreased balance.

One has to keep in mind that an increase in pain and contractures, especially in the shoulder, can lead to a dramatic decrease in function. Even a small decrease in range of motion can affect activities of daily living (ADL), such as pulling a shirt over one's head or rolling the wheelchair.

Traumatic brain injury survivors also have a prevalence of arthritis, as studied by Colantonio, Ratcliff, Chase, and Vemich (2004). The authors speculated that the mechanism of injury, which included motor vehicle crashes, can lead to multiple injuries, as well as prevalence of heterotopic ossification, both of which can lead to arthritic changes. Thirty percent of 286 clients with moderate to severe traumatic brain injury interviewed identified arthritis as a major problem, as compared to 15% of the general U.S. population (Colantonio et al., 2004).

FATIGUE

As interfering as pain can be, fatigue is also a function-robber. Fatigue in the general population is reported at 15% to 20%. Fatigue that interferes with the performance of ADL is three times higher in the disabled vs the nondisabled population. There are several types of fatigue: central, peripheral, and mental.

- Central: Characterized by exhaustion and a lack of energy
- Peripheral: Characterized by muscle weakness
- Mental: An inability to focus or stay alert

The Rehabilitation Research and Training Center (RRTC) on Aging with a Disability identified that between 62% and 78% of people with CP, rheumatoid arthritis, postpolio syndrome, and SCI experienced central fatigue. Two thirds of those with CP and SCI and 25% of those with postpolio syndrome said that this central fatigue interfered with their duties (Thompson, 2004). Cook, Molton, and Jensen (2011) looked at 1836 people in Washington State using the Patient Reported Outcome Measurement Information System. They found that not only did individuals with a disability have a greater risk for fatigue, but this risk also increased with age.

Fatigue is insidious and can slowly lead to debility. Clients report giving up a little here and a little there, until their activities consist only of the basics necessary to function day to day. They report that they give up extras, like social activities, so they can stay on track.

FUNCTIONAL IMPAIRMENT SYNDROME

In 2001, Thompson and Yakura postulated a functional impairment syndrome to describe clients who appeared to have developed a constellation of pain, fatigue, and weakness. The RRTC studied more than 600 people with varied diagnoses who complained of these symptoms. They concluded that these symptoms occur as a syndrome and usually lead to major changes in function (Thompson & Yakura, 2001). In addition, they found that of 150 people with SCI who were at least 3 years postinjury, 11% of the people recognized that they were having changes in

strength only after they were no longer able to perform an ADL or functional skill (Thompson & Yakura, 2001).

SKIN INTEGRITY

Another area affected by aging is skin integrity. This area has been studied in those who have SCI, but not as much in those with other diagnoses. Clinically, clients often come into clinic surprised that they have developed impaired skin integrity after having no pressure problems for many years. As one ages with SCI, sweating and fat decrease, and the capillary walls grow thinner and are more prone to rupture. This can lead to decreased sitting tolerance and increased need for pressure relief (or development of the habit of shifting weight) and the need for protective equipment (Shea, 2013).

Chen, Devivo, and Jackson (2005) looked at 3361 people from the SCI database. The sample included about the same number of those with tetraplegia and paraplegia. This review showed that the incidence of pressure injuries was steady for about the first 10 years postinjury, with an increase in incidence noted at about 15 years postinjury. By 20 years postinjury, there was a 30% increase.

EVALUATION

Armed with information, the seating clinician can assist in educating and problem solving with clients. The clinician evaluates someone who has been living with a disability differently from a client with a recent injury or diagnosis. The process of evaluation is the same: interview, mat evaluation, observation, functional evaluation, and use of trial equipment to meet the client's goals. The clinician must listen, look, and feel. Listening is paramount. No one knows the client's function like the client does. The clinician should assist clients in anticipating and identifying changes due to aging with a disability based on common problems that have been identified by research and anecdotal experience of the clinician in working with others.

Interview

The General Interview

The general interview for the seating evaluation is covered in Chapter 1. A primary question for the client aging with a disability is, "Why are you here?" Is this a routine visit or is there a special problem? Is there an ongoing problem that has reached a critical stage? Many times, symptoms have gotten so bad that the client comes into clinic hoping to address these issues. Medical history, including diagnoses and onset of the primary diagnosis as well as secondary diagnoses, is collected. Surgical history, including skin and musculoskeletal procedures, as well as neurological interventions, such as baclofen pumps is reviewed. History of and current pressure injuries are discussed.

Equipment History

Obviously, the clinician and supplier need to determine the age of the equipment. Often, the equipment that the client is using is no longer available, so exact replacement is impossible. Also, it may be that the client's current funding is more restrictive than the funding used previously. It is important to discuss these issues with the client because he or she may need to allow time to get used to something very different. Observe the current equipment and how it is used. For example, does the client require back canes at a certain height to hook his or her arms around for balance? Observe the wear patterns of parts, because that can provide information about how the client sits and functions on his chair and seating. For example, deep wear marks in the armpads may indicate that the client is heavily reliant on his or her arms for balance. Lastly, overall measurements of equipment determine environmental access.

Lifestyle Factors

Just as with any other seating evaluation, strategies the client and caregiver use for ADL and instrumental ADL is discussed with an emphasis on where and how the chair and seating are used. This includes any of the client's environments, including home and work. If the client or caregiver have a van or car, it is necessary to trial any equipment with this vehicle.

Mat Evaluation

In addition to the way a mat evaluation is typically performed, it is necessary to elicit feedback on how hands-on support from the clinician affects the client's postures and ability to balance from the head and neck through the trunk and pelvis. One can learn a lot from just observing how someone sits and moves, with or without support. For example, people become so used to sitting and moving in a certain way that they may not realize the compensatory movements to which they have grown accustomed can affect pain and level of fatigue. The level of support needed can increase as the client ages, so increasing the support may not have been brought up to the client previously. While introducing hands-on support during the mat evaluation, the clinician must elicit feedback on how much support is too much and pay close attention to the amount of pressure required to achieve and maintain a posture. Nonverbal cues from the client, such as an awkward posture at the neck, can tell the clinician that the level of support applied may be too aggressive.

Functional Evaluation

The clinician should observe as many transfers as possible—independent, assisted, or dependent—to view what methods and what parts of the wheelchair are used.

In these areas, the clinician should probe for details on how skill performance has changed over time, such as change in abilities or in performing a task that was once routine.

Trial Equipment

Trial equipment is, of course, necessary in all evaluations. Even if replacement equipment is being recommended, styles and the features of the equipment change over the years. As indicated earlier, this must be included in the conversation. Any postural intervention must be tried with the client, specifically with the client performing functional skills, such as transferring, propelling the wheelchair, or accessing controls on a powered wheelchair. Often, clients do not realize how much effort they have been putting into balancing and functioning until adequate support is provided. In the study by Thompson and Yakura (2001), 78% of 54 clients with a functional decline required new equipment after assessment, whereas only 10% of these clients thought new equipment was needed.

On the basis of client feedback over the years, it can be a relief to the client to have someone who is aware of the issues around aging with a disability listen and understand that changes are difficult. The clinician should remember that change is difficult for anyone, particularly someone who totally relies on the functional environment of a wheelchair and seating. Many clients are also relieved to hear that these are common problems and that solutions are possible. One must encourage the client to trial equipment without judgment. How suggestions are made is as important as the suggestions themselves. The clinician is there to provide the information and opportunity. Assure the client that there are tools that can be used to help him or her to make the final decision and that the final decision is his or hers alone. The client is there for an evaluation; he or she might as well see what is new.

SIDE NOTES

In summary, there is a great deal of available information on aging with a disability. This information should be incorporated into the clinical practice of the seating and mobility clinician. The clinician and the client need to consider the fact that there may be equipment and support surface changes over time. With this type of evaluation, everyone is in it for the long haul. It is not that unusual for an evaluation and trials to happen over months and even years before the client decides it is time to make a change.

The client, however, cannot make that kind of decision without information.

It is important to know when seating and mobility options cannot solve an issue and when referral to a physician is indicated. Appropriate situations may include new onset of weakness, new skin injury, or a collapsing spinal curve.

Successful aging begins in childhood. Now that there is information about changes that occur over time, particularly from overuse, many therapists have begun to apply this in pediatrics. Specifically, to look at what is expected from children and taking an approach that includes multiple ways of accomplishing tasks like mobility. The goal is to lessen the effects of aging as the child grows into adulthood.

Barry Corbet, SCI survivor and editor of *New Mobility Magazine* (1991-2000) made a statement many years ago that can be applied beyond those with SCI. An edited version follows: "The SCI survivor must balance quality of life costs over the ability to stay independent. Bodies are abused far more by overuse than disuse. The use it or lose it maxim no longer washes … instead of doing what's possible, do what is feasible."

A delicate balance indeed. Fully educated consumers are the ones who can make the best decisions for themselves. As health care professionals, we must understand and integrate past into present.

CASE EXAMPLE

Aging with a disability affects each person differently, although, as discussed in this chapter, there are some commonalities.

The person described in this case study is now in his early 50s. He injured his spinal cord in 1980, playing rugby as a junior in high school. When initially injured, he did not have functional use of either upper extremity. He was in inpatient rehabilitation for 4 months at a time when most people at his level of injury stayed about 6 months, but he wanted to get back to school and graduate on time.

The first equipment he used as an inpatient was a power wheelchair with sip-and-puff driving controls. In about 6 months, he developed enough right arm movement to use a joystick. He used a power wheelchair solely for 18 months, but then added a manual wheelchair. He clearly remembers being told "no pain, no gain" and was determined to maximize his abilities. For 5 years, he used a manual wheelchair as his primary means of mobility, although he could only propel on flat, level surfaces, so he often had to have the assistance of a caregiver. At the time, the available manual wheelchairs had very heavy steel frames. His frame also had handrim projections, a Jay Active cushion, and no back support (just the sling upholstery). He was functioning at a weak C6 level on the right and C5 on the left.

He went to Loyola College in Chicago for 3 years; then was accepted into the University of Chicago graduate business school in his junior year. During this time, he lived at home. He did get a license to drive a modified van but quickly gave it up because he did not feel confident in his driving skills. He was accepted to Tufts University in Boston for a second master's degree in International Law Diplomacy. While at Tufts, he had a team of caregivers and the school made an accessible suite for him. In 1998, he received a fellowship in Geneva, Switzerland, for 4 to 5 months, then came back to live in Washington, DC, where he worked until 2005.

In the 1990s, he took up handcycling. He stated that it is his favorite activity and he receives a great deal of joy from it. With assistance over hills and other uneven terrain, he has completed one full marathon, two half marathons, and two 7-mile bridge races in the Florida Keys. The last event he was able to participate in was more than 5 years ago. By now, the reader must have a picture of a highly motivated and directed individual.

He has a tethered cord in the cervical area, which was diagnosed about 10 years ago. In the past, he experienced intermittent pain; however, his current pain ranges from 5 to 8 on a scale of 10 with neck movement, as well as shoulder movement, that moves toward extension. His sternocleidomastoid muscles are very sensitive bilaterally, and anything that pulls on them creates significant pain.

When I first met him in clinic in 1999, he was using a power wheelchair with a Jay 2 cushion and a scapular relief back that allowed him to hook his arm around the backpost for truncal stability as he used the opposite arm for function (Figure 22-1). He also used this hooking as his pressure relief method. This was not an effective weight shift, so education was provide about using powered seating for pressure relief. After several years, he received a power wheelchair with a powered tilt. After a few more years, he was developing neck pain. It was clear that he was overusing his neck muscles to accommodate for the fact that he had no trunk balance. However, he could not tolerate trunk supports because these seemed to increase his neuropathic pain and prevented him from moving side to side for function.

In the mid-2000s, the skin over his buttocks became sensitive. He was prescribed a ROHO Quadtro Select cushion and a new Permobil power wheelchair with powered tilt and recline. We hoped to use lateral trunk supports to stabilize him better and reduce the neuropathic pain, but this did not work.

Finally, he was unable to bear weight on his buttocks at all without redness and pressure injury development, so he was transitioned to an off-loading cushion, a Ride Designs Custom cushion. He tilts back fully and then reclines just a few degrees to complete the pressure relief (Figure 22-2). On the way back up, he reverses the tilt and recline in combination to maintain his position on the cushion. This has greatly reduced redness and pressure injury development.

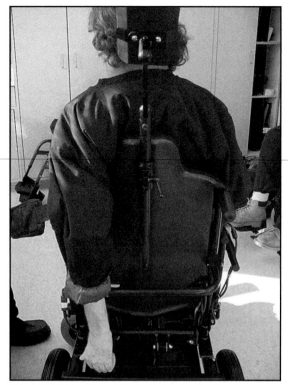

Figure 22-1. Hooking on the back support for function.

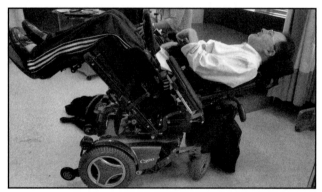

Figure 22-2. Complete pressure relief.

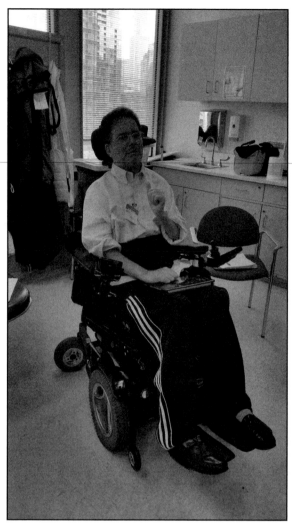

Figure 22-3. Front view of newest chair with Ride Designs back.

About a year later, he was provided with a Ride Designs custom back with an abdominal panel to provide lateral, posterior, and anterior support of his trunk (Figures 22-3 and 22-4). He decided that trunk stability was more important now than the mobility of his trunk. In addition, adjustable posterior elbow supports were recently added to limit the movement of his upper extremities and shoulders (Figure 22-5). The exact position required to provide upper extremity support and alleviate pain varies, and so this is adjusted as needed.

He has had a long equipment journey, requiring changes to meet his changing physical needs. All along the way, education was provided about how the equipment might help his physical needs. Suggestions were made, equipment was trialed, and he made the decisions that he felt would suit him best at the time. His neuropathic pain has worsened, and he will be seeing the neurosurgeon again, although he is reluctant to pursue surgery. From a seating clinician's viewpoint, only so much can be accomplished through equipment—sometimes medical interventions are also required.

SUMMARY

When we as seating professionals are seeing clients who are aging with a disability, we need to be prepared with knowledge of their condition and the anticipated progression and be prepared to trial equipment and ideas over a long period of time.

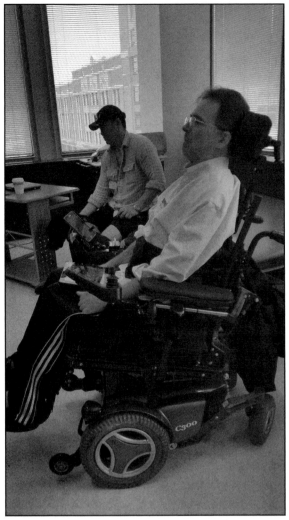

Figure 22-4. Full lateral view, joystick now on left side due to pain, phone accessed on the right.

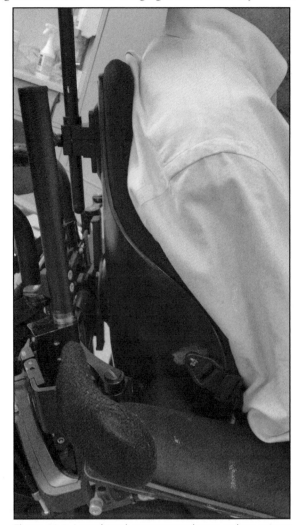

Figure 22-5. Lateral trunk supports are low to reduce contact near armpits due to pain.

REFERENCES

Andersson, C., & Mattson, E. (2001). Adults with cerebral palsy: A survey describing problems, needs and resources with special emphasis on locomotion. *Developmental Medicine and Child Neurology, 43,* 76-87.

Chen, Y., Devivo, M. J., & Jackson, A. B. (2005). Pressure ulcer prevention in people with spinal cord injury: Age-period-duration effects. *Archives of Physical Medicine and Rehabilitation, 86,* 1208-1213.

Colantino, Ratcliff, G., Chase, S., & Vemich, L. (2004). Aging with traumatic brain injury: Long term health implications. *International Journal of Rehabilitation Research, 27,* 209-214.

Cook, K. F., Molton, I. R. & Jensen, M. P. (2011). Fatigue and aging with a disability. *Archives of Physical Medicine and Rehabilitation, 92,* 1126-1137.

Haak, P., Lensik, M., Cooley Hidecker, M. J., Li, M., & Paneth, N. (2009). Cerebral palsy and aging. *Developmental Medicine and Child Neurology, 51*(Suppl. 4), 16-23.

Hitzig, S. L., Eng, J. J., Miller, W. C., Sakakibara, B. M., & the SCRIE Research Team. (2011). An evidence-based review of aging and the body systems following spinal cord injury. *Spinal Cord, 49*(6), 684-701.

Kemp, B. J., & Mosqueda, L. (Eds.). (2004). Introduction. *Aging with a disability: What the clinician needs to know* (pp. 1-8). Baltimore, MD: Johns Hopkins University Press.

Klingbeil, H., Baer, H. R., & Wilson, P. E. (2004). Aging with a disability. *Archives of Physical Medicine and Rehabilitation, 83*(Suppl. 3), 68-73.

Moore, C. D., Craven, B. C., Thabane, L., Laing, A. C., Frank-Wilson, A. W., Kontulainen, S. A.,...Giangregorio, L. M. (2015). Lower-extremity muscle atrophy and fat infiltration after chronic spinal cord injury. *Journal of Musculoskeletal and Neuronal Interactions, 15*(1), 32-41.

Pentland, W. E., & Twomey, L. T. (1994). Upper limb function in persons with long term paraplegia and implications for independence. Part II. *Paraplegia, 32,* 219-224.

Rowe, J. W., & Kahn, R. L. (1998). *Successful aging.* New York, NY: Pantheon.

Shea, M. (2013, March). Presentation notes, "Aging With a Disability." Presented at the International Seating Symposium, Vancouver, British Columbia, Canada.

Sie, I. H., Waters, R. L., Adkins, R. H., & Gellman, H. (1992). Upper extremity pain in the post rehabilitation spinal cord injury patient. *Archives of Physical Medicine and Rehabilitation, 73,* 44-48.

Thompson, L. (2004). Functional changes affecting people aging with disabilities. In: B. J. Kemp, & L. Mosqueda (Eds.), *Aging with a disability: what the clinician needs to know* (pp. 115-116). Baltimore, MD: Johns Hopkins University.

Thompson, L., & Yakura, J. (2001). Aging related functional changes in spinal cord injury. *Topics in Spinal Cord Injury Rehabilitation, 6,* 69-82.

Voglte, L. (2009). Pain in adults with cerebral palsy: Impacts and solutions. *Developmental Medicine and Child Neurology, 51*(Suppl. 4), 113-121.

Waters, R., & Sie, I. (2001). Upper extremity changes in spinal cord injury contrasted to common aging in the musculo-skeletal system. *Topics in Spinal Cord Injury, 6,* 61-68.

23

Environmental Assessment

Cindi Petito, OTR/L, ATP, CAPS

We experience all types of environments in which we engage throughout our life span. When individuals become dependent on wheelchairs, assessing and recommending the most appropriate wheelchair and seating system encompasses more than just the ability to sit in a sufficient functional posture; it also includes their ability to engage in their environments. Within these environments, clients will need to carry out their daily self-care routines, participate in social and cultural activities within their communities, and fulfill their life roles, which may include being a student, an employee, a parent, or caregiver for a parent or spouse.

Individuals interact in their social and physical environments and create meaningful representations of the self within the environment (Gamache et al., 2016). Depending on their individual needs and goals, people create a sense of meaning with their environments and life experiences and attach psychological, social, and cultural significance to these environments. Recommending the most appropriate wheelchair allows clients to continue building (or rebuilding) their relationships with their environments, engaging in life experiences, and carrying out their social and cultural activities and life roles.

This chapter reviews the most common environments that need to be considered and assessed when recommending a wheelchair and seating system. It also discusses how to measure both clients and their environments, assess the most common environmental barriers that challenge clients after they become wheelchair dependent, and use the standards of the Americans With Disabilities Act (ADA, 1990) as a guide to reduce or eliminate environmental barriers.

TYPES OF ENVIRONMENTS

Home Environment

The home is where most clients will use their wheelchair primarily for daily self-care routine activities, such as grooming, dressing, bathing, toileting, meal preparation, and household chores. Older dwellings typically have narrow doors and smaller hallways unless modifications have been completed to address wheeled mobility and accessibility. Newer homes will still have minimal wheelchair accessibility built into the new construction unless the homeowner made a conscious effort to include specifications that meet accessibility standards.

The aging-in-place movement in the United States is attempting to address the building standards and code changes needed for new home construction, which will address accessibility throughout the life span of individuals. Currently, this aging-in-place movement has increased home remodeling businesses throughout communities in the United States to address the aging population over 65 years of age. In addition, people with disabilities are living longer and the home accessibility industry has grown significantly to meet the demands of this population growth.

Within the home, the most common areas to assess are entrances and egresses, doorways, flooring, hallways, and bedroom, bathroom, and kitchen spaces. Other persons living or working in this environment must be a part of the assessment and included in the wheelchair and seating recommendations. Family members and caregivers may be assisting or operating the wheelchair for clients

Lange, M. L., & Minkel, J. L.
Seating and Wheeled Mobility: A Clinical Resource Guide
(pp. 373-384). © 2018 SLACK Incorporated.

with significant physical and cognitive impairments. For example, a caregiver may have to operate a manual tilt-in-space wheelchair inside the home to carry out daily care for an aging client with dementia who is dependent.

The most common types of home environments include a house, condominium, townhome, mobile home, or apartment. Other types of home environments include a group home, independent retirement community, assisted living facility, or skilled nursing facility.

Work and School Environments

For clients who attend school or work, it is important to assess the type of school, work, or career task demands, workspace, building accessibility, and school or work hours.

School and work hours and type of transportation are important for clinicians to assess for safety. For example, a client may work nightshifts and needs reflectors or lights on his wheelchair if he has to travel to a dark parking lot or bus stop. In addition, accessibility in commercial buildings and public facilities may not meet ADA standards. Clinicians may find the ramp access and entrances for commercial or public buildings to be limited. An example would be where a client has to travel a long distance between the ramp and the entrance of the building. In this situation, if the client uses a manual wheelchair, the distance of travel to enter into the building may be problematic if the client does not have the strength and endurance to self-propel the distances demanded. If the client works outdoors, the type of terrain being negotiating throughout his or her workday will need to be assessed, especially for clients who are farmers or work in rural environments.

Clients who attend school or college may have long distances to travel on campus. It is important to ask about the type of terrain students have to negotiate from the parking lot or bus stop to the campus. Do not assume all schools have flat concrete walkways. Some schools in rural environments have packed gravel or rock walkways.

When assessing a client's workspace, clinicians will need to know if he or she sits at a desk. If so, the clinician will have to assess how much knee clearance is needed under the desk and what are the upper body reach ranges in order to access his or workspace.

Community and Social Environments

Clients will need their wheelchairs to carry out community-based activities. These activities may include going to the bank or grocery store. Clinicians will need to consider situations such as reach ranges and heights while grocery shopping and banking. For example, a client who lives alone and does not have caregiver support may need a wheelchair that allows her to access narrow grocery store aisles. Reach ranges and heights of shelving in the grocery store may also be problematic. It is important to consider how clients will manage reaching grocery items on higher shelves and how they will carry grocery bags into the home.

Attending church, social events, and participating in meaningful leisure activities are also an important part of the environmental assessment. Clinicians need to assess client and caregiver goals and recommend a wheelchair that will not only be conducive for use in the home environment, but also to help the client participate in activities that support his or her cultural and social needs.

ENVIRONMENTAL FACTORS

When assessing a client's environments, the most common factors to consider in each environment are as follows:

- Accessible entryways and egresses
- Width of actual user space ("clear width") of doorways
- Clear width of hallways and accessible routes
- Turning radius
- Transfer surface heights
- Surface heights, clearances, and foot space
- Reach ranges
- Type of flooring
- Outside terrain
- Distance of travel within each of the environments

The assessment should reflect current accessibility and barriers in each of the environments, as well as the client's task demands and activities in each of the environments. Lastly, the type of transportation used to access these environments need to be considered when recommending a wheelchair (discussed further in Chapter 24).

INDOOR ENVIRONMENTS

Doorways and Thresholds

Clients will need a minimum 32 inches of user space, or *clear width* to access doorways safely (U.S. Department of Justice Civil Rights Division, 2010) (Figure 23-1). Clear width is measured from the face of the door (hinged side) to the doorstop (inside doorframe) when the door is fully opened at 90 degrees (Marinelli & International Code Council, 2012) (Figure 23-2). For bariatric clients, doorway clear widths may need to be 34 to 36 inches depending on the type of wheelchair recommended. For pediatric clients where the overall width of a wheelchair is smaller, a 30- to 32-inch clear width may be sufficient.

The most common mistake when measuring the actual user space (clear width) of a doorway is not taking into

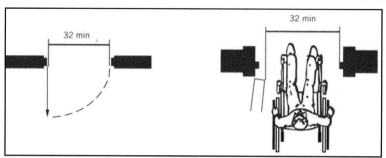

Figure 23-1. Door-clear width 32 inches.

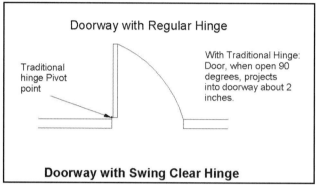

Figure 23-2. Swing-clear hinge diagram.

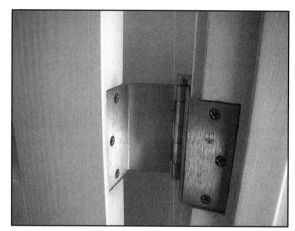

Figure 23-3. Swing-clear hinge.

account the hinged side of the door face, which can take up 1 to 2 inches of clear width.

When recommending a wheelchair, it is important to know the overall width of the manual or power wheelchair. With bariatric clients using power mobility, the seating system may be the widest part of the wheelchair. For those clients using manual wheelchairs, overall width is measured outside of the wheel rims from floor level to take into account wheel camber. Any camber in the wheels will make the overall width of the manual wheelchair wider.

Swing-clear (offset) door hinges may be added to increase the clear widths of doors without having to modify the doorframe (Figure 23-3). Replacing the door's standard hinges with swing-clear hinges can add up to 2 inches of clear width. The swing-clear hinges allow the inside door face to open flush with the doorframe at 90 degrees (Marinelli & International Code Council, 2012) (see Figure 23-2).

Accessible door thresholds are important for manual wheelchair clients. Any threshold or rise greater than 1/4-inch will be difficult for a manual wheelchair client to negotiate. A threshold between 1/4-inch and 1/2-inch should be sloped to help propel over the door threshold (U.S. Department of Justice Civil Rights Division, 2010). Clients who use power mobility will not have difficulty negotiating 1/4- to 1/2-inch door thresholds because the motor and suspension provides adequate power to overcome this obstacle. Power wheelchairs designed to climb low obstacles with adequate suspension can overcome door thresholds greater than 1/2-inch.

Sliding doors with door tracks, such as sliding glass patio doors, will be difficult for both manual and power wheelchair users because of the amount of rise and the track itself. When door thresholds are too high, threshold ramps can provide accessibility. Manufactured threshold ramps are made of rubber, aluminum, or plastic materials (Figures 23-4 and 23-5).

Flooring

When assessing clients for wheelchairs, the type of flooring being negotiated is important for both manual and power mobility users. Carpet creates challenges depending on the thickness of the carpet and padding. Thick carpet and plush padding creates the greatest amount of difficulty for manual wheelchair propulsion and power mobility. The thicker the carpet and padding, the greater amount of resistance is placed on the wheels. The energy required to maneuver on carpeting is increased exponentially with pile thickness for both manual wheelchair clients and power wheelchairs alike. Manual wheelchair users need more upper body strength to endurance to self-propel the wheelchair on carpet. Power wheelchair casters may stall and resist movement on thick-pile carpeting.

Low-pile carpet has a flatter finish than sculptured, frieze, cable, shag, or looped types. Originally used in commercial and retail buildings with heavy foot traffic, low-pile carpet is frequently chosen by builders and homeowners for

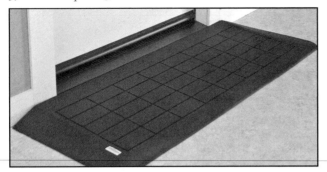

Figure 23-4. Rubber threshold ramp.

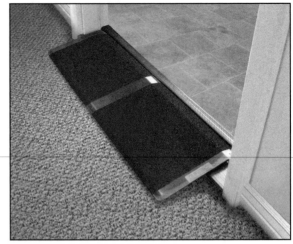

Figure 23-5. Aluminum threshold ramp.

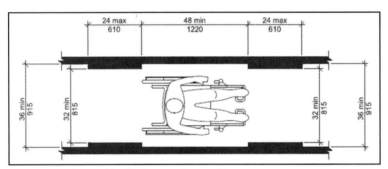

Figure 23-6. Clear width of hallways and accessible routes.

flooring in busy rooms and hallways of houses. Whether thick- or low-pile carpet, it is important to complete mobility trials. Laminate and vinyl flooring present the least challenge for both manual and power mobility users. Hardwood flooring can create maintenance problems for a homeowner because hardwood can be scratched or damaged. Throw rugs are common in homes and can create safety hazards for both manual and power mobility users and should be removed. Throw rugs can get caught and wrapped in the wheels and casters of both manual and power wheelchairs.

Hallways and Accessible Routes

According to the ADA Standards, accessible routes consist of one or more of the following: walking surfaces with a running slope not steeper than 1:20, doorways, ramps, curb ramps excluding the flared sides, elevators, and platform lifts (U.S. Department of Justice Civil Rights Division, 2010).

When assessing environments, hallways and accessible routes should consist of 36 inches of clear width per ADA standards; however, some homes may have 32 to 34 inches of clear width in hallways inside the home, which is sufficient for small to standard size wheelchairs (U.S. Department of Justice Civil Rights Division, 2010) (Figure 23-6). When assessing a home, narrow hallway widths and

small turning radius into bedrooms and bathrooms may limit accessibility. It is important to complete in-home or on-site wheelchair trials to ensure the wheelchair being recommended is conducive for use in the related areas of the home and their environments.

Turning Radius

Evaluating the environment for turning space is important and critical to the type of wheelchair frame or base being recommended. As power mobility devices vary in their turning radius abilities, it is important to know the space available and turning pathways the client will have to negotiate. For example, the turning radius of a rear-wheel drive power wheelchair will be larger than a mid-wheel drive power wheelchair because of the configuration of the drive wheel and casters. The difference between a mid-wheel and front-wheel drive power wheelchair may be a critical factor in a home with small hallways and tight 90-degree turning spaces. For example, a front-wheel drive power wheelchair may provide smaller turns around tight corners from the hallway into a bedroom where turning space is limited.

Manual wheelchairs also vary in their turning radius depending on the configuration of the wheels, frame, and front riggings. The turning radius of a rigid

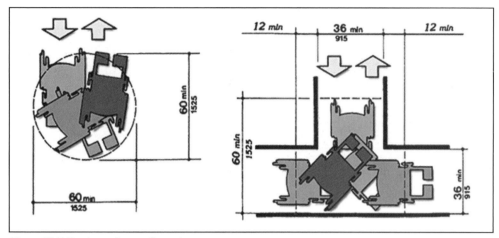

Figure 23-7. Turning radius configuration.

manual wheelchair for an individual who is 5 feet 2 inches (62 inches tall) with 80-degree front riggings will be smaller than the turning radius of a person who is 6 feet (72 inches tall) with the same degree of front-rigging configuration, because the length of the frame will be longer for the taller individual. Standard turning radius space required for wheelchairs is 5 feet x 5 feet (U.S. Department of Justice Civil Rights Division, 2010) (Figure 23-7). When recommending a wheelchair, the configuration of the manual wheelchair frame or power wheelchair base and seating system can create barriers in environments if not properly assessed.

Transfer Surfaces and Heights

Transfer surfaces and transfer heights from a wheelchair need to be assessed to ensure the client can carry out functional transfers throughout their daily routine. The most common transfer surface heights to assess include the bed, toilet, shower chair, and vehicle seat. Clients who complete multiple transfers throughout the day will need their wheelchair's seating system at the proper floor to seat height. For example, a common floor to seat height of a handicapped accessible toilet is 17.5 inches. However, the client's bed may be 20 inches high. In this situation, the optimal overall floor to seat height (including seat cushion) of the wheelchair may be 18 inches, because the bed mattress will compress approximately 2 inches during a transfer. Completing trials to assess transfers and floor to seat heights are critical for both clients and caregivers.

When assessing the environment, it is important to measure all of the client's transfer surfaces and heights to avoid creating barriers and limitations in his or her physical abilities. An inadequate seat height can create a barrier and also hinder the caregiver's ability to carry out daily routine care for the client. It is also important to assess transfer heights for safety and to avoid injury to the client and the caregiver. For example, if a client is transferred by a caregiver using a

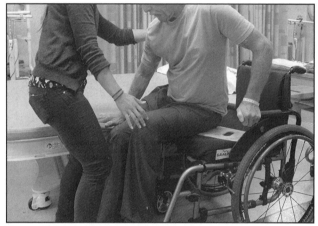

Figure 23-8. Side transfer using a sliding board.

sliding board from a power wheelchair to his or her bed and has a bed height of 21 inches, the seating system's overall seat height to the top of the seat cushion should also be 21 inches for safe side transfers with a sliding board (Figure 23-8).

Reach Ranges and Reach Heights

Assessing reach ranges from a wheelchair is important to ensure clients can access table and countertops, appliances, sinks, cabinets, wall switches, and work spaces. Figures 23-9 and 23-10 show the types of reach ranges that need to be assessed within clients' environments. Reach ranges depend on the client's physical abilities, such as trunk control, joint range of motion, and strength. If the reach range forward is limited, the client's foot placement may need to be more tucked in (knees in more flexion, closer to 90 degrees) while sitting in the wheelchair. The user space under the work surface may also need to be lengthened in depth to accommodate the overall length of the wheelchair and foot placement.

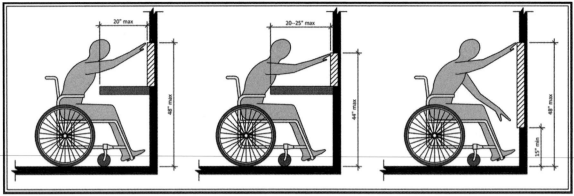

Figure 23-9. Forward reach ranges and heights.

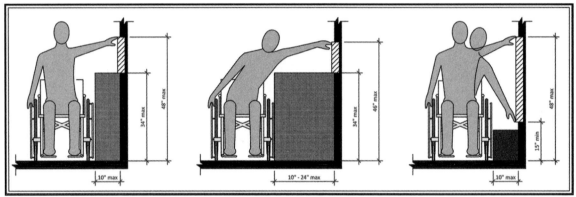

Figure 23-10. Side reach ranges and heights.

Surface Heights, Clearances, and Foot Space

Tabletop, countertop, and sink heights need to be considered and assessed in all the environments where the wheelchair will be used. The average knee clearance under tables and sinks is 27 to 30 inches for both manual and power mobility. Individuals who use hemiheight wheelchairs will need less clearance due to lower floor to seat heights. It is important to assess the overall knee height and thigh height clearances when recommending a wheelchair and seating system. For example, a client who is 6 feet 4 inches (76 inches tall) with a lower leg length of 21 inches and a thigh height of 4 inches may need 30 to 32 inches of clearance under a dining room table. In this situation, the height of the foot placement has to be included in this measurement and can be as much as 3 to 4 inches from the floor. When recommending seating systems, it is important to measure the client and the environment, which is addressed further later this chapter.

Foot space and toe clearance under tables, sinks, countertops, and around toilets is one area that is often missed during an environmental assessment (Figures 23-11 and 23-12). Inadequate foot space and toe clearance can hinder the client's transfer abilities. When wheelchair casters obstruct transfer space and foot clearance is limited, clients can be at risk for falls and injuries. A common barrier with toilet transfers that is often not addressed is when the casters of a manual or power wheelchair touch the toilet base causing a longer transfer distance. Another example of a transfer barrier is when the fixed front end of a rigid manual wheelchair is placed to far out in front of the frame, causing greater transfer distance for the client.

Wheelchair trials in clients' environments can ensure the proper mobility base and configuration is recommended to maximize independence.

Elevators

Clients will negotiate elevators in their own homes, retirement facilities, and the community. Elevators in private homes can be indoor or outdoor elevators.

Negotiating elevators may pose challenges for clients when operating a wheelchair. Clients who live in high-rise condominiums, apartment buildings, and retirement community buildings need to be able to negotiate elevators safely. However, not all elevators are large enough to accommodate both ambulatory individuals and wheelchair users. In addition, not all elevator controls are easily reached from a wheelchair level. Assessing clients' abilities to maneuver their wheelchairs on and off the elevator, operate the elevator controls, and negotiate around other people on the elevator is important to ensure safety.

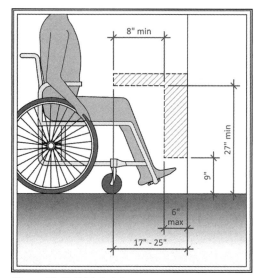

Figure 23-11. Table height.

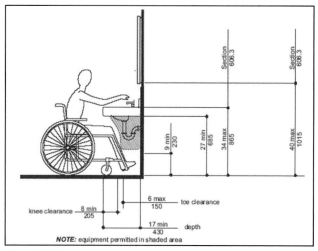

Figure 23-12. Sink height.

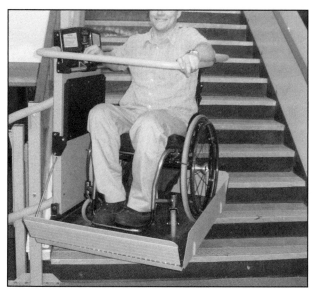

Figure 23-13. Wheelchair platform stair lift.

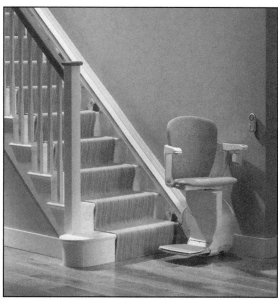

Figure 23-14. Standard stair lift.

Stair Lifts

Wheelchair platform stair lifts allow manual and power wheelchairs to maneuver safely up and down stairs inside multilevel homes and public facilities. A client should be assessed for safe maneuvering skills on and off the stair lift (Figure 23-13).

More often, clients will purchase a standard stair lift for their multilevel home that requires them to transfer to the lift seat (Figure 23-14). Usually, clients will purchase a second wheelchair, one to use on each level of the home. In this situation, the client's transfer skills from the wheelchair to the stair lift chair needs to be assessed with use of all of their mobility devices, whether a cane, walker, manual wheelchair, scooter, or power wheelchair.

OUTDOOR ENVIRONMENTS

Entryways and Egresses

An accessible entryway and safe egress should be identified in all the environments when a wheelchair is being recommended. An *egress* is a place or means of exiting or leaving. When assessing the home environment for those who use wheelchairs, it is important to ensure clients can safely enter and exit the home in case of emergencies. The clinician or the equipment provider can complete the in-home trial. It is standard practice for home accessibility specialists to recommend two means of egress in the event of a fire or other dangerous situation.

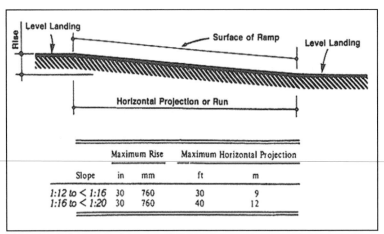

Figure 23-15. Ramp rise and run configuration.

Slope	Maximum Rise		Maximum Horizontal Projection	
	in	mm	ft	m
1:12 to < 1:16	30	760	30	9
1:16 to < 1:20	30	760	40	12

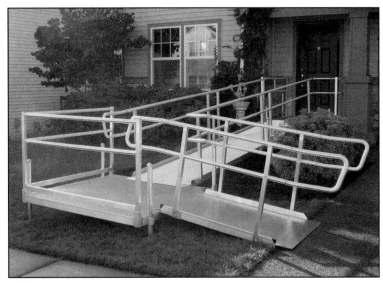

Figure 23-16. Aluminum modular ramp.

Ramps and Wheelchair Lifts

When wheelchair ramps already exist in the environment, mobility trials can identify possible barriers present and if the client is able to negotiate the ramp. Ramps should be a 1:12 slope for most wheelchairs per ADA guidelines (Figure 23-15). In some situations, a manual wheelchair user cannot propel up a 1:12 slope ramp due to upper body weakness. In this case, the ramp recommendations may need to include a 1:16 or 1:20 slope. If there is not enough landscape for a longer ramp, a wheelchair platform lift is considered, or other wheelchair configurations need to be assessed. The longest run of a slope should not be more than 30 feet.

Most ramps are designed from either wood or aluminum. They may be custom built from pressure-treated wood or prefabricated out of aluminum in modular sections of different lengths (Figure 23-16). For shorter ramp needs, aluminum ramps come in either folding or platform (nonfolding) styles (Figure 23-17).

Clinicians will find barriers that may exist with ramps with high transition rises greater than 1/4-inch from concrete to wood (Figure 23-18). In Figure 23-18, a manual wheelchair user would not be able to negotiate this rise. Ramp transitions from one surface to another should be level (Figure 23-19). Another barrier includes the use of aluminum folding ramps where the slope is too steep or the wheel space is too narrow. When ramps are too steep, the footplates of the wheelchair may hit and scrape the ramp when negotiating up the ramp. Negotiating down a steeply sloped ramp can cause unsafe forward pitching, making the client at risk for falling forward.

Folding and platform aluminum ramps can pose barriers when used as the primary means of accessibility into the environment. Folding aluminum ramps have limited clear widths (wheel space) of 28 to 29 inches. This can present safety issues with standard wheel bases of 25 to 27 inches wide because there is not enough wheel space for casters to turn or for the client to make corrections in steering. In this situation, if there is not enough clear width for the

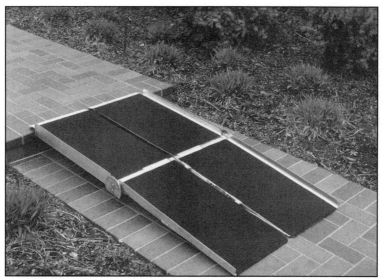

Figure 23-17. Aluminum folding ramp.

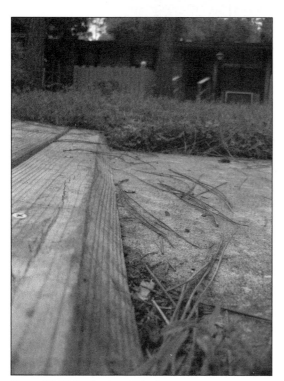

Figure 23-18. Barrier rise of 2 inches.

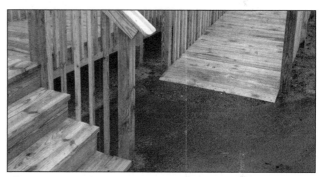

Figure 23-19. Level transition concrete to wood.

purchases a 2-foot folding ramp. In this situation, the ramp would be too steep and unsafe.

Wheelchair lifts, such as vertical platform lifts, give plenty of space for manual and power wheelchairs to maneuver safely (Figure 23-20). Vertical platform lifts typically allow for 5 x 5-feet or 3 x 4-feet clear widths.

Outdoor Terrain

When recommending a wheelchair, the client's outside terrain of all the environments need to be part of the clinician assessment. Clients who live in rural areas, such as a farm, will have challenges if the proper wheelchair is not recommended to accommodate both the terrain outdoors and flooring indoors.

With technology advancements, power wheelchair bases and wheel configurations can accommodate multiple types of terrain and can negotiate climbing up to 2 inches of rise and uneven ground. The advancements in suspension and wheel tracking of power wheelchairs allow clients to negotiate both rural and suburban communities.

wheels and casters to pivot, the client risks maneuvering the wheelchair off the ramp's edge and tipping over the wheelchair. A safer option would be a platform aluminum ramp offering 30 to 32 inches of clear width. Often, individuals buy folding aluminum ramps that are not 1:12 slope and are too steep because they have not consulted with a contractor or home accessibility specialist. For example, a home may have a 5-inch step up into the entryway; however, the client

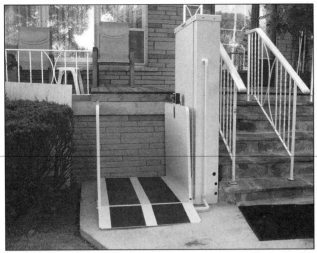

Figure 23-20. Platform lift.

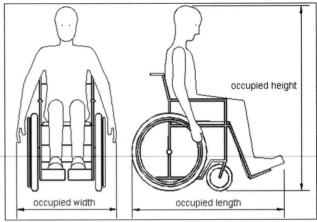

Figure 23-21. Measuring the occupied wheelchair.

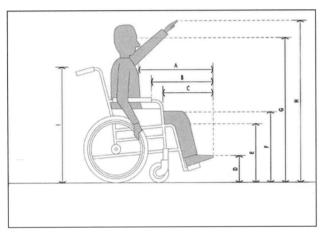

Figure 23-22. Measuring the client and the environment.

MEASURING THE CLIENT AND ENVIRONMENT DURING MOBILITY TRIALS

In Chapter 6, anthropometric measurements taken during the wheelchair assessment were discussed. When completing mobility trials in the client's environment, other measurements need to be taken while the client is sitting in the wheelchair. Measuring the occupied wheelchair will assist clinicians with determining accessible pathways, turning radius, and clearances needed (Figure 23-21).

Earlier in this chapter, surface heights, knee, foot and toe clearances, and reach ranges were discussed. This should be completed while the client is sitting in the wheelchair. Figure 23-22 is a diagram of measurements needed to ensure compatibility between the occupied wheelchair and clients' environments (Ainsworth & De Jonge, 2011). This diagram is especially handy when the wheelchair evaluation is performed in a clinic and the home assessment

cannot be completed. In these situations, the family and caregivers can provide information about the home environment, such as table, bed, and toilet heights, to properly configure the wheelchair.

In the diagram, measurements A, B, and C are important when the client is using a wall-mounted sink or will be sitting at a desk or surface against a wall (see Figure 23-22). An example of a possible barrier would be if a client is over 6 feet (72 inches tall) and has a long thigh length (seat depth). Taller individuals may have their footplates and feet placed far out in front of the wheelchair. When attempting to reach a sink or surface mounted against a wall, the reach range may be outside their normal arm length. In addition, the client's feet would hit the wall before he or she is close enough to access the space. An example of a recommended ADA sink for tall clients would be an extra-long bathroom sink where the reach range would be within his or her functional arm length (Figures 23-23 and 23-24).

Measurements D, E, and F are necessary to ensure clients' knees will clear under table surfaces, and to clear toe kicks under cabinets.

Reach ranges for upper cabinets and clothes closets can be determined by measurements G and H. Measurement G gives the clinician the client's level eye gaze range while sitting in a good upright posture. This is important for both daily activities and for operation of the wheelchair (see Figure 23-22).

MOBILITY TRIALS, FITTING, AND TRAINING

Completing mobility trials in the environments where the wheelchair will be used ensures the proper wheelchair has been recommended by (1) allowing assessment for client and caregiver safety, (2) maximizing independence, (3) allowing individuals to carry out daily activities in their home and communities, and (4) ensuring clients are able

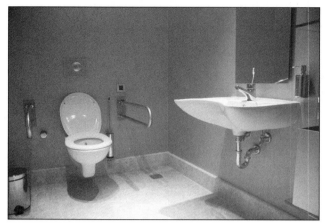

Figure 23-23. Standard wall-mounted sink.

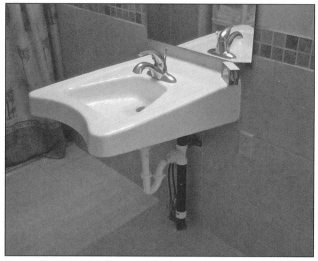

Figure 23-24. Long wall-mounted sink.

to engage in social and cultural activities and life roles (Figure 23-25).

During the assessment period, mobility trials are completed before making the final wheelchair recommendations. During or after delivery of the wheelchair, wheelchair fitting and training visits may be completed depending on the complexity of the wheelchair and seating system. After the wheelchair fitting, training and follow-up visits are made as needed to complete training in the following skill areas: (1) manual wheelchair propulsion, (2) power wheelchair drive control operation, (3) transfer training, (4) ADL and instrumental ADL retraining from the wheelchair, and (5) caregiver training.

During these visits within the client's environment, the equipment provider may be present to complete minor modifications as needed to the seating system, wheel configurations, and power drive control programing.

MAKING ACCESSIBILITY RECOMMENDATIONS AND FINDING A CONTRACTOR

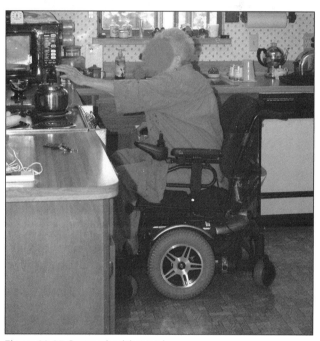

Figure 23-25. Power wheelchair trial.

Clinicians can make recommendations for home safety and environmental modifications to ensure compatibility with the client's functional capabilities, the wheelchair, and caregiver needs. Recommendations may include removing throw rugs, rearranging furniture and appliances, widening doorways, installing swing-clear hinges, and installing ramps. Environmental modifications that require structural changes and remodeling will require a licensed contractor or remodeler. Licensed handyman companies can often complete small construction jobs.

The National Association for Home Builders (NAHB; n.d.) has a website directory where an accessibility specialist

can be found. This site lists clinicians, contractors, and remodelers who are certified accessibility specialists.

Clinicians who are interested in becoming a home accessibility specialist can contact NAHB and their professional organizations. The Certified Aging-in-Place Specialist designation program teaches the technical, business management, and customer service skills including home modifications for aging-in-place and universal design. If a client is in need of home modifications, it is important to refer the client to a clinical specialist who works with specialized licensed contractors in the area of accessibility.

FUNDING

Environmental modifications and remodeling are currently not covered by Medicare or commercial insurances. Funding comes from private pay, foundations, grants, and some state-funded programs. Some organizations such as Habitat for Humanity, Rebuilding Together, Lowes, Home Depot, and local churches, offer donations and volunteers for those individuals in need of home modifications.

Currently, Medicare and Medicaid require the recommended wheelchair be conducive for use in the client's home and a home assessment report be documented by the durable medical equipment supplier; however, they do not cover environmental modifications.

AMERICANS WITH DISABILITIES ACT AND THE FAIR HOUSING ACT

In 1991, ADA Standards for Accessible Design was printed as Appendix A of the title III regulation in the Code of Federal Regulations for public and commercial construction. The Department of Justice's revised regulations for Titles II and III of the ADA of 1990 and were published in the Federal Register on September 15, 2010. These revised regulations, called the 2010 ADA Standards for Accessible Design, were implemented March 15, 2012.

The ADA does not apply to residential housing. However, certain ADA issues arise with the accessibility of common-use areas in residential developments if the facilities are open to persons other than owners, residents, and their guests (the public). Examples include sales and rental offices, sales areas in model homes, pools and clubs open to the general public, and reception rooms that can be rented to nonresidents.

Many builders, contractors, and remodelers believe that if they are using the ADA standards, then they are meeting the needs of all individuals with physical limitations. This is not necessarily true because clients will have their own individual physical challenges based on their abilities and limitations. Clinicians and remodelers should use the ADA standards as a guide only, and home modifications recommendations should be based on clients' individual needs specific to their home environment. For example, a client who is 5 feet (60 inches tall) and a client who is 7 feet (84 inches tall) may need grab bar placement different from the ADA standard of 33 to 36 inches from the floor next to the toilet.

The Fair Housing Act covers most housing. In some circumstances, the Act exempts owner-occupied buildings with no more than four units, single-family housing sold or rented without the use of a broker, and housing operated by organizations and private clubs that limit occupancy to members.

Under the Fair Housing Act, the accessibility provisions apply to the following types of housing:

- New buildings designed for first occupancy after March 13, 1991
- All housing, including privately financed housing
- Buildings with four or more units
- All units in elevator buildings; ground floor units in nonelevator buildings
- Single-story townhouses/patio homes
- Timeshares, dormitories, homeless shelters
- Existing buildings with additions of four or more units

SUMMARY

This chapter has described the most common environments clients will engage throughout their life span. During the wheelchair assessment, clinicians will need to consider both indoor and outdoor environments where clients will be using their wheelchairs to ensure there are no barriers in their mobility and performance in daily living skills. Measuring the client in the occupied wheelchair and measuring their environment will maximize mobility and independence. When an accessibility specialist is needed, clinicians should refer clients to a clinical specialist or contractor who has the knowledge and skills to complete an accessibility and home modifications assessment.

REFERENCES

Ainsworth, E., & De Jonge, D. (2011). *Measuring the person and the home environment. An occupational therapist's guide to home modification practice.* Thorofare, NJ: SLACK Incorporated.

Americans With Disabilities Act of 1990. Pub. L. No. 101-336, § 2, 104 Stat. 328.

Gamache, S., Vincent, C., Routhier, F., McFadyen, B. J., Beauregard, L., & Fiset, D. (2016). *Development of a measure of accessibility to urban infrastructures: A content validity study.* Walnut, CA: Medical Research Archives.

Marinelli, D., & International Code Council. (2012). *Code source accessibility: Codes, standards, and guidelines.* Clifton, NY: Delmar Cengage Learning.

National Association of Home Builders. (n.d.). Certified aging-in-place specialists (CAPS). Retrieved from www.nahb.org/en/learn/designations/certified-aging-in-place-specialist.aspx

U.S. Department of Justice Civil Rights Division. (2010). *2010 ADA standards for accessible design.* Retrieved from https://www.ada.gov/2010ADAstandards_index.htm

24

Wheelchairs and Transportation

Mary Ellen Buning, PhD, OTR/L, ATP/SMS, RESNA Fellow

Transportation becomes an important issue for all people who need to use a wheelchair when they travel beyond their residence. Those who require the postural support of a wheelchair often have limitations that prevent them from easily or safely transferring into the safety engineered seat of a family car; whether sedan, van, or pickup truck. Those who live in suburban areas may need to travel by way of wheelchair accessible minivan, paratransit, or adapted pickup truck. Even for those who live in an urban setting where they can meet most of their needs using city sidewalks, bus or taxi transportation is needed at times.

TYPICAL ROLE AND PERFORMANCE REQUIREMENTS OF A WHEELCHAIR

Wheelchairs are valued for their capacity to restore the ability to move easily within typical daily environments. However, this runs counter to the engineering requirements for a seat within a motor vehicle. Within the field of transportation engineering; the strength, stability, and crashworthiness of a vehicle seat is the foundation for occupant protection. Occupant protection ratings are a key selling feature in family-owned vehicles. Manufacturers of today's passenger vehicles take care to meet and exceed the National Highway Traffic Safety Administration (NHTSA) standards for performance when it comes to designing and testing the performance of seats within the vehicle frame. Within this compartment, lap shoulder belts, air bags, and side curtain airbags are added to ensure that the passenger

stays safely seated in that seat. The standard impact test pulse for confirming performance of these automotive components is a 30-mph/20-g load. Although it may not sound strict, this load represents the 95th percentile for severity in frontal impact crashes. Only 5% of accidents are more severe (Bertocci & Evans, 2000; Schneider, Hobson, & Bertocci, 2003).

WHY DO WE NEED WHEELCHAIRS READY FOR TRANSPORTATION?

The chapters in this text are intended to provide the rationale for all the ways that a wheelchair and its features can and should be selected and customized to meet the needs of each client. In the world of complex rehabilitation technology, it is hard to find any two wheelchairs that are configured alike. Add to this the complexity of clients who vary by age, body size, diagnosis, orthopedic/neurological frailty, human occupations, and personal interest in or need for community transportation. How do you begin to take all of this variation into account and come up with a best practice in securing an individual wheelchair and its occupant during transportation? It may come as a relief to learn that all of this variation can be dealt with by learning from the science of transportation engineering and applying wheelchair transportation safety (WTS) standards. The Rehabilitation Engineering and Assistive Technology Society of North America (RESNA) Assistive Technology Standards Board has recently completed

Lange, M. L., & Minkel, J. L.
Seating and Wheeled Mobility: A Clinical Resource Guide
(pp. 385-395). © 2018 SLACK Incorporated.

Volume 4: Wheelchairs and Transportation, which contains the following standards:

- WC18: Wheelchair tie-downs and occupant restraint systems for use in motor vehicles
- WC19: Wheelchairs used as seats in motor vehicles
- WC20: Wheelchair seating systems for use in motor vehicles
- Section 10: Rear-facing spaces in large, accessible transit vehicles. (RESNA, 2012)

WHEELCHAIR TRANSPORTATION SAFETY IS CREATED BY IMPLEMENTING A SYSTEM

It is beyond the skills and scope of a single professional group to create wheelchair transportation safety situations. For that reason, the standards in *Volume 4* (RESNA, 2012) affect the following:

- People with physical disabilities who remain seated in their wheelchairs when traveling in motor vehicles, as well as their families and caregivers
- Manufacturers of wheelchairs and seating, tie-down/restraints, and vehicle manufacturers
- Transit providers, including paratransit, public transit, school transportation, and families
- Wheelchair clinicians/rehab suppliers who prescribe wheelchairs and seating for clients
- Rehabilitation and auto safety engineers and researchers
- Federal, state, and local governments and policy makers who establish the expectation of equivalent safety for those who ride seated in their wheelchairs

As public policy and legislation have increased society's expectations for equivalent community access for education, employment, and participation, accessible transportation has become a necessity. Under the Public Accommodations title of the Americans with Disabilities Act (U.S. Department of Justice, 1998), transportation service providers must accommodate persons who wish to travel while seated in their wheelchairs. Today, individuals who use wheelchairs utilize transportation options that range from public fixed-route buses and door-to-door paratransit vehicles to independent driving or travel in an adapted, personally owned vehicle. Although great strides have been made, a critical need still exists for accessible transportation, especially in small and rural communities. The director of the Easter Seal's Project Action reported that one third of the 25 million transit-dependent people with disabilities have inadequate transportation and find it a significant barrier to community integration (Prohaska et al., 2012).

THE KEY ELEMENTS OF OCCUPANT PROTECTION

In the general U.S. population, motor vehicle accidents are the leading cause of death for Americans aged 3 through 33 years (Subramanian, 2005). Frontal impact crashes are the most common type of serious and fatal injury. Using pelvic-shoulder occupant restraint belts reduces by 45% the risk of fatal injury to front-seat occupants of passenger cars (for ages 5 and older). Using these safety belts reduces by 50% the risk of moderate to critical injury. Safety belts make an even more significant safety impact (NHTSA, 2003). Standards development started with frontal impact protection. Clinicians who are typically concerned about the use of the word *restraint* when used in regard to wheelchairs and seating should realize that it is a common descriptor for belts used to prevent occupant injury in motor vehicle accidents.

Limiting the risk of death or injury in motor vehicle accidents requires a systems approach that takes into account the characteristics of the vehicle, the vehicle seat and its securement to the vehicle, occupant restraints (i.e., pelvic and shoulder belt, air bags) and occupant characteristics (i.e., size, weight, posture, position). Federal Motor Vehicle Safety Standards (FMVSS) regulate the vehicle seat, its anchorage to the vehicle, and occupant restraints for typical (non-wheelchair seated) passengers (U.S. Department of Transportation, 1999). However, no federally mandated FMVSS regulations apply to wheelchairs when these are used as seats in vehicles.

In fact, the features that make a wheelchair a good mobility aid may make it a poor vehicle seat. A vehicle seat must provide a secure seating support surface for an occupant in case of a crash. This means that the vehicle seat must be securely anchored to the vehicle, and the seat structure must maintain its integrity. This stable support surface allows properly positioned occupant restraints, like lap and shoulder belts, to provide effective occupant protection. In cases when the seat support surface fails, injury may occur through a phenomenon known as *submarining*. Submarining occurs when seat failure allows the pelvis to drop downward and the lap belt to ride upward over the iliac crests causing injury to soft abdominal tissue (MacLaughlin, Sullivan, & O'Connor, 1988; Severy, Blaisdell, & Kerkoff, 1976).

Occupant restraints are critical to protecting an occupant as these prevent forward motion during emergency driving maneuvers and crashes. These also prevent occupant ejection from the vehicle and secondary collisions inside the vehicle. Occupant restraints are designed to

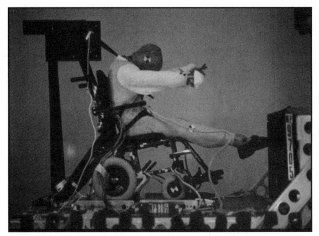

Figure 24-1. A clip taken from a video at the point of impact within a dynamic crash test on a sled simulating the effects of a 30-mph/20-g crash at a lab at University of Michigan Transportation Research Institute.

increase the amount of time over which a wheelchair rider comes to a stop, thereby reducing the deceleration experienced by the occupant. Proper belt fit and position—the belt should be over bony structures of the body—is key so that crash level forces are transmitted to structures capable of withstanding such forces.

As wheelchairs are primarily designed for ease of performance of mobility related activities of daily living, the safest means of transport for any wheelchair-using passenger or driver is sitting in an original equipment manufacturer's (OEM) occupant seat (Bertocci, Manary, & Ha, 2001). This motor vehicle seating is required to be designed and tested to meet rigorous FMVSS standards.

Wheelchair Securement

Use of OEM seating is not possible for those who are unable to transfer to a vehicle seat due to weakness, paralysis, or conditions that make them vulnerable to falls and injury during transfer. This applies to most individuals who use power wheelchairs, because this form of mobility device is used when upper extremity weakness or a significant physical impairment is present. This also applies to clients who may be able to transfer or be lifted by a caregiver but require more postural support than is provided by the OEM seat.

All standards related to the transportation of wheelchair-seated passengers are voluntary industry standards. These standards are developed with the leadership of engineers who take seriously their commitment to the transportation safety of those who use wheelchairs. Due to the frequency and severity of frontal impact, standards development started with frontal impact protection. The focus is now moving toward using these voluntary industry standards to properly secure mobility devices for transportation.

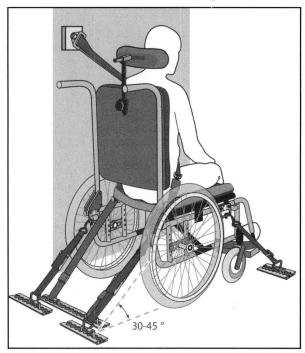

Figure 24-2. Four-point, strap-type wheelchair securement. Note the specification for the angles of the rear strap angles.

Four-Point Securement

Four-point, strap-type securement is the most commonly used form of wheelchair securement. It was first developed in the early 1990s to accommodate all types of wheelchairs and to be useable in all types of motor vehicles, from buses to minivans. The standards for wheelchair tie-down and occupant restraint systems (WTORS) use the same 30-mph/20-g test pulse that is used in FMVSS standards. The WTORS standards define the design, testing, performance, labeling, and instructions for use of products that comply with this standard. The WTORS standard requires that the securement straps successfully restrain a surrogate wheelchair (187 pounds) used by a 50th percentile male (168 pounds) crash test dummy in a 30-mph/20-g frontal impact (Figure 24-1).

The four-point, strap-type tie-down standard describes WC18-compliant webbing straps with end fittings that anchor to the vehicle on one end and to the forward facing wheelchair frame on the other (Figure 24-2). The advantage of four-point straps is the ability to safely secure most types of wheelchairs and stabilize a wheelchair and its passenger in normal driving as well as in a crash or emergency maneuvers. The disadvantage of this securement system is that these are time-consuming to attach, the wheelchair rider must rely on others for four-point attachment, it is difficult to know where to attach these on a wheelchair frame, people without technical training may decide where to attach these, and in public vehicles, the four straps may become dirty, missing, or damaged and likely to

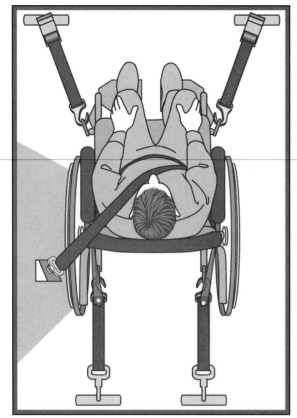

Figure 24-3. In this overhead view, notice that the front straps are angled outward to add lateral stability, and the rear straps are parallel to the direction of vehicle travel.

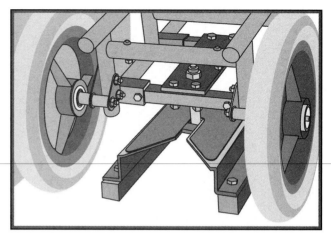

Figure 24-4. Wheelchair docking system with the pin interface that is added to a wheelchair's manual frame or power base for use in a personally owned vehicle.

malfunction. Note the presence of the vehicle anchored lap/shoulder safety occupant restraint, as it is often part of an integrated system.

Docking Systems in Personal Vehicles

Automated docking systems are another type of commercially available wheelchair securement system. These are primarily used in personally owned transportation vehicles, because both the wheelchair and the vehicle must be modified with custom hardware before use. Docking systems use a latching mechanism installed in the floor of the vehicle and a pin system that extends down from the base of the wheelchair (Figure 24-3). A powered release is also installed so that the wheelchair rider can release the locking mechanism when leaving the vehicle.

When someone drives the vehicle while seated in a wheelchair or wishes to ride in the front right passenger position, docking is the preferred method of wheelchair securement. It is essential to adapt the OEM lap/shoulder belt as an occupant safety restraint when using a docking system. The dock addresses wheelchair securement, but crash-tested occupant restraint belts are still needed.

The advantage of docking systems is that clients can dock easily and can manage the securement system

independently. The disadvantage of this system is that unique hardware must be attached to the underside of the wheelchair, which can make a manual wheelchair heavier and reduce ground clearance for both manual and powered wheelchairs. These systems are also more costly and require mechanical maintenance. Just like strap-type securement, the docking system must successfully restrain a surrogate wheelchair (187 pounds) used by a 50th percentile male (168 pounds) crash test dummy in a 30-mph/20-g frontal impact (Figure 24-4).

The Low G, Rear-Facing Passenger Station

To simplify the process of securing wheelchair passengers in large accessible transit vehicles, a new standard for wheelchair securement has been developed. These are the buses that traverse our cities and which must maintain time schedules to allow riders to make transfers to other routes.

This securement standard allows a wheelchair rider to board a bus and enter a rear-facing compartment that does not require strap-type securement. Instead, the wheelchair backs up to a narrow backrest for head and neck protection and a safety arm on the aisle side of the compartment is lowered to prevent the wheelchair from pivoting out of the compartment (Figure 24-5).

OCCUPANT RESTRAINT

Wheelchair securement is only half of WTORS challenge. The other half is occupant protection. In the world of transportation engineering today, the systems for protecting passengers commonly include safety belts or belt restraints, air bags, and crumple zones that surround the occupant. In the world of wheelchair-seated passengers,

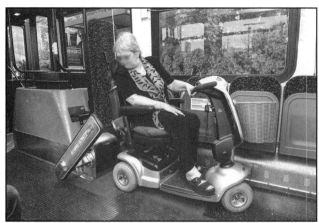

Figure 24-5. A rear-facing passenger station designed for use only in a large accessible transit vehicle or fixed-route bus. (Reprinted with permission from Q'Straint.)

occupant protection is typically limited to use of lap/shoulder belts.

Lap/Shoulder Belts for Three-Point Occupant Restraint

WC18 also describes in detail the design, performance, testing, and labeling of occupant protection products. Just like wheelchair-securement systems, compliant occupant restraint systems are crash-tested in dynamic conditions with a surrogate wheelchair and a 50th percentile male crash test dummy in a 30-mph/20-g crash test simulation. Occupant restraint systems are designed to attach to D-rings on the four wheelchair securement straps or directly to anchor points on the floor of the vehicle. The torso or shoulder belt portion is always attached to the vehicle sidewall above and slightly behind the occupant (Figures 24-6 and 24-7).

Five-Point Occupant Restraints for Children Under 25 Pounds

In a recent update of WC18, the standard was amended to include wheelchair-seated passengers who weigh under 25 pounds. Travelers in these smaller wheelchairs—often in the form of a stroller base—are best protected by five-point belt harness systems, which are able to distribute crash loads over more body segments and limit forward excursion. It is important to remember that anterior chest supports or harnesses are only compliant with this standard if they are so labeled. Labeling is an important aspect of compliance with transportation standards.

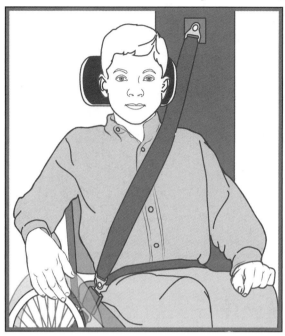

Figure 24-6. Shoulder belt placement should travel across the clavicle between the neck and acromion process and across the sternum.

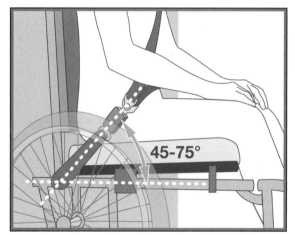

Figure 24-7. Note that the lap or pelvic belt placement should be low and snug in front of the bony prominence of the anterior pelvis, not over soft abdominal tissue.

This modification to the WC18 standard creates an alternative to the use of a child passenger safety seat that may be helpful in some transit situations. Of note, the American Academy of Pediatrics (2014) recommends the use of a car seat for a clients under 40 pounds. More specific information about child passenger safety seats is located at www.HealthyChildren.org

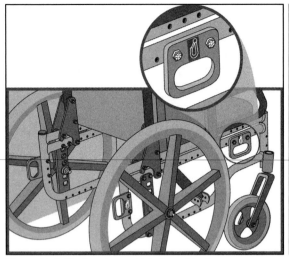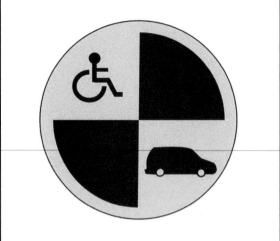

Figure 24-8. The location and labeling of the four securement points on a wheelchair frame or power base.

Wheelchair Tie-Down and Occupant Restraint Systems: One Without the Other Equals Absence of Safety

In an effort to create safety for wheelchair-seated passengers, many believe that securing the wheelchair to the floor of the vehicle is the most important component. Many also assume that the passenger is protected if a pelvic positioning belt or anterior trunk support is present. Unless a secondary postural support has been crash-tested in a 30-mph/20-g simulation and labeled as such, it should not be trusted for safety in transportation. Velcro and plastic buckles are unable to withstand a crash load. These important positioning or postural supports do have a role when used to support optimal posture and enable occupant restraints to be effectively placed over bony prominences.

CRASH-TESTED WHEELCHAIRS

Securing a wheelchair in a vehicle and routing a passenger's lap/shoulder belt so that it makes contact with his or her body at the bony prominences can be complicated in real-life practice. The individuals we work with are not typical and use customized manual, tilt-in-space, and power wheelchairs, along with postural supports and after-market components. These variations may require modification of the typical practices for applying WTORS. When engineers became aware of all the issues surrounding the wide variety of wheelchairs coming on the market in the 1990s, the need for a wheelchair designed with transportation came to mind. This started the work that became the RESNA WC19 standard.

The work of Canadian and U.S. engineers has always occurred under the auspices of the American National Standards Institute (ANSI). Like-minded engineers in Europe developed transportation standards through the International Standards Organization (ISO). In most cases, the standards developed by these two distinct organizations are harmonized and do not oppose each other.

FEATURES OF REHABILITATION ENGINEERING AND ASSISTIVE TECHNOLOGY SOCIETY OF NORTH AMERICA WC19-COMPLIANT MANUAL AND POWER WHEELCHAIRS

As a wheelchair frame supports the primary seating surface for individuals who travel in wheelchairs, it must provide stable support and the structural integrity sufficient to withstand crash forces. Additionally, wheelchairs must offer optimal securement of the frame to the vehicle floor and allow proper routing of lap/shoulder belts for effective belt fit for the occupant. For this reason, the WC19 standard focuses on wheelchair design requirements, instructions for use, test methods, and product labeling. A WC19 wheelchair is tested with a crash test dummy that matches the size of the wheelchair.

A key design feature is the correct location of the four labeled and easily accessible securement points that are geometrically compatible with the end fitting of strap-type securement systems (see Figure 24-6). This eliminates the possibility of error that arises when trying to identify where to attach tie-downs on the wheelchair frame. The ease of use should increase correct placement and use of all four securement straps (Figure 24-8).

Additionally, wheelchairs are rated for their ability to accommodate proper placement of vehicle anchored occupant restraints. These belts must make contact with the skeletal structures of the passenger's body. To accomplish this, both the lap and shoulder portion of the belts need to travel unimpeded by the armrest or back support.

A WC19 wheelchair must pass crash testing while a wheelchair-anchored pelvic belt is present. This is a much more strenuous strength and integrity test for the wheelchair frame and has led some manufacturers to opt out of complying with the WC19 standard. As a further requirement, the manufacturer must make it possible for the end user to purchase this tested pelvic belt. The addition of this belt to the WC19 standard makes it possible for any wheelchair seated passenger to have a basic level of occupant protection during transportation. This pelvic belt has a pin bushing that mates easily with the shoulder portion of the lap shoulder belt (see Figure 24-6). This greatly reduces the invasion of personal space often required to properly route a full lap/shoulder belt system.

Today, many commercially available wheelchairs comply with ANSI RESNA WC19. There is a regularly updated list of products that meet transit standards on the web at http://wc-transportation-safety.umtri.umich.edu. The list is managed at the University of Michigan Transportation Research Institute, where most of the product testing occurs.

The list informs clinicians and suppliers about wheelchairs and seating systems that comply with standards. It will indicate those wheelchairs that offer the wheelchair-anchored pelvic belt restraint, thus indicating that these have passed the more stringent test. WC19 has also been improved to require a passing grade for the chair's ability to accommodate vehicle-mounted occupant restraints. This proved to be an important update as previously products without a passing grade on this important feature were allowed to be labeled as WC19-compliant.

WHAT ABOUT THE DIFFERENCE BETWEEN AMERICAN NATIONAL STANDARDS INSTITUTE WC19 AND INTERNATIONAL STANDARDS ORGANIZATION 7176-19 STANDARD?

RESNA WC19 and ISO 7176-19 were developed with significant coordination between the RESNA working group and the ISO subcommittee. In fact, much of the leadership and authorship for the two standards came from the same individuals. Although every effort was made to harmonize the two standards, there are some differences.

The ISO 7176-19 allows frontal impact crash testing to use either a commercial tie down or the surrogate tie down. A surrogate tie down is one designed exclusively for the purpose of testing. It withstands repeated use and eliminates

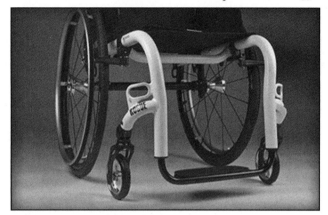

Figure 24-9. A cantilevered frame on a Ki Mobility Rogue provided with WC19 securement points.

the bias of a commercial product. The RESNA test requires the use of the surrogate tie down for comparable performance and requires that wheelchairs provide the occupant with the option of using a wheelchair-anchored pelvic belt restraint. A wheelchair-anchored pelvic belt restraint must be used instead of a vehicle-anchored pelvic belt in the frontal impact test. Clinicians and suppliers will most likely encounter wheelchairs and stroller-bases labeled with ISO 7176-19 on products that originate in Europe.

Differences Between Manual and Power Wheelchairs

The WC19 standard applies to both manual and power wheelchairs. Given the great difference in equipment weight, it is easier to successfully crash test a lighter wheelchair because the load forces are less. As the Centers for Medicare & Medicaid Services (CMS) imposes an *in the home* restriction on payment for wheelchairs, this allows disregard of the WC19 standard for the majority of standard manual and Group 2 power wheelchairs, even though these wheelchairs are often used as seats in transportation vehicles.

Although the frame strength of these standard wheelchairs may be less than is needed to survive crash testing, it is still possible to attach four-point tie-down straps to the wheelchair frame to improve safety. The addition of four crash-tested webbing loops to each corner of a wheelchair frame or base encourages the use of strap-type wheelchair securement to provide some level of transportation safety (Figure 24-9). These straps/loops are inexpensive and sold by van modifiers and forward-thinking rehab technology suppliers.

Attaching a crash-tested webbing loop (Figure 24-10) allows S-hooks to attach to the tubing on each corner of a wheelchair without crash-tested securement points. Presence of the straps also encourages transporters to respect rules for securement of wheelchairs for ensuring transportation safety.

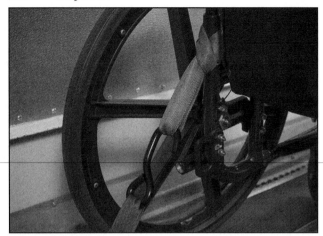

Figure 24-10. Crash-tested transportation webbing loops attached to appropriate parts of the wheelchair base (available from several suppliers of ANSI/RESNA WC18-compliant wheelchair securement products) can help with wheelchairs not equipped with four wheelchair securement points.

When we think of the clients who will benefit most from transportation safety technologies, we think of those who use power wheelchairs. These clients often have motor impairments that limit safely transferring to an OEM vehicle seat. A vehicle is required that can transport a 200- to 400-pound power chair. Heavier wheelchairs increase the forces that must be counteracted in small mass vehicles traveling at highway speeds. Access to fixed-route public or paratransit buses is a valuable, if temporary, transportation option for many.

The clinicians and suppliers who serve clients with more significant needs owe them the professionalism to be extra vigilant when recommending mobility products and to be aware of WTS standards and community transportation options and services. State Vocational Rehabilitation agencies are one of the only sources of funding for van modifications, although many companies who offer modifications are able to provide a wide range of price points. Low-interest loans from State Tech Act projects are another funding resource.

Pairing WC19 Wheelchairs With Rehabilitation Engineering and Assistive Technology Society of North America WC20-Compliant After-Market Seating

The third, and newest, transportation standard in *Volume 4: Wheelchairs and Transportation* (RESNA, 2012) is the WC20. This standard, which applies to after-market wheelchair seats and backs, will continue to develop over the coming years. WC19, as it is written, only applies to the wheelchair frame and the typical or company-provided seating system. Clinicians who work with clients who need

complex rehabilitation technologies know that standard seating is rarely adequate for that patient. Seating specialists recommend wheelchairs with after-market or specialized seating systems to meet their client's needs. The website referenced previously will also include the seating products that comply with WC20.

WC20 describes the design, performance, test procedures, and labeling requirements for wheelchair seat and back supports to withstand the 30-mph/20-g test pulse forces generated by a crash test dummy. To develop WC20, engineers first had to develop a surrogate wheelchair frame that would allow independent crash testing of seats and/ or backs. Further work is required to develop the surrogate backs and seats that will allow independent testing of wheelchair frames. This kind of incremental process is inherent in the development of standards. At the current stage of development, the standard should allow a WC19 wheelchair frame that meets the postural support and pressure management needs of a client to be mated with a successfully crash-tested WC20 seat or back. This will allow the provision of a crash-tested mobility device for individuals with complex rehabilitation technology needs.

DEALING WITH CLINICAL PROBLEMS

Although the standards can make the process of WTS appear straightforward, it is useful to present some additional information in the form of best practices. This will help clinicians and suppliers make better decisions when dealing with clients and everyday realities, including funding, attitudes, and variations in vehicles and wheelchairs.

Why Does the Size or the Speed of a Vehicle Matter?

When a wheelchair-seated passenger is traveling in a large, slow-moving vehicle that is suddenly stopped, it will take the vehicle longer to come to a halt and the forces of deceleration will be absorbed by the mass of the vehicle and the elongation of the period of time that this force is transmitted to its passengers. This is a key reason that city and school buses provide excellent passenger safety.

In contrast, when a wheelchair-seated passenger is traveling in a small vehicle (e.g., a family minivan) at interstate highway speeds and is suddenly stopped, the forces of deceleration are instantly transmitted from the smaller mass of the vehicle to its passengers. This is the reason that highway accidents so often exceed the 95th percentile of severity. Rollovers as well as passenger ejection with death or serious injuries often follow this deceleration.

The risk for death and injury will be lower in a large-mass vehicle. This means that wheelchair-seated passengers using personally owned passenger vehicles are at greater risk for death and injury. Travel in the small-mass vehicle creates a greater reliance on a strong and stable seat, effective occupant restraint, and other safety technologies, such as air bags and crumple zones. This information is key in helping clients make mobility equipment decisions, as well as working with National Mobility Equipment Dealers Association (NMEDA) certified van modifiers.

Wheelchair Users and Driving

Some wheelchair users will be able to drive a motor vehicle. In this situation, the seating team needs the assistance of both a Certified Driver Rehabilitation Specialist and a NMEDA-certified van modifier. The driver specialist will assess the client's ability to drive and will both specify the adaptive driving equipment to be installed in the vehicle and provide training in its use. NMEDA modifiers always take their installation instructions from these adaptive driving specialists.

Manual wheelchair users often prefer to slide into the driver's seat of a vehicle, if possible. Hand controls can be specified and installed in the vehicle, along with any other adaptations needed, such as a spinner knob or alternate controls for wipers.

Often, an initial decision is choosing a full-size or minivan. Full-size vans are less common these days than minivans. Full-size vans, because of height, always require a hydraulic lift system, rather than a ramp. Many of these vans also require a pop-top to allow room for head clearance.

Minivans are widely available and preferred because of their gas economy and maneuverability. An optional conversion process to lower the vehicle floor increases headroom and allows the use of a simple ramp for wheelchair loading.

When a van or minivan is the best option, the wheelchair driver uses the same hand controls available for other vehicles. For the driver who cannot transfer to the height of a van seat, an adaptive driver's seat, often called a *five-way seat*, is an option. These are powered seats that move back and forth from the steering wheel and pivot, elevate, or lower to make transfer from wheelchair to driver's seat easier. This option allows others to drive the adapted van using the same driver's seat.

Other clients drive seated in their wheelchair, often if transferring to another seat is too difficult or if the standard driver's seat does not provide adequate postural support or pressure relief. This requires removing the driver's seat and installing a docking system to enable independent wheelchair securement. The lap/shoulder belt on the driver's side will need adaptation so that the tongue part can insert into a receptacle that is elevated from the vehicle floor, placing it within reach. Driving from a wheelchair requires selecting a cantilever armrest, which allows the lap portion of the belt to make positive contact with the driver's anterior superior iliac spine while simultaneously fitting across his or her clavicle and sternum. Of course this setup requires careful planning so that hand controls and other modifications are properly aligned. Some clients will also need an anterior chest strap or lateral trunk supports to provide adequate postural support, particularly during vehicle movement.

Other Methods for Transporting Wheelchairs and Their Attachments

Not everyone can afford a wheelchair-accessible van, although there is a thriving market in secondhand equipment. When a client is not riding in his or her wheelchair, the mobility device should still be secured for its protection and the safety of others. Van modifiers have many devices to help with this task. Unoccupied wheelchairs may be transported inside a van, in the bed of a pickup truck using four-point strap securement, or with a docking system. Another option is a bumper lift, which mounts on a class 3 hitch, lowers to the ground, and allows securement of a wheelchair or scooter on a trailer hitch or platform behind the vehicle. Small lifts are available to help with placing small wheelchairs and scooters (with forward-folding backs) into the back section of an SUV. Some still use a roof top carrier to lift a folding-frame wheelchair into its own compartment. Some clients have limited walking ability and are able to manage such systems independently; others will require the assistance of a family member or caregiver.

Many individuals who want to travel with their own vehicle find it useful to purchase a suitcase ramp. These easily portable, lightweight ramps cost between $100 and $300 and can solve many access problems. These can create access to a vehicle, a relative or friend's home, and help avoid disappointment when arriving at a destination with one or two steps.

Reimbursement

Since the WC19 standard was adopted in 2000, it has been challenging to increase awareness and knowledge of and about the standard and its benefits for the end user. Initially, the additional cost of adding the WC19 securement points to the frame of a wheelchair (about $250 to $300) was considered a major barrier, because Medicare and other funding sources would not pay for it. Gradually, this barrier is beginning to collapse as more manufacturers integrate the securement points into the design of the wheelchair frame or include it as a standard feature of the product.

Advising the Wheelchair Selection Process

When a manufacturer crash tests a mobility product, it is placing its engineering reputation on the line. For the prescribing team, testing ensures provision of a mobility device that has passed a rigorous test that is equivalent to the 95th percentile of crash severity. Staying up to date with changes and improvement in standards is essential for clinicians and suppliers working with mobility technologies.

Non-Compliant Wheelchair Models

Many clients are attracted to the appearance of a wheelchair frame. Ultralight wheelchairs offer a sleek appearance, a reputation for responsiveness, and the appeal of speed and ease of movement. However, many ultralight manual wheelchairs are not crash-tested. Many individuals who use ultralight wheelchairs have no difficulty transferring into an OEM vehicle seat, so tie-downs are not required. However, ultralights are often useful for individuals with marginal strength who require the lightweight and frame adjustments to move under their own power, with or without a power add-on. This individual may need to ride in his or her wheelchair.

Many young clients are unimpressed by reports about wheelchair transportation safety. We can only do our best to educate the clients with whom we work. Many attractive ultralight wheelchair designs are available that are equipped with securement points and have met testing standards.

An ultralight manual wheelchair may not be safe for a client to sit in during transport, such as on a bus, because of a low back height or the absence of head support. Even with the use of occupant restraints, this seating configuration does not provide adequate support during transport. Transporters need to be educated about the appropriateness of such a mobility device for daily mobility independence but the lack of appropriateness as a transport system. School bus policy should be flexible enough to allow these students to transfer to the compartmentalized safety of a typical school bus seat with additional seat belt, if needed.

Ultralight Frame Design: Box Versus Z-Frame

Another strategy for increasing the safety of an ultralight manual wheelchair user is to guide the client toward a box frame. This allows the use of crash-tested webbing loops on the frame, even if the chair is not crash-tested. The majority of ultralights that have been crash-tested do have box-type frames. The use of a box frame chair offers good looks while offering the greater stability of an additional welded tubing structure. Welded junctions are the strongest areas on the wheelchair frame. An increasing number of cantilevered or Z-frame ultralight manual wheelchairs are meeting crash testing requirements (see Figure 24-10).

Adding Crash-Tested Securement Loops

The WC19 standard does allow for the postsale addition of WC19-compliant securement points to the wheelchair frame. Manufacturers vary in their approach to this request. Some will supply the loops but refuse to label it as safe for transportation. Others will require that the wheelchair be shipped back to the factory at significant cost to the end user. Basically, it is best to consider transportation safety upfront when choosing a wheelchair.

What to Do After a Crash

After a 30-mph/20-g crash, a careful inspection of the wheelchair frame and the occupant restraint system is required. If damage is found, this should be noted in the accident report, and the equipment should be replaced.

When Upright Sitting Is Not Possible

The tilt-in-space wheelchair has benefited greatly from the development of the WC19 standard. Before this standard, transporters were required to use securement straps on both the wheeled base and the seat structure. The linkage between the two segments that allowed tilting was considered too weak to survive the 30-mph/20-g loading sustained in a crash or during emergency driving. Now these wheelchairs are consistently available in crash-tested versions with a single set of four securement points.

Transportation is now limited only by the degree of tilt that is allowed during vehicle movement. The wheelchair occupant should be positioned at no more than 15 degrees of tilt. This amount of tilt should still allow the torso occupant restraint to make continuous contact with the clavicle and sternum. This correct fit prevents the forces of a frontal impact from throwing the passenger forward into the belt restraint. This sudden forward acceleration could cause head and neck injuries.

Resources for Secondary Postural Supports

Although no standards exist for head supports, lateral and anterior trunk supports, and lateral and medial thigh supports, among other supports, a best practices document was developed by engineers at the University of Pittsburgh (Rehabilitation Engineering Research Center [RERC] on Wheelchair Transportation Safety, 2006). This document suggests strategies based on occupant protection and crash dynamics. Secondary postural supports should be used as a second layer of protection or in harmony with the occupant restraint belt during transportation. For example, it is clear that anterior trunk supports are not crash-tested, but these may enable upright sitting that will allow the crash-tested lap/shoulder belt to make effective contact with the client's clavicle and sternum.

This document also includes information about using items that attach to wheelchairs or clients during transportation. Some individuals rely on wheelchair lap trays to support their upper body during transit. The document recommends purchasing a lightweight rigid foam tray that will perform the same function but not cause injury to the client or others in a sudden stop or crash. A wooden or Lexan tray should be removed and stowed. Similarly, speech-generating or augmentative alternative communication devices should be removed with their mounts and stowed. Perhaps a low-tech communication board with transit-oriented symbols or words can be provided for use during transport. Oxygen tanks need to be secured as well. Using these types of equipment will often guide the selection of a student's securement location on a school bus. The *Secondary Postural Supports* document (RERC on Wheelchair Transportation Safety, 2006) also addresses the topic of head support and encourages the use of a soft support such as a Hensinger head support. Avoid forehead straps during transportation or the use of any item that might create a fulcrum under the client's chin.

Although the standards only apply to seated transportation, clinicians, and suppliers will meet situations in which a passenger needs to lie down during transit. E-Z-On of Florida manufactures transit vests that link with vehicle safety belts, allowing transport of clients who must lie down in family vehicles, school buses, and medical transport.

Future Strategies Being Considered

In my experience with the development of transportation technologies, rehabilitation engineers and product designers include appropriate care and concern for safety while respecting independence, autonomy, and self-determination. However, this is a difficult balance to achieve. Universal docking systems, stabilizing arms controlled by clients, and wheelchair-anchored occupant restraint systems have been proposed to this end. Only now are the first commercial products being marketed to bus manufacturers (see Figure 24-5). An ongoing issue is the use of three-wheeled scooters as seats in large accessible transit vehicles. With their narrow wheelbase and the rider's high center of mass, they are inherently tippy and unsafe for typical four-point securement. Standards do exist for design and testing of scooters, but no compliant products have reached the marketplace. A more immediate solution may lie in the adoption of the rear-facing passenger compartment approach. Development issues always seem to revolve around ease of use, universal access, and cost. There is still plenty of room for innovation in the WTS field.

Summary

This information may seem complicated and technical; however, it is critical to create a level of safety that is equivalent to what you experience in your own vehicle. In your vehicle, the seat is well-designed with head protection, is solidly anchored to the floor, and your ability to remain in that seat is ensured with the help of an occupant restraint system. In cars, millions of dollars have been spent to provide crumple zones and front and side curtain air bags. Let's do our best to create safety for our wheelchair-seated fellow travelers. As always, education and good clinical decision making is the key.

References

American Academy of Pediatrics. (2014). *Car seats: Information for families.* Retrieved from http://www.healthychildren.org/English/safety-prevention/on-the-go/Pages/Car-Safety-Seats-Information-for-Families.aspx

Bertocci, G., & Evans, J. (2000). Injury risk assessment of wheelchair occupant restraint systems in a frontal crash: A case for integrated restraints. *Journal of Rehabilitation Research & Development, 37,* 573-590.

Bertocci, G., Manary, M., & Ha, D. (2001). Wheelchairs used as motor vehicle seats: Seat loading in frontal impact sled testing. *Medical Engineering and Physics, 23,* 679-685.

DOJ 36 CFR Part 1192. ADA accessibility guidelines for transportation vehicles (ADAAG) 1192 C.F.R. § 36 CFR Ch. XI (1998).

MacLaughlin, T. F., Sullivan, L. K., & O'Connor, C. S. (1988). *Rear seat submarining investigation: Final report.* Washington, DC: National Highway Traffic Safety Administration.

National Highway Traffic Safety Administration. (2003). *Traffic safety facts.* Washington, DC: U.S. Department of Transportation.

Prohaska, T., Ragland, D., MacLeod, K., Hughes, S., Smith, M., Satariano, W.,...Dabbous, F. (2012). Data analyses: Assessing the intersection between health and transportation. In *Accessible community transportation in our nation.* Washington, DC: Easter Seals Project Action,.

Rehabilitation Engineering and Assistive Technology Society of North America. (2012). *RESNA wheelchairs: Volume 4: Wheelchairs and transportation RESNA standards.* Washington, DC: RESNA Press.

Rehabilitation Engineering Research Center on Wheelchair Transportation Safety. (2006). *Guidelines for use of secondary postural support devices by wheelchair users during travel in motor vehicles.* Retrieved from http://www.riskcontrolservices.com/aol/Wheelchair/RERC_WTS_032_06.pdf

Schneider, L. W., Hobson, D. A., & Bertocci, G. E. (2003). *Development of voluntary standards for improved transportation safety of wheelchair-seated occupants.* Paper presented at the Annual RESNA Conference, Atlanta, GA.

Severy, D. M., Blaisdell, D. M., & Kerkoff, J. F. (1976). *Automotive seat design and collision performance.* Paper presented at the Twentieth Stapp Car Crash Conference, Warrendale, PA.

Subramanian, R. (2005). Motor vehicle traffic crashes as a leading cause of death in the United States, 2002. In National Highway Transit Safety Administration National Center for Statistics and Analysis (Ed.), *Traffic safety facts* (p. 2). Washington, DC: U.S. Department of Transportation.

U.S. Department of Transportation. (1999). *Federal motor vehicle safety standards and regulations* (DOT HS 808 878). Washington, DC: US Government Printing Office.

Application of Wheelchair and Seating Standards
From Inside the Test Lab and Beyond

Kay Ellen Koch, OTR/L, ATP, RESNA Fellow and
Anita Perr, PhD, OT/L, FAOTA, RESNA Fellow

WHAT ARE WHEELCHAIR AND SEATING STANDARDS?

Who Uses Standards?

Standards are developed and managed by both private and governmental organizations and are applied to many things in our lives, including Underwriters Laboratory (UL) standards for electronic equipment (UL, 2014), American Kennel Club standards for dog breeds (American Kennel Club, 2014), and building codes for environmental accessibility (U.S. Department of Justice, Civil Rights Division, 2010). Standards are developed for a variety of reasons, including safety and uniformity. By standardizing objects and procedures, it is possible to use combinations of devices manufactured by different companies. For example, because plugs and outlets are standardized, hair dryers, blenders, power saws, and other electronic devices that are made according to UL standards can plug into outlets that also comply with UL standards. In certain circumstances, standards also give people information about how a given device is expected to perform. You can think about this similarly to the way you might compare the performance of a few different cars based on the miles/gallon they attain. That information gives you an idea about which car might go farthest on a gallon of gas. Of course you also have to think about what the roads are like, such as hills or muddy surfaces and what you are carrying, such as a trunk full of playground sand. So, like cars, where the actual mileage

might differ from that reported by the manufacturer, wheelchair performance standards might vary in real-life settings from the laboratory findings. One area of performance, for example, regards the capacity of the wheelchair battery. The actual energy consumption in real-life use will differ from the laboratory findings. The laboratory findings let us compare various manufacturers and models of equipment because the test setup is the same in each case.

Some of the standards have minimal performance levels to pass. For example, there are standards that identify the flammability allowed for wheelchair upholstery. This safety measure is in place so that wheelchair users can be protected from extensive damage and injury from upholstery that ignites and burns easily. Similar flammability standards have been used for many years in the manufacture of clothing (U.S. Consumer Product Safety Commission, 2008). These standards are in place in an attempt improve the safety of the products. This is a good example of how standards developed in other industries carryover and have been adapted to wheelchair seating. This not only helps improve product safety and development but provides guidelines for manufacturers.

Some standards are voluntary and some are mandatory. Wheelchair and seating standards are voluntary. This means that wheelchair and wheelchair seating manufacturers can choose whether to comply with the standards. Manufacturers that choose to comply with wheelchair and wheelchair seating standards perform tests that are set out by the standards and disclose the results in the manner prescribed in the standards. There are a number of reasons that manufacturers might choose not to comply with wheelchair

Lange, M. L., & Minkel, J. L.
Seating and Wheeled Mobility: A Clinical Resource Guide
(pp. 397-408). © 2018 SLACK Incorporated.

and seating standards. For example, standards testing can be very expensive. Some manufacturers perform the testing within their own companies. Others hire testing facilitates to perform the tests. Still others use a combination of in-house and contracted testing. Whether the tests are performed within the company or by an outsider contractor, expenses reflect the cost of testing equipment and space as a well as the manpower involved in performing the tests and documenting the results. The cost of standards may be especially difficult to manage for small, start up companies or for companies that have many devices requiring testing. Other reasons may also prevent a company from volunteering to comply with wheelchair and seating standards. When wheelchair users, clinicians, and payers consider the options for the most appropriate equipment, they should ask manufacturers their reasons for not complying or disclosing testing results. The answers to these questions can be part of the information gathered for the decision-making process when selecting equipment.

Most manufacturers have adopted standards testing because they can help when developing new products. The standards that apply to durability and performance, for example, may assist with a prototype of a new product by identifying design strengths or weaknesses. The testing performed on the prototype could also help identify whether the design of the product or its components could create a risk of injury. Manufacturers keep these test results because they can also be beneficial when changing the design of a product or the manufacturing process. Manufacturers use the information they report in two ways. The first purpose is to provide objective information about their products in their marketing literature or websites. The second way this disclosed information is used assists in identifying and providing objective data for classification of their products by regulatory and government or funding agencies.

Seating and Mobility Standards

There are three sets of standards directly related to seating and wheeled mobility. They are (1) Wheelchair Standards, including requirements and test methods for wheelchairs (including scooters); (2) Additional Requirements for Wheelchairs With Electrical Systems; and (3) Wheelchair Seating Standards. A listing of the sections of these standards can be found in Table 25-1.

As is evident in Table 25-1, wheelchair and seating standards address performance issues that directly relate to everyday wheelchair use. Some standards simply require disclosure of testing results, whereas others require minimum acceptable performance parameters. Standards that have minimum acceptable performance parameters are those that have safety implications for the user. Disclosure standards are used, identifying characteristics and features of the device being tested.

An example of a disclosure standard is the standard Determination of Static Stability of Wheelchair. As in all the standards, this describes the wheelchair setup to be used during the testing, which usually means factory settings with armrests and footrests in place. A test dummy, as defined elsewhere in the standards, is put in the wheelchair to simulate a rider. The test dummy is built in accordance to International Organization for Standardization (ISO) standards that specify the weight of the rider (25 kg, or 55 pounds; 50 kg, or 110 pounds; 75 kg, or 165 pounds; or 100 kg, or 220 pounds) and are designed to simulate the same center of gravity as a person seated in a wheelchair (ISO, n.d.c). The wheelchair is placed on a tilting surface in the uphill, downhill, and sideways positions. For any wheelchair to be stable, all of the wheels have to be in contact with a surface. When the testing surface is titled to the point where two wheels lift off the surface, this is an indication that the wheelchair is no longer stable (Figure 25-1).

This angle is not the same angle that any wheelchair user might tip. Real life is much more complicated than that. The tipping angle of an individual will be influenced by the person's size, body makeup, ability to compensate for wheelchair tippiness, setup of the wheelchair, his or her center of gravity, and myriad other factors. The test data for this standard tells wheelchair users, clinicians, designers, and payers that, with all else being equal, a certain wheelchair has a certain level of stability or "tippiness." This information can also be used to compare multiple wheelchairs that have each been tested using the same standard test methods.

The results from the testing are disclosed, and, in most cases, there is no judgment on passing or failing. Remember the discussion of the standard that measures tipping angle? This information, for example, is of little importance to a person who only uses the wheelchair on flat surfaces and does not propel it at high speeds. There is no minimum acceptable performance level for this person. It would be a disservice to eliminate devices based on factors that are not important to specific users.

That is not the case in all circumstances, however. There are few standards that identify a minimum passing rate of performance. These are related to safety and include standards for durability, fire retardation, and equipment to be used with a tie-down in a vehicle.

Let's look at two more test standards:

1. Energy Consumption of Power Wheelchairs and Requirements

2. Test Methods for Static, Impact, and Fatigue Strengths of Wheelchairs

The Energy Consumption test is a performance test standard that focuses on the maximum speed of a power wheelchair and the range (or how far) the wheelchair will travel on a fully charged battery. This information is useful, when combined with knowledge about the environment, to estimate how the power wheelchair will perform for a given individual.

TABLE 25-1

WHEELCHAIR AND SEATING STANDARDS

TITLE OF THE STANDARD	DESCRIPTION
Determination of Static Stability Of Wheelchairs	This section identifies the test methods to determine the ability of a wheelchair to remain stable on a sloped surface, or how tippy is a chair.
Determination of Dynamic Stability of Electrically Powered Wheelchairs	This section identifies the test methods to determine the stability of the wheelchair when: • Starting to move up a hill • Braking while moving up or down a hill • Turning on a level or sloped surface
Determination of Effectiveness of Brakes	This section identifies the test methods to determine the effectiveness of wheel locks (parking brakes). This refers to the wheel lock's ability to prevent the wheelchair from rolling on a sloped surface. This section also identifies the methods used to determine the minimum stopping distance of a power wheelchair moving at its maximum speed.
Energy Consumption of Electrically Powered Wheelchairs and Scooters for Determination of Theoretical Distance Range	This section identifies test methods that use a measured course to determine how much energy is consumed by a power wheelchair. This theoretically relates to how far a power wheelchair can travel on a single charge, although actual performance will vary based on the environment and user characteristics.
Determination of Dimensions, Mass, and Maneuvering Space	This section identifies the test methods to determine the amount of space the wheelchair occupies and the smallest amount of space needed to maneuver.
Determination of Maximum Speed, Acceleration, and Deceleration of Electrically Powered Wheelchairs	This section identifies the test methods to determine the maximum speed of a power wheelchair in forward and reverse on level and sloped surfaces. It also identifies the methods to determine the fastest rates at which a power wheelchair can: • Achieve top speed (accelerate) • Come to a stop (decelerate)
Method Of Measurement of Seating and Wheel Dimensions	This section identifies the test methods to determine the linear measurements and angular orientations of the seating system.
Requirements and Test Methods for Static, Impact, and Fatigue Strengths	This section identifies the test methods to determine the strength and durability of a wheelchair.
Climatic Tests for Electrically Powered Wheelchairs	This section identifies the test methods to determine the impact that moisture and temperature have on a power wheelchair.
Determination of Obstacle-Climbing Ability of Electrically Powered Wheelchairs	This section identifies the test methods to determine the height of obstacles the wheelchair can climb and descend safely.
Test Dummies	The test dummy simulates an occupant in the wheelchair. This standard identifies the configuration to be used in testing the other standards. A standardized test dummy allows results to be compared.
Determination of Coefficient of Friction of Test Surfaces	This section identifies the surfaces that are used during testing in the other standards. It describes the level of resistance to slip off the testing surface.

(continued)

TABLE 25-1 (CONTINUED)	
WHEELCHAIR AND SEATING STANDARDS	
TITLE OF THE STANDARD	**DESCRIPTION**
Power and Control Systems For Electrically Powered Wheelchairs—Requirements And Test Methods	This section identifies the test methods to determine the electrical safety of power wheelchairs.
Requirements for Information Disclosure, Documentation, and Labeling	This section identifies how manufacturers should label and identify testing results in their literature.
Resistance to Ignition of Upholstered Parts Requirements and Test Methods	This section identifies the test methods to determine the extent to which wheelchair upholstery withstands burns. It is a measure of the material's ability to retard fire.
Wheeled Mobility Devices for Use as Seats in Motor Vehicles	This section addresses how the wheelchair seat and frame are secured to a vehicle, as well as how the design supports the wheelchair user during impact. It also addresses the position and security of the restraints used to secure the wheelchair (RESNA Technical Standards Board, 2008).
Requirements and Test Methods for Electromagnetic (EM) Compatibility of Electrically Powered Wheelchairs and Motorized Scooters	EM compatability refers to the compatibility with EM energy in the environment and ensures that the power wheelchair and charger do not emit levels of EM energy that cause EM interference with other devices in the vicinity. One example would be to ensure that cell phone transmissions do not cause the power wheelchair to move or stop without the user's control.
Setup Procedures	This standard defines the setup of the testing space and the wheelchair configuration.
Batteries and Chargers for Powered Wheelchairs	This section defines specific test methods and the requirements for batteries and battery chargers used in power wheelchairs and scooters.
Wheelchair Seating	
Vocabulary, Reference Axis Convention, and Measures for Body Segments, Posture, and Postural Support Surfaces	This section identifies the unified set terms relating to seating and seating devices. (See Chapter 6 for specific information about this standard.)
Determination of Physical and Mechanical Characteristics of Devices Intended to Manage Tissue Integrity—Seat Cushions	This section identifies the test apparatus and the methods used to determine performance. It also identifies the disclosure requirements for wheelchair seat cushions intended to maintain tissue integrity and prevent tissue trauma (ISO, n.d.b).
Determination of Static, Impact, and Repetitive Load Strengths for Postural Support Devices	This section identifies the test methods to determine the strength and durability of the seating device.
Seating Systems for Use in Motor Vehicles	This section identifies the test methods to determine the specific test methods and requirements for design and performance, for instructions and warnings, and for product marking and labeling of seating systems intended to be used as a forward-facing seat in a motor vehicle when fitted to a manual or powered wheelchair. It evaluates the frontal crashworthiness performance of complete seating systems for occupancy by adults or children of mass equal to or greater than 22 kg.

(continued)

TABLE 25-1 (CONTINUED)

WHEELCHAIR AND SEATING STANDARDS

TITLE OF THE STANDARD	DESCRIPTION
Resistance to Ignition of Nonintegrated Seat and Back Support Cushions	This section identifies the test methods to determine the extent to which wheelchair seat and back support cushions withstand burns. It is a measure of the material's ability to retard fire. This standard is one of the few standards that set a minimum performance level.
Determination of Perspiration Dissipation Characteristics of Seat Cushions Intended to Manage Tissue Integrity	This section identifies the test methods to determine the moisture-wicking ability of the seat and back support cushion.

This table represents a list and brief description of the standards relating to wheelchairs and wheelchair seating. The information is derived from a variety of sources and combines information from American National Standards Institute (ANSI)/Rehabilitation Engineering & Assistive Technology Society of North America (RESNA) and International Organization for Standardization (ISO) standards. (Axleson, Minkel, & Chesney, 1994; RESNA Standards Committee on Support Surfaces, 2014; ISO, n.d.a, n.d.b, n.d.c). Additional input from William Ammer, ammerconsulting.com.

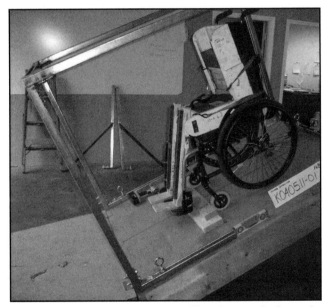

Figure 25-1. Static stability test rig. This photograph shows the wheelchair loaded with the test dummy on the tilting surface. In this test, the surface is tilted until the two rear wheels lift off the surface. That angle is reported. (Reprinted with permission from Bill Ammer, ammerconsulting.com)

The group of tests for Static, Impact, and Fatigue strength includes setting the wheelchair in a testing device that repeatedly pushes against specific parts of the wheelchair either a certain number of times or until the part fails, or breaks. For instance, in Figure 25-2, the testing device is set to repeatedly press against the footrest to determine its durability. This is meant to represent the wear and tear of the footrest from daily use.

Another test in this group of durability tests requires that the wheelchair be placed on equipment comprising two large rollers. This is often referred to as the *double drum test* (Figure 25-3). Each roller is fitted with slats. As the

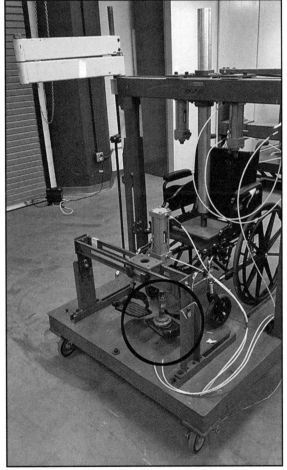

Figure 25-2. Footrest durability testing. Testing device that can be used to measure wheelchair strength and fatigue. Note the plunger pushing on the footplate. This may simulate the forces a wheelchair user applies when pressing his or her feet into the footrests. (Reprinted with permission from Gebrosky, B. G., Pearlman, J., Cooper, R. A., Cooper, R., & Kelleher, A. (2013). Evaluation of lightweight wheelchairs using ANSI/RESNA testing standards. *Journal of Rehabilitation Research & Design, 50,* 1373-1390.)

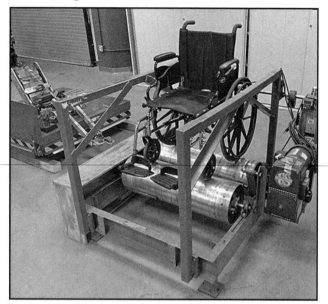

Figure 25-3. Double-drum testing: Wheelchair on double-drum roller. Slats on each roller simulate the uneven terrain that wheelchair users encounter in their daily wheelchair use. Note the motor on the right side that turns the rollers at the speed identified in the testing methods for the standard. (Reprinted with permission from Gebrosky, B. G., Pearlman, J., Cooper, R. A., Cooper, R., & Kelleher, A. (2013). Evaluation of lightweight wheelchairs using ANSI/RESNA testing standards. *Journal of Rehabilitation Research & Design, 50*, 1373-1390.)

wheelchair rides on the spinning rollers, the slats make the wheelchair bounce in a manner that simulates riding over rough terrain. The purpose of this test is to see whether parts dislodge or break as the wheelchair rolls over surfaces designed to simulate rough roads.

Again, this information does not directly correlate with any given person's experience with a wheelchair braking down, because each wheelchair user has his or her own set of unique circumstances. It does, however, allow wheelchair users, clinicians, designers, and payers to compare durability performance between different wheelchairs tested using the same method. This information can then be included in the decision-making process such that a person who frequently travels over rough terrain might need a more durable wheelchair than a person who only uses the wheelchair on smooth surfaces. Standards focusing on durability are important because they provide information about the differences between acquisition costs and life-cycle costs. Sometimes the wheelchair with a higher purchase price may actually be less costly over time than ones with lower initial purchase prices (Cooper et al., 1996).

Standards Organizations

The development and review of standards related to wheelchairs and positioning equipment are managed on both the national and international levels. At the national level, the standards are governed by a collaboration between ANSI and RESNA. These are called ANSI/RESNA

Standards. At the international level, the standards are governed by ISO. Newly developed standards are voted on to be accepted as ISO and/or ANSI/RESNA Standards. These are reviewed every 5 years for revisions or updating. The wheelchair and seating standards were developed by experts from each constituent group interested in the equipment including equipment users; manufacturers and suppliers; engineers from manufacturing, academic institutions, and government agencies; product developers; and clinicians including occupational and physical therapists. These groups collaborated to identify the items in need of testing and possible regulation. They developed the testing and reporting methods to address the concerns that were raised. Testing facilities evaluate the procedures to insure that the methods are reliable and valid. In a commentary to the *Journal of Spinal Cord Medicine*, Cooper (2006) called for more involvement from equipment users and clinicians to strengthen the standards and to increase their use in clinical decision making.

Seating and wheeled mobility standards play a number of roles in the lives of people with disabilities. Standards are used to disclose product information in a uniform way so that people who need to select equipment can compare the equipment and select the specific device that is most useful to them. Specifically, people who use wheelchairs and seating equipment, clinicians who recommend equipment, and funders who pay for equipment all can use information derived as a result of standards to make the best selections (Ferguson-Pell et al., 2005). Additionally, designers use the standards as they develop new devices and change existing ones. Most of the wheelchair and seating standards describe methods to test the performance relative to a specific feature of the chair or seating support device—for example, the durability of the device or top speed of a power chair.

HOW DO WHEELCHAIR AND SEATING STANDARDS PERTAIN TO ME?

Using Standards to Match User Needs With Equipment

Since June 1979, the ANSI/RESNA Wheelchair Standards Committee has worked to provide consumers with objective information about the characteristics and performance of wheelchairs. The committee includes rehabilitation engineers, wheelchair manufacturers, representatives from the Department of Veterans Affairs (VA) and the Food and Drug Administration, wheelchair users, and clinicians, such as occupational and physical therapists. Manufacturers use standards to help shape product components and equipment designs. Often the standards are created with certain product needs in mind, such as durability and life expectancy of the device. Testing is completed that provides the information needed to match needs identified in a clinical assessment and specific model selection.

Wheelchair and seating standards should also be used by wheelchair users, clinicians, prescribers, and payers to inform the selection process. Information about the performance, safety, and dimensions is needed in order to make the best match between the client's needs and the equipment. The following case studies illustrate how information from the wheelchair standards test results were used in the selection process. Similar strategies can be used when selecting seating equipment as well.

CASE EXAMPLE

Rex is an independent, manual wheelchair user. He schedules an appointment in a seating clinic because he needs a new wheelchair, and wants to make sure that he makes the best choice. He is a full-time wheelchair user, using his wheelchair for all mobility inside his house and the community. Rex is able to transfer from his wheelchair to all surfaces, including his bed and toileting equipment, the floor, and his car. Rex is not currently working but is hoping that he will be able to find a job once he has a reliable wheelchair. He would also like to hike and camp because these were interests before he started using a wheelchair. Rex is 32 years old, was a football player in college, and has a strong upper body and trunk. He is unable to move or feel his legs.

Information from at least three of the manual wheelchair standards is especially useful in determining the best equipment for Rex.

Determination of Static Stability

Testing of static stability provides information on the relationship of the center of gravity in relation to the position of the rear wheel and regarding the stability of the wheelchair. This is important so that the rear wheel position can be positioned for efficient propulsion and to unweight the casters, so that Rex can pop a wheelie easily and navigate his wheelchair over uneven terrain and environmental obstacles. He is looking for a chair with a relatively small tipping angle, indicating that the chair will be easier for him to pop into a wheelie

Overall Dimensions, Mass, and Turning Radius

Information gained from testing of this standard will provide information about how much space the wheelchair takes up when it is moving and when it is still. Clearance through Rex's bathroom door is 24 inches, and there is no space inside the bathroom or in the adjacent hallway to make the door opening wider. Rex can use the overall dimensions to select a wheelchair that is narrow enough to fit through the space. His kitchen is small, and he likes to cook. The space inbetween the stove, sink, and refrigerator is tight, so Rex can use the turning radius information to make sure the equipment he selects will not only fit in this space but allow him to turn around as well. A smaller turning radius will allow easier access to appliances and cabinets. Knowing the mass (weight) of the equipment is important because after Rex transfers into his car, he lifts his wheelchair over his body and puts it in the passenger seat. By using the results of wheelchair standards testing, he can determine whether he will be able to manage that process with the equipment he selects.

Guidelines for Information Disclosure

This standard identifies the information that manufacturers must disclose. As all manufacturers who comply with wheelchair standards disclose information in the same format, Rex and his clinicians can compare similar wheelchairs from multiple manufacturers to match the client's needs with the best technology and options from the information provided.

CASE EXAMPLE

Rexanne is an active power wheelchair user who is scheduled in the seating clinic to determine whether there is another power wheelchair that will work better for her. She is having difficulty managing her current power wheelchair, and it "conks out" in the middle of her day. Rexanne works in a large office complex and has to move between buildings for meetings several times each week. Some people drive their cars between the buildings, but Rexanne finds it easier to use her power wheelchair rather than take the bus. She uses the chair up to 10 hours a day. There is varying terrain at home and at work that needs to be considered because the power wheelchair is used on smooth flat surfaces, inside her home and office, and outside on grassy terrain. While in the home and office settings, Rexanne needs to navigate in small spaces. Rexanne lives in an accessible apartment on a bus line; the bus stop is close to the entrance to her apartment building. The bus stop at work, however, is about a half mile from her office building. She loves the walkway that leads from the bus stop to the office and enjoys this part of her commute even when it is raining or snowing.

Information from at least three wheelchair standards is especially useful in determining the best equipment for Rexanne.

Dynamic Stability

Dynamic stability is an important area to consider because Rexanne uses her power wheelchair over all sorts of surfaces, including ramps and grassy slopes. She is looking for a chair that has a higher tipping angle so that she can safely use her power chair to go up steeper ramps and across a grassy slope while being confident that all the wheels will stay in contact with the surface.

Energy Consumption

Rexanne knows that her wheelchair performance is based in part on the batteries she uses and on how she cares for the batteries. She also knows that the when she carries heavy loads, her wheelchair may consume more energy. Given these variations, Rexanne can still get an idea about how well her wheelchair will perform by comparing the energy consumption of the models she considers. Results of energy consumption testing provide information on how long the power wheelchair will last on a charge and approximately how far it will go. This is important to Rexanne because she is out of the house for about 10 hours each day and drives her power wheelchair long distances.

Determination of Max Speed, Acceleration, and Deceleration

Rexanne likes to drive fast in open areas. She is adept at using the joystick control and demonstrates good problem solving and safety judgment. She has good reaction time, and although her trunk balance is somewhat impaired, she uses a chest strap for external support and can maintain her balance well, even when the wheelchair stops quickly.

The cases featuring Rex and Rexanne demonstrate how wheelchair and seating standards can inform the decision process in selecting the most appropriate wheelchair. Remember that this is only part of the information used to make the best match for each individual. A comprehensive assessment including sensory motor function, cognitive abilities, and environmental consideration must also be performed.

In addition to the standards mentioned in the case studies, information from many of the other standards could also be used in the decision-making process. It should be clear how the information derived from wheelchair and seating standards can inform equipment choices by wheelchair users in and out of seating clinic settings. The information derived from standards can also be used to strengthen the justifications for why a specific product is

being recommended over another. Funding agents may see why certain equipment is recommended when information regarding performance, safety, and durability data from standards testing is included in the justification for funding.

HOW ARE WHEELCHAIR STANDARDS DISCLOSED?

Wheelchair and seating standards also describe how the information should be disclosed. Each manufacturer that complies with the standards provides the testing results in its product literature. A sample of such product literature can be found in Table 25-2.

Using Standards Inside the Test Lab for Research

Research in seating and mobility is ultimately performed so that people who use wheelchairs can participate to their optimal level in the environments of their choice. Seating and mobility research includes both qualitative and quantitative studies and varies from investigations of the materials used to manufacture seating equipment and mobility devices, to investigations of the effect of wheelchair configuration on performance, to investigations of peoples' opinions of how their own mobility and seating equipment influences their performance of daily activities. New technologies, methods, or processes are developed as a result of this research.

Much valuable research that contributes to our knowledge of device performance was completed in the process of developing wheelchair and seating testing methodologies (Cooper et al., 1997; Cooper, et al., 1994; Sprigle, Dunlop, & Press, 2003). Not only was this research instrumental in developing the wheelchair and seating standards, it has also given researchers the opportunity to think about the role of standards in the new product development, and further understand how currently available equipment is being used by people with disabilities. For instance, while developing standards for seat cushions, the development team had to think about how to uniformly describe and measure what happens to a wheelchair user's buttocks tissue when it is compressed and capillary blood flow is decreased, when a person sits on a wheelchair seat cushion, designed to redistribute pressure and protection the skin from a pressure injury. It is important to understand the deformation of the buttock tissue when testing the effectiveness of a seat cushion to provide skin protection.

Wheelchair and seating standards can be used in clinical research far beyond the development of standards. In general terms, the value of research is increased when the test methods are strong. For example, researchers who

TABLE 25-2

TECHNICAL SPECIFICATIONS

Sample folding frame: manual wheelchair. This chart shares some of the product information that wheelchair manufacturers provide. This information is used in the selection process to determine whether a specific wheelchair will be appropriate for a specific person.

MANUAL WHEELCHAIR SPECIFICATION SHEET

Frame Style	Folding
Healthcare Common Procedure Coding System Code	K0005
Wheelchair Weight	27.2 lb (folding frame) 28.9 lb (folding frame with swing-away footrests in place) 26.0 lb (folding frame with fixed front end)
Material	Aluminum
User weight capacity	250 lb (regular frame) 350 lb (heavy-duty frame)
Transit Approved	Yes*
Shipping Dimensions	33" L x 38" H x 13" W
Average Shipping Weight	50 lbs.

FRAME AND FEATURE MEASUREMENTS

Seat Widths	12" to 22"
Seat Depths	12" to 20"
Frame Angle	Fixed Front: 70° or 80° Swingaway Front: 70° or 80° or 90°
Front Seat to Floor Height	13.5" to 22"
Rear Seat to Floor Height	13" to 22" (adjustable)
Lower Leg Length Setting	5.5" to 20.5" (adjustable)
Back Height	9" to 21" (adjustable)
Angle Adjustable Backrest Adjustment Range	-15° to +3°
Camber	0°, 2°, 4°, 6°
Center of Gravity Adjustment (axle-plate adjustments)	-1" to 4.5"**

*The test related to this standard results in either a "yes" or a "no." "Yes" indicates that the wheelchair has the needed equipment to interface with tie-downs in vehicles.

** The center of gravity is adjusted by moving the rear wheel forward or backward by adjusting the axle plate. This adjustment makes the wheelchair more or less stable. Moving the axle position back (reflected as a negative measurement, here 1") puts the axle of the rear wheel behind the center of gravity making the wheelchair more stable. Moving the axle position forward (reflected as a positive measurement, here 4.5") puts the axle of the rear wheel in front of the center of gravity, lightening the load on the casters (front wheel), making the wheelchair less stable (more tippy) and easier to maneuver around and over obstacles.

tested the durability of manual wheelchairs use wheelchair standard's fatigue testing methods (Cooper et al., 1996). By using the testing methods describe in wheelchair standards, these researchers were able to compare performance of various wheelchairs, and readers could use this information in the selection process. Using wheelchair and seating standards can strengthen the methods in research—not just specifically in this area but also in other areas of rehabilitation. Clinical research that uses standards as part of their methodology may have a stronger study design than a similar project that does not use wheelchair standards. This is because the methods used in wheelchair and seating standards have been used repeatedly across different labs and have been shown to be effective. As more and more research is done on participation, there should be an effort to ensure that wheelchair testing standards are used in researchers' methodology to build the evidence on which effective practice is based.

Wheelchair standards have been used as the test criteria to compare performance of various manual and powered wheelchairs. Research is being done that uses wheelchair standards identified where performance differences existed between specific wheelchair models. These findings can be used in a number of ways, including the selection process for specific wheelchair users. In one study, the authors reported the critical dimensions and masses of ultralight manual wheelchairs, as well as the results of fatigue testing, which gives readers information on device durability and tilt angle that is potentially relevant to navigation of wheelchairs in real-life settings (Cooper, Boninger, & Rentschler, 1999).

Performance differences in powered wheelchairs, reported in a more recent article, included findings of clinically relevant testing, such as dynamic stability. Clinically, this type of research result give wheelchair users and clinicians an idea of the stability of powered wheelchairs when they are moving, braking distance, or how far a powered wheelchair rolls before stopping in three conditions: when the joystick is released, when the joystick is moved from forward to reverse, and when the wheelchair is powered off (Rentschler et al., 2004).

Wheelchair standards were used as the testing procedures to compare performance in durability among powered wheelchairs (Fass et al., 2004). Using ANSI/RESNA test procedures, researchers studied the displacement of seating surfaces when the reclining and tilting seating systems were used on a wheelchair (Cooper, Dvorznak, Rentschler, & Bonniger 2000). They also used the test dummy required for testing rather than using human subjects. By using standardized procedures and a standardized dummy, findings for individual equipment can be compared. The findings of the research described here are important in and of themselves. Further, by using standardized procedures and equipment, the findings of these studies can be joined with those from other studies using the same standard procedures, thus building the available evidence.

Wheelchair and seating standards can also be used in combination with other standards in practice and in research. For example, in her chapter in this volume on transportation (Chapter 24), Buning describes safety standards for transporting wheelchairs, and Waugh and Crane describe the use of body measures and seating standards in Chapter 6 on measurement. By performing research that uses standards regarding wheelchairs, wheelchair seating, and transportation, wheelchair users may be able to participate in their chosen activities more fully and safely. Research continues to elevate the development of new seating and wheeled mobility technologies and products. Position papers, which reflect a consensus, opinion or viewpoint about an issue or trend is also used by organizations to make public the official beliefs of the group, are also used along with research to highlight the importance of these new technologies or products.

Using Standards in Coverage Policies and Coding

In the United States, governmental organizations oversee just about every aspect of our lives, including health and product safety-related issues. Provision of wheelchairs and wheelchair seating equipment is usually paid by medical insurance. In the United States, there are four main groups of insurance providers that provide seating and wheeled mobility products as part of their covered benefit package:

1. Private insurance companies, used by many employed adults and their families

2. Medicare, used by people over age 65 and, in certain circumstances, by people with long-term disabilities who are under age 65

3. Medicaid, used by people with limited incomes who are unable to pay for private insurance

4. The VA, used by veterans

Each of these funding sources has policies outlining coverage criteria and funding limitations of medical equipment including wheelchairs and wheelchair seating.

The VA is one of the largest purchasers of the wheelchair in the United States, and was a large supporter of the development of the original wheelchair standards work in the 1980s. Currently, the VA requires the submission of wheelchair standards test results as part of the procurement process. Manufacturers who want their products to be available for purchase by the VA must test their products and submit the results.

The Centers for Medicare & Medicaid (CMS) oversees the Medicare and Medicaid programs, including the determination of Medicare coverage policies. Before 2001, CMS was known as the Health Care Financing Administration (HICFA, pronounced hick-fa). In 1978, HICFA developed a coding system for describing the specific items and services provided in the delivery of health care. Such coding is necessary for Medicare, Medicaid, and other health insurance programs to ensure that insurance claims are processed in an orderly and consistent manner. The coding system is called Healthcare Common Procedure Coding System (HCPCS; pronounced hick-picks). Initially, use of the codes was voluntary, but with the implementation of the Health Insurance Portability and Accountability Act of 1996 (HIPAA), use of the HCPCS for transactions involving health care information became mandatory. Initially there were very broad descriptions of seating and mobility products under the HCPCS system. For example, there was only one HCPC code (E0192—Low pressure and positioning equalization pad, for wheelchair) to describe any cushion to use while sitting in a wheelchair. As a result of the Medicare Modernization Act of 2003, Congress mandated CMS and its contractors to revise the HCPC coding system to represent more closely the range of products in the seating and mobility marketplace. CMS chose to use the standards testing results to outline new product descriptions and to categorize them into a much wider range of HCPC codes. For example, general use cushions were differentiated from skin protection cushions, and Group 2 power wheelchairs, which are designed for indoor use, were differentiated from Group 4 power wheelchairs, which are designed for active outdoor use. Through this differentiation of products by their materials and intended uses, it was possible to identify and assign specific HCPC codes to products that have been designed to meet different intended uses. Manufacturers who want their products coded and covered by Medicare are now required to submit their standard test results to get a HCPC code assigned for the product. CMS and private insurance companies have looked at performance and safety requirements as they relate to the coding attached to wheelchairs using the standards to ensure quality as well as matching user's needs to the wheelchair.

Although private insurance may also use codes, they are used primarily by Medicare and Medicaid for reporting services, equipment, and supplies purchased using Medicare or Medicaid funds. Congress passed HIPAA in 1996, which required that CMS adopt standardized systems for reporting and billing health care transactions. CMS reports that Medicare alone pays 4.4 million claims on any given day (Medicare Newsgroup, 2012). These claims are for all covered benefits that were provided, not just wheelchairs and wheelchair seating equipment. This number represents the claims that are paid, not all of the equipment and services that are submitted for payment. If you imagine all the billing requested throughout the country for Medicare and other providers, you should be able to see how overwhelming the process would be if standardized coding systems were not in place. Standardized coding helps ensure that claims are processed in an orderly and uniform fashion. These codes have been adopted by state Medicaid programs and private insurances across the United States. In his commentary, Cooper stated, "CMS announced requirements for testing of electric-powered wheelchairs as part of efforts to modernize coding. In this century, CMS, in what might be classified by some as an uncharacteristic move, has provided leadership in evidence-based classification of wheelchairs" (Cooper, 2006, p. 93).

There are two sets of codes. The first set of codes, or Level I, is a set of five-digit numbers, developed by the American Medical Association, that represents diagnoses, procedures, and services used by physicians and other health care providers. These codes are used in medical documentation and billing.

The second set of codes, or Level II, is a code set for medical services, procedures, and products not included in Level I, such as durable medical equipment, including wheelchairs and wheelchair seating equipment. These codes begin with a letter, such as an E or K in the case of durable medical equipment or wheelchairs, followed by four numbers. This system is evolving, and it is possible for wheelchair and positioning product manufacturers to request HCPC codes for new products they develop. CMS (2014) requires that the manufacturers submit wheelchair and seating standard testing in this process.

SUMMARY

This chapter has sought to describe what wheelchair and seating standards are and how they are used clinically, in research, and in public policy. How these standards affect the variety, quality, and development of future products was also discussed. Standards provide uniform, reliable information with a consistent reporting system that allows wheelchair users, clinician's, designers, payers, researchers, and others to compare and select products. Two case studies illustrated how information derived from standards testing can be used clinically to make the best match between a wheelchair user and the wheelchairs available. Standards are a uniform and useful way for people in various disciplines to describe product features and to inform the selection process.

In addition to wheelchair and seating standards, other standards are also useful to wheelchair users. Measurement standards are discussed in Chapter 6, and Transportation standards are discussed in Chapter 24 of this book. There are standards for adaptive sports equipment including winter sports equipment like sit-skis and adapted golf carts (RESNA Standards Committee on Adaptive Sports Equipment, 2014). These devices are used by people with mobility impairments and may be useful to wheelchair users. There are also standards for equipment that can be used in emergencies to evaluate wheelchair users and other people with mobility impairments from buildings (RESNA Standards Committee on Emergency Stair Travel Devices for Individuals with Disabilities, 2014). All of these related standards should also be of interest to wheelchair users and clinicians. As discussed in this chapter, information from these other standards is useful in clinical practice, research, and in policy development.

We hope this will pique your interest in learning more or joining one of the working groups involved in the revision and development of wheelchair and seating standards. For more information about joining standards working groups, visit www.resna.org/at-standards.

REFERENCES

American Kennel Club. (2014). *Breed matters*. Retrieved from https://www.akc.org/breeds

Axleson, P., Minkel, J., & Chesney, D. (1994). *A guide to wheelchair selection: How to use the ANSI/RESNA wheelchair standards to buy a wheelchair*. Washington, DC: Paralyzed Veterans of America.

Centers for Medicare & Medicaid. (2014). *Application and checklist for PDAC HCPCS coding verification request manual wheelchairs*. Retrieved from https://www.dmepdac.com/docs/review/manual_wheelchairs.pdf

Cooper, R. A. (2006). Wheelchair standards: It's all about quality assurance and evidence-based practice. *Journal of Spinal Cord Medicine, 29*, 93-94.

Cooper, R. A., Boninger, M. L., & Rentschler, A. (1999). Evaluation of selected ultralight manual wheelchairs using ANSI/RESNA standards. *Archives of Physical Medicine and Rehabilitation, 80*, 462-467.

Cooper, R. A., Dvorznak, M. J., Rentschler, A. J., & Boninger, M. L. (2000). Displacement between the seating surface and hybrid test dummy during transitions with a variable configuration wheelchair: a technical note. *Journal of Rehabilitation Research and Development, 37*(3), 297-303.

Cooper, R. A., Gonzalez, J., Lawrence, B., Renschler, A., Boninger, M., & VanSickle, D. P. (1997). Performance of selected lightweight wheelchair on ANSI/RESNA tests. *Archives of Physical Medicine and Rehabilitation, 78*, 1138-1144.

Cooper, R. A., Robertson, R. N., Lawrence, B., Heil, T., Albright, S. J., VanSickle, D. P., & Gonzalez, J. (1996). Life-cycle analysis of depot versus rehabilitation manual wheelchairs. *Journal of Rehabilitation Research and Development, 33*, 45-55.

Cooper, R. A., Stewart, K. F., VanSickle, D. P., Albright, S., Heil, T. A., Robertson, R. N., Flannery, M.,...Ensminger, G. (1994). Manual wheelchair ISO-ANSI/RESNA fatigue testing experience. Proceedings of the RESNA '94 Annual Conference: *Tuning in to the 21st Century Through Assistive Technology: Listen to the Music*.

Fass, M. V., Cooper, R. A., Fitzgerald, S. G., Schmeler, M., Boninger, M. L., Algood, S. D.,...Duncan, J. (2004). Durability, value, and reliability of selected electric powered wheelchairs. *Archives of Physical Medicine and Rehabilitation, 85*, 805-814.

Ferguson-Pell, M., Nicholson, G., Bain, D., Call, E., Grady, J., & deVries, J., (2005). The role of wheelchair seating standards in determining clinical practices and funding policy. *Assistive Technology: The Official Journal of RESNA, 17*,1-6.

International Organization for Standardization. (n.d.a). *Search: Wheelchair*. Retrieved from http://www.iso.org/iso/search.htm?qt=wheelchair&sort_by=rel&type=simple&published=on&active_tab=standards

International Organization for Standardization. (n.d.b). *Wheelchair seating—Part 2: Determination of physical and mechanical characteristics of devices intended to manage tissue integrity—Seat cushions*. Retrieved from http://www.iso.org/iso/home/store/catalogue_ics/catalogue_detail_ics.htm?ics1=11&ics2=180&ics3=10&csnumber=40980

International Organization for Standardization. (n.d.c). *Wheelchairs: Test dummies*. Retrieved from http://www.iso.org/iso/iso_catalogue/catalogue_tc/catalogue_detail.htm?csnumber=13787

Medicare Newsgroup. (2012). *Medicare FAQs: How many Medicare claims are processed by the Centers for Medicare & Medicaid Services (CMS) per year?* Retrieved from http://www.medicarenewsgroup.com/news/medicare-faqs/individual-faq?faqId=780e2daa-e758-4a7c-9ada-eba5a32f2102

Rentschler, A. J., Cooper, R. A., Fitzgerald, S. G., Boninger, M. L., Guo, S., Ammer, W. A.,...Algood, D. (2004). Evaluation of selected electric-powered wheelchairs using the ANSI/RESNA Standards. *Archives of Physical Medicine and Rehabilitation, 85*, 611-619.

Rehabilitation Engineering & Assistive Technology Society of North America Standards Committee on Adaptive Sports Equipment. (2014). *Adaptive sports equipment*. Retrieved from http://www.resna.org/adaptive-sports-equipment

Rehabilitation Engineering & Assistive Technology Society of North America Standards Committee on Emergency Stair Travel Devices for Individuals with Disabilities. (2014). *Emergency stair travel devices for individuals with disabilities*. Retrieved from http://www.resna.org/standards/emergency-stair-travel-devices-individuals-disabilities/emergency-stair-travel-devices

Rehabilitation Engineering & Assistive Technology Society of North America Standards Committee on Support Surfaces. (2014). *Support surfaces*. Retrieved from http://www.resna.org/support-surfaces

Sprigle, S., Dunlop, W., & Press. L. (2003). Reliability of bench tests of interface pressure. *Assistive Technology, 15*, 49-51.

Underwriters Laboratory. (2014). *Understanding standards*. Retrieved from http://ulstandards.ul.com/about/understanding-standards

U.S. Consumer Product Safety Commission. (2008). 16 CFR Part 1610 Standard for the Flammability of Clothing Textiles; Corrections. *Federal Register, 73*(203), 62187-62189

U.S. Department of Justice, Civil Rights Division. (2010). *Information and Technical Assistance on the Americans with Disabilities Act: ADA Standards for Accessible Design*. Retrieved from http://www.ada.gov/2010ADAstandards_index.htm.

Financial Disclosures

Atli Ágústsson has no financial or proprietary interest in the materials presented herein.

Michael Babinec is an employee of Invacare.

Theresa F. Berner has no financial or proprietary interest in the materials presented herein.

Sheila N.R. Buck has no financial or proprietary interest in the materials presented herein.

Dr. Mary Ellen Buning has no financial or proprietary interest in the materials presented herein.

Jo-Anne Chisholm has no financial or proprietary interest in the materials presented herein.

Elizabeth Cole is an employee of Permobil.

David Cooper is an employee of Priority Posture Systems.

Dr. Barbara A. Crane has no financial or proprietary interest in the materials presented herein.

Dr. Carmen P. DiGiovine received a research grant from Invacare.

John "Jay" Doherty an employee of Quantum Rehab.

Jan Furumasu has no financial or proprietary interest in the materials presented herein.

Dr. Deborah A. Jones has no financial or proprietary interest in the materials presented herein.

Guðný Jónsdóttir has no financial or proprietary interest in the materials presented herein.

Kay Ellen Koch has no financial or proprietary interest in the materials presented herein.

David Kreutz has no financial or proprietary interest in the materials presented herein.

Michelle L. Lange is a consultant for Stealth Products and AbleNet.

Elizabeth McCarty has no financial or proprietary interest in the materials presented herein.

Jean L. Minkel has no financial or proprietary interest in the materials presented herein.

Amy M. Morgan is an employee of Permobil.

Dr. Anita Perr has no financial or proprietary interest in the materials presented herein.

Cindi Petito has no financial or proprietary interest in the materials presented herein.

Julie Piriano is an employee of Pride Mobility Corporation.

Joanne Rader has no financial or proprietary interest in the materials presented herein.

Lauren E. Rosen has no financial or proprietary interest in the materials presented herein.

Dr. Mark Schmeler has not disclosed any relevant financial relationship.

Jill Sparacio has no financial or proprietary interest in the materials presented herein.

Maureen Story has no financial or proprietary interest in the materials presented herein.

Sharon Sutherland is an employee of Seating Solutions, LLC.

Melissa Tally has no financial or proprietary interest in the materials presented herein.

Stephanie Tanguay is and employee of Motion Concepts.

Susan Johnson Taylor has no financial or proprietary interest in the materials presented herein.

Kelly Waugh has no financial or proprietary interest in the materials presented herein.

Joanne Yip has no financial or proprietary interest in the materials presented herein.

Index